610 HIG

Clinical Reasoning in the
Health Professions

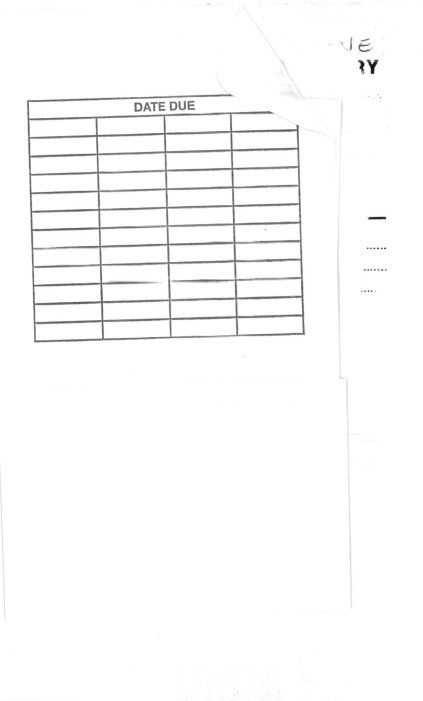

DATE DUE

For Elsevier:

Publisher: Heidi Harrison
Associate Editor: Siobhan Campbell
Development Editor: Veronika Watkins
Project Manager: Gail Wright
Senior Designer: George Ajayi
Illustration Manager: Merlyn Harvey
Illustrator: Richard Morris

Clinical Reasoning in the Health Professions

THIRD EDITION

Joy Higgs BSc GradDipPhty MHPEd PhD AM

Strategic Research Professor in Professional Practice, and Director, Education for Practice Institute, Charles Sturt University, Australia

Mark A. Jones BSc(Psych) PT MAppSc

Program Director, Postgraduate Coursework Masters Programs, School of Health Sciences, University of South Australia, Australia

Stephen Loftus BDS MSc PhD

Pain Management Research Institute, Royal North Shore Hospital, Sydney, Australia; Senior Lecturer, Education for Practice Institute, Charles Sturt University, Australia

Nicole Christensen MAppSc PT

Assistant Professor, Doctor of Physical Therapy Program, Samuel Merritt College, USA, PhD candidate, University of South Australia, Australia

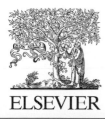

ELSEVIER

AMSTERDAM • BOSTON • HEIDELBERG • LONDON
NEW YORK • OXFORD • PARIS • SAN DIEGO
SAN FRANCISCO • SINGAPORE • SYDNEY • TOKYO

Focal Press is an imprint of Elsevier

ELSEVIER
BUTTERWORTH
HEINEMANN

First edition 1995
Second edition 2000
Third edition 2008

ISBN: 978-0-7506-8885-7

British Library Cataloguing in Publication Data
A catalogue record for this book is available from the British Library

Library of Congress Cataloging in Publication Data
A catalog record for this book is available from the Library of Congress

Notice
Neither the Publisher nor the Editors assume any responsibility for any loss or injury and/or damage to persons or property arising out of or related to any use of the material contained in this book. It is the responsibility of the treating practitioner, relying on independent expertise and knowledge of the patient, to determine the best treatment and method of application for the patient.

The Publisher

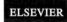

ELSEVIER your source for books, journals and multimedia in the health sciences

www.elsevierhealth.com

Working together to grow libraries in developing countries

www.elsevier.com | www.bookaid.org | www.sabre.org

ELSEVIER   BOOK AID International   Sabre Foundation

The publisher's policy is to use **paper manufactured from sustainable forests**

Printed in China

Contents

Contributors

Rola Ajjawi BAppSci(Physiotherapy)Hons PhD
Associate Lecturer in Medical Education, Centre for Innovation in Professional Health Education and Research (CIPHER), Faculty of Medicine, University of Sydney, Australia

Suzanne Alder MAPS
Senior Psychologist, Mental Health Project Officer, NSW Central West Division of General Practice, Bathurst, Australia

José F. Arocha
Associate Professor and Associate Chair of Graduate Studies, Department of Health Studies and Gerontology, University of Waterloo, Canada

Sue Atkins MSc DipNEd RN
Principal Lecturer, School of Health and Social Care, Oxford Brookes University, UK

Alexandra Barratt MBBS MPH PhD
Associate Professor, Epidemiology, School of Public Health, University of Sydney, Australia

Henny P.A. Boshuizen PhD
Professor of Education and Educational Technology; Dean of the Master Programme on Educational Design for Active Learning, The Netherlands

Stephen D. Brookfield PhD
Distinguished University Professor, University of St Thomas, Minneapolis-St Paul, USA

Mary E. Cahill BNS RN
Staff Nurse, Department of Oncology, Rhode Island Hospital, Providence, Rhode Island, USA

Christine Chapparo DipOT MA PhD FAOTA
Senior Lecturer, Faculty of Health Sciences, University of Sydney, Australia

Cathy Charles PhD
Professor, Department of Clinical Epidemiology and Biostatistics, McMaster University, Hamilton, Canada

Nicole Christensen MAppSc PT
Assistant Professor, Doctor of Physical Therapy Program, Samuel Merritt College, USA; PhD candidate, University of South Australia, Australia

Sheila A. Corcoran-Perry PhD FAAN
Professor Emeritus, formerly University of Minnesota, USA

Linda de Cossart PhD
Consultant Vascular and General Surgeon, Countess of Chester NHS Foundation Trust and Council Member, Royal College of Surgeons of England, UK

Anne Croker BAppSc(Physio) GradDipPublicHealth
PhD Candidate, Charles Sturt University, Australia

Clare Delany BApplSciPhysio MPhysio(manip) MHlth MedLaw PhD
School of Physiotherapy, University of Melbourne, Australia

Helen Edwards MA PhD
Consultant Higher Education, Melbourne, Australia

Ian Edwards BAppScPhysio GradDipPhysio(Ortho) PhD
Lecturer, School of Health Sciences, University of South Australia; Physiotherapist, Brian Burdekin Clinic, Adelaide, Australia

Elizabeth Ellis PhD
Honorary Senior Lecturer, Faculty of Health Sciences, The University of Sydney, Sydney, Australia

Arthur S. Elstein PhD
Professor Emeritus Department of Medical Education, University of Illinois at Chicago, USA

Steven J. Ersser BSc(Hon) CertTHEd PhD(Lond) RN
Professor of Nursing Development and Skin Care Research, Institute of Health and Community Studies, Bournemouth University, UK

Michael J. Field BS BSc(Hons) MD FRACP
Professor of Medicine, Associate Dean and Head, Northern Clinical School, Faculty of Medicine, University of Sydney

Della Fish PhD
Professor (Postgraduate Studies), School of Health Sciences, University of Wales, UK

Maureen Hayes Fleming EdD OTR FAOTA

Marsha E. Fonteyn RN PhD
Professor, School of Nursing, University of San Francisco, USA

Amiram Gafni PhD
Professor, Department of Clinical Epidemiology and Biostatistics; Member, Centre for Health Economics and Policy Analysis, Canada

Jill Gordon MB BS, BA, MPsychMed, PhD
Associate Professor in Medical Humanities, Centre for Values, Ethics and the Law in Medicine, The University of Sydney, Australia

Janet Grant MSc PhD CPsychol FBPsS FRCGP(Hon) FRCP (Hon) MRCR(Hon) MIoD
Professor of Education in Medicine; Director, Open University Centre for Education in Medicine, UK

Karen Grimmer-Somers BPhty MMedSc PhD CertHealthEc LMusA
Professor of Allied Health; Director, Centre for Allied Health Evidence, a Collaborating Centre of the Joanna Briggs Institute, University of South Australia, Australia

Amy M. Haddad BSN MSN PhD
Director, Centre for Health Policy and Ethics and the Dr. C. C. and Mabel L. Criss Endowed Chair in the Health Sciences, Omaha, Nebraska, USA

Elizabeth C. Henley BSc BPT MCISc
Former Educational Consultant, Doonan, Australia

Joy Higgs BSc GradDipPhty MHPEd PhD AM
Strategic Research Professor in Professional Practice and Director, Education for Practice Institute, Charles Sturt University, Australia

Debbie Horsfall BEd MA PhD
Senior Lecturer Social Research and Gender Studies, School of Social Sciences, University of Western Sydney, Australia

Gail M. Jensen PT PhD FAPTA
Dean, Graduate School and Associate Vice-President in Academic Affairs; Professor of Physical Therapy; Faculty Associate, Center for Health Policy and Ethics; Creighton University, USA

Mark A. Jones BSc(Psych) PT MAppSc
Program Director, Postgraduate Coursework Masters Programs, School of Health Sciences, University of South Australia, Australia

David R. Kauffman BA, MA, PhD
Assistant Professor, Cognition and Development, School of Education, University of California at Berkeley, USA

Shiva Khatami DDS
PhD Candidate, Department of Oral Health Sciences, Faculty of Dentistry, University of British Columbia, Canada

Richard K. Ladyshewsky BMR(PT) MHSc PhD
Associate Professor, Graduate School of Business, Curtin University of Technology, Australia

Dale Larsen BAppSc MAppSc PhD
Principal, Macquarie St Physiotherapy Centre, Sydney, Australia; Independent Physiotherapy Consultant, Work Cover, New South Wales, Australia; Research Associate, Education for Practice Institute, Charles Sturt University, Australia

Stephen Loftus BDS MSc PhD
Pain Management Research Institute, Royal North Shore Hospital, Sydney, Australia; Senior Lecturer, Education for Practice Institute, Charles Sturt University, Australia

Lindy McAllister BSpThy MA PhD
Associate Professor of Speech Pathology, School of Community Health, Charles Sturt University, Australia

Kirsten J. McCaffery BSc(Hons) PhD
Senior Research Fellow, School of Public Health, University of Sydney, Australia

Michael I. MacEntee LDS(I) DipProsth FRCD(C) PhD
Professor of Prosthodontics and Dental Geriatrics, Faculty of Dentistry, University of British Columbia, Canada

Cheryl Mattingly PhD
Associate Professor, Department of Occupational Therapy, University of Illinois at Chicago, USA

Suzanne M. Narayan PhD RN
Professor, School of Nursing, Metropolitan State University, USA

Geoff Norman BSc MA PhD
Professor, Department of Clinical Epidemiology and Biostatistics, McMaster University, Canada

Vimla L. Patel PhD DSc
Professor and Chair, Departments of Biomedical Informatics and Medical Psychology; Director, Laboratory of Decision Making and Cognition, Columbia University, USA

Margo Paterson PhD OTReg(Ont)
Associate Professor and Chair Occupational Therapy Program, Queen's University, Canada

Judy L. Ranka BSc MA
Lecturer, Faculty of Health Sciences, University of Sydney, Australia

Linda Resnik PT PhD OCS
Research Health Scientist, Providence VA Medical Center, Assistant Professor, Department of Community Health, Brown University Medical School, USA

Barbara J. Ritter RNC EdD MS FNP CNS PHN
Instructor and Coordinator Advanced Practice Programs, Department of Family Health and Nursing Systems, School of Nursing, University of San Francisco, USA

Darren A. Rivett BAppSc(Phty) GradDipManipTher MAppSc(ManipPhty) PhD
Associate Professor and Deputy Head, School of Health Sciences, Faculty of Health, University of Newcastle, Australia

Miranda L. Rose GradDip Health Research Methodology GradDip Communication Disorders Neurological Origin BAppSci(Speech Pathology) PhD
Senior Lecturer, School of Human Communication Sciences, La Trobe University, Australia

Rodd Rothwell MA PhD
Honorary Senior Lecturer, School of Behavioural and Community Health Sciences, Faculty of Health Sciences, University of Sydney, Australia

Susan Ryan BAppSc MSc PhD
Professor and Head of Occupational Therapy Department, University College Cork, Ireland

Henk G. Schmidt PhD
Professor of Psychology, Dean of the Faculty of Social Sciences, Erasmus Medical Center, Rotterdam, The Netherlands

Lambert Schuwirth MD PhD
Professor for Innovative Assessment, Department of Educational Development and Research, University of Maastricht, The Netherlands

Alan Schwartz PhD
Associate Professor, Department of Medical Education, University of Illinois at Chicago, USA

Ann Sefton MBBS BSc(Med) PhD DSc
Formerly Professor in Physiology and Associate Dean, Faculty of Medicine; Emeritus Professor, University of Sydney, Australia

Megan Smith BAppSc(Physiotherapy) MAppSc (Cardiopulmphysio) GradCertUT&L PhD
Senior Lecturer, School of Community Health, Charles Sturt University, Australia

Angie Titchen MSc DPhil(Oxon)
Clinical Chair, Knowledge Centre for Evidence Based Practice, Fontys University for Applied Science, The Netherlands

Franziska Veronika Trede PhysDip MHPEd PhD
Senior Research Fellow, Education for Practice Institute, Charles Sturt University, Australia

Lyndal Trevena MBBS(Hons) MPhilPH
Lecturer, School of Public Health, University of Sydney, Australia

Robyn Twible
School of Occupation and Leisure Sciences, Faculty of Health Sciences, University of Sydney, Australia

Cees van der Vleuten PhD
Scientific Director School of Health Professions Education, Chair Department of Educational Development and Research, Maastricht University, The Netherlands

Timothy Whelan BM BCh
Professor, Department of Oncology, McMaster University and Juravinski Cancer Centre Hamilton, Canada

Gail Elizabeth Whiteford BAppSc MHSc PhD
Professor and Chair, Occupational Therapy, Charles Sturt University, Australia

Preface

The third edition of this book includes a significant quantum of new research, theorization and practice-based knowledge of the nature of clinical reasoning, practice knowledge and the teaching of clinical reasoning. Of the 47 chapters 30 are new. We have added 30 new authors to our writing team. This demonstrates the significant growth that has occurred in clinical reasoning research in recent years.

There are six sections in the book, expanding the scope of the previous edition with a greater emphasis on research trends, the context of clinical decision making, the participants in this complex activity, the place of communication of reasoning and the nature of practice knowledge and the epistemology of practice. The sections are:

1. Clinical reasoning and clinical decision making – nature and context
2. Reasoning, expertise and knowledge
3. Clinical reasoning research trends
4. Clinical reasoning and clinical decision-making approaches
5. Communicating about clinical reasoning
6. Teaching and learning clinical reasoning.

From the perspective of the participants in clinical decision making, we have increased our emphasis in this edition on the place of interests and motivations in shaping the behaviour and decisions of practitioners and patients in relation to collaborative decision making, patient-centred care, multidisciplinary decision making, shared decision making, language, communication, and decision aids that involve clients.

As our understanding of clinical reasoning in the health professions grows, more questions emerge that require further research across a range of both traditional and more innovative research methodologies. From our first edition of this book to this third edition we have recognized that producing a definitive portrayal of clinical reasoning in the health professions is both undesirable and unfeasible. Rather, by drawing on the latest research, practice, teaching and theory we have attempted to provide readers with an evolving update to stimulate further research, sound professional practice and high-quality education grounded in the context and needs of the student group with the core aim of maximizing students' clinical reasoning capabilities.

Australia 2007

Joy Higgs
Mark A. Jones

SECTION 1

Clinical reasoning and clinical decision making– nature and context

SECTION CONTENTS

Chapter 1

Clinical decision making and multiple problem spaces

Joy Higgs and Mark A. Jones

In the second edition of this book we drew on our initial view of clinical reasoning as a process incorporating the elements of cognition, knowledge and metacognition, expanding this to place a greater emphasis on patient-centred care as the context for clinical reasoning. Practitioners were presented as interactional professionals (Higgs & Hunt 1999) whose effectiveness required interaction with their immediate and larger work environment, with the key players in that context, and with the situational elements pertinent to the patient and case under consideration. Health care was presented via a social ecology model as occurring within the wider sphere of social responsibility of professionals which requires practitioners to be proactive as well as responsive to changes in healthcare contexts (Higgs et al 1999).

In this opening chapter of the third edition we extend our previous examination of the nature of clinical reasoning and its context, drawing on our own research and that of colleagues and co-authors. We expand our interpretation of clinical reasoning from a process view, to explore clinical reasoning as a contextualized phenomenon (see also Chapters 2, 8). We extend consideration of the decision-making context from a focus on the immediate task environment of case management acting in the wider healthcare context to explore the multiple levels of the clinical decision-making space, or rather the multiple decision-making spaces, within which interactive reasoning and decision making occur (see Higgs 2006a, b).

In relation to clinical reasoning expertise, we extend the notion of an expert to encompass capability, professional artistry and patient-centredness; expertise is a journey rather than a point of arrival (see also Chapters 11, 16). In examining and making explicit these aspects of clinical reasoning our goal is to make clinical reasoning more accessible for novices to learn, for experienced practitioners to portray, for educators to teach, for clinicians to practise and for researchers to explore.

UNDERSTANDING CLINICAL REASONING

In the 10 years since we produced the first edition of this book, we have retained our view that clinical reasoning is both simple and complex. Simply, clinical reasoning is the sum of the thinking and decision-making processes associated with clinical practice; it is a critical skill in the health professions, central to the practice of professional autonomy, and it enables practitioners to take 'wise' action, meaning taking the best judged action in a specific context (Cervero 1988, Harris 1993). Despite being straightforward and 'simple' this view is very broad; clinical reasoning is seen as permeating throughout clinical practice and as being the core of practice. The importance of understanding the complex nature of clinical reasoning is emphasized in the goal of developing tolerance of ambiguity and a reflexive understanding of practice artistry during health sciences education, as suggested by Bleakley et al (2003).

The complex view of clinical reasoning is embedded in its simplicity and breadth (Higgs 2006b). By encompassing so much of what it means to be a professional (autonomy, responsibility, accountability and decision making in conditions of uncertainty), clinical reasoning gains an inherent mystique. This complexity lies in the very nature of the task or challenge, faced by novice and expert alike, which is to process multiple variables, contemplate the various priorities of competing healthcare needs, negotiate the interests of different participants in the decision-making process, inform all decisions and actions with advanced practice knowledge, and make all decisions and actions in the context of professional ethics and community expectations. The mystique is most evident in the skill of the expert

diagnostician who makes difficult decisions with seeming effortlessness, and in the professional artistry of the experienced practitioner who produces an individually tailored health management plan that addresses complicated health needs with humanity and finesse. To address and achieve these professional attributes clinical reasoning is much more a lived phenomenon, an experience, a way of being and a chosen model of practising than it is simply a process. To this end we adopt the following definition of this complex phenomenon:

> Clinical reasoning (or practice decision making) is a context-dependent way of thinking and decision making in professional practice to guide practice actions. It involves the construction of narratives to make sense of the multiple factors and interests pertaining to the current reasoning task. It occurs within a set of problem spaces informed by the practitioner's unique frames of reference, workplace context and practice models, as well as by the patient's or client's contexts. It utilises core dimensions of practice knowledge, reasoning and metacognition and draws on these capacities in others. Decision making within clinical reasoning occurs at micro, macro and meta levels and may be individually or collaboratively conducted. It involves metaskills of critical conversations, knowledge generation, practice model authenticity and reflexivity. (Higgs 2006b)

Of note in this definition is the term 'clinical'. For some health professionals their workplace is not 'clinical', their clients are not patients, the focus of their role may be on health rather than illness, and the term 'consultant' rather than 'practitioner' may be more appropriate. To avoid clumsy expression of these alternative terms we use the terms clinical reasoning and clinical decision making below.

CLINICAL REASONING AND METASKILLS

Our previous model of clinical reasoning (Higgs & Jones 2000) was presented as an upward and outward spiral, a cyclical and a developing process. Each loop of the spiral incorporated data input, data interpretation (or reinterpretation) and problem formulation (or reformulation) to achieve a progressively broader and deeper understanding of the clinical problem. Based on this deepening understanding, decisions are made concerning intervention, and actions are taken. The process was described as including:

a) the core dimensions of
- Knowledge. A strong discipline-specific knowledge base, comprising propositional knowledge (derived from theory and research) and non-propositional knowledge (derived from professional and personal experience), is necessary for sound and responsible clinical reasoning.
- Cognition or reflective inquiry. Cognitive or thinking skills (such as analysis, synthesis and evaluation of data collected) are utilized to process clinical data against the clinician's existing discipline-specific and personal knowledge base in consideration of the client's needs and the clinical problem.
- Metacognition. Metacognition or reflective self-awareness serves to bridge knowledge and cognition. It enables clinicians to identify limitations in the quality of information obtained, inconsistencies or unexpected findings; it enables them to monitor their reasoning and practice, seeking errors and credibility; it prompts them to recognize when their knowledge or skills are insufficient and remedial action is needed.

b) the additional dimensions of
- mutual decision making, or the role of the client or patient in the decision-making process
- contextual interaction, or the interactivity between the decision makers and the situation or environment of the reasoning process
- task impact, or the influence of the nature of the clinical problem or task on the reasoning process.

These additional dimensions were included in recognition of the growing expectation by and of consumers that they play an active role in their own health care. The image of compliant, dependent patients is replaced by one of informed healthcare consumers who expect their needs and preferences to be listened to, who increasingly want to participate in decision making about their health, and who expect to take action to enhance their health. Alongside this 'health rather than illness' focus on the part of the consumer, there are increasing expectations of service and of quality and ownership of health programmes, due to economic factors such as an increasing reliance on 'user pays' funding strategies, within which consumers are indeed purchasing health care. Similarly, caregivers need and wish to play a greater role in health management and decision making.

To these dimensions we now add four meta-skills:

- the ability to derive knowledge and practice wisdom from reasoning and practice (see Chapter 14). Reasoning plays a significant role in the acquisition of knowledge (Lawson et al 1991)
- the location of reasoning as behaviours and strategies within chosen practice models, each with an inherent philosophy of practice (see Chapters 3, 11)
- the reflexive ability to promote positive cognitive, affective and experiential growth, not only in the well-being of patients but also in the capabilities of oneself as practitioner (see Chapters 16, 29)
- the use of critical, creative conversations (Higgs 2006a) to make clinical decisions.

It is preferable to view clinical reasoning as a contextualized interactive phenomenon rather than a specific process. The practitioner responsible for making the decisions interacts both with the task and informational elements of decision making and with the human elements and interests of other participants in the decision making. Such interactions can be called critical creative conversations that involve interactions based on critical appraisal of circumstances and, where possible, critical interests in promoting emancipatory practice, and the creation and implementation of particularized, person-centred healthcare programmes (Higgs 2006a).

THE ADEQUACY OF DIFFERENT INTERPRETATIONS

There is no single model of clinical reasoning that adequately represents what clinical reasoning is in the context of different professions and different workplaces. The reason for this lies in several factors:

- the complex nature of the phenomenon of clinical reasoning and the consequent challenges of understanding, researching, assessing and measuring it
- the context-dependent nature of clinical decision making in action
- the inherent individuality of expertise
- the changing conceptions of quality and error in clinical reasoning
- the challenge to novices in developing clinical reasoning skills and to educators in facilitating this development.

THE NATURE OF CLINICAL REASONING AS A PHENOMENON

Consider the real world of clinical decision making. Orasanu & Connolly (1993) have described the characteristics of decision making in dynamic settings as follows:

- Problems are ill-structured and made ambiguous by the presence of incomplete dynamic information and multiple interacting goals.
- The decision-making environment is uncertain and may change while decisions are being made.
- Goals may be shifting, ill-defined or competing.
- Decision making occurs in the form of action–feedback loops, where actions result in effects and generate further information that decision makers have to react to and use in order to make further decisions.
- Decisions contain elements of time pressure, personal stress and highly significant outcomes for the participants.
- Multiple players act together, with different roles.
- Organizational goals and norms influence decision making.

To work within this practice world we need an approach to clinical reasoning that accommodates these complexities. Higgs and colleagues (2006, p. 1) described a number of key characteristics of clinical reasoning as follows:

- Clinical reasoning as a solo process is a complex mostly invisible process that is often largely automatic and therefore not readily accessible to others in practice or research

- Clinical reasoning is linked with more visible behaviours such as recording diagnoses and treatment plans in patient histories and communicating treatment rationales in team meetings, case conferences and teaching novices
- Clinical reasoning and practice knowledge are mutually developmental; each relies on the other, gives meaning to the other in the achievement of practice and is the source of generation and development of the other
- Clinical reasoning can be implemented as a sole practitioner process or a group process
- Clinical reasoning may be understood as both cognitive and collaborative processes; however, in either case there is a growing imperative, linked to increasing demands for evidence-based practice and public accountability, to make reasoning more explicit
- As well as core reasoning abilities, language and interactive behaviours are required for understanding and developing practice knowledge and clinical reasoning
- Recent research has emphasised the importance of understanding clinical reasoning behaviours and effectiveness (including the communication of reasoning) in relation to contextual influences and chosen or required practice models
- Clinical reasoning requires a range of capabilities including cognitive, metacognitive, emotional, reflexive and social capabilities
- Clinical reasoning is, and for the purposes of quality assurance, should be, a reflexive process which involves practitioner(s) in critical self-reflection and ongoing development of their reasoning abilities, knowledge and communication (of reasoning) abilities.

DIFFERENT INTERPRETATIONS OF CLINICAL REASONING

In various chapters of this book a number of interpretations of clinical reasoning are discussed from the perspective of different disciplines, the history of clinical reasoning research, and models of practice within which clinical reasoning occurs. In Table 1.1 we present an overview of key models,

Table 1.1 Models and interpretations of clinical reasoning (CR)

View	Model	References	Related terms	Description
CR as cognitive process	*Hypothetico-deductive reasoning*	Barrows et al 1978; Elstein et al 1978; Feltovich et al 1984	*Procedural reasoning* (OT) Fleming 1991; *diagnostic reasoning* (N) Padrick et al 1987; (PT) Edwards et al 1993; *induction-related probabilistic reasoning* Albert et al 1988	The generation of hypotheses based on clinical data and knowledge, and testing of these hypotheses through further inquiry. It is used by novices, and in problematic situations by experts (Elstein et al 1990) Hypothesis generation and testing involves both inductive reasoning (moving from a set of specific observations to a generalization) to generate hypotheses and slower, detailed deductive reasoning (moving from a generalization – if – to a conclusion – then – in relation to a specific case) to test hypotheses (Ridderikhoff 1989). Procedural reasoning identifying the patient's functional problems and selecting procedures to manage them (Fleming 1991)
	Pattern recognition	Barrows & Feltovich 1987	*Pattern interpretation* Inductive reasoning Categorization	Groen & Patel (1985) identified that expert reasoning in non-problematic situations resembles pattern recognition or direct automatic retrieval of information from a well-structured knowledge base. New cases are categorized, i.e. similarities are recognized (signs, symptoms, treatment options, outcomes, context), in relation to previously experienced clinical cases (Brooks et al 1991; Schmidt et al 1990). Through the use of inductive reasoning, pattern recognition/interpretation is a process characterized by speed and efficiency (Arocha et al 1993; Ridderikhoff 1989)
	Forward reasoning; backward reasoning	Patel & Groen 1986; Arocha et al 1993	*inductive reasoning Deductive reasoning*	*Forward reasoning* describes inductive reasoning in which data analysis results in hypothesis generation or diagnosis, utilizing a sound knowledge base. Forward reasoning is more likely to occur in familiar cases with experienced clinicians, and backward reasoning with inexperienced clinicians or in atypical or difficult cases (Patel & Groen 1986) Backward reasoning is the re-interpretation of data or the acquisition of new clarifying data invoked to test a hypothesis
	Knowledge reasoning integration	Schmidt et al 1990; Boshuizen & Schmidt 1992		Clinical reasoning requires domain-specific knowledge and an organized knowledge base. Boshuizen and Schmidt (1992) proposed a stage theory which emphasizes the parallel development of knowledge acquisition and clinical reasoning expertise. Clinical reasoning involves the integration of

(Continued)

Table 1.1   Models and interpretations of clinical reasoning (CR)—cont'd

View	Model	References	Related terms	Description
CR as cognitive process cont'd	*Intuitive reasoning*	Agan 1987; Rew 1990; Rew & Barrow 1987	*Instance scripts* *Inductive reasoning* *Heuristics* *Pattern matching*	knowledge, reasoning and metacognition (Higgs & Jones 1995) 'Intuitive knowledge' is related to 'instance scripts' or past experience with specific cases which can be used unconsciously in inductive reasoning. Fonteyn & Fisher (1992) linked nurses' experience and associated intuition to the use of advanced reasoning strategies or heuristics. Such heuristics include pattern matching and listing (or listing items relevant to the working plan) (Fonteyn & Grobe 1993)
CR as interactive process	*Multidisciplinary reasoning*	Loftus 2006	*Interprofessional reasoning* *Team decision making*	Members of a multidisciplinary team working together to make clinical decisions for the patient, about the patient's condition, e.g. at case conferences, multidisciplinary clinics
	Conditional reasoning	Fleming 1991; Hagedorn 1996; Edwards et al 1998	*Predictive reasoning* *Projected reasoning*	Used by practitioners to estimate patient responses to treatment and likely outcomes of management and to help patients consider possibilities and reconstruct their lives following injury or the onset of disease
	Narrative reasoning	Mattingly & Fleming 1994; Edwards et al 1998; Benner et al 1992		The use of stories regarding past or present patients to further understand and manage a clinical situation. Telling the story of patients' illness or injury to help them make sense of the illness experience
	Interactive reasoning	Fleming 1991; Edwards et al 1998		Interactive reasoning occurs between therapist and patient to understand the patient's perspective
	Collaborative reasoning	Coulter 2005; Edwards et al 1998; Trede & Higgs 2003; Beeston & Simons 1996; Jensen et al 1999	*Mutual decision making*	The shared decision-making that ideally occurs between practitioner and patient. Here the patient's opinions as well as information about the problem are actively sought and utilized
	Ethical reasoning	Barnitt & Partridge 1997; Edwards et al 1998; Gordon et al 1994; Neuhaus 1988	*Pragmatic reasoning*	Those less recognized, but frequently made decisions regarding moral, political and economic dilemmas which clinicians regularly confront, such as deciding how long to continue treatment
	Teaching as reasoning	Sluijs 1991; Edwards et al 1998		When practitioners consciously use advice, instruction and guidance for the purpose of promoting change in the patient's understanding, feelings and behaviour

OT=Occupational therapy, N=Nursing, PT=Physiotherapy

strategies and interpretations of clinical reasoning. These have been divided into two groups: cognitive and interactive models. This division reflects three trends: changes in the focus of research and theoretical understandings of clinical reasoning (see Chapters 18, 19); changes in society and expectations of health care (see Chapter 2); and a major shift in emphasis (as outlined above) from the second to the third edition of this book.

EXPERTISE AND CLINICAL REASONING

In a review of clinical reasoning literature in medicine, Norman (2005) suggested that there may not be a single representation of clinical reasoning expertise or a single correct way to solve a problem. He noted that 'the more one studies the clinical expert, the more one marvels at the complex and multidimensional components of knowledge and skill that she or he brings to bear on the problem, and the amazing adaptability she must possess to achieve the goal of effective care' (p. 426).

Clinical reasoning and clinical practice expertise is a journey, an aspiration and a commitment to achieving the best practice that one can provide. Rather than being a point of arrival, complacency and lack of questioning by self or others, expertise requires both the capacity to recognize one's limitations and practice capabilities and the ability to pursue professional development in a spirit of self-critique. And it is – or at least we should expect it to be – not only a self-referenced level of capability or mode of practice, but also a search for understanding of and realization of the standards and expectations set by the community being served and the profession and service organization being represented. Box 1.1 presents these characteristics and expectations of experts.

We have deliberately added the idea of expectations to this discussion to emphasize that any human construct is sociohistorically situated. Beyond the research-driven science view of technical expertise there is a need for any professional – but particularly experts, with their claim to superior service and performance – to address the needs of society. Today there is a growing expectation of patient-centred humanization (including cultural competence, information sharing, collaborative decision making, virtuous practice) of expert practice that turns health professional expertise into a collaborative professional relationship rather than an expert-empowered, technically superior, practitioner-centred approach. As highlighted in the research findings of Jensen et al (2006), this patient-centred approach is grounded in a strong moral commitment to beneficence or doing what is in the patient's best interest. This manifests in therapists' non-judgemental attitude and strong emphasis on patient education, with expert therapists being willing to serve as patient advocate or moral agent in helping them be successful.

Box 1.1 demonstrates an evolution in thinking about expertise, beginning with the classic research by Glaser & Chi (1988) into expert attributes (a). In 2000 we added to this view ideas of patient-centredness, collaboration, metacognition, mentoring, effective communication and cultural competence (Higgs & Jones 2000) (b). We have added the third group (c) to reflect ideas highlighted in this book.

We propose that clinical expertise, of which clinical reasoning is a critical component, be viewed as a continuum along multiple dimensions. These dimensions include clinical outcomes, personal attributes such as professional judgement, technical clinical skills, communication and interpersonal skills (to involve the client and others in decision making and to consider the client's perspectives), a sound knowledge base, an informed and chosen practice model and philosophy of practice, as well as cognitive and metacognitive proficiency.

A concept related to expertise is professional artistry, which 'reflects both high quality of professional practice and the qualities inherent in such artistic or flexible, person-centred, highly reflexive practice' (Paterson & Higgs 2001, p. 2). Professional artistry refers to 'practical knowledge, skilful performance or knowing as doing' (Fish 1998, p. 87) that is developed through the acquisition of a deep and relevant knowledge base and extensive experience (Beeston & Higgs 2001). Professional artistry reflects a uniquely individual view within a shared tradition involving a blend of practitioner qualities, practice skills and creative imagination processes (Higgs & Titchen 2001). Rogers (1983, p. 601) spoke of the artistry of clinical reasoning that is 'exhibited in the craftsmanship with which the therapist executes the series of steps that culminate in a clinical

Box 1.1 Characteristics and expectations of expert practitioners

a) General characteristics of experts
(Glaser & Chi 1988)
- Experts excel mainly in their own domains
- Experts perceive large meaningful patterns in their domain
- Experts are fast: they are faster than novices at performing the skills of their domain, and they quickly solve problems with little error
- Experts have superior short-term and long-term memory
- Experts see and represent a problem in their domain at a deeper (more principled) level than novices; novices tend to represent a problem at a superficial level
- Experts spend a great deal of time analysing a problem qualitatively
- Experts have strong self-monitoring skills (Glaser & Chi 1988, p. xvii–xx)

b) Particular characteristics and expectations of health professional experts (Higgs & Jones 2000)
- Experts need to pursue shared decision making between client and clinician if 'success' is to be realized from the client's perspective
- Experts need to monitor and manage their cognitive processes (i.e. to use metacognition) to achieve high-quality decision making and practice action
- Experts critically use propositional and experience-based up-to-date practice knowledge to inform their practice

- Expertise requires the informed use and recognition of patient-centred practice
- Expert practitioners are mentors and critical companions (see Titchen 2000) to less experienced practitioners
- Experts are expected to communicate effectively with clients, colleagues and families and to justify clinical decisions articulately
- Experts should demonstrate cultural competence

c) Emerging characteristics and expectations of expert professionals
- Experts demonstrate information and communication literacy
- Experts value and utilize the expertise of other team members
- Experts own and embody their practice model
- Expertise goes beyond technical expertise in pursuit of emancipatory practice
- Expert practice is community-oriented
- Expertise is informed by reflexive practice as well as research
- Experts are informed of the health and demographic trends in the communities they serve
- Experts' behaviour demonstrates a strong moral commitment to beneficence through such behaviours as patient advocacy and non-judgemental attitudes

decision'. The concept of professional practice judgement artistry is discussed in Chapter 16.

ERRORS AND QUALITY: COGNITIVE DIMENSIONS

Errors in clinical reasoning are frequently linked to errors in cognition (Kempainen et al 2003, Rivett & Jones 2004, Scott 2000). Examples of such errors include over-emphasis on findings that support an existing hypothesis, misinterpretation of non-contributory information as confirming an existing hypothesis, rejection of findings which do not support a favoured hypothesis and incorrect interpretation related to inappropriately applied inductive and deductive logic (Elstein et al 1978, Kempainen et al 2003). These errors are commonly associated with habits of thinking and practice which themselves are a potential risk of pattern recognition. That is, in adopting a pattern recognition approach the novice or unreflective practitioner might focus too much on looking for the presence or absence of specific patterns and overlook other potentially important information, or might find it difficult to see anything outside the most familiar patterns (De Bono

1977). Patterns can become rigid, making it difficult to recognize variations. This excessive focus on favourite patterns also leads to patterns being identified on the basis of insufficient information, where one or several key features in a presentation are prematurely judged to represent a particular pattern. Metacognitive skills are the key to protecting against errors associated with pattern recognition.

ERRORS AND QUALITY: INTERACTIVE DIMENSIONS

Within the changing face of health care and the trend towards interactive reasoning there is a need not only to look beyond the cognitive processes of reasoning but also to see matters of quality and errors beyond simply cognitive abilities. Practitioners who wish to adopt a patient-centred approach or a team approach may make errors related to inauthentic implementation of espoused models of practice, lack of valuing or inclusion of the knowledge and reasoning input of team members or patients, and limitations in interpersonal communication, including cultural incompetence. The matter of ethical reasoning also becomes more prominent in interactive reasoning, in terms of choosing to share decision-making responsibilities while yet retaining individual responsibility for one's actions. Also, in determining to share decision making with patients the practitioner faces the dilemma of dealing with patient's wishes, informed position and power, which may be in conflict with what the practitioner considers to be in the patient's best interests.

A MODEL OF INTERACTIVE REASONING AND THE PROBLEM SPACE

Health care is not a decontextualized implementation of protocols, scientific evidence or intellectual information processing. Instead, whether at the level of individual patient or system, health care and decision making operate in context. This is true not only of decision making but also of the store of practice wisdom that the practitioner draws upon as the professional frame of reference

for decision making. Practice experiences are gained in context; they are stored in the context of the settings and happenings which they comprise, and they are recalled for future application and contemplation as contextualized meaning chunks (see e.g. Boshuizen & Schmidt 2000, Gordon 1988, Schön 1983).

One of the greatest challenges of clinical reasoning is to harmonize generally accepted healthcare practices and evidence for practice with person-centred practice. This means that *best practice* should be particularized, not generic. Many people today are recognizing the importance of firmly embedding thinking and reasoning in context (Whiteford & Wright-St Clair 2005). In recent significant research on the impact of context on clinical decision making, Smith (2006) identified that clinical decision making in actual practice is a context-dependent process that is socially and culturally determined. Smith developed a model of factors influencing clinical decision making (see also Chapter 8) in which three levels of context impact on clinical decision making: the immediate patient care context, the practitioner context and the workplace context.

According to Schön (1983), clinical reasoning involves the naming and framing of problems based on a personal understanding of the client's situation. Two forms of scientific reasoning identified by researchers in occupational therapy are diagnostic reasoning (Rogers & Holm 1991) and procedural reasoning (Mattingly & Fleming 1994). These processes involve a progression from problem sensing to problem definition and problem resolution. These tasks give rise to the idea of the problem space. The notion of the problem space in clinical reasoning has been used by a number of authors. Elstein et al (1978), for example, considered the size of the problem space in relation to the number of hypotheses generated by students and physicians. They found that early in the patient encounter students and physicians generated a limited number of hypotheses (three to five) from limited patient data, and that these guided subsequent data collection. The authors postulated that this was a way of coping with the problem of information overload by reducing the size of the problem space that must be searched for a solution to the problem. Patel & Arocha (2000) examined the theory of protocol analysis that is based on the idea that verbalizations in problem solving are interpreted as a search through a problem space of hypotheses and data.

We use the term *problem space* in a broader way than described above, to reflect the multiple contexts of clinical reasoning. Problem spaces comprise the immediate clinical problem and task environment of clinical decision making embedded in the interests and frames of references of the practitioner(s) and the patient/client. These problem spaces, in turn, are located in the broader clinical reasoning context that encompasses the many local, organizational, sociocultural, global factors that influence clinical decision making (see Figure 1.1).

THE CLIENT'S PROBLEM SPACE

The role for the healthcare consumer is radically different in many respects from the dependent patient role of traditional medicine, where 'autonomy' of health professionals was defined as complete control over clinical decision making and clinical intervention. Consumers of health care are becoming increasingly well informed about their health and about healthcare services. Terms such as *self-help* and *holistic health care* are becoming

more central to health care, and the goal of achieving effective participation by consumers in their health care is widespread, requiring health professionals to involve their clients actively in clinical decision making wherever possible. Increasingly, clients' choices, rights and responsibilities in relation to their health are changing. Payton et al (1990) advocated client involvement in decision making about the management of their health and well-being. They argued that this process of client participation is based on the 'recognition of the values of self-determination and the worth of the individual' (p. ix). Using understanding of their clients' rights and responsibilities, clinicians need to develop their own approaches to involving the client in reasoning and decision making. Mutual decision making requires not only a sharing of ownership of decisions but also the development of skills in negotiation and explaining, to facilitate effective two-way communication. Professional autonomy becomes redefined as independence in function (within a teamwork context) combined with responsibility and accountability for one's actions (including the sharing of decision making).

The problem space of clients plays an important role in the process of clinical reasoning since it impacts on framing, naming and dealing with their healthcare needs and concerns; it comprises:

- The *personal context* of individual clients, which incorporates such factors as their unique cultural, family, work and socioeconomic frames of reference and their state of health. Each of these factors contributes to clients' beliefs, values and expectations, and to their perceptions and needs in relation to their health needs and problems.
- The *unique multifaceted context of clients' healthcare needs*. This includes clients' health conditions as well as their unique personal, social and environmental situation. Clinical problems can be 'confusing and contradictory, characterised by imperfect, inconsistent, or even inaccurate information' (Kassirer & Kopelman 1991, p. vii). Similarly, for clients who are seeking health promotion solutions, health professionals face the task of identifying and dealing with multiple personal and environmental

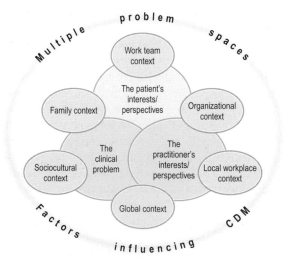

Figure 1.1 Clinical decision making (CDM) in multiple problem spaces (based on Higgs 2006a)

variables to produce an optimal client-centred solution.

- The *specific context of health care for the client under consideration*. Health care settings are many and varied, ranging from programmes of mass media health promotion to high-technology intensive care hospital units. Despite this diversity, a number of commonalities exist. Firstly, in each case the focus is on the health of people. Secondly, since the services provided occur in human contexts, the healthcare environment is typically characterized by complexity, uncertainty and subjectivity. These factors have a strong influence on the nature of reasoning and on the impact of decisions made.

An important aspect of involving patients or clients in clinical decision making is determining and facilitating an appropriate level of participation and responsibility. A level of participation in clinical reasoning appropriate for the individual has been demonstrated to contribute to the patient's sense of control; in this process it is important to ensure that the patient's input is voluntary and the patient is informed of the inherent uncertainties of clinical decision making (Coulter 2002).

THE PRACTITIONER'S PROBLEM SPACE

Practitioners bring their personal and professional selves to the task of clinical decision making; these selves frame their problem space. As well as functioning within their personal frames of reference, clinicians operate within their professional frameworks (e.g. the ethical and competency standards/ requirements of the profession) and within a broader context of professionalism. The term *health professional* implies a qualified healthcare provider who demonstrates professional autonomy, competence and accountability (Higgs 1993). Professional status incorporates the responsibility to make unsupervised and accountable clinical decisions and to implement ethical, competent and person-centred practice. This requires health professionals to consider the patient's problem space, as described above, and to make decisions about the patient's level of involvement. Dealing with ill-structured healthcare problems requires high-level clinical

reasoning abilities, increasingly refined and elaborated medical knowledge (Schmidt et al 1990) and judgement (Round 2001). In relation to ethical issues, practitioners need the ability to deal with these matters in person-centred, professional ways. In addition, practitioners' problem spaces include their choice of practice model (see Chapter 3), their clinical reasoning capability, and clinical reasoning expertise (see Chapter 11).

THE COLLABORATIVE PROBLEM SPACE OF THE TEAM

Most health professionals work in collaboration with other team members, either directly or indirectly via referral. This includes work across mainstream and complementary and alternative medicine. Byrne (1999) suggested that a coordinated and integrated approach to care is particularly important in the management of chronic and complex health problems. Similarly, Grace et al (2006) identified an increasing preference in patients with chronic health problems, particularly those dissatisfied with mainstream medicine, for practices that directly integrate complementary and alternative medicine with general practice; such models worked best for the patients when both practitioners worked in collaboration. Another area where multidisciplinary health care has been found to be beneficial and widespread is chronic pain management (Loftus & Higgs 2006).

The level of collaboration in clinical decision making in these settings varies considerably. Practitioners may make decisions separately and report decisions to others (e.g. via patient records); they may refer patients to others to take over patient care or to receive advice; they may operate as a decision-making team, making decisions on behalf of their patients (see Chapter 26); or they may work with patients as members of the decision-making team (see Chapters 4, 34).

THE PROBLEM SPACE OF THE WORKPLACE AND THE LOCAL SYSTEM

Clinicians frequently face ill-defined problems, goals that are complex and outcomes that are difficult to predict clearly. Many aspects of the workplace (see Chapter 9) influence clinical decision making, particularly levels of available human, material and economic resources. Many factors in the workplace frame our approaches to our practice of clinical reasoning. Funding pressures create 'clinical practices whose explicit demands are heavily weighted toward management and productivity rather than diagnosis and understanding' (Duffy 1998, p. 96). Such practices are not conducive to reflecting on our understanding of practice. Further, misinterpretations of what evidence-based practice really requires (see Reilly et al 2004), means that some clinicians do not use clinical reasoning critically and wisely to assess evidence for its applicability to individual patients (Jones et al 2006a, b).

One way of thinking about healthcare systems is to conceptualize them as 'soft systems', a term introduced by Checkland (1981) to refer to systems in which goals may be unrecognizable and outcomes ambiguous. Professional judgement and decision making within the ambiguous or uncertain situations of health care is an inexact science (Kennedy 1987) which requires reflective practice and excellent skills in clinical reasoning (Cervero 1988, Schön 1983). These skills reflect the importance of individual perspectives rather than a priori criteria (Jungermann 1986). Skills of professional judgement and critical self-evaluation are needed to cope with information processing constraints or 'bounded rationality' (Newell & Simon 1972) which result in limitations on the individual's ability to access knowledge and solve problems (Bransford et al 1986, Feltovich 1983, Hassebrock & Johnson 1986). One way to interpret the way in which professionals cope with the uncertainties and challenges of clinical reasoning is to look beyond science. Harris (1993), for instance, presents the concept of professional

practice as comprising a blend of art, craft and technology.

THE PROBLEM SPACE OF THE GLOBAL SYSTEM WITH ITS HEALTHCARE DISCOURSE, KNOWLEDGE AND TECHNOLOGY

Many factors of the wider healthcare environment need to be taken into consideration in clinical reasoning. Health professionals need to develop a broad understanding of the environment in which they work, including knowledge of the factors influencing health (e.g. the environment, socioeconomic conditions, cultural beliefs and human behaviour). In addition, they need to understand how the information age and the technological revolution impact on healthcare demands, provision and expectation. They need to be able to work confidently and effectively with an increasing body of scientific, technical and professional knowledge. Developing a sound individual understanding of clinical reasoning and a capacity to reason effectively will facilitate the clinician's ability to manage complex and changing information.

CONCLUSION

Whether understanding clinical reasoning is for knowledge generation or research (what is it like?), education (how can it be learned?), or practice (how can we use it? how can we do it well?), the central need is to understand what it is and how it can be developed. In this chapter we have portrayed clinical reasoning as a complex set of processes occurring within multiple and multidimensional problem spaces.

References

Agan R 1987 Intuitive knowing as a dimension of nursing. Advances in Nursing Science 10:63–70

Albert A D, Munson R, Resnik M D (eds) 1988 Reasoning in medicine: an introduction to clinical inference. Johns Hopkins University Press, Baltimore

Arocha J F, Patel V L, Patel Y C 1993 Hypothesis generation and the coordination of theory and evidence in novice diagnostic reasoning. Medical Decision Making 13: 198–211

Barnitt R, Partridge C 1997 Ethical reasoning in physical therapy and occupational therapy. Physiotherapy Research International 2:178–194

Barrows H S, Feltovich P J 1987 The clinical reasoning process. Medical Education 21:86–91

Barrows H S, Feightner J W, Neufield V R et al 1978 An analysis of the clinical methods of medical students and physicians. Report to the Province of Ontario Department of Health. McMaster University, Hamilton, Ontario

Beeston S, Higgs J 2001 Professional practice: artistry and connoisseurship. In: Higgs J, Titchen A (eds) Practice knowledge and expertise in the health professions. Butterworth-Heinemann, Oxford, p 108–117

Beeston S, Simons H 1996 Physiotherapy practice: practitioners' perspectives. Physiotherapy Theory and Practice 12:231–242

Benner P, Tanner C, Chesla C 1992 From beginner to expert: gaining a differentiated clinical world in critical care nursing. Advances in Nursing Science 14:13–28

Bleakley A, Farrow R, Gould D et al 2003 Making sense of clinical reasoning: judgement and the evidence of the senses. Medical Education 37(6):544–552

Boshuizen H P A, Schmidt H G 1992 On the role of biomedical knowledge in clinical reasoning by experts, intermediates and novices. Cognitive Science 16:153–184

Boshuizen H P A, Schmidt H G 2000 The development of clinical reasoning expertise. In: Higgs J, Jones M (eds) Clinical reasoning in the health professions. 2nd edn. Butterworth-Heinemann, Oxford, p 15–22

Bransford J, Sherwood R, Vye N et al 1986 Teaching thinking and problem solving: research foundations. American Psychologist 41:1078–1089

Brooks L R, Norman G R, Allen S W 1991 Role of specific similarity in a medical diagnostic task. Journal of Experimental Psychology: General 120(3):278–287

Byrne C 1999 Interdisciplinary education in undergraduate health sciences. Pedagogue (Perspectives on Health Sciences Education) 3:1–8

Cervero R M 1988 Effective continuing education for professionals. Jossey-Bass, San Francisco

Checkland P B 1981 Systems thinking: systems practice. John Wiley, New York

Coulter A 2002 The autonomous patient: ending paternalism in medical care. Nuffield Trust, London

Coulter A 2005 Shared decision-making: the debate continues. Health Expectations 8.95–96

De Bono E 1977 Lateral thinking. Penguin, London

Duffy J 1998 Stroke with dysarthria: evaluate and treat; garden variety or down the garden path. Seminars in Speech and Language 19:93–98

Edwards I C, Jones M A, Carr J et al 1998 Clinical reasoning in three different fields of physiotherapy – a qualitative study. In: Proceedings of the Fifth International Congress of the Australian Physiotherapy Association, Melbourne, p 298–300

Elstein A S, Shulman L S, Sprafka S A 1978 Medical problem solving: an analysis of clinical reasoning. Harvard University Press, Cambridge, MA

Elstein A S, Shulman L S, Sprafka S A 1990 Medical problem solving: a ten year retrospective. Evaluation and the Health Professions 13:5–36

Feltovich P J 1983 Expertise: reorganizing and refining knowledge for use. Professions Education Researcher Notes 4:5–9

Feltovich P J, Johnson P E, Moller J H et al 1984 LCS: the role and development of medical knowledge in diagnostic expertise. In: Clancey W J, Shortliffe E H (eds) Readings in medical artificial intelligence: the first decade. Addison-Wesley, Reading, MA, p 275–319

Fish D 1998 Appreciating practice in the caring professions: refocusing professional development and practitioner research. Butterworth-Heinemann, Oxford

Fleming M H 1991 The therapist with the three track mind. American Journal of Occupational Therapy 45:1007–1014

Fonteyn M, Fisher S 1992 The study of expert nurses in practice. Paper presented at: Transformation through unity: decision-making and informatics in nursing, 17 October, University of Oregon Health Science Centre, Portland, OR

Fonteyn M, Grobe S 1993 Expert critical care nurses' clinical reasoning under uncertainty: representation, structure and process. In: Frisse M (ed) Sixteenth annual symposium on computer applications in medical care. McGraw-Hill, New York, p 405–409

Glaser R, Chi M T H 1988 Overview. In: Chi M T H, Glaser R, Farr M J (eds) The nature of expertise. Lawrence Erlbaum, Hillsdale, NJ, p xv–xxviii

Gordon D 1988 Clinical science and clinical expertise: changing boundaries between art and science in medicine. In: Lock M, Gordon D R (eds) Biomedicine examined. Kluwer Academic, Dordrecht, p 257–295

Gordon M, Murphy C P, Candee D et al 1994 Clinical judgement: an integrated model. Advances in Nursing Science 16:55–70

Grace S, Higgs J, Horsfall D 2006 Integrating mainstream and complementary and alternative medicine: investing in prevention. In: Proceedings of the University of Sydney From Cell to Society 5 conference, 9–10 November, p 18–25

Groen G J, Patel V L 1985 Medical problem-solving: some questionable assumptions. Medical Education 19 (2):95–100

Hagedorn R 1996 Clinical decision making in familiar cases: a model of the process and implications for practice. British Journal of Occupational Therapy 59:217–222

Harris I B 1993 New expectations for professional competence. In: Curry L, Wergin J F and Associates (eds) Educating professionals: responding to new expectations for competence and accountability. Jossey-Bass, San Francisco, p 17–52

Hassebrock F, Johnson P E 1986 Medical knowledge and cognitive effort in diagnostic reasoning. Paper presented at the annual meeting of the American Educational Research Association, San Francisco

Higgs J 1993 Physiotherapy, professionalism and self-directed learning. Journal of the Singapore Physiotherapy Association 14:8–11

Higgs J 2006a Realising hermeneutic dialogues: creating spaces for critical, creative conversations in learning, research, clinical decision making and practice advancement. CPEA Occasional Paper no. 5. Collaborations in Practice and Education Advancement, University of Sydney, Australia

Higgs J 2006b The complexity of clinical reasoning: exploring the dimensions of clinical reasoning expertise as a situated, lived phenomenon. Seminar presentation at the Faculty of Health Sciences, 5 May, University of Sydney, Australia

Higgs J, Hunt A 1999 Rethinking the beginning practitioner: introducing the 'interactional professional'. In: Higgs J, Edwards H (eds) Educating beginning practitioners: challenges for health professional education. Butterworth-Heinemann, Oxford, p 10–18

Higgs J, Jones M 1995 Clinical reasoning. In: Higgs J, Jones M (eds) Clinical reasoning in the health professions. Butterworth-Heinemann, Oxford, p 3–23

Higgs J, Jones M 2000 Clinical reasoning in the health professions. In: Higgs J, Jones M (eds) Clinical reasoning in the health professions. 2nd edn. Butterworth-Heinemann, Oxford, p 3–14

Higgs J, Titchen A 2001 Towards professional artistry and creativity in practice. In: Higgs J, Titchen A (eds) Professional practice in health, education and the creative arts. Blackwell Science, Oxford, p 273–290

Higgs C, Neubauer D, Higgs J 1999 The changing health care context: globalization and social ecology. In: Higgs J, Edwards H (eds) Educating beginning practitioners: challenges for health professional education. Butterworth-Heinemann, Oxford, p 30–37

Higgs J, Trede F, Loftus S et al 2006 Advancing clinical reasoning: interpretive research perspectives grounded in professional practice, CPEA Occasional Paper no. 4. Collaborations in Practice and Education Advancement. University of Sydney, Australia

Jensen G M, Gwyer J, Hack L M et al 1999 Expertise in physical therapy practice. Butterworth-Heinemann, Boston

Jensen G M, Gwyer J, Hack L M et al 2006 Expertise in physical therapy practice, 2nd edn. Saunders-Elsevier, St Louis

Jones M, Grimmer K, Edwards I et al 2006a Challenges in applying best evidence to physiotherapy. Internet Journal of Allied Health Sciences and Practice 4(3). Online. Available:http://ijahsp.nova.edu/18 June 2007

Jones M, Grimmer K, Edwards I et al 2006b Challenges in applying best evidence to physiotherapy practice: part 2 – reasoning and practice challenges. Internet Journal of Allied Health Sciences and Practice 4(4):Online. Available:http://ijahsp.nova.edu/18 June 2007

Jungermann H 1986 The two camps on rationality. In: Arkes H R, Hammond K R (eds) Judgment and decision making: an interdisciplinary reader. Cambridge University Press, New York, p 627–641

Kassirer J P, Kopelman R I 1991 Learning clinical reasoning. Williams and Wilkins, Baltimore

Kempainen R R, Migeon M B, Wolf F M 2003 Understanding our mistakes: a primer on errors in clinical reasoning. Medical Teacher 25(2):177–181

Kennedy M 1987 Inexact sciences: professional education and the development of expertise. Review of Research in Education 14:133–168

Lawson A E, McElrath C B, Burton M S et al 1991 Hypothetico-deductive reasoning skill and concept acquisition: testing a constructivist hypothesis. Journal of Research in Science Teaching 28:953–970

Loftus S 2006 Language in clinical reasoning: learning and using the language of collective clinical decision making. Unpublished doctoral thesis. University of Sydney, Australia. Online. Available:http://ses.library.usyd.edu.au/handle/2123/1165

Loftus S, Higgs J 2006 Clinical decision-making in multidisciplinary clinics. In: Flor H, Kalso E, Dostrovsky J O (eds) Proceedings of the 11th World Congress on Pain. International Association for the Study of Pain, IASP Press, Seattle, p 755–760

Mattingly C, Fleming M H 1994 Clinical reasoning: forms of inquiry in a therapeutic practice. F A Davis, Philadelphia

Neuhaus B E 1988 Ethical considerations in clinical reasoning: the impact of technology and cost containment. American Journal of Occupational Therapy 42:288–294

Newell A, Simon H A 1972 Human problem solving. Prentice-Hall, Englewood Cliffs, NJ

Norman G 2005 Research in clinical reasoning: past history and current trends. Medical Education 39:418–427

Orasanu J, Connolly T 1993 The reinvention of decision making. In: Klein G A, Orasanu J, Calderwood R et al (eds) Decision making in action: models and methods. Ablex, Norwood, NJ, p 3–20

Padrick K, Tanner C, Putzier D et al 1987 Hypothesis evaluation: a component of diagnostic reasoning. In: McClane A (ed) Classification of nursing diagnosis: proceedings of the seventh conference. CV Mosby, Toronto, p 299–305

Patel V L, Arocha J F 2000 Methods in the study of clinical reasoning. In: Higgs J, Jones M (eds) Clinical reasoning in the health professions, 2nd edn. Butterworth-Heinemann, Oxford, p 78–91

Patel V L, Groen G J 1986 Knowledge-based solution strategies in medical reasoning. Cognitive Science 10:91–116

Paterson M, Higgs J 2001 Professional practice judgement artistry. CPEA Occasional Paper no. 3. Centre for Professional Education Advancement, University of Sydney, Australia

Payton O D, Nelson C E, Ozer M N 1990 Patient participation in program planning: a manual for therapists. FA Davis, Philadelphia

Reilly S, Douglas J, Oates J 2004 Evidence-based practice in speech pathology. Whurr, London

Rew L 1990 Intuition in critical care nursing practice. Dimensions of Critical Care Nursing 9:30–37

Rew L, Barrow E 1987 Intuition: a neglected hallmark of nursing knowledge. Advances in Nursing Science 10: 49–62

Ridderikhoff J 1989 Methods in medicine: a descriptive study of physicians' behaviour. Kluwer Academic, Dordrecht

Rivett D A, Jones M A 2004 Improving clinical reasoning in manual therapy. In: Jones M A, Rivett D A (eds) Clinical reasoning in manual therapy. Butterworth-Heinemann, Edinburgh, p 403–431

Rogers J C 1983 Clinical reasoning: the ethics, science, and art. Eleanor Clarke Slagle Lecture, American Journal of Occupational Therapy 37:601–616

Rogers J C, Holm M 1991 Occupational therapy diagnostic reasoning: a component of clinical reasoning. American Journal of Occupational Therapy 45:1045–1053

Round A P 2001 Introduction to clinical reasoning. Journal of Evaluation in Clinical Practice 7:109–117

Schmidt H G, Norman G R, Boshuizen H P A 1990 A cognitive perspective on medical expertise: theory and implications. Academic Medicine 65:611–621

Schön D A 1983 The reflective practitioner: how professionals think in action. Temple Smith, London

Scott I 2000 Teaching clinical reasoning: a case-based approach. In: Higgs J, Jones M (eds) Clinical reasoning in the health professions, 2nd edn. Butterworth-Heinemann, Oxford, p 290–297

Sluijs E M 1991 Patient education in physiotherapy: towards a planned approach. Physiotherapy 77:503–508

Smith M C L 2006 Clinical decision making in acute care cardiopulmonary physiotherapy. Unpublished doctoral thesis. University of Sydney, Sydney

Titchen A 2000 Professional craft knowledge in patient centred nursing and the facilitation of its development. Ashdale Press, Oxford

Trede F, Higgs J 2003 Re-framing the clinician's role in collaborative clinical decision making: re-thinking practice knowledge and the notion of clinician–patient relationships. Learning in Health and Social Care 2(2):66–73

Whiteford G, Wright-St Clair V (eds) 2005 Occupation and practice in context. Elsevier, Sydney

Chapter 2

The context for clinical decision ... century

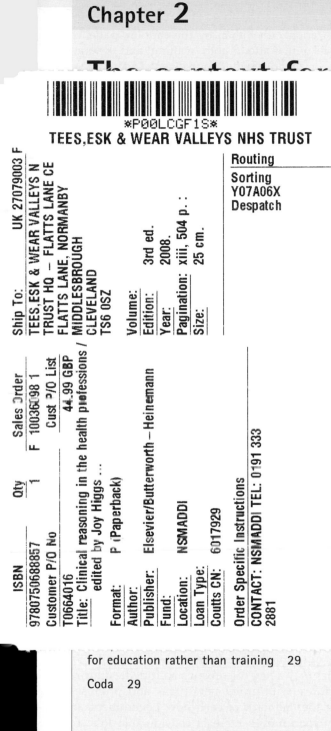

INTRODUCTION

In this chapter we consider the broad context of the 21st century within which professionals think and act. We look specifically at trends and patterns that have significance for clinical reasoning and decision making. We illustrate the current clashes of values and therefore of discourse in use by government, by health care, in education, in health management, in the media and by the public.

LIQUID MODERNITY: THE NATURE OF 21ST CENTURY LIFE

It seems to be commonly accepted that the world of the early 21st century is characterized by fragmentation and uncertainty. The global village that we all now inhabit enables on a daily basis the rapid spread of intimate knowledge of both current and potential major disasters. This frequent reminder of our vulnerability is distinctly destabilizing and anxiety-generating. Increasingly blurred national boundaries, problems of world aid and the complexity of balancing economic demands with the decreased resources of the public purse all have implications for consumers and providers (Higgs et al 1999). The major implication of these factors is our inability to cope with anything but 'now' and anyone but ourselves. This increasingly drives professionals to seek answers to such questions as 'Why?', 'Why not?', 'Why now?', 'Who is to blame?', and is reason enough for professionals to be ready with explanations of their clinical reasoning and decision making and able to articulate their explanations in a language appropriate to the listener or situation.

The terrible imbalances between the needy and impoverished developing world and the wealthy and self-absorbed West are clear. (And the Third World is not entirely located geographically separately from the Western world, but rather is often inside it.) Bauman (2000, 2005) has caught the spirit of life in the West in the 21st century in his term 'liquid modernity'. This mercurial 'liquid modern age' metaphor captures well the values and desires that are the current mark of the prosperous West. These values and desires involve considerable opposition to and rejection of the attitudes that predominated in the second half of the 20th century (such as the vision that puts others first, the sense of mystery of things beyond us, and recognition of the fallibility of human knowledge). They also challenge the ideals of service and moral responsibility that many professionals still have and, we would argue, should cling to, since exploring our clinical thinking is helped by having ideals to aspire to and a standard of expertise for which to strive.

Bauman's ideas, though extreme, certainly highlight current trends. In the liquid modern world, shortcuts are sought in order to do away with avoidable and resented chores or pass them on to others (outsourcing, delegation, restricted job specifications). A focus on – indeed an obsession with – the enjoyment of present goals and desires obscures the importance of the short term and obliterates the significance of the long term. Even consumerist values have changed. Durable and long-lasting products and possessions which used to be seen as attractive are now rather seen as liabilities. Long-term employment is increasingly considered an entanglement or a pipe dream. Solidity (including the strength of human bonds) is resented as a threat. Commitment augurs 'a future burdened with obligations'; and 'the prospect of being saddled with one thing for the duration of life is downright repulsive and frightening' (Bauman 2005, p. 40–41).

In this liquid modern age, things are expected to last for a fixed term only. Motives are characterized by impatience for the fulfilment of self-gratification rather than by the caution, patience and delay that attend both 'waiting' and the concern for others beyond ourselves. Today, these things somehow suggest inferiority. 'Rise in social hierarchy (status) is measured by the rising ability to have what one wants (whatever one may want) *now* – without delay … time is a bore and a chore, a pain, a snub to human freedom and a challenge to human rights, neither of which must or needs to be suffered gladly' (Bauman 2005, p. 38). Today's consumerism is not about the accumulation of things but their one-off enjoyment. As Neuberger (2005, p. xviii) writes: 'we have become demanders, not citizens; we look to ourselves rather than to society as a whole … the idea of an obligation to society, beyond the demands we ourselves wish to make, has become unfashionable.'

Where health care is still concerned with commitment – to patients, to best possible care, to persistence, to resilience, to carefulness and to obligations arising from and through multiprofessional teamwork – the liquid modern age seeks instant gratification and constant movement (which goes beyond fluency and flexibility to volatility, fragmentation and short life span of knowledge, tasks, work groups, etc.). Indeed, it apparently values not only the meretricious but also the ability to skate swiftly on thin ice rather than conduct oneself with the steadfastness of careful attention to detail or consideration for others.

It also seeks to foster 'loose knit organizations that could be put together, dismantled and reassembled as the shifting circumstances require – at short notice or without notice' (Bauman 2005, p. 44). Consider, for example, the independent treatment centres in the UK and how these are diminishing the role of NHS (National Health Service) hospitals (see Ribero, in Sylvester 2005). Politics play a key role in such shifting healthcare structures, with grand new plans and promises being the hallmark of each new government. In many such moves there is considerable loss: of institutional wisdom that avoids repeated errors and ill-advised quick fixes; of human motivation based in shared ownership of decision making and goal pursuit; and a clear, at least mid-term, sense of direction.

Thus, in the liquid modern world, established knowledge and know-how have a short life, and tradition and experience are no longer valued. Indeed, in the UK, for example, successive governments have declared history as of no importance and have uncritically pursued 'modernization' as a mantra for compulsive and impulsive change. In this atmosphere, hardly any form keeps its shape long enough to warrant trust and to gel into long-term reliability. 'In the volatile world of instant and erratic change the settled habits, solid cognitive frames and stable value preferences' (Bauman 2005, p. 44) are cast as handicaps.

Yet the fundamental relationship that enables healthcare practitioners to manage patient care is trust. The 'fiduciary relationship' which establishes trust is fostered by the ability of practitioners to explain professional matters articulately and clearly to all parties and to take proper account of their own values as well as the needs and values of all those involved or influential in patient/client care (including those providing services to other clients beyond the direct clinical context, e.g. in schools, community settings and industry). It is particularly hard to maintain this standard, given the general failure of trust and aversion to risk that occurs, in a world where health professionals 'do not trust the politicians not to blame them when things go wrong' and where society believes that 'politicians lie when they ... [promise] various services for all of us' (see Neuberger 2005, p. xix). But trust is essential, and professionals have to have the integrity to do all they can to earn it, even if they feel undervalued.

We believe that, ironically, the current drive for 'modernization' combined with a distorted bureaucratic form of 'political correctness' are bringing with them a world-wide drive for sameness or cloning which is using management control mechanisms to ensure that everyone is treated the same, behaves the same, adheres to the same ideas and which therefore has little room for creativity and individuality. There is something deeply undemocratic about bureaucrats imposing their values, their endless anxieties about 'conflicts of interest', their rule-book ways of working and their watchdog approach to accountability on professionals. As responsible members of a profession, their role is precisely to

argue their moral position, utilize their abilities to wear an appropriate variety of hats on different occasions with proper transparency and integrity, and exercise their clinical thinking and professional judgement in the service of differing individuals while making wise decisions about the relationship between the privacy of individuals and the common good.

However, the new capitalism of the West is certainly set to impose this bureaucratic approach on ever wider realms, fuelling both avarice and a demand for a dubious 'transparency' that renders everything about us relevant to the world at large and which arises from a distorted view of equality and diversity. As Bauman writes, quoting Dany-Robert Dufour: 'Capitalism dreams of not only pushing the territory in which every object is a commodity ... to the limits of the globe, but also to expand it in depth to cover previously private affairs once left to the individual charge (subjectivity, sexuality)' (Bauman 2005, p. 45). A recent ePress Kit, *The Future of Health Care*, by Deloitte & Touche USA (2006) stated 'The outlook among U.S. hospital administrators is more positive about the financial future of their facilities. At the same time ... [the report writers noted] that thin margins translate to a need for closer scrutiny of all hospital operations to boost revenues and reap cost savings through enhanced efficiencies.'

THE DOT.COM MENTALITY: MODERNIZATION A MAJOR THEME

The new 'modernized' world of work in the West is seated firmly within the liquid modern age and mirrors its values. It is, as Sennett points out, based on a very unrepresentative business model, that of internet startups and dot.com. entrepreneurs (see Garner 2006).

Sennett, who has studied society and culture for several decades in Britain and America, writes of the challenges facing us all today that 'only a certain kind of human being can prosper in unstable, fragmentary conditions' (Sennett 2005, p. 3). He argues persuasively that in Britain in the 21st century, the Labour government has been seduced by the superficial glamour of hot-desking and the short-term, no ties mentality of dot.com companies and is trying to impose it wholesale on the public sector. He adds: 'There is something bizarre about taking the conditions of an IT [information technology] startup firm and thinking you can run a hospital or a university that way. He notes that when New Labour talks about reforming the public sector – and they are endlessly bringing in one new policy after another without allowing anything to bed in – they are not talking about making it do what it does better. As he points out, it takes time to learn how to make things work through trial and error, but if you change it constantly you never find out what works and what does not. It is like a form of ADHD (attention deficit hyperactivity disorder) (see Sennett 2005, Garner 2006).

O'Neill (2002) made the same point when she suggested that the particular system of accountability that has been foisted on us by what we would call the human resources industry 'actually damages trust'. 'Plants', she wrote, 'don't flourish when we pull them up too often to check how their roots are growing: political, institutional and professional life too may not flourish if we constantly uproot it to demonstrate that everything is transparent and trustworthy' (p. 19).

Both 'liquid modernity' and the 'dot.com mentality' emphasize short-term fixes in the abstract, rather than long-term relationships with people. Lack of stability is par for the course, and there is endless shifting around of both ideas and products to make them catch the eye and sell better. Further, as Sennett points out, the business world favours young people who have no commitment and no sense of commitment, and encourages a culture that does little to bind community together. Under the pressure of more vested and glamorous priorities, calm rational and humane thinking are sidelined. Society's 'managed' acceptance of the diminishing importance of maintaining the continuity of care for a given patient is a major example of how the climate of the times seduces us to go along with ideas and values that we could not actually defend in cold blood.

Thus we see that the modernization of everything that moves has produced a system geared up to institutions shedding their responsibilities to employees and not making long-term commitments (such as pensions). It is all about how quick you can be rather than how seriously you take the problem. And as Sennett shows, in Britain (unlike Finland and Sweden) there is no political discussion of what is happening. However, we are optimistic that this is a 'self-limiting disease'. With Sennett, as quoted in Garner, we believe that this new capitalism is ultimately doomed because more and more people will come to understand that it is not about reforming the system but deforming it. As Sennett says perspicaciously, 'This [realization] will be the drama of the coming decades' (Garner 2006, p. 12).

Coincidentally with all this, healthcare professionals will need to maintain their integrity and their moral commitment to their patients, and will thus take a lead in establishing and enacting important values in health care. To do so they will need to understand better both the importance of their clinical reasoning and its role in developing that essential core of professional practice, namely professional judgement, and they will need to engage actively in continuing education. But initially at least they are likely to find the climate of health care in the Western world less than comfortable and encouraging.

CHANGING PATTERNS OF HEALTH CARE AND GOVERNMENT HEALTH AGENDAS

The context of clinical decision making in the 21st century is strongly influenced by changing policies and patterns of health care. The Fourth European Consultation on Future Trends, held in London in 1999, considered the prospects for implementing the WHO HEALTH21 policy framework (Barnard 2003). Two key practical issues were identified. Firstly, there is a need to break down the barriers between the curative services of clinical medicine and the services provided by many other health workers under the heading of 'public health'. Secondly, there is a recognition that while endeavouring to build policies, service development and professional practice on strong knowledge foundations, it is important to remember that policy and service provision environments are never static and the knowledge context of health care is highly dynamic. The consultation predicted a complex, volatile and stressful future for policy makers and implementers.

But while these ideas are unquestionably important, the language which presents them as 'workforce' issues and systems problems reveals priorities that are far from sympathetic to professionals' humanistic values. For example, the UK Pathfinder report of the 'Policy futures for UK health' project has identified six issues to inform UK health policy to 2015 (Barnard 2003):

1. People's expectations of health and health services are rising and the long-term financial sustainability of health services needs to be addressed.
2. Demography and ageing: the population is ageing and the working population is decreasing. An integrated policy for older people is required that properly addresses the individual experience of older people.
3. Information and knowledge management requires an effective strategy with an international focus.
4. The consequences of scientific advances and new technology need to be addressed in policy and management.
5. Workforce education and planning need to address the increasing pressures on health professionals and their changing roles.
6. Evaluation and improvement of system performance and quality (efficiency, effectiveness, economy and equity) are required with international benchmarking.

Healthcare systems in many countries face changing patterns of disease and disability, changing locations for health services provision, an increased focus on chronic diseases, and an increase in the need for complex disease management strategies. The pattern and location of healthcare provision is changing, with shorter hospital stays, an increase in outpatient/short-stay surgery, and an increasing percentage of healthcare expenditure (over 75% in Australia) on health care outside of hospitals (Horvath 2005). Horvath argues that medical education is not keeping up with

these trends. In conjunction with these trends are demographic changes (e.g. ageing populations, an increase in multicultural populations) which bring concomitant challenges and demands to healthcare provision.

The healthcare needs of society are also changing. Patients' expectations are shifting from wanting to be told what to do to wanting to be involved and informed about treatment options (Lupton 1997). Trede (2000) argues that more patients want to be taken seriously as people, rather than 'conditions', and this shift in patient role and expectations requires a parallel shift in clinicians' roles. Given the rise in incidence of chronic illnesses, with no cure commonly available in the near future, the role of clinicians is being and needs to be transformed from that of technical expert and authoritarian advisor to that of collaborative partner (Trede & Higgs 2003). This may prompt a return to a 'therapeutic relationship' in which the true value of each patient is the central motivator for care (Fish & de Cossart 2007), and where 'the power of medicine [and all health care] then becomes the power letting go control, [and] using knowledge of the limitations of medical work to encourage the patient to take part in the shared task of trying to understand and deal with the illness that affects his or her personal being' (Campbell 1984, p. 28).

THE IMPORTANCE OF DISCOURSE

By *discourse*, we mean 'the [choice of] vocabulary and language structures that we all use to refer to the world as we see it, or to shape the meanings we make of it. The discourse we use daily indicates our mindset and our particular ways of thinking about, or seeing, "reality"' (see Fish & Coles 2005, p. 62). Discourse is shaped by our personal and professional values. But these ways of seeing our world are tacit, and are rarely subjected to critical scrutiny. As a result they can exercise a hidden and potentially subverting influence over our lives and work. This is evident in the section above where the language of policy sounds familiar and apparently unquestionable.

Indeed, as Niblett (2001, p. 206) has pointed out, in order to understand a particular period or era, we need to be acquainted not, as one might expect, with its widely stated public opinions, but rather with the doctrines which have in everyone's minds become unchallengeable facts and an inevitable part of the life of the time. The problem is that people not only cease to 'see' these 'doctrines' as mere ideas, but they come habitually to view most other things *through* them, and this then leads to routine acceptance of certain metaphors as the only way to characterize the current world.

We suggest, for example, that management discourse has clandestinely taken over and is now quite inappropriately dominating how professionals see their practice. Metaphors from the world of industry, manufacturing and training (rather than images that conjure up professionalism, commitment to service, to human care, and to education rather than training) have become so familiar that we no longer challenge them. Indeed, we fail to notice their power in describing one thing in terms of another, until eventually we employ them quite unthinkingly as 'the given', even while with another voice we would roundly reject their implications once they were pointed out. Here are some examples: delivering health care and the management of care; health care as a product or package to be purchased; outcomes-related care; testing the product against specification; risk management; stakeholders; and cost efficiency and effectiveness.

Much of the thrust of this trend comes from recasting health care as an industry, and from managers' over-protective response to the current 'risk-aversion climate in society'. Neuberger (2005, p. vii–viii) offers this phrase as a signal that the world has unthinkingly embraced 'rules and regulations, well founded, well meant, even theoretically sensible that yet lead to an extraordinary situation in which a care worker cannot change a light bulb for fear of the consequences', which in turn makes the lives of vulnerable people more difficult than they need to be. She adds later: 'It is as if we are trying to create a risk-free society, which we know in our heads and hearts is impossible. The result is that we restrict and regulate, hoping to make terrible things impossible whilst knowing we cannot, and in the process, deterring the willing and kind' (p. xi–xii). Risk-aversion, she argues persuasively, 'will make for bad services, where no

one will do what seems natural and kind in case they get accused of behaving improperly or riskily' (p. xix).

What is lost here are these ideas: *care*-centred health care; health care as a process rather than a product; compassion for the individual; responsibility for more than just ourselves; sympathetic and humane decision making rather than patient management; well-founded trust between patient and professional; and an acceptance by all involved that life cannot be risk-free and will remain complex and uncertain. This would constitute what Campbell (1984, p. 114), in an earlier discourse, called 'a tipping of the balance away from predominantly self-satisfying motives … towards a gratuitous concern for the welfare of others which does not deny self-interest but which from time to time at least, breaks through egotistical boundaries.'

Management discourse drives and sustains the same pattern of ideas at the level of governmental control of the professions. In addition to using the above terminology, government documents now refer to professionals as 'manpower', 'human resources', and 'the workforce', and encourage the notion that clinical practice is the 'shop-floor' of 'the health industry'. What these metaphors (which arise from the *apparently* ubiquitous but unexamined desire to see health care in consumerist terms) are leading to is well captured by Tallis (2004, p. 243) in terms of medicine but applying equally across health care:

> The patient as client or customer in the shopping mall of medical care will see the doctor as a vendor rather than as a professional. There will be an increasing emphasis on the accoutrements that make the first experience, or the first encounter, customer-friendly. The key to the doctor-as-salesman will be the emphasis on those aspects of customer care that give the patient a feeling of 'empowerment'.

But what of those who cannot assert their rights so robustly? Will they be forced to receive whatever the system sells them? How does that fit with high-sounding healthcare goals such as the UK NHS philosophy of 'the best possible care for the greatest number of people' (see Neuberger 2005, p. xvii)?

Indeed, society in the Western world at the beginning of the 21st century seems to prioritize (value) uncritically only that which is superficially evident, measurable and able to be speedily executed. It has fallen into the trap that MacNamara's fallacy illustrates (Broadfoot 2000, p. 219):

> The first step is to measure whatever can easily be measured. This is OK as far as it goes. The second step is to disregard that which cannot easily be measured or to give it an arbitrary quantitative value. This is artificial and misleading. The third step is to presume that what can't be measured easily really isn't important. This is blindness. The fourth step is to say that what can't easily be measured really doesn't exist. This is suicide.

A key example of an important 'immeasurable' in health care is the real experience and goals people have for their own health:

> Health potential can be best achieved when patients' personal integrity remains intact, their quality of life is enhanced, and when they gain an improved sense of control over their health with long-term sustainability wherever possible. (Trede & Higgs 2003, p. 67)

The world of commerce thrives on manipulating numbers and on clever advertising using witty and memorable catchwords. These disarm criticism, gain our passive acceptance and absorption, and create the climate the *market* needs while pretending it is responding to consumers' wishes. In health care now it is interesting to note how consumerist catchphrases, initially advanced by bureaucrats, have been so quickly accepted as unchallenged and unalterable 'facts'. All this poses questions about the nature of health professionals' expertise, autonomy and responsibility.

HEALTHCARE EXPERTISE AND THE CURRENT CLIMATE

As several writers have argued, recognition of their membership of a profession obliges healthcare workers to seek to serve the public in ways that properly acknowledge their moral and ethical responsibilities (see Fish & Coles 2005; Freidson 1994, 2001; Higgs 1993). In concurring with this, we see the work of a professional as involving far more than visible skills. It frequently involves making difficult and complex clinical decisions that result from extensive but invisible exploration and weighing of apparently equal but seemingly incompatible priorities. It also demands that professionals take account in this of their own values and preferences and may even have to set these aside for the greater good of the patient.

The arguments in respect of not merely behaving like a professional, but actually being a member of a profession, are well illustrated by the statement in Box 2.1 of what membership of a profession entails. We see here the challenges that professionals face, the expectations that the public should be able to have of professionals in the provision of services, and the demands that need to be met in order to reach high levels of professional status and performance.

This statement highlights the commitment to high-quality health care expected of all health professionals. But such commitment and the integral clinical reasoning of which it is a part are commonly hidden from view. Some aspects of professionalism may be inferred from visible behaviour, but much of it is not in the public domain unless the professional places it there. This invisibility puts health professionals at a considerable disadvantage in a world where there is a strong tendency for patients, managers, the media and the public to see and unhesitatingly judge quality solely on the basis of the observable. Professionals are indeed 'under siege' (see Fish & Coles 1998). And ironically, this hidden realm is a place where incompetence, deception and unethical behaviour can remain unchallenged.

Responses to these contradictory dilemmas include increasing levels of bureaucratic scrutiny in the form of programme and institution accreditation (with an emphasis on counting the easily countable) and moves by professional organizations to rethink their roles and responsibilities in this changing world. For example, this is why we welcome the recent report from the British Royal College of Physicians (2005) on medical professionalism in a changing world. Their arguments (with which we concur and would apply across the health professions) might be summarized thus:

Box 2.1 Membership of a profession (adapted from Fish & Coles 2005, p. 110, with acknowledgement to Freidson 1994)

A profession is an occupation. It is *specialized work* by which a living is gained.

But it is more than an occupation. It is *work for some good in society* (education, health, justice).

A member of a profession *exercises 'good' in the service of another*, and engages in *specific activities which are appropriate to the aims of the service*.

The service that a member of a profession renders a client *cannot entirely be measured by the remuneration given*.

Members of a profession have a *theoretical basis* to their practice and draw upon a *researched body of knowledge*.

Work by a member of a profession is *esoteric, complex, and discretionary*. It requires *theoretical knowledge, skill and professional judgement that ordinary people do not possess, may not wholly comprehend, and cannot readily evaluate*.

Professionals have an *ethical basis* to their work. This is about much more than having a code of conduct to follow. It is about having to make on-the-spot judgements and engage in actions which are *immediate responses to complex human events, as they are experienced*. (That is, professionals create meaning *on the spot in response to complex situations*.)

This brings with it the *moral duty* for professionals to be aware of the values (personal and professional) *that drive their judgements and actions* and the duty to recognize *and take account of them as part of their on-the-spot responses*.

Being aware of one's *personal and professional values is therefore vital*.

It also brings with it the need for *some autonomy of action*. This needs to be *circumscribed by the traditions within which professionals are licensed to practise*.

The capacity to perform this service depends upon retaining *a fiduciary relationship with clients* ('fiduciary' means that it is necessary for the client to put some trust in the judgement of the professional).

In the public interest, professionals also need to have *a commitment to lifelong education*.

Medical practice is characterized by the need for judgement in the face of uncertainty. A doctor's medical knowledge and skill may provide the explicit scientific and experiential base for such judgement. But medicine's considerable unpredictability and complexity calls for wisdom as well as technical ability. Since this is invisible, doctors' decisions are neither transparent nor easily accountable. This means that they must be clearer about what they do, and how and why they do it; must show a commitment to inquire into and review their clinical thinking and decision making; and must be aware of the qualities that make up their professionalism and its implications for their own practice.

But such endeavours will not be easily accomplished. The climate of the 21st century is distinctly unfriendly to members of professions. It has, for example, erected considerable barriers to the very humane approaches to caring that probably brought professionals into health care in the first place. Neuberger (2005, p. xii–xiii) refers to nurses 'being unwilling to offer a dying person a drink in case they choke, thereby risking legal action against themselves, or, more likely, the hospital … . Because of the requirements of the Health and Safety Executive, nurses cannot even lift an elderly person who has fallen out of bed … [having instead to wait until] suitable hoists have been found.' She points out that although none of this 'is necessarily wrong in itself', the 'cumulate effect of a risk-averse culture results in an erosion of simple kindness … pushes out common sense … [and] has increased a natural human reluctance to get involved.'

This context sharply illustrates why there is now a greater need than ever before for health-care professionals to be able to unearth and consider all the priorities in each patient case, to come up with good clinical decisions and sound professional judgements, and to explain how they have been reached. In short, it now requires them to make explicit and explore both the implicit and tacit in their practice, and to be able to articulate them (often on the spot) to a wide variety of audiences.

THE IMPORTANCE OF PATIENT CONTEXT

In professional practice, context is paramount. Every patient encounter is individual. Each case, while not being unique, is certainly particular to the one patient and all those involved. How the practitioner(s) are influenced by and read the context will affect their interpretation of the case (see Fish & de Cossart 2007). Thus, 'the activities that practitioners engage in are intelligible *only* by reference to their own understandings of what they are doing and the tradition of conduct of which they are a part' (Golby & Parrott 1999, p. 9). Good practice is thus context-specific (and as we shall see later, professionals' understanding of this situation is more significant than the level of their skill).

Thus, making sense of health professionals' clinical reasoning (both for themselves and those with whom they share it) depends both on the individual context of the case and on the broader climate in which it has occurred.

DELIVERING THE NHS PLC: AN EXAMPLE FROM THE UK

In the UK (as across healthcare systems in much of the rest of the world) politicians have for the last 25 years, under successive governments, progressively dismantled and privatized the UK National Health Service, gradually turning it from a welfare system into a public limited company (see Dyson 2003, Pollack 2005). This has involved orchestrating a huge change in values, and it has by and large been achieved by stealth.

Pollack argues, with thoroughness and persuasiveness, that health care has become once again a commodity to be bought rather than a right to be demanded. She declares: 'the dismantling

process and its consequences are profoundly anti-democratic and opaque' (Pollack 2005, p. i). She points out that the catchphrases endemic to the political discourse ('public–private partnerships'; 'modernization'; 'value for money'; 'local ownership') conceal the complexity of [the NHS's] transformation into a market. She demonstrates how the complexity of health care allows this transformation 'to be buried under a thousand half-truths', while the systematic nature of the change is 'hidden in the rhetoric of "diversity" and "choice".' She illustrates this process both at an overall level and in detail in terms of three core sectors of health care: hospitals; primary care and long-term care for the elderly.

In similar spirit, but employing a rather more managerial perspective, Dyson (2003) analyses the failings of the NHS and proposes a more durable system for health care in the UK. He proposes six underpinning premises:

1. NHS care should be free at the point of delivery.
2. The health service should be funded out of taxation and borrowing.
3. The Secretary of State for Health should be responsible for public health provision.
4. Equality of provision is a fundamental value.
5. Clinical provision in hospital needs to be based on a partnership of specialists and generalists across professions.
6. There should be a boundary between health and social care.

This last point brings us to another of the major characteristics of UK health care in the 21st century: the increase in working across professions in partnership, the increasing development of new professions, and the increased demand for interprofessional or multidisciplinary teamwork. These developments give healthcare practitioners yet another reason for improving their articulation of all those invisible elements of their practice, in the interests of being better understood by those whose profession uses different language and may embrace different values, and also by those in professions that abut each other's territory.

As a major and flourishing 'industry', the NHS is already attracting glances from the big capitalists from America and Europe who could well asset-strip the current system and may leave the 'customer' having to travel vast distances for the range of care that the NHS used to provide in nearby hospitals, centres and surgeries. While healthcare professionals are required to base all their work on evidence-based practice, governments bring in change after change, untested, unresearched, undebated. And alongside this, many members of the public and the media persist in their expectations of clinicians providing perfect solutions and maintain unintelligent or unrealistic ideas about the nature of clinical practice (see e.g. Fish & Coles 2005, Tallis 2004).

Despite all that, there is a profound (if unthinking) affection in the UK for the NHS:

> Despite the worries about quality and standards, and worries as to whether the service will be there for us when we it need it most, the NHS is still highly trusted and much loved ... The welfare state may have its difficulties, but the UK population still believes in it ... The way it works may change ... But by providing health services relatively cheaply and efficiently to the whole population, the NHS is part of the glue that holds British society together. (Neuberger 2005, p. vii).

Healthcare professionals need to know where they stand in all this. They need as never before to be able to explain their values and philosophy, and they need to be able to do so in a variety of ways to meet the needs of a variety of listeners.

IMPLEMENTING THE NATIONAL CHRONIC DISEASE MANAGEMENT STRATEGY (AN AUSTRALIAN EXAMPLE)

Chronic disease currently accounts for more than 80% of Australia's overall disease burden (Horvath 2005). To address this shift in emphasis from infectious disease to chronic disease management, a National Chronic Disease Strategy is being developed to serve as a framework for healthcare management across a broad range of diseases, including asthma, cardiovascular disease, diabetes, cancer and arthritic conditions. This strategy incorporates:

- building workforce capacity by providing skills needed to work effectively in multidisciplinary teams

- strategic partnerships between government and key industry bodies to facilitate work across current funding and service delivery boundaries
- enhanced investment and funding opportunities that allow multidisciplinary and integrated care, self-management and health promotion
- investment in information systems and technology to allow efficient electronic management of patients' records and information systems.

Health professionals working with patients with chronic diseases face changes in their practices:

- Patients will be older and sicker because of co-morbidities.
- Care will need to be provided across a range of different settings that includes community care clinics, private specialist rooms, general practice and residential aged care as well as inpatient acute facilities.
- More service providers will be involved in the care of each patient and a team approach to case management will be essential.
- There will be an increased focus on delivering interventions to address the major risk factors for chronic disease, including smoking, poor nutrition, risky and high alcohol use and physical inactivity.

All these factors have significant implications for the education and practice of health professionals. A major consideration is the development of clinical reasoning capacity and strategies that are suited to this population. Collaborative decision making has an important part to play in this context (Edwards et al 2004), building both on the principle of *the right of persons and communities* to participate in decision making affecting their health as outlined by the World Health Organization in its global strategy of 'Health for All' (WHO 1978) and on the demonstrated improvement in outcomes from genuine collaborative approaches to health care (Lorig et al 1999, Neistadt 1995, Shendell-Falik 1990, Werner 1998).

Evidence-based medicine is another aspect of medicine that provides a high motive for professionals needing to be able to explain their clinical reasoning and decision making. A highly distorted but commonly held version of evidence-based practice has given rise to absolutist expectations from patients about treatment. This ignores the original intentions, as stated by those who introduced the concept of evidence-based medicine, that medicine (and by association, health care generally) still depends crucially on the judgement of the professional. This:

> requires a bottom-up approach that integrates the best external evidence with individual clinical expertise and patient choice, [and] it cannot result in slavish cook-book approaches to individual patient care. External evidence can inform, but never replace, individual clinical expertise and it is this expertise that decides whether external evidence applies to the individual patient at all, and if so, how it should be integrated into a clinical decision. (Sackett et al 1997, p. 4)

The processes of clinical thinking and decision making are the centre of the expertise of health care professionals, who need to be ready to respond on the spot to questions and challenges to their decisions and actions. Time and thought need to be routinely available for them to explore the tacit and the implicit in their practice. Unearthing these invisible elements is an important part of their work, not a luxury add-on.

THE PRICE OF FALSE ECONOMY: HEALTH CARE'S NEED FOR EDUCATION RATHER THAN TRAINING

Because the demands for visible, measurable outcomes and accountability are ubiquitous, competencies are assumed to be the proper basis of training and assessment for healthcare professionals. Competencies are skills, and skills are visible. This emphasis on the visible and measurable has been further supported by the demands of health care's risk management industry and its proliferation of protocols in response to the

encouragement by the media and lawyers that the public should rush to litigation whenever possible. But although skills are necessary, they are not a sufficient basis for professional conduct. And their inculcation in professionals is short-term and overly expensive. Fish and de Cossart (2006) argue that an approach to the development of the practice of healthcare professionals that is based only on improvement in and extension of their skills is short sighted, morally bankrupt, dangerous and a false economy.

The myth that underpins training in the health professions is the idea that skills are generic, and once learned in one place can be unproblematically applied (will 'transfer') to all others. Were this so, training in skills *would* be the perfect (and cheap) long- and short-term solution to 'continuing professional development'. But good practice in a profession is context-specific. Skills need to be adapted every time they are used. And what aids their appropriate adaptation is adherence to sound principles that have been thought out and understood. So the preparation and development of professionals must include changing their understanding (education). *Understanding* involves the capacity to reflect on and apply reasoning to new problems; the capacity to modify skills to deal with similar but significantly different problems; and an awareness of why this modification is appropriate (Wilson 2005, p. 69).

CODA

By engaging in clinical reasoning and exploring the invisible dimensions of their practice, professionals extend their own education. Intelligent managers should see the economy and value in such pursuits as this; patients should recognize their gain from it; and the public should be reassured by it.

References

Barnard K 2003 The future of health – health for the future. Fourth European Consultation on Future Trends, published on behalf of the WHO Regional Office for Europe by the Nuffield Trust, London

Bauman Z 2000 Liquid modernity. Polity Press, Cambridge

Bauman Z 2005 The liquid modern challenges to education. In: Robinson S, Katulushi C (eds) Values in higher education. Aureus and the University of Leeds, Leeds, p 36–50

Broadfoot P 2000 Assessment and intuition. In: Atkinson T, Claxton G (eds). The intuitive practitioner: on the value of not always knowing what one is doing. Open University Press, Buckingham

Campbell A V 1984 Moderated love: a theology of professional care. SPCK, London

Dyson R 2003 Why the NHS will fail: and what should replace it? Mathew James Publishing, Chelmsford

Edwards I, Jones M, Higgs J et al 2004 What is collaborative reasoning? Advances in Physiotherapy 6:70–83

ePress Kit: The future of health care by Deloitte & Touche USA 2006. Online. Available: http://www.deloitte.com/dtt/press_release/0,1014 11 Oct 2006

Fish D, Coles C (eds) 1998 Developing professional judgement in health care: learning through the critical appreciation of practice. Butterworth-Heinemann, Oxford

Fish D, Coles C 2005 Medical education: developing a curriculum for practice. Open University Press in association with McGraw Hill, Maidenhead

Fish D, de Cossart L 2006 Thinking outside the (tick) box: rescuing professionalism and professional judgement. Medical Education 40(5):403–404

Fish D, de Cossart L 2007 Developing the wise doctor. Royal Society of Medicine Press, London

Freidson E 1994 Professionalism reborn: theory, prophesy and policy. Polity Press, Cambridge

Freidson E 2001 Professionalism: the third logic. Polity Press, Cambridge

Garner M 2006 Craftsmanship is laid low by quick-fix fever. Times Higher Educational Supplement, 10 Feb:18–19

Golby M, Parrott A 1999 Educational research and educational practice. Fair Way Press, Exeter

Higgs J 1993 Physiotherapy, professionalism and self-directed learning. Journal of the Singapore Physiotherapy Association 14:8–11

Higgs C, Neubauer D, Higgs J 1999 The changing health care context: globalization and social ecology. In: Higgs J, Edwards H (eds) Educating beginning practitioners: challenges for health professional education. Butterworth-Heinemann, Oxford, p 30–37

Horvath J 2005 The future of health care and the role for medical leaders, Australian Government Department of Health and Aging Media Release. Online. Available: http://www.dhac.gov.au/internet/wcms/publishing.nsf/Content/health-mediarel-yr2005 8 June 2006

Lorig K R, Sobel D S, Stewart A L et al 1999 Evidence suggesting that a chronic disease self-management program can improve health status while reducing utilization and costs: a randomized trial. Medical Care 37:5–14

Lupton D 1997 Doctors on the medical profession. Sociology of Health and Illness 19(4):480–497

Neistadt M E 1955 Methods of assessing clients' priorities: a survey of adult physical dysfunction settings. American Journal of Occupational Therapy 45:428–436

Neuberger J 2005 The moral state we're in. HarperCollins, London

Niblett W R 2001 Life, education, discovery: a memoir and selected essays. Pomegranate Books, Bristol

O'Neill O 2002 A question of trust. Polity Press, Cambridge

Pollack A 2005 NHS plc: the privatization of our health care. Verso Books, London

Royal College of Physicians 2005 Doctors in society: medical professionalism in a changing world. Royal College of Physicians, London

Sackett D L, Richardson W S, Rosenberg W et al 1997 Evidence-based medicine: how to practice and teach EBM. Churchill Livingstone, New York

Sennett R 2005 The culture of the new capitalism. Yale University Press, New Haven

Shendell-Falik N 1990 Creating self-care units in the acute care setting: a case study. Patient Education and Counselling 15:39–45

Sylvester R 2005 The man who thinks NHS funding needs radical surgery. The Telegraph 13 Aug. Online. Available: http://www.telegraph.co.uk/news/main.jhtml?xml=/news/2005/08/13/nrib113.xml 5 June 2007

Tallis R 2004 Hippocratic oaths: medicine and its discontents. Atlantic Books, London

Trede F V 2000 Approaches physiotherapists take in low back pain education. Physiotherapy 86(8):427–433

Trede F, Higgs J 2003 Re-framing the clinician's role in collaborative clinical decision making: re-thinking practice knowledge and the notion of clinician–patient relationships. Learning in Health and Social Care 2(2):66–73

Werner D 1998 Nothing about us without us: developing innovative technologies for, by and with disabled persons. HealthWrights, Palo Alto, CA

Wilson A 2005 Values in higher education: a social and evolutionary perspective. In: Robinson S, Katulushi C (eds) Values in higher education. Aureus and the University of Leeds, Leeds

World Health Organization 1978 Declaration of Alma Ata. International Conference on Primary Health Care, Alma-Ata. World Health Organization, Geneva, 6–12 September

Chapter 3

Clinical reasoning and models of practice

Franziska Trede and Joy Higgs

INTRODUCTION

Clinical reasoning occurs within models of practice. These models can be tacit (understood and largely unquestioned), controversial (known and debated), hegemonic (dominant and widely supported) and chosen (knowingly adopted). Practice models occur at different levels: they identify the broad strategy (such as the biomedical model) which operates at the level of a system, organization or workplace; they frame the interactions of team members (such as patient-centred care); and they give meaning and direction to the actions of individual practitioners (such as a humanistic or evidence-based orientation). In each case they reflect or challenge the interests (benefits and motivations) of the people working within the systems in which these models operate. In this chapter we report on doctoral research (Trede 2006) investigating interests underlying models of practice, and the impact of these interests on the model(s) that practitioners adopt, and the behaviours, particularly clinical reasoning, that are associated with these models.

The key issue addressed in this chapter is the impact of practitioners' interests on the construction of their practice models and thus their clinical reasoning. Of particular interest is how these interests are shaped and to what extent the practitioners are conscious of the interests that determine their decision making and behaviour. We discuss in this chapter a framework that illuminates current practice models from an interest-driven practice perspective and present a critical practice model, considering how such a perspective could redefine clinical reasoning.

Clinical reasoning is a challenging undertaking. It is influenced by a complex interplay between different interests and priorities that can range from wanting to assert professional authority and control over healthcare situations, to wanting to negotiate common ground with patients and create meaning, to striving to learn, transform and change oneself and patients. This discussion is framed by Habermas's (1972) theory of cognitive interests, in which he argued that ideas shape our interests and actions. In this chapter we explore the link between interests and the actions of clinical reasoning and clinical practice. Interests can be thought of as the motivation for wanting to think and act in certain ways. Such motivation can be internally driven by values, attitudes and desires, such as a humanistic perspective, valuing rationality, or the desire to be patient-centred. It can also be shaped by external interests such as pressures to adhere to the dominant healthcare practice model, system imperatives such as economic rationalism, society and peer expectations of professional behaviour, and trends or discourse in health care.

Health professionals are accountable and accept responsibility for their decisions and actions. What values, assumptions and reasons underpin and guide their thinking and decisions? Often such interests are subconscious and have been acquired through the pervasive and often osmotic process of professional socialization (Eraut 1994) rather than being consciously learned and adopted through critical self-appraisal and informed choice of a desired model of practice. Once practitioners are aware of their interests and understand what motivates these interests they are in a better position to make critically conscious choices as to how they seek to frame their clinical reasoning and consequent actions.

OVERVIEW OF THE RESEARCH

The doctoral research (Trede 2006) that informs this chapter was conducted with physiotherapy practitioners using an integrated research approach involving descriptive, critical and action-learning oriented strategies. The research methodology was guided by hermeneutic traditions including principles of question-and-answer dialogue. These dialogues were critically analysed to illuminate unreflected assumptions, professional ideology and any hidden professional authority adopted by the participants or their workplaces.

MODELS OF PRACTICE

The first phase of the research involved examination of the literature and different practice models and their underlying interests. Models of practice are abstract ideas of what practice should look like if it followed a given framework. These frameworks comprise a variety of interests, criteria, norms, practice principles and strategies and behavioural expectations that inform clinical reasoning and practice. Models can be thought of as mental maps that assist practitioners to understand their practice. They serve to structure and to fine-tune practitioners' clinical reasoning. Whether they are learned, chosen or unconsciously acquired through professional socialization, practice models generate the principles that guide practice, create the standards practitioners strive towards and the behavioural expectations that determine performance. Participants in this research had commonly acquired a biomedical science or medical practice model, the dominant physiotherapy practice model, through their educational and practice acculturation, with limited critique or questioning of this model. In such cases practitioners are commonly unaware of their practice model since it represents the unquestioned norm, and they are consequently unaware of how this model influences the way they reason. They reason within their adopted practice model without challenging the values and interests their practice model may entail.

THE SHAPING OF PRACTICE MODELS: THE PLACE OF IDEOLOGY

Professional ideology and interests, whether consciously or unconsciously enacted, inform practice models and professional practice (Newman 1994). Professional ideology is made up of the values, assumptions and prejudgements that guide our thinking (Therborn 1999). The type of practice we aspire to enact, the type of knowledge and evidence we value and utilize in practice, the way we justify our way of practising, and our clinical reasoning are all informed by interests that guide our curiosity in the first place.

We tend to interpret and justify our clinical reasoning processes with theoretical knowledge and research findings without acknowledging the interests and assumptions that inform our practice. Practice is justified with theories, guidelines and professional training. The ideology behind these theories and training remains hidden. To bring the assumptions out of hiding and question our way of reasoning enhances our practice awareness and provides us with real choices to practise optimally in each given clinical context.

It would be simplistic and limiting for a profession to define its practice purely on the basis of technical knowledge and skills (Schön 1987). This would reduce practice to the aspects that can be measured with empirico-analytical evidence only. What we observe, what we do, needs to be interpreted to make sense for us and to be communicated to others. Measurements and numbers on their own are meaningless. As professions develop and mature they become more involved with questions of expertise development and knowledge growth. Higgs et al (1999) claimed that a mature profession is one that enters into dialogue about its practices, is self-reflective, and pro-actively transforms with global changes.

CATEGORIZING PRACTICE MODELS

Professional practice models can be categorized in a number of ways. One such categorization is based on the theory of knowledge and human interest (Habermas 1972). According to this theory there are three types of interest, technical, practical and critical, each of which generates a certain type of knowledge. Each interest directs the types of question that can be asked, in turn dictating the type of knowledge that is generated and the way we practise. These interests not only shape the professional practice we adopt and determine which

modes of practice we see as valuable, they also influence the identity we adopt as professionals, how we see the role of patients, how we believe clinical decisions should be made, and how we justify and argue our professional roles and actions. Table 3.1 presents the illness, wellness and capacity practice models and their inherent interests, based on the three Habermasian interests.

Table 3.1 illustrates how interests shape practice models, knowledge and clinical reasoning in practice. Some aspects are of particular relevance in this discussion of clinical reasoning:

- The focus and definition of health influences healthcare goals. When health care focuses on illness and biomedical pathology, the goal of care is limited to reducing deficit or merely helping patients cope with current situations. When health is seen as a potential, the focus of reasoning and health care is on building capacity. A capacity practice model transcends the dualism of an illness and wellness model.
- The relative power of the clinician and patient varies significantly across different practice models and is reflected in clinical reasoning strategies. For instance, in an emancipatory model collaboration, inclusiveness and reciprocal facilitation of responsibility are embedded in clinical decision making.
- The type(s) of knowledge that practitioners value is grounded in their professional socialization. Practice knowledge is inclusive of hierarchical scientific (empirico-analytical) and psycho-socio-cultural (ethnographic, phenomenological) constructs of knowledge.
- The relative roles of practitioners and patients are significantly influenced by practice approaches, whether chosen or unconsciously adopted. Biomedical practice models speak of providers and recipients of practice. In an emancipatory/capacity model, patients and practitioners engage in dialogues and learn from each other, both accepting the roles of listening and negotiating.
- The level of critique and reflexivity that practitioners bring to their practice is grounded in practice and reasoning approaches. Critical self-awareness of professional or personal interests is the key to consciously choosing a practice model.

Table 3.1 Three frameworks for professional practice models in health

Practice model	Illness model	Wellness model	Capacity model
Kind of interest	Technical	Practical	Emancipatory
Approach	Clinician-centred	Patient-centred	Patient-empowered
Philosophical paradigm	Empirico-analytical	Interpretive	Critical
Health definition	Reductionist	Holistic	Holistic
Focus of health	Technical	Practical	Political
Clinician power	Clinician has power	Clinician may share some power	Equal power sharing
Patient power	Disempowered	Empowered	Empowered in a way that can be sustained
Practice knowledge	Propositional-technical	Propositional-technical and experiential	Propositional-technical, experiential and political
Stance towards status quo	Taking things for granted, accepting, reinforcing	Being aware of taken-for-granted things	Challenging status quo and changing frameworks
Role of patient	Passive, obedient, not asked to think for self	Interactive, participative but obedient, encouraged to think a bit for self	Interactive, participative, contributing, self-determining, learn to think for self
Role of clinician	Teacher/provider	Listener	Facilitator
Context of decision-making	Out of context	Psychocultural context (definitely not political)	Historical-political context
Clinician as helper	Helping to survive	Helping to cope	Helping to liberate
Clinicians helping patients	To comply	To cope	To liberate
Clinician self-awareness	Unreflective	Reflective with the aim to empower	Reflective with the aim to transform

CRITIQUING CURRENT PRACTICE MODELS

In the second phase of the research, the participants (physiotherapists) were asked to reflect on their way of practising, how they thought about their practice, and how they communicated with patients. The interview and discussion questions were categorized into issue questions and topical questions.

Issue questions were:

- What does it mean to be a physiotherapist? Can you describe the kind of physiotherapist that you could identify with?
- What are the aims and principles that guide your treatments and patient management?
- What factors influence the way you practise physiotherapy?
- What are the aims and guidelines that you set yourself?

What is it like to be a physiotherapist?

Topical questions were:

- How would you describe your role as a physiotherapist? (Why, do you think, did you end up in this area?)
- What components make up your professional knowledge?
- How do you know what your patients need?
- How do you build trust in your clinician–patient relationship?
- What is your biggest challenge as a physiotherapist?

The aim was to critically understand how practitioners made sense of their practice and how they interpreted what happened in practice. There was a wide range of practice models that this participant group adopted. Participants were commonly unclear about their practice model and the values that underpinned it, and had difficulty articulating those factors. Most said at one stage in the interview that they found these questions difficult to answer, they had not thought about these questions, and they had to think more about them.

The interviewees' responses revealed that practice is complex and that the practitioners in this study unknowingly adopted practice models. Much of their practice was unreflected and taken for granted. We concluded from the analysis that practice approaches are diverse and depend on context. Unsurprisingly, there was a preference for the biomedical practice model, as the hegemonic system and educational model of the participants' workplaces and professional socialization.

All interviewees claimed that it was important to listen to patients and they stated that they were somewhat patient-centred. However, in practice, when experiencing interest clashes they reinforced their therapist-centred approach on the basis of technical interests. Felix (pseudonym), for instance, was convinced that his treatment plans were the right ones. Herein lies a fundamental contradiction: he described exercises as promoting independence but in reality his approach was actually prescriptive and fostered dependence on his power and control. Felix displayed purely instrumental, technical values that underpinned his understanding of his professional role and power. Felix critiqued his patients' beliefs but he did not critique his own beliefs. He chose selective reasoning or professional power over negotiated clinical reasoning.

Another key finding of the research was the importance of external context factors on the preferred or existing practice model of the practitioners and the workplace. Where the environment was 'hi-tech' and healthcare delivery relied on advanced technology, and in acute care or emergency situations where patients were very ill or required critical care, the level of acceptability of the technical, biomedical model was high. There was an unchallenged focus on pathological diagnoses and biomedical intervention approaches, with the expectation of patient compliance. In less acute and less technology-dependent healthcare settings participants considered that there was greater opportunity for patient-centred care that involved patient participation in clinical decision making. The notion of emancipatory practice

was foreign to most of the participants, and in early discussions they considered that in their workplace situations, with high workloads, time pressures, medical model frameworks, traditional approaches to professional hierarchies and an emphasis on evidence-based practice and cost efficiency, moves to treat patients on an equal footing in terms of clinical decision making were not particularly feasible, expected or needed.

DEVELOPING A CRITICAL SOCIAL SCIENCE MODEL FOR PRACTICE

The primary goal of the research (see Trede 2006, Trede & Higgs 2003) was to understand how a critical social science (CSS) perspective, with its inherent emancipatory interests, might influence and transform healthcare practice. The development of the CSS model for practice involved four cycles of critical transformative dialogues based on critique and reflexivity and the pursuit of change that led to liberation. The dialogues involved two-way conversations with self and others (including other participants, patients, colleagues) using critical reasoning. The first dialogue described the status quo of the CSS and health-related literature and developed a conceptual approximation of a CSS model for healthcare practice. The second dialogue involved critique and interpretation of the related physiotherapy literature followed by a critical dialogue with the first group of physiotherapist participants to critique the status quo of physiotherapy practice. In the third dialogue a group of practitioners trialled a CSS approach using action-learning strategies. The fourth dialogue, with another physiotherapy participant group, envisioned a CSS approach to practice.

In discussion of the status quo of practice a few participants, either through dissatisfaction with their model or prompted by further education, consciously chose to adopt an alternative model based in humanistic philosophy or, less frequently, a critical social science perspective. The more conscious the choice of practice model and the more this model differed from hegemonic practices, the more likely it was that the practitioners adopted a heightened level of awareness into their reasoning and behaviour. Instead of reasoning against scientific knowledge, evidence, established practice guidelines, or learned behaviour expectations set by their professions, workplaces or society at large, these practitioners sought to critically construct their own set of practice standards and ways of being in the world of practice, and they monitored their behaviour against these standards. These participants, without theoretical understanding of CSS theory, had created a critical practice model.

A critical practice model starts with the assumptions that practice is complex, outcomes are uncertain, and perceptions and interpretations of patient presentations are diverse. This means that a patient with an arthritic knee is not simply an arthritic knee – an object of treatment. Instead, practitioners need to consider patients holistically, thus including age, gender, attitude towards pain and physical activity, expectations of practitioners and themselves. Gaining a critical perspective means becoming aware of the interests that collide in practice, and questioning these interests.

A CRITICAL SOCIAL SCIENCE PERSPECTIVE

Critical social science is distinguished from the natural and social sciences in that it focuses on critique that leads to change and emancipation (Fay 1987). Critique is raising awareness about interests that have arisen in the sociocultural, historical worlds that influence clinical reasoning and practice approaches. From a CSS perspective, critical thinking means being able to take a sceptical stance towards self, culture, norms, practices, and institutions, as well as policy and regulations. CSS starts from the assumptions that all these dimensions are human-made and therefore can be changed. Before these dimensions are accepted and adopted they should be challenged and checked for their intentions and assumptions. CSS separates truth from ideology, reason from power and emancipation from oppression. The agenda of CSS is to critique, engage in dialogue and transform the status quo at an individual as well as a collective level, working towards transformation through professional development and maturity to become a self-aware and articulate professional who works with patients, policy and institutions that respect diversity and social justice. The focus is on transforming unnecessarily constraining policies and oppressive practices that restrict workforce development as well as patient empowerment.

TRIALLING A CRITICAL PRACTICE MODEL

We conducted action-learning research with a second participant group, trialling what it was like to transform their practice into (or towards) a critical practice model. This dialogue cycle included a pre-implementation workshop, an action-learning phase and a critical appraisal workshop. Participants were informed about the findings from the first phase of the research investigating the status quo of physiotherapy practice models. They were educated about the dimensions of critique, power and emancipation of CSS, and they were invited to critically discuss our critique of current practices. All participants designed an action plan that identified what aspects of their practice they were willing to change towards a more CSS-oriented approach. During the action-learning phase participants were interviewed on two or three occasions to discuss their progress and experiences of CSS practice.

The findings from this phase indicated that the practitioners had varied levels of readiness (cognitive, emotional and pragmatic) to engage in practice reflection and change, and different perceptions of the value of CSS as a basis for practice. Different levels of engagement with CSS were identified. These are discussed below, in conjunction with the findings of phase four of the research.

CRITIQUING AND VISIONING THE CRITICAL SOCIAL SCIENCE PRACTICE MODEL

In the final phase of the research we identified a group of participants who practised a patient-centred model closely related to our emerging model. The prime purpose of these discussions was to provide a 'reality check' of the emerging CSS model. These participants were explicitly requested as practising physiotherapists to provide critique of the draft model, as well as a self-critique of their own practice models, including their practice dilemmas.

A CRITICAL PRACTICE MODEL

This model for practice has two core dimensions:

(A) AN EMANCIPATORY DIMENSION

The emancipatory dimension entails recognition that to adopt a CSS or emancipatory model in a world of practice where such practice is a minority view requires a journey of emancipation for the practitioner. We have labelled this a journey of critical transformative dialogues. We recognize that to journey towards practice that is informed by CSS can start with a small degree of change. The research identified five modes of engagement with CSS as a practice model. These were labelled:

1. *The Uninformed* Those who had not heard of CSS
2. *The Unconvinced* Those who trialled CSS but did not change their current practice, which remained in the biomedical model
3. *The Contemplators* Those who trialled CSS and thought that some aspects of CSS were convincing but encountered too many perceived barriers to transform their practice substantially
4. *The Transformers* Those who were convinced of CSS and were transforming aspects of their practice
5. *The Champions* Those who were convinced of the value of CSS and embodied CSS in their practice.

In this study the participants in this group were called *impending* champions, to recognise their adoption of CSS practices and their learning about CSS theory. They have come a long way from their traditional medical model backgrounds but have some way to go towards fully embodying CSS principles in their practice.

Table 3.2 details the interests, practices and characteristics of each of these modes. Of particular relevance here are the changing patterns of interaction, power use and reasoning approaches, ranging from therapist-centred and therapist-empowered decision making *for* patients to patient-centred and mutually empowered decision making dialogues *with* patients.

(B) A CRITICAL, LIVED DIMENSION

Practitioners bring their assumptions, values and prejudgements and professional experiences to the clinical situation. Practitioners with a critical perspective are aware of the interests that collide in practice, and they question these interests.

To practise within a CSS model rather than journeying towards CSS is to live or embody CSS in practice. Figure 3.1 illustrates Trede's (2006) critical practice model. In the centre are critical transformative dialogues that enable practitioners to make practice model choices (on the lower left-hand side) and list all the requirements for critical practice (right-hand side).

Practising within a CSS model requires practitioners to:

- challenge models of practice, practice cultures and taken-for-granted practice interests
- be accountable to self as well as to those influenced by their professional practice
- analyse what is valuable practice knowledge
- critically and responsibly exercise choice about courses of action
- adopt a critical pedagogy approach to teaching and learning. Such an approach involves and enhances learners' capacity to question existing assumptions and current practices
- engage patients (and carers) in transformative dialogue
- imagine alternatives
- be willing to question self, their professional identity and their chosen model of practice.

In advocating consideration and adoption of a CSS practice model we recognize that critical practice has variable relevance and potential across the range of practice contexts, and that other models (as discussed above) may be preferable or more feasible in certain contexts. We see critical practice as the practice model of choice in situations of emancipatory need, predilection and support. That is, critical practice is an accessible and acceptable choice when four situations coincide: (a) when there is a perceived need for patients and physiotherapists to collaborate in clinical decision making and to liberate practice; (b) when it is the preferred practice model of a practitioner (or group) who is a champion of critical practice; (c) when other

Table 3.2 Five prototypical engagements with CSS (Trede 2006, with permission)

Practice dimension	The uninformed	The unconvinced	The contemplators	The transformers	The champions
Definition	Those who have not heard of CSS	Those who have trialled CSS but do not change their current practice	Those who have explored CSS in their practice and have chosen to adopt some aspects of CSS in their practice	Those who are convinced of critical practice and are transforming their practice to this model	Those who are convinced of the value of critical practice and advocate it
Practice model	Typically the biomedical model	Typically the biomedical model	Mixed biomedical and critical model	Approximating a critical practice model	Critical model
Interests	Technical/practical	Technical/practical	Practical/technical/ Emancipatory	Emancipatory (+technical/ practical)	Predominantly emancipatory
Self-appraisal	Mastering technical application	Mastering technical application	Mastering technical application and acknowledging patients' interests	Acknowledging own assumptions and unreflected ideology	Seeking critical self-understanding, reflexive
Mode of critique	Critiquing practice from an empirico-analytical, technical perspective	Critiquing practice from an empirico-analytical, technical perspective	Critiquing practice from practical perspectives working within systems that are taken-for-granted or at least assumed unchangeable	Critiquing practice by starting with self-critique and awareness of system challenges	Being open, sincere, curious, avoiding making generalizations and unreflected judgements, paying attention to detail [rethinking practice dimensions through relational thinking]
Approach to reasoning	Linear, cause and effect, minimal contextual consideration	Linear, cause and effect, minimal contextual consideration	Appreciate critical reasoning without adopting it	Adopting critical reasoning in aspects of practice	Critical, dialogical reasoning
Approach to knowledge	Propositional-technical	Propositional-technical	Propositional-technical and experiential	Propositional-technical, experiential and critical	Propositional-technical, experiential and critical
Patient relationships	Therapist is the expert and dominates	Therapist is the expert and dominates	Therapist is the expert but acknowledges patient experience	Democratizing patient-therapist relationship	Dialogical, reciprocal relationship where expertise of therapist and patient are both acknowledged

Power/authority	Owned by physiotherapist's propositional knowledge	Owned by physiotherapist's propositional knowledge	Owned by propositional knowledge and some non-propositional knowledge	Shift from propositional to critical knowledge. System propositional knowledge dominant	Shared as critical knowledge
Context interpretation	Within biomedical domain	Within biomedical domain	Within biopsychosocial domain	Within cultural and biopsychosocial domain	Within critical cultural biopsychosocial domain
Professional identity and role	Technical and telling patients what they need	Technical and telling patients what they need	Technical, practical and empathic, guiding patients	Moving to a facilitating role of emancipatory learning in self. Asking patients what they need	Moving to a role of facilitating emancipatory learning in self and patients, and chosen and self-owned identity
Goals	Achievement of positive technical, biomedical outcomes	Achievement of positive technical, biomedical outcomes	Achievement of functional and practical outcomes	Achievement of negotiated outcomes	Emancipation of self, others and the system for enhancement of patient outcomes in a critical framework

CSS=critical social science

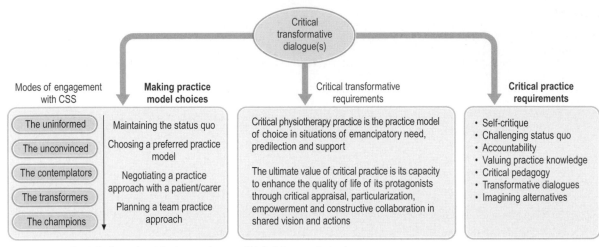

Figure 3.1 Trede's (2006) critical practice model (with permission)

team members are supportive of this approach and keen to embody authentic critical practice; and (d) where management and organizational systems support rather than restrict critical approaches. These four situations create a facilitative and supportive environment for embedding a critical practice perspective in the existing discourse. Critical practice would then be the practice model of choice because marginalized voices of patients and practitioners are heard and acted upon in a system-based environment that is sensitive, supportive and responsive to critique and emancipation.

The relevance of CSS for health professional practice is that such a practice model:

- builds the capacity of practitioners for critical self-reflection as a tool for practice development
- democratizes professional relations and ensures inclusive, appropriate and ethical practice that empowers patients
- raises awareness of interests and values that inform clinical reasoning
- redefines professional identity within a constantly changing world to empower practitioners and liberate them from restrictive hegemonic practice rules
- encourages rethinking of the boundaries and inclusions of the practice context.

A critical practice model is challenging because practitioners must constantly question their clinical reasoning and maintain a critical stance to current practices. This critical stance to self and others can only be sustained within a supportive environment that facilitates such emancipatory learning. Adopting a CSS perspective requires advanced clinical reasoning skills that allow critical reflection about self, patients and the wider practice context and open yet sceptical professional relationships with patients.

CONCLUSION

Healthcare practice operates in increasingly more complex, diverse and uncertain environments. Patients are better informed, technology is advancing, and healthcare practice is constantly changing. It is important in this context to adopt an informed and critical stance to practice. Being aware of the interests that drive and frame practice and practice models, and understanding the way these models influence practice actions and clinical reasoning, are necessary aspects of being a responsible and critically competent practitioner in a demanding work environment. We have examined different practice models and have proposed advantages in relevant contexts of adopting a critical practice model. The relevance of critique in today's challenging and dynamic healthcare environments is for practitioners to reclaim their human agency and critical self-reflective capacity. Critical thinking based on technical and practical interests is important but incomplete in meeting the challenging demands of current practice.

References

Eraut M 1994 Developing professional knowledge and competence. Falmer Press, London

Fay B 1987 Critical social science. Cornell University Press, Ithaca

Habermas J (trans J J Shapiro) 1972 Knowledge and human interest. Heinemann, London

Higgs J, Hunt A, Higgs C et al 1999 Physiotherapy education in the changing international healthcare and educational contexts. Advances in Physiotherapy 1:17–26

Newman M 1994 Defining the enemy: adult education in social action. Stewart Victor Publishing, Sydney

Schön D A 1987 Educating the reflective practitioner. Jossey-Bass, San Francisco

Therborn G 1999 The ideology of power and the power of ideology. Verso, London

Trede F V 2006 A critical practice for physiotherapy Unpublished PhD thesis, University of Sydney, Australia

Trede F, Higgs J 2003 Re-framing the clinician's role in collaborative clinical decision making: re-thinking practice knowledge and the notion of clinician–patient relationships. Learning in Health and Social Care 2(2):66–73

Chapter **4**

Collaborative decision making

Franziska Trede and Joy Higgs

INTRODUCTION

One of the great debates in health care in the 21st century centres on the tension between patient-centred health care and evidence-based practice. Within this debate lies an important clinical reasoning issue, namely the patient's role in clinical decision making. This chapter explores Franziska Trede's doctoral research (supervised by Joy Higgs and Rodd Rothwell), which investigated explorations and experiences of emancipatory practice and collaborative decision making involving patients (or clients), relevant others (families, carers, advocates) and practitioners (Trede 2006, Trede & Higgs 2003, Trede et al 2003). (Please note that although we acknowledge the importance of the term *client* in many fields of health practice and health promotion, and to clients themselves, in order to probe into the need for a critical perspective – or at least its consideration and challenge – we use the term *patient* in most of this chapter, it being the common term used in traditional healthcare settings.)

Of particular significance in this research was the consideration of the interests of participants in the decision-making process. Healthcare practitioners participating in this study were asked to reflect on how they made decisions, what criteria they used to justify their approach to decision making and what role they assigned to, or encouraged in, their patients in the decision-making process. A critical hermeneutic approach was used to interpret interview transcripts and identify interests, assumptions, motivations and biases that the practitioners brought to their decision-making practice. In this chapter we report on a critical practice perspective on collaborative decision making.

WHY COLLABORATE IN THE DECISION-MAKING PROCESS?

Practitioners make numerous daily decisions about their patients: which questions to ask, which label or diagnosis to assign, which treatment options to discuss, which information to share or not share with patients, which treatment interventions and care plans to pursue. The way decisions are made impacts on patients' persistence with treatment, sense of ownership, control and perceptions of healthcare outcomes. For many patients, the more they participate in decision-making processes the more likely they are to be well informed, involved, satisfied and feeling valued (Trede & Higgs 2003).

Many factors support the case for collaboration in decision making (Hall & Visser 2000), including ethical issues related to quality of life (Mueller et al 2004), legal issues regarding informed consent (Braddock et al 1997), the patient's right to self-determination (Snapshot 2004), patient safety and the duty to prevent and do no harm (Winokur & Beauregard 2005), and cultural safety in terms of respecting and valuing diversity (Richardson & Carryer 2005). Patient dissatisfaction with communication aspects of health care has been shown to contribute to 40% of health complaints, implying that decisions were not collaborative but were imposed (NSW Health Care Complaints Commission 2005). Collaboration and communication are now considered as important as delivering care (Department of Health and Ageing 2000). These expectations are influenced by such factors as changing societal attitudes to health and patients' rights, cultural variations in attitudes towards health care, the advocacy of community support and patient groups, increasing litigiousness, improved patient education and greater availability of health information.

AGREEING ON DECISIONS DOES NOT NECESSARILY EQUATE WITH COLLABORATION

Patients may indicate their agreement with health professionals' decisions explicitly or implicitly through actual or apparent compliance with treatment or healthcare programmes. However, practitioners need to consider whether this agreement is genuine. Patients enter healthcare situations with a wide range of preparedness for the events that will unfold during their journey of ill-health or disability and for the processes of decision making they encounter. They may or may not have had time to investigate the nature of their condition or its medical management, to prepare mentally, physically or emotionally for the health situation they are facing, and to develop a position on what they would like their health outcome to be. In addition, they commonly do not have the relevant medical knowledge or expertise adequately to understand the nature of the condition, the treatment options and potential health outcomes. So, when it comes to the point of agreeing with a health professional or healthcare team in decision making, the patient's agreement could be influenced by many 'entry' factors. Any agreement or otherwise could also be influenced by factors within the communication or interaction, such as the relationship built up with the practitioner(s), language or cultural familiarity or barriers, aspects of behaviour such as intentions, motivations and practitioners' practice models (e.g. biomedical, biopsychosocial and emancipatory models). In addition, decision-making processes are influenced by professional authority, professional roles, and expectations held by professional groups and the community.

When clinicians and patients share the same values, intentions and interests, agreement is more likely. However, agreement or compliance that is unarticulated or unquestioned may not be true agreement at all. It is tempting to assume that patients adopt the role that practitioners assign to them, without checking with patients either at the point of decision making or during subsequent treatment programmes. Are patients reporting honestly on their perceptions of progress or their pain levels, etc? A critical perspective to decision making reminds us that commonality of values and interests between patients and practitioners should not be taken for granted.

SHARED OR MUTUAL DECISION MAKING

It is interesting to note that most of the literature on decision making has a tendency to use the term *shared* decision making rather than *collaborative* decision making. Makoul & Clayman (2006), in a systematic review of the literature on shared decision making, found great fluidity in what was understood by the term, ranging from clinician-led to patient-led decision making. The authors listed essential elements of shared decision making as: defining the problem, presenting the options, identifying patient values and preferences as well as doctor knowledge, and clarifying understanding. This checklist reflects the transactional procedures in decision making but it falls short of considering how various interests and motivations influence the reasoning behind decision making. Instead it is useful to consider a series of questions that helps to clarify assumptions about knowledge and how knowledge is generated (Edwards et al 2004). When is it appropriate to be practitioner-centred and when patient-centred? Who has permission to define the problem? Who is authorized to identify and legitimize what all the options are? How are patients invited and encouraged to share their values? Whose understanding needs clarification? What counts as knowledge and evidence?

To adopt a critical perspective towards answering the above questions and to pursue collaborative decision making in a critical frame of reference requires also pursuing awareness of 'self', 'the other', and the wider clinical and patient context. To understand this perspective we turn to the work of Habermas, a prominent critical social scientist and philosopher who developed a theory of knowledge and human interest (1972). Interests are the motivations, intentions and goals that guide behaviours.

Habermas divided interests into three categories, technical, practical and emancipatory. He argued that technical interest has a scientific bias and aims for technical success, practical interest has a pragmatic bias and aims for consensual understanding, whereas emancipatory interest is directed towards critique and emancipation, and aims for critical understanding. We discussed and illustrated the relationship between interest and practice in Chapter 3 (see especially Table 3.1).

COLLABORATIVE DECISION MAKING FROM A CRITICAL PERSPECTIVE

Many scholars have delineated the dualism between practitioner-centred and patient-centred care (e.g. Arnetz et al 2004), leaving the reader and practitioner appreciating differences between these terms but not helping them to communicate and transcend this dualism. A critical perspective in this context starts with critical self-awareness of what motivates professional bias, professional authority and professional roles, and illuminates the various interests and interpretations underpinning practice approaches, especially those interests that pursue and drive power rather than reason. For example, adopting a critical perspective means seeking first to understand the historical and social factors and influences that have led practice to be accepted and valued the way it is (in a given context) and then to challenge and change this practice with the goal of emancipating those who are restricted or disempowered by it. Within this framework, practitioner-centred practice is typically practice that favours technical rationalism and those in power (commonly the practitioners), whereas in truly (critical) patient-centred practice the practitioner seeks to share knowledge and power with the patient and to respect the input the patient can make to clinical decision making and healthcare management.

People who reason with scientific rationality and objectivity risk silencing emotional, cultural and self-determining rationality. Such communication occurs when practitioners are firmly entrenched in the biomedical model, see evidence-based practice as driven by and contained within scientific method research, and seek an objective and authoritarian pattern of interaction and communication with patients. This practice approach can be highly altruistic, or it can be focused on other interests such as practitioner authority, economic and technical rationalism, and income generation. In each case it is practitioner-centred rather than patient-centred in a critical sense.

Those who reason with cultural and historical rationality tend to silence science and objectivity. Their practice is more patient-centred and can react in an anti-science manner to biomedical model practices. Wellness model advocates and practitioners fit into this category. They have questioned the values and cultural norms of the hegemonic practice model and favour greater levels of person- and patient-centredness. These practitioners embrace subjectivity and holistic approaches to health care but retain their position of authority. This is patient-centredness within a 'caring for' (rather than an egalitarian) frame of reference.

Both these perspectives neglect the goal of emancipating patients from the dualism between practitioner-centred and patient-centred care and its potential manipulation and coercion. By comparison, the ideology of a critical perspective to collaboration is a commitment to critical rationality (Habermas 1972).

This leads to consideration of what a collaborative decision-making approach that is informed by a critical perspective would be like. Habermas developed his theory of communicative actions based on a critical perspective of intersubjective communications and interpretations (1984, 1987). This theory describes ideal speech situations (in our case collaborative decision making) as undistorted, open, egalitarian debates that silence unwarranted authority and tradition. Making the intentions and arguments for decisions transparent is seen as the key to making truly collaborative decisions. In addition, collaborative decision making requires critique (including self-critique) and moderation of interests, values and expectations of all parties involved in the decision-making process, and safe, democratizing and caring environments to foster open transparent collaboration where patients feel they are listened to and taken seriously.

In ideal decision-making processes, all involved are aware of their own interests and motivations; this clarifies the reasoning process and enables collaborators to reach critical decisions that include objective, emotional, political, cultural and other factors. The interests of critical rationality and collaborative decision-making processes are emancipatory in that the goal is to find consensus free from traditions, domination and hidden motives. Decisions that are based on critical self-reflection, mutual respect and interest in emancipation are collaborative decisions and are differentiated from false consensus (Roderick 1986).

The arguments in favour of adopting a critical perspective on collaborative decision making are as follows:

- Not all parties involved in the decision-making process necessarily share the same values, intentions and interests about health beliefs and health behaviours. Decisions need to be negotiated free of coercion and power imbalances.
- Decision-making roles of practitioners and patients are dynamic and change as the health condition of patients progresses from acute and life-threatening to subacute and chronic conditions. Therefore it is important to make conscious choices about which approach to decision making is appropriate.
- Patients are increasingly better informed and they (or at least many of them) want to know their options and be involved in decision making and self management.
- Given appropriate opportunity and inclusive environments, most patients can be empowered to collaborate in decision making and have a say in their health management.

The way practitioners define themselves as professionals informs the way they make decisions. Practitioners who see themselves as the expert authority who knows best might find it confronting to have patients collaborate and 'contaminate' their decisions based on best practice. They assume that patients come to them to get advice and comply with it. Healthcare practice today remains predominantly influenced by the biomedical model discourse that assigns decision-making power to healthcare professionals. Practitioners who locate themselves in the medical model may describe decision making as a practitioner-led, transactional, linear process in which periodic checking of understanding is recommended. The focus of decision making in the medical model is traditionally based on certainty and prediction of biomedical aspects (Whitney 2003). The implication is that collaboration is necessary only when outcomes of decisions are unpredictable and uncertain. There is a place for practitioner-led decision making, especially in acute situations; however, there is also a place for patient-led decisions. Collaboration is based on the conviction that inclusiveness and critical self-reflection produce better outcomes for patients than empirico-analytical precision. Collaborative decision making is based on inclusive evidence that entails embracing uncertainty and recognizing diversity of patients, clinicians and therapeutic environments (Jones et al 2006). A critical approach helps practitioners to become conscious of their choices in decision making because hidden agendas and bias are made explicit.

OPERATIONALIZING COLLABORATIVE DECISION MAKING FROM A CRITICAL SOCIAL SCIENCE PERSPECTIVE

Shifting towards collaborative decision making requires a capacity to redefine professional practice knowledge, professional authority and professional relations between clinicians and patients. In some fields of health professional practice (e.g. occupational therapy, nursing, speech pathology, physiotherapy) there have been moves away from professional authority models in terms of such issues and strategies as:

- Replacing the term 'patient' with the term 'client', along with a change in the role of that person from receiver of health care, expected to adopt a passive role in decision making but an active role in compliance, to informed customer seeking to purchase the best (for their needs and circumstance) available healthcare options.
- Moving (philosophically and behaviourally) from the 'clinical' context with inherent ideas of objectivity, disease and detachment to a 'professional' context with a broader focus on dual community and professional expectations of a more market-based approach to service provision. Both contexts expect professional

behaviour such as ethical conduct, duty of care and commitment to high levels of competence and best practice. The differences lie in relationship patterns and the emphasis on a received view of best practice versus a negotiated view of the most situationally appropriate practice.
- Moving (geographically) out of traditional healthcare settings to work in community arenas (such as schools) and in well population contexts (such as fitness programmes for the elderly).
- Shifting towards a critical model that includes practitioner and patient emancipation. Silenced voices are heard and oppressive structures are transformed.

AN EXPLORATION OF A CRITICAL SOCIAL SCIENCE PERSPECTIVE IN CLINICAL PRACTICE: IMPLICATIONS FOR COLLABORATIVE DECISION MAKING

As authors and researchers, our interest in examining collaborative decision making lies in fostering and employing critique and emancipation from both unreflective and intentional dominance in decision making. We see collaborative decision making as a strategy enabling practitioners to liberate themselves from unnecessary constraints, to work authentically with patients, to empower patients to reclaim responsibility for their health, autonomy, dignity and self-determination. The intention of collaboration in critical practice is to engage in dialogue and to democratize roles. Collaboration starts with critique, scepticism and curiosity to deepen understanding and to identify the scope of common ground for change. In our research, critique of decision making focused on four closely interrelated dimensions:

1. capacity for critical self-reflection
2. rethinking professional roles
3. rethinking professional power relations
4. rethinking rationality and professional practice knowledge.

Franziska explored these four dimensions by engaging in critical transformative dialogues with three physiotherapist practitioner groups. In Chapter 3 we reported on five prototypes (the uninformed, the unconvinced, the contemplators, the transformers and the champions) who represented the way the research participants engaged (or did not engage) with a critical social science perspective in their practice. Here we take each of these prototypes in turn and consider their implications for collaborative decision making.

STUDY GROUP 1

The uninformed

The first group of participants had no prior experience with critical social sciences as a field of study or practice approach and were not involved in education sessions on this topic during the study. To be uninformed about particular approaches to practice does not imply the absence of an approach in one's practice. However, it is likely that practitioners who have received no education or information about practice approaches that differ greatly from the status quo will tend to adopt the approved, hegemonic approach of the professional or workplace setting. In Franziska's research, participants who were uninformed about a critical practice approach were not aware of their interests and how those interests influenced their decisions; they often said they did not know what their patients really wanted and what their goals were. The uninformed group's practice interests were blurred. Practitioners did not think in terms of models or interests but reacted to presenting challenges. There seemed to be a lack of reflexivity. The uninformed had unknowingly adopted the mainstream approach to decision making. However, there was a tendency towards technical rather than emancipatory interests. Figure 4.1 illustrates the continuum and the extreme ends of the various practice models. Collaboration with patients in decision making was limited. In the following accounts of the study, pseudonyms are used for all participants to preserve anonymity.

When Hilda, one of the participants in the study, was asked to describe how she negotiated with patients who did not want to comply with her treatment, she provided a typical example of well-intended but unreflective decision-making processes when she replied:

Unconscious	Known
Tacit	Knowing
Minimal capacity development	Explicit capacity development
Detached from self	Being self
Safe replication	Calculated risk
Single perspective	Multiple perspectives
Telling	Listening and responding

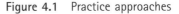

Practice interests

Technical	Practical	Emancipatory

Figure 4.1   Practice approaches

You have to just keep talking to them and just keep explaining; and by telling them what bad things are going to happen, which isn't a very nice thing to do, but, if they're still not complying then you just, I mean, you can't treat them. (Hilda)

Patients' needs were equated with a need to bring abnormal medical symptoms back as close to normal as possible. Although she would ask patients how they felt and what they thought they needed, Hilda would use technical, clinical findings to determine (without consulting with the patient) which treatment approach was appropriate. There appeared to be little incorporation of patient perspectives into her needs assessment and treatment plans. Collaboration seemed to be equated with compliance. Felix, another participant, started to think more deeply about how he negotiated decision making with his patients:

You try to get the patient involved as much as possible, definitely. Explain to them the possible strategies that are involved. And, of course, then you ask them are they okay with it – are they willing to go through with all that – be it some form of manual treatment or some form of exercise. You tell them how long you expect them to be coming for, so you ask them are they willing to put up with that, are they going to participate in the treatment exercises and so on. So, in that way, do you think that means they're participating? Do you think that's actually getting them actively involved? It's not really, is it? Not really, now that I'm thinking more about it. It's almost like you're telling them what to do, really, aren't you? But you're informing them about what you're doing, though ... I thought I was trying to get them involved by informing them as much as possible. That's all. That's the way I do it. I don't actually ask them 'what do you think we should do about this?' and get them to sort of come up with it. (Felix)

Felix first portrayed himself as a patient-including physiotherapist, but he noticed that he was not really engaging patients in the decision-making process. His professional relations emphasized his professional status and claimed professional power over patients. Physiotherapists need patients at least to cooperate, especially for exercise therapy. There is a difference between patient participation as a result of egalitarian negotiations and patient participation arising from imposed management strategies based on the therapist's technical reasoning. The difference lies in the interest and motivation that guides communication between the therapist and patient. Felix showed little interest in the patient's perspective. He was keen to operationalize his technical interests. Another participant learned about collaborative reasoning by reflecting upon a critical incident that made her question the way she tended to make clinical decisions:

The penny dropped for me only after 10 years of clinical experience. I had [a patient with] an above-knee amputation and he had a prosthesis. He walked perfectly in the gym. I had him walk without a limp. I was really pleased with all this. Then I met him downtown in the shopping centre: he had his knee locked, he was walking on the inner quarter of his foot, foot stuck out at right angle and he was perfectly happy. I stood and looked at him and thought 'I can make you walk perfectly without a limp but you don't want to do that'. And you know when he came to treatment he would do it but obviously he wasn't feeling safe and he didn't want to do it that way and that is that. I think I wanted him to do what I wanted. I was trying to be a perfectionist. And it has also to do with all the other physiotherapists. They are checking on you that you are doing it all properly. (Jill)

Seeing her patient mobilizing in a non-ideal way but with confidence and seeing him integrated into a social community life made Jill start to question her goal-setting practices and her professional interests. Why should she make patients walk without a limp if all they wanted was to walk safely? Jill became aware of clashes between professional and patient goals. She was aware of peer expectations and she felt pressured to comply with the professional physiotherapy culture. Collaborative decision making is influenced not only by the stakeholders of decisions but also by the practice culture and the workplace environment.

STUDY GROUP 2

The second participant group received education about critical social science as part of a pre-implementation workshop. They were asked to trial changing self-selected aspects of their practice towards a more critical approach. Table 4.1 lists the strategies participants wrote down in their action plans to identify their focus of change. These strategies addressed concerns relating to the therapist, the patient and their professional relationship. Strategies focused on therapist interest, on patient interest, or on collaboration and dialogue. Participants who chose to focus on self appeared to be more willing to critique self than those who chose to focus on patients, colleagues or the healthcare system. Different levels of engagement characterize the unconvinced, the contemplators, the transformers and the champions.

The unconvinced

Dorothy, who fitted the unconvinced prototype, equated collaboration with compliance. She felt that patients had to understand physiotherapy reasoning but she did not think that physiotherapists had to understand the way patients reasoned. She did not challenge the biomedical interests that influenced the way she reached decisions.

Giving the patients options is definitely making them feel more in control and you get a better response out of them. They don't just feel like sitting there having things done to them. They are having a bit more of a say what is happening to them. So it is good for both. (Dorothy)

Table 4.1   Strategies that participants had planned

Aspects of practice participants sought to change

Patient focused	Self focused	Professional relationship focused	Systems focused
• Explore what patients want from therapy • Give patients more information • Increase patient education • Give patients a more active role • Empower patients so they can take responsibility • Let patients feel more involved • Explore how to tell patients in acute settings what to do • Make better use of patient feedback • Listen better to patients • Achieve patients' goals and relate short-term to long-term goals	• Gain insights into decision making • Explore how patient-centred I really am • Increase understanding of my role as physiotherapist • Explore the difference between being a therapist and being a friend • Explore my practice and how to change it • Explore my own practice patterns	• Be an advocate for patients • Collaborate with patient and family in goal setting • Learn from my patients in any areas that empower me to improve my skills as a therapist • Explore compliance issues • Educate with the aim of giving more power to patients in professional relationships and to foster collaboration	• Increase awareness of others' professional decision-making patterns that I want to emulate or avoid • Look at our [physiotherapy department] report writing documents and look at the questions we ask and see which way they are slanted [therapist- or patient-centred] and see if I can add some questions that will allow both ends of the model to be used

Dorothy experienced working in collaboration with patients as positive. However, her understanding of collaboration was narrowly defined because she limited the patients she chose to collaborate with. She noticed that patients who shared her values and expectations made her more relaxed and she was able to give them choice. These patients did not challenge her practice. What Dorothy described as collaboration was patient compliance. With *difficult* patients she felt she had to be more forceful.

> You get a few people that you need to push or you are not going to get anywhere with them. Patients with stubborn personality won't do anything no matter what reason you give them. (Dorothy)

Dorothy categorized patients who did not agree with her as difficult people with stubborn personalities. It appeared that either patients worked with her or she had to use professional power to get patients to comply. She did not acknowledge her motivations and interests and she did not practise self-critique.

The contemplators

This group of therapists struggled with the concept of collaboration and patient emancipation. They interpreted collaboration as allowing patients to dominate them and they rejected this approach to decision making. However, they could see some benefits in trying to work with patients by 'making practice suitable to patient's background, as much as their biomedical illnesses allowed'.

> I am trying to turn the patients' concerns around to mine. I guess that is what I would like so that we are working together. So it's all about educating them about what they need to do. (Petra)

Petra understood collaborative decision making as persuading patients to adopt the physiotherapist's perspective. It was not based on egalitarian principles; the biomedical perspective prevailed unchallenged. Petra's practice values remained firmly grounded in the acute medical model despite appreciation of patients' individual fears and needs. Petra believed that once patients were familiar with their acute conditions they could be empowered to take more control and determine their own treatment routine in consultation.

> Doing-to patients saves lives and prevents complications. Doing-to is simple and straightforward. It means following my duty of care. In acute [settings] you focus on biomedical signs and you cannot always develop a relationship with the human being. In chronic settings you have time to develop a professional/personal relationship. In long-term rehabilitation you need to consider the human being more. It is more relaxing, working slower with patients. (Petra)

This quote succinctly describes the attitude of the contemplators who saw collaboration as optional and not suitable in some settings. The attitude was that practitioners have permission to assume professional power over their patients due to their professional status and knowledge. Thus professional relationships in the healthcare context start with uneven power relationships, where practitioners have more power than patients. When the participants were asked to rethink and democratize their relationships with patients, the implication was that patients had to be taken more seriously as people with a role to play in clinical decision making and self-management. In exploring collaboration the participants were challenged to listen critically to patients and develop open dialogue with patients.

The transformers

Those participants who trialled democratizing their relationships with patients and who were willing to challenge their use of professional power were classified as transformers. Jocelyn, for example, became more attentive to interests and to her patients' expectations of physiotherapy. She found that some patients had clear expectations and knew what they wanted. When comparing these with her own professional expectations and goals Jocelyn experienced conflict. She described an incident with an 80-year-old patient who could not carry her shopping home but otherwise was able to be fully independent. Jocelyn noted the decreased range of motion in her shoulder joint and she wanted to work first on increasing range of motion and then on strengthening muscles. However, her patient was not interested in increasing range of motion.

> I could see that [this] patient was not interested in my plan. I thought this wasn't particularly functional [wanting to increase strength before increasing range of motion] but she was able to do everything: cook, clean etc. The only thing she couldn't do was go shopping because she couldn't carry anything. So, that was really glaring in my face. This is what she wants to do. I am not sure if I always pick that up. (Jocelyn)

In this situation Jocelyn appeared comfortable going along with her patient's goals. Her decision was influenced by her patient's age. Had her patient been younger she might have insisted on improving range of motion as well. Jocelyn made decisions in the context of her patient's age and function and with a critical stance to self. She was willing to reconsider, in this situation. However, generally speaking, Jocelyn was not content to allow patients to lead treatment plans.

> I am not so comfortable [with that]. I feel it takes away some of my authority or professional expertise when I say to them, 'what would you like to do in physiotherapy?' because they don't know physiotherapy technique and they say 'I don't know. You should know, you are the physiotherapist'. (Jocelyn)

Jocelyn could see that professional power is a flexible commodity. Simply handing it over was not a useful and critical approach. She would need to use it wisely and with critical awareness in each clinical situation. Jocelyn developed critical awareness of her patients' expectations, their ideas and their capacity to contribute and participate. This insight enabled her to make more appropriate use of professional power and expand her skills to build more democratic professional relationships.

Corinne displayed a capacity for critical self-reflection in relation to her issues around professional authority and power relations. Corinne had over 30 years of clinical experience and her area of expertise was outpatient physiotherapy. She questioned her practice and surprised herself:

> After the pre-implementation workshop I have been taking more notice of what I am doing with people and I was very surprised to find that I do tend to use quite a lot of physiotherapy [practitioner] power. I was actually very surprised to notice that. I had an incident the other day: I was doing something with a quite young lady and I was palpating her knee and she pushed my hand away and said 'you are hurting me'. I considered this palpation was appropriate for her age, health and all that. Well it was funny, it was more a – 'think of my feelings' reaction – rather than – 'Oh dear [sorry]' – but I thought 'how dare you'. I am not used to being treated like that (laughter). I didn't consider my palpation being too severe and I was thinking, 'oh, I don't like this'. The way she said it did not sit well with me. (Corinne)

Corinne did not like to be told that her professional judgement about touch was wrong from the patient's perspective. Corinne was reminded that she had no control over her patient's pain perception. However, the patient's manner conveyed an assertiveness that Corinne was not used to. Collaboration means working together and includes listening and talking as well as giving and taking. Corinne viewed each treatment as a learning process for herself as well as for her patients:

> I want to learn from patients so that I can improve my own skills. I think that every treatment session is a learning session for me. (Corinne)

Corinne learned to recognize that she was not the only expert or the professional who should know all the answers. She could appreciate that patients had relevant knowledge as well. Corinne learned to reframe herself as a facilitator of collaborative decision making. She not only transformed her approach to practice and her view of herself as a professional, but she also learned about practice as a collaborative transformation.

The champions

Participants who had operationalized collaborative decision making and endorsed the values of inclusion and power-sharing were labelled champions or advocates of the critical social science approach. These participants were sceptical and critical of professional authority that was taken for granted and automatically assumed. Raymond, one of this group, saw himself as a scientist, a critical self-reflector and a patient collaborator.

> Is physiotherapy a social science? To me it is, and my colleagues will hit me over the head. I think there are the arts and the sciences. It is somewhere between the two. You have to oscillate all the time to facilitate an outcome for the patient. So I have this pulling force in me all the time. I value the scientific and searching for the evidence but I am worried about the patient. (Raymond)

Raymond saw himself as integrating biomedical facts with patients' perceptions of their healthcare needs and condition. He defined his practice as 'doing qualitative medicine'. He recognized that a collaborative approach to decision making did not exclude propositional or scientific knowledge but it also required non-propositional knowledge to achieve emancipatory outcomes. Champions do not make decisions without continually checking their impact with individual patients; they regard patients as social, cultural and political human beings.

> You cannot tell a teenager to stop smoking. You need to look at their social issues. I practise physiotherapy like that. First [I consider] scientific knowledge and then social beliefs and patient knowledge. (Raymond)

In analysing the interviews with the champion group a number of factors that indicated participants' capacity or inclination for participating in collaborative decision making were identified. These included:

- appreciating patients' perspectives (e.g. fear, lack of knowledge)
- becoming self-aware of personal bias
- actively providing opportunities for patients to participate
- being willing to reconsider treatment choices
- exploring options with patients
- establishing reciprocal relationships (by being open and enabling patients to be open)
- facilitating a reciprocal process of teaching and learning from each other
- recognizing clearly the values that inform decision making.

The champions in this study were distinguished from the other groups in that they used their human agency to facilitate change in their patients. This change was greater than biomedical improvement because it was initiated in collaboration with patients, so that treatment interventions were appropriate and meaningful for both physiotherapist and patient.

CONCLUSION

Collaboration can be improved and better understood when people start being more open to learning and understanding the other party's interests and goals, and when they ask questions to enable others to elaborate on their perspective and values. Understanding the other person by illuminating their interests and biases and doing the same with oneself is part of gaining a critical perspective. Beyond listening more attentively and respecting diversity, it is important to act on this increased understanding and move towards collaboration. Cultivating curiosity and addressing one's limits of collaboration is a starting point to becoming more aware of when, how, what and why decision making needs to be collaborative. A critical perspective fosters practitioners' confidence to communicate democratically with patients with the goal of making appropriate decisions. It helps clinicians to make conscious choices about the degree of collaboration that is appropriate in each clinical situation.

References

Arnetz J E, Almin I, Bergström K et al 2004 Active patient involvement in the establishment of physical therapy goals: effects on treatment outcome and quality of care. Advances in Physiotherapy 6:50–69

Braddock C H III, Fihn S D, Levison W et al 1997 How doctors and patients discuss routine clinical decisions: informed decision making in the outpatient setting. Journal of General Internal Medicine 12(60):339–345

Department of Health and Ageing 2000 Public health practice in Australia today: a statement of core functions. Online. Available: www.nphp.gov.au/publication/phpractice/phprac/pdf 24 July 2006

Edwards I, Jones M, Higgs J et al 2004 What is collaborative reasoning? Advances in Physiotherapy 6:70–83

Habermas J (trans J J Shapiro) 1972 Knowledge and human interest. Heinemann, London

Habermas J 1984 The theory of communicative action. Vol 1. Reason and the rationalization of society (trans. T McCarthy). Polity Press, Oxford

Habermas J 1987 The theory of communicative action. Vol 2. The critique of functionalist reason (trans. T McCarthy). Polity Press, Oxford

Hall J A, Visser A 2000 Health communication in the century of the patient. Patient Education and Counseling 41(2):115–116

Jones M, Grimmer K, Edwards I et al 2006 Challenges in applying best evidence to physiotherapy. Internet Journal of Allied Health Sciences and Practice 4(3). Online. Available: http://ijahsp.nova.edu/9 June 2007

Makoul G, Clayman M L 2006 An integrative model of shared decision making in medical encounters. Patient Education and Counseling 60(3):301–312

Mueller P S, Hook C C, Fleming K C 2004 Ethical issues in geriatrics: a guide for clinicians. Mayo Clinic Proceedings 79:554–562

NSW Health Care Complaints Commission 2005 Annual Report 2004–5. Online. Available: www.hccc.nsw.gov.au/downloads/ar/04-05pdf 24 July 2006

Richardson F, Carryer J 2005 Teaching cultural safety in a New Zealand nursing education program. Journal of Nursing Education 44(5):201–208

Roderick R 1986 Habermas and the foundations of critical theory. St Martin's, New York

Snapshot 2004 Empowered patients are more satisfied with their care. Snapshot: An Electronic Newsletter 3(3):1–3

Trede F V 2006 A critical practice model for physiotherapy. Unpublished PhD thesis, University of Sydney, Australia

Trede F, Higgs J 2003 Re-framing the clinician's role in collaborative clinical decision making: re-thinking practice knowledge and the notion of clinician–patient relationships. Learning in Health and Social Care 2(2): 66–73

Trede F, Higgs J, Jones M et al 2003 Emancipatory practice: a model for physiotherapy practice? Focus on Health Professional Education: A Multidisciplinary Journal 5(2):1–13

Whitney S N 2003 A new model of medical decisions: exploring the limits of shared decision making. Medical Decision Making 23:275–280

Winokur S C, Beauregard K J 2005 Patient safety: mindful, meaningful and fulfilling. Frontiers of Health Services Management 22(1):17–32

Chapter 5

Action and narrative: two dynamics of clinical reasoning

Maureen Hayes Fleming and Cheryl Mattingly

Research in clinical reasoning emerged from the medical problem-solving tradition which emphasized the hypothetical deductive method. Recently many theorists have argued that this strictly cognitive view is too narrow to encompass the myriad ways in which health professionals devise solutions for clients' needs. We have found that the desire to conduct effective treatment, especially in the rehabilitation professions, directs the clinician to understand the client as a person who makes meaning of the illness or injury in the context of a life. By emphasizing the social dimension of clinical reasoning we are highlighting a quality of expert judgement which is by nature improvisational, flexible, and highly attuned to the specifics of the person, the condition and the context.

We discuss two streams of reasoning, active judgement and narrative. Working out narrative possibilities and making active judgements are two dynamic processes which intertwine while the clinician carries out the best treatment with and for the individual patient. We further submit that through making and reflecting on these active judgements and narrative possibilities clinicians develop their own stock of tacit knowledge and enhance their expertise. We draw upon ethnographic research projects we have conducted over the past decade, primarily (but by no means exclusively) among occupational therapists. This chapter is not a report of findings. We refer to these studies in a general way to illustrate and support a conceptualization of clinical reasoning and expertise grounded in the complexities and nuances of everyday practice in the world of rehabilitation.

ACTION AND JUDGEMENT

Action is the essence of clinical practice. In occupational, physical and speech therapy the patient *must* act. Without the patient's participation there is no therapy. One common view of action is that action takes place after one has carefully thought about the problem and its possible resolution. The assumption is that one thinks carefully about the problem, decides what the central issue is, determines the best solution, and takes action. This sequence may often be the case, but not always. Some philosophers, particularly phenomenologists, claim that thought and action occur in a rapid dynamic relation to one another, not in a fixed sequence. The word 'judgement' is often used to express this dynamic relationship. Buchler (1955), following on the work of John Dewey, C. S. Pierce and others, pointed out that action not only expresses the results of a judgement, it can be a judgement itself. Buchler (p. 11) commented, 'every action is itself a judgement'. Schön (1983) submitted that reflective practitioners act first and judge the results afterward. Architecture students develop their expertise by looking at an area of land and sketching out versions of the structure they envision for that space. This action (sketching) is a way of seeing and a way of thinking. It is an act of both imagination and production, in which an image becomes visible and can be judged. The imagined building comes briefly to life in the form of a drawing. The structure is 'built' in imagination, action, and judgement long before the bulldozers arrive. Between the imaginative eye and the artful hand the practitioner negotiates the route between the creative image and the concrete restrictions of the size, slope and orientation of the site, using a dynamic process of active judgement.

Healthcare practitioners also use imagination and action to make professional judgements about clients' problems and potential solutions. The patient is a 'site' where the best structure must be not constructed but reconstructed. Healthcare practitioners work with people in crisis, with whom action must be taken immediately. Many judgements are made before, during and after action. In professional work, action and judgement merge. The practitioner often has the advantage of having the patient – the person – as a partner, or at least informant, in the endeavour. Usually the patient trusts the clinician and is willing to respond to requests for action. The actions that the patient executes give the practitioner a great deal of information. Conversely, the clinician might take action on the patient, which provides another source of information. The clinician and patient become involved in a coordinated set of actions and interactions which many observers have characterized as a therapeutic dance.

Many professional judgements are based on observations and interpretations of patients' actions. Clinicians want to see if and how a patient can perform an action. The practitioner judges the quality of a motion in order to make clinical judgements regarding the current level of strength or range of motion and to estimate the possible functional gains the patient may make during treatment. By judging today's action the clinician can gauge the potential for future functional performance. The patient is asked to perform specific motions or sets of movements often and with frequent repetitions. Isolated motions, such as elbow flexion or thumb–finger prehension, are requested. Every day the therapist asks for more repetitions, more weight, more concentration, etc. Therapists remind patients that they could not do this last week or yesterday, and point out what they can do today and where they could be tomorrow or next week. The story of progress towards reconstruction is played out in increasingly better and more functional actions. Therapists want the patient's movements to match the image in the therapist's mind – to meet the perceived potential. Eventually the motions are combined into actions or sets of motions with a motive, such as shoulder rotation, elbow extension, wrist stabilization, finger extension and flexion to reach for an object. Later these and other motions and actions are combined so that desired functional activities, such as eating, may be performed. In a sense it is not the professional who is the therapist, but rather the patient and his or her ability to invest in meaningful action. Through this investment the patient rebuilds the body and reconstructs a sense of self as a person who can function in the world, an actor.

Practitioners take many actions while treating their patients. They also gain information from their interpretations of the sensations they receive from the patient and they learn from their own actions. The therapist tests muscle tone, adjusts the position of finger and thumb in a tenodesis grasp, or balances a child in her lap while he works with a toy. In the interest of improving patients' potential for future action, experts evaluate patients' actions, guide their own actions, make interpretations simultaneously, make rapid judgements, and change actions smoothly and rapidly. Action is both a concrete event and a reasoning strategy that mediates the flow of therapy from image to result. Simultaneously, clinicians learn if and how their own actions work as effective treatment strategies. In this way a wealth of personal/professional expertise is developed.

TACIT KNOWLEDGE AND PROFESSIONAL JUDGEMENT

When we conducted our first study we were confident that we would discover that therapists had a great deal of professional knowledge and skill and had a great stock of tacit knowledge. We did not anticipate the degree to which they were unaware of the amount of knowledge they had. Polanyi (1966, p. 4) coined the term 'tacit knowledge' and described it as the stock of professional knowledge that experts possess that is not processed in a focused cognitive manner but rather lies at a not quite conscious level, where it is accessible through acting, judging or performing. This level of awareness is what Polanyi called 'the tacit dimension'. It is a type of knowledge that is acquired through experience. Polanyi called it tacit knowledge because experts were able to act on it but could not always verbalize exactly what they were doing or why. He expressed this concisely with the words, 'we know more than we can tell'.

In daily practice the clinician encounters a new situation, takes action, perhaps several variations of a set of actions, and reflects on them to evaluate whether the action 'worked'. Was it effective in

solving a problem with this particular patient who, in some ways, was subtly different from the last patient of the same age, gender and diagnosis? Through this action and reflection the therapist builds a stock of tacit knowledge which becomes increasingly nuanced with further experience. Tacit knowledge has some advantages and disadvantages. It contributes to efficiency. The expert can do what is required, quickly and smoothly in much less time than it takes to explain. Since tacit knowledge is developed in action, it remains accessible to immediately guide action. Clinicians often literally act before they think. This is not mindless action, it is an automaticity of expertise which does not have to be processed through the lengthier channels of formal cognition. However, the inability to explain all that one knows can cause others to question the credibility of the professional's knowledge. Occupational therapists in our study had a particular problem with this credibility issue because they had a wealth of practical tacit knowledge and confidence in their clinical skills but did not have a rich language to explain or describe their practice, as do physicians and some other practitioners in the clinical environment. Giving language to some aspects of their practice (Mattingly et al 1997) gave the therapists a clearer perspective on their practice and a vehicle to examine and advance it.

Tacit knowledge works in the immediate situation owing to its development in the past. It can also work to help a clinician formulate an image of the potential future situation, both as an image and a guide to plan treatment. Below is an example of a clinician whose tacit knowledge was copious, and who could also articulate that knowledge given just a little prompting.

A Norwegian therapist we know read a transcript of an American therapist's report on her work with a man with a crush injury to his hand. The report was basically a long list of abbreviations about distal and proximal interphalangeal and other joints and various soft tissue injuries. This therapist looked up from the notes and sighed. When we asked what the matter was she replied:

> I can just see it all now. This man is going to get very depressed, lose his job, probably become an alcoholic, and his wife will divorce him. He will probably have bad contractures, more surgery, be

> committed to therapy for a while and cycle back
> and forth between depression and attempts to get
> his life and therapy back on track.

We looked at her in astonishment, for that was exactly what had happened to him. 'How did you know?' we asked. She said:

> I've seen it all before. I have been a hand therapist
> for several years. As soon as I read the description
> of his injuries, his hand just lit up in my mind. I
> could just see it. Then his life just rolled along in
> my mind as well. I knew just how it was going to
> be. This is a very difficult injury and very
> devastating to the person.

This experienced therapist had known similar people with similar injuries in the past and was able to envision this man's situation. The strong imagistic quality, to say nothing of the accuracy, of her comments demonstrates more than simple memory. Her capacity to suddenly see this patient in her mind's eye is part of her expertise. The image is a vivid and powerful portrayal of the person's future life. This therapist's ability to create vivid images of a patient's life, to take a minimal description of a hand injury and envision a host of life consequences, including how they might affect the emotions and motives of the patient, also reveals well developed skills in narrative reasoning.

NARRATIVE REASONING

One might assume that narrative reasoning is related strictly to telling and interpreting stories. However, it has come to be associated with a much broader human capacity. It constitutes a form of meaning making which is pervasive in human activity (Bruner 1986, 1990, 1996; Carr 1986; MacIntyre 1981; Nussbaum 1990; Ricoeur 1984). In recent years, narrative thinking has been recognized as important in clinical judgement (Frankenberg 1993; Good 1994; Hunt 1994; Hunter 1991; Mattingly 1991, 1998a, b; Mattingly & Fleming 1994). Narrative reasoning is necessary to interpret the actions of others and to respond appropriately to the social context. Bruner (1986, 1996) referred to it as a capacity to 'read other minds,' that is, to make accurate inferences about

the motives and intentions of others based on their observable behaviour and the social situation in which they act. When we try to make sense of what another person is up to, we ask, in effect, what story is that person living out? Narrative thinking, as the anthropologist Michael Carrithers (1992, pp. 77–78) observed, 'allows people to comprehend a complex flow of action and to act appropriately within it ... narrative thinking is the very process we use to understand the social life around us'.

When occupational therapists reason narratively, clinical problems and treatment activities are organized in their minds as an unfolding drama (Mattingly 1998b). A cast of characters emerges. Motives are inferred or examined. Narrative reasoning is needed when clinicians want to understand concrete events that cannot be comprehended without relating an inner world of desire and motive to an outer world of observable actions and states of affairs. Narrative reasoning concerns the relationship among motives, actions, and consequences as they play out in some specific situation (Bruner 1986; Dray 1954; Ricoeur 1980, 1984). However, attention to the specifics of context is not sufficient to distinguish narrative reasoning from other modes of clinical thinking. As Hunter (1991, p. 28) noted: 'The individual case is the touchstone of knowledge in medicine.' The hallmark of narrative reasoning is that it utilizes specifics of a very special sort: it involves a search for the precise motives that led to certain key actions and how those critical actions produced some further set of consequences. Although narrative reasoning is evidently a generic human capacity, it is prone to tremendous misjudgement. As we all know, it is quite easy to misinterpret the motives and intentions of others, especially if they are strangers and come from unfamiliar social or cultural backgrounds. In some cases, and for some practices, interpretive errors are not especially important. One can make a splint, for example, without needing to have tremendous skill in interpreting the meaning of splint wearing for one's client. But one cannot make a good decision about when to give a client a splint, or figure out how to get that client to wear it, without developing a capacity to assess the beliefs, values, and concerns of the client.

There are practical reasons why expert rehabilitation professionals in particular hone their narrative reasoning skills. The most obvious reason is that effective treatment depends upon highly motivated patients. As occupational therapists often say, in therapy, patients are not 'done to' but are asked to 'do for themselves'. This 'active healing' process means that patients cannot passively yield their bodies to the expert to receive a cure; rather they need to become highly committed participants in the rehabilitation process. This presents a special challenge to the professional: 'How do I foster a high level of commitment in my patients?' This task calls upon narrative reasoning as the practitioner tries to design a treatment approach which will appeal to a particular patient. Occupational therapists refer to this as 'individualizing treatment'. Narrative reasoning figures centrally in those health professions – such as rehabilitation therapies – where efficacious practice requires developing a strong collaboration with clients. When motives matter, narrative reasoning is inevitable, and poor narrative reasoning skills will mean that therapy is likely to fail.

PROSPECTIVE STORIES: THERAPY STORIES AND LIFE STORIES

In occupational therapy at least, narrative reasoning is not merely directed at the problem of obtaining the cooperation of a patient during a particular clinical encounter. The therapist's ability to employ narrative reasoning sensitively is essential to another clinical task, helping patients link their past (often a time before illness or disability) both to the present and to a future worth pursuing. When therapists ask themselves, 'Who is this patient?' they are asking a fundamentally narrative question. They are wondering what might motivate this particular patient in treatment, and beyond that, which treatment activities and goals would be most appealing and useful, given the life this person will likely be living once therapy is completed. Therapists routinely struggle to develop images of their patients as individuals with unique needs and commitments, and with singular life stories. 'Curing' is rare in the world of rehabilitation and in any case it is not

possible to transport a patient back in time to younger and healthier years. Instead, occupational therapists work to connect with patients in order to judge which treatment goals are most fitting and which treatment activities make most sense given the patient's conceptions of what is important in life. In fact, collaboration with patients is so central, it is probably more accurate to speak of the co-construction of treatment goals and activities.

The power of narrative as an ongoing, largely tacit, reasoning process which guides action becomes most evident in clinical situations when things break down – when it is difficult for the practitioner to make narrative sense of the clinical encounter or the patient. When practitioners confront patients who are incomprehensible in some significant way, the whole direction of treatment may falter. The tacit narrative reasoning which practitioners carry into clinical encounters is likely to turn into explicit storytelling as they try to discern what is going on and 'what story they are in' with a particular client. For instance, a patient may insist that he wants to return to his job, show up to all his clinical appointments faithfully, comply with all the tasks set before him during his therapy hour, but never manage to 'get around' to doing the exercises he is supposed to be carrying out at home. Without these home exercises, the therapist may explain several times, treatment will not be successful. He will not be able to use his hand. He will not be able to return to work. And yet, nothing helps. Things continue just as before. Perhaps he has been lying, or deceiving himself. Perhaps he does not want his job back after all. But if he were merely non-compliant, uninterested in returning to work, why does he show up to every appointment so faithfully, even arriving early? Why does he try so hard during therapy time? Such mysteries are common. Therapists become increasingly unclear about how to proceed in their treatment interventions, even when the 'good' (outcome) for a patient (say, maximal return of hand function) remains fixed in an abstract sense.

Narrative reasoning is a guide to a therapist's future actions because it provides images of a possible future for the client. When employing narrative reasoning, practitioners are trying to assess how to act in particular clinical situations, taking into consideration the motives and desires of themselves, their clients, and other relevant actors. The ongoing construction of a narrative framework provides clinicians with historical contexts in which certain actions emerge as the inevitable next steps leading to the most promising future. Although the question of what the good future is for any particular patient may never be explicitly asked, the process of treatment itself is very often a process of exploring and negotiating a vision of the future good. When clinicians assess how they can help patients reshape their situation for the better, this assessment is often informed by a 'prospective story', an imagined future life story for the individual. Thus, clinicians contemplate how to situate their therapeutic interventions (a kind of 'therapeutic present') in light of a patient's past and some hoped-for vision of what will follow in the future when the patient is discharged.

Narrative reasoning is directed to the future in the sense that it involves judgements about how to act in order to 'further the plot' in desirable directions and to subvert, as far as possible, undesirable ones. While our traditional concept is that stories recount past events, stories in the clinical world are often directed to future possibilities. How are such 'prospective stories' communicated to patients or negotiated with them? Generally, it is not by telling the stories in detail. Rather, the stories are sketched through subtle hints or cues, or enacted in clinical dramas that prefigure life after therapy. The prospective story is offered, like the architect's sketch, as a possibility, something to be looked at, viewed from different angles, something to make a judgement about. When therapists offer short stories to their patients about what their life will be like 'in a few weeks' or 'when the halo comes off' or 'when you are home with the kids', they are offering images and possibilities of a meaningful future. Therapists hope that a commitment to these narrative images, images that point towards a future life story, will carry the patients through the long, tedious, often painful routines of treatment.

ACTIVE JUDGEMENTS, TACIT KNOWLEDGE AND NARRATIVE IMAGES: A CASE STORY

The interplay of actions, judgements, tacit knowledge, and narrative image making is dauntingly intricate to describe in the abstract, but becomes easily visible when examining concrete instances of practice. The following case story, written by an experienced occupational therapist (see acknowledgements), illustrates how image, action and narrative come together in expert therapeutic practice.

THE STORY OF ANN

Maureen Freda
Ann was a 26-year-old woman who had had a stroke following childbirth. She was admitted to a rehabilitation hospital with right hemiparesis. When I first met Ann, she was very depressed about being separated from her new baby and her main fear was that she would not be able adequately to care for the baby on her own. Adding to this fear was the knowledge that her insurance would not cover any in-home services. Her husband was her only family. He worked in construction every day and they lived in a trailer park. In order to go home with the baby, she would need to be very independent.

The initial therapy sessions were centred around tone normalization, with an emphasis on mat activities, along with traditional ADL (activities of daily life) training in the mornings. Ann's husband visited daily and usually brought the baby with him. At first this was extremely frustrating to Ann, since she could not hold the baby unless she was sitting down with pillows supporting her right arm. She continued to voice anxiety around the issue of going

(Continued)

THE STORY OF ANN *cont'd*

home and being able to care for the baby. Her husband was also very worried about how this transformation would take place – from Ann as a patient to Ann as wife and mother. I spent a lot of time talking to both Ann and her husband about the necessity of normalizing the tone and improving the movement of the upper extremity as a sort of foundation to the more complex functional skills Ann was so anxious to relearn.

Eventually it was time to spend the majority of the treatment time on functional skills. The two areas we focused on were homemaking and child care. The homemaking sessions were fairly routine and traditional in nature. However, it proved to be a bit more difficult to simulate some of the child care activities.

Our first obstacle was to find something that would be like a baby. We settled on borrowing a 'resusc-a-baby' from the nursing education department. We used this 'baby' for the beginning skills such as feeding and diaper changing. Ann had progressed to a point where she had slight weakness and incoordination in the right arm and she was walking with a straight cane. The next step was to tackle walking with the baby. We of course practised with a baby carrier. We also had to prepare for the event of carrying the baby without the 'carrier'. I wrapped weights about the 'baby' to equal the weight of the now 3-month-old infant at home. Ann walked down the hall carrying the 'baby' and I would be following behind jostling the 'baby' to simulate squirming (we became the talk of the hospital with our daily walks!). Ann was becoming more and more comfortable and confident with

these activities, so it was time to make arrangements to have the real baby spend his days in the rehab with his mother. This was not as easy as it might seem. The administration of the hospital was not used to such requests. But with the right cajoling in the right places this was eventually approved. The real baby now replaced 'resusc-a-baby' on our daily walks and in the clinic. While these successes were comforting to Ann and her husband, the fact remained that we were still in a very protective environment. The big question was yet unanswered – would these skills hold up under the stresses of everyday life – alone – in a trailer for 8 hours daily?

Never being one to hold to tradition, I decided to go to administration with one more request. I wanted to do a full-day home visit with Ann and her baby. This too was approved and a week before Ann's scheduled discharge, she and I set out for a rigorous day at the home front. Once there all did not go smoothly. Ann fell once and practically dropped the baby. She was very anxious and stressed, but we managed to get through the day. We talked and problem-solved every little real or perceived difficulty. Both Ann and the baby survived the fall and the 'almost' dropping. When we got back to the hospital, Ann, her husband, the social worker and I sat down and realistically discussed and decided what kind of outside help was a necessity and what Ann could really accomplish in a day. Ann's husband adjusted his schedule, a teenage neighbour was brought in for 2–3 hours a day and Ann was able to do the majority of the care for her baby.

ACTION, JUDGEMENT, NARRATIVE AND EXPERTISE IN THE STORY OF ANN

In the above story an experienced clinician orchestrates a therapy programme for a somewhat unusual patient. Maureen begins her story with a typical medical case history approach but it quickly becomes evident that the patient's particular life situation shapes Maureen's judgements about how to design treatment. It matters, for

instance, that one of the primary consequences of Ann's stroke is that Ann is fearful about her ability to care for her newborn baby. Maureen also immediately takes into account key elements that will be at play in Ann's 'future story'. Maureen notes the particular situation to which Ann will be returning as a mother unable to afford child care, with no family to turn to except her husband, who works all day.

Maureen judges what actions Ann will need to relearn and selects and invents therapeutic activities based on her perception of the social context and personal goals of Ann and her husband. Maureen is sensitive to the husband's insight about the need for Ann's transformation from patient to wife and mother. She situates her treatment goals within the notion of transformation. Her treatment approach develops as a powerful 'short story' which aids in Ann's transformation from fearful patient to confident mother, able to handle even the difficult task of carrying her baby in her arms. Maureen makes continual judgements about how to shift treatment from safer and easier tasks to those more closely approximating Ann's 'real world' life situation.

In creating this unique treatment story, Maureen relies on her accumulated tacit knowledge culled from years of experience. She draws upon a typical treatment sequence, from building individual motions, to actions, to coordinated functional skills. She clearly has a great deal of tacit knowledge regarding how to help patients build their ADL skills. While this occupational therapist can draw upon a wealth of tacit knowledge, in many ways she faces a singular situation which requires her to make judgements specifically tailored to Ann's needs.

The symbolic plays a powerful role in this treatment. Maureen sees the need for a substitute or symbolic baby, not just a pretend baby in the form of a pillow. She borrows a model from another clinical department and this seems to do the trick. Maureen moves on with Ann from sedentary baby care activities to the more challenging, complex and risky activity of walking with the baby. She rises to this challenge by developing novel therapeutic activities, such as adding weights and simulating the baby's squirming. These increasingly active qualities of the 'resusc-a-baby' are proxy for the real baby, who now enters the picture as a more viable image. The more realistic the 'baby's' actions become, the more Ann becomes prepared to make the transition from patient to mother.

Maureen judges when it is time for the real baby to make an appearance on the rehabilitation floor. Maureen's confidence in her judgements prepares her to make and win the case with administration for the baby to participate in his mother's therapy.

The therapy works. It is clear to everyone that this move beyond conventional practice has reaped benefits far greater than would have been obtained had Maureen stuck to conventional exercise and routine ADL activities.

Finally, the therapist determines that it is time to take what they have learned and see how they work in the real-life situation of Ann's home. Here we see that Maureen's perceptions of her own judgement and her tacit knowledge differ. She is thoroughly confident that the home visit is the right thing to do. However, she is somewhat less confident regarding the potential success that Ann will have in some of the specific activities of baby care. Ann and Maureen now have enough trust in each other and in the plan to believe that this practice session is well worth any potential risks. Although she does not say so, we can infer that Maureen is constantly attentive to the small details of the activities that she asks Ann to carry out in the home and has set up subtle safety features, including her heightened attention and undoubted physical closeness to mother and child.

This confluence of image and action is typical of experienced therapists who are able to see opportunities in the midst of action to gradually or dramatically change their treatment plan in response to particular details of a patient's skills and needs. Notably, this capacity for flexible plan development is central because, as Ann illustrates, a patient's needs and concerns often change over the course of therapy. Maureen, through her sensitivity to this patient and her personal and social context, was able to both speed up and individualize treatment in order to maximize her ability to act and return Ann to her desired social roles.

We have described this treatment process as the creation of a 'short story' within the larger life story of the patient, Ann (and, of course, the life stories of her husband and baby as well). Notably, this is a short story which not only connects to Ann's past, as a young woman who has recently given birth, but to a future – that is, to events and experiences which have not yet taken place. With the careful guiding of treatment activities, the therapist is able to steer Ann towards her hoped-for future, the one in which she can independently care for her child, and steer her away from a very undesirable future, in which she remains depressed and fearful of her capacities to take on such care.

The power of any therapeutic short story is its capacity to help patients and their families realize some future story which deeply matters to them. The therapist cannot simply impose this desired future upon Ann, even if it is a future Ann dearly wants. She must look for signals that Ann is ready to move towards it. This requires the therapist's continual judgement about what constitutes the 'just right challenge' (Csikszentmihalyi 1975) for Ann at any moment in therapy. Such judgements involve assessing Ann's physical capabilities but also require narrative reasoning, assessing the state of Ann's inner world of emotions, desires and beliefs, as they are expressed in her outward actions and words.

Narrative reasoning is also utilized when Maureen helps to create symbolically potent images for Ann, helping her to envision what life will be like with her baby. Maureen creates dramatic situations in which Ann can test her abilities and face her fears. This dramatic play even allows Ann to face one of her worst nightmares, as she nearly drops her child upon returning home for a trial run with Maureen. Notably, these experiences help Maureen to talk with Ann, her husband and a social worker in order to make a more realistic plan about how Ann might care for her child upon discharge, including changes in the husband's work schedule and bringing in a neighbourhood babysitter to help out.

CONCLUSION

We have found that clinical reasoning is not just one cognitive process and is not limited to the task of making decisions about concrete biological problems. We claim that to be truly therapeutic, clinicians must understand their patients and the ways in which they make meaning in lives that are changed by illness or injury. Two of the ways practitioners perceive patient's perceptions of their past and future lives and orchestrate treatment programmes to achieve that future vision have been briefly discussed. These strategies are narrative reasoning and active judgement. These forms of reasoning serve to enlarge clinicians' stock of tacit knowledge and expand their expertise.

Acknowledgements

This chapter is an edited version of a chapter of the same title from the second edition of this book.

'The Story of Ann' is by Maureen Freda, MA, OTR.

References

Bruner J 1986 Actual minds, possible worlds. Harvard University Press, Cambridge, MA

Bruner J 1990 Acts of meaning. Harvard University Press, Cambridge, MA

Bruner J 1996 The culture of education. Harvard University Press, Cambridge, MA

Buchler J 1955 Nature and judgement. Grosset and Dunlap/ Solidus Columbia University Press

Carr D 1986 Time, narrative, and history. Indiana University Press, Bloomington

Carrithers M B 1992 Why humans have cultures. Oxford University Press, Oxford

Csikszentmihalyi M 1975 Beyond boredom and anxiety: the experience of play in work and game. Jossey-Bass, San Francisco

Dray W 1954 Explanatory narrative in history. Philosophical Quarterly 23:15–27

Frankenberg R 1993 Risk: anthropological and epidemiological narratives of prevention.

In: Lindenbaum S, Lock M (eds) Knowledge, power and practice: the anthropology of everyday life. University of California Press, Berkeley, p 219–242

Good B 1994 Medicine, rationality, and experience: an anthropological perspective. Cambridge University Press, New York

Hunt L 1994 Practicing oncology in provincial Mexico: a narrative analysis. Social Science and Medicine 38(6):843–853

Hunter K M 1991 Doctors' stories: the narrative structure of medical knowledge. Princeton University Press, Princeton, NJ

MacIntyre A 1981 After virtue: a study in moral theory. University of Notre Dame Press, Notre Dame, IN

Mattingly C 1991 The narrative nature of clinical reasoning. American Journal of Occupational Therapy 45:998–1005

Mattingly C 1998a Healing dramas and clinical plots: the narrative structure of experience. Cambridge University Press, Cambridge

Mattingly C 1998b In search of the good: narrative reasoning in clinical practice. Medical Anthropology Quarterly 12 (3):273–297

Mattingly C, Fleming M H 1994 Clinical reasoning: forms of inquiry in a therapeutic practice. F A Davis, Philadelphia

Mattingly C, Fleming M H, Gillette N 1997 Narrative explorations in the tacit dimension: bringing language to clinical practice. Nordiske Udkast 1(1):65–77

Nussbaum M 1990 Love's knowledge. Oxford University Press, New York

Polanyi M 1966 The tacit dimension. Doubleday, Garden City, NY

Ricoeur P 1980 Narrative time. In: Mitchell T J (ed) On narrative. University of Chicago Press, Chicago, p 165–186

Ricoeur P 1984 Time and narrative, vol 1. University of Chicago Press, Chicago

Schön D A 1983 The reflective practitioner: how professionals think in action. Basic Books, New York

Chapter 6

Clinical reasoning and generic thinking skills

Stephen Brookfield

THE ROLE OF THINKING IN CLINICAL REASONING

Clinical practice, as most clinicians know, is frequently located in a zone of ambiguity. The reality of clinical experience often stands in marked contrast to the patterns of practice laid out in introductory texts and pre-service education. Indeed, the contrast between the neatness of professional education programmes and the apparent chaos of clinical experience calls into question the usefulness of pre-service education. If the world refuses to conform to the models, concepts and research studied in professional education, what use is it to study theory and read professional literature? If the techniques acquired in school are constantly distorted or rendered irrelevant by the exigencies of practice, why should we bother learning them?

In this chapter I argue that pre-service education still plays a crucial role in professional development, but only if pre-service curricula place acquisition of the thinking skills of clinical reasoning – particularly the skill of critical appraisal – at their centre. Such skills might be regarded as the metacognition of clinical practice. They shape the way practitioners approach, analyse and respond to the multiple contexts and idiosyncrasies of practice. They do not displace the learning of specific skills or protocols, but they do frame how we determine the appropriateness of these protocols for different situations and how we modify the application of these skills in practice.

One can be technically proficient to a high level, but if one is unable to think in the way clinical reasoning demands then this proficiency is exercised haphazardly. A reliance on protocol and habitual responses works well as long as the world does not trip you up by refusing to conform to the shape you anticipate. Since the one constant of clinical practice is that nothing stays the same, it follows that the best form of pre-service clinical education develops generic skills of analysis that can increase the likelihood of clinicians taking informed clinical action.

At the heart of clinical reasoning are three interrelated skills that might be described as 'scanning', 'gathering' and 'critical appraisal'. These skills are thinking skills – they stress analysis rather than instrumental competence.

Scanning is an act of apprehension. It describes the ways we identify the central features of a clinical situation. In scanning a situation we decide what its boundaries are, which patterns of the situation are familiar and grounded in past experience, and which are in new or unusual configurations. We also decide which of the cues that we notice should be attended to. Scanning is the initial sweep, the experiential trawl we conduct to construct the big picture.

In the *gathering* phase of clinical reasoning we explore the interpretive resources and analytic protocols available to help us understand the situation correctly. These include the general clinical guidelines we have learned as part of our professional preparation or through in-service development. We remember superiors' instructions regarding what to do in such situations and also colleagues' suggestions we have heard, or practices we have seen. Finally, we call on our own intuition. We attend to the instinctive analyses and responses that immediately suggest themselves as relevant.

In the *appraisal* phase we sort through the interpretations we have gathered. We decide which seem to fit most closely with the situation we are reviewing and, on the basis of these, we take informed action. Contextually appropriate reasoning is central to this phase. Scanning and gathering involve looking for patterns and broad similarities between a new situation and previous experiences. But in appraisal we judge the accuracy and validity of the assumptions and

interpretations we have gathered. This occurs through a number of interconnected processes: by sifting through past experiences and judging the closeness of their fit to the current situation; by intentionally following prescribed clinical protocols and introducing experimental adaptations of these when they suggest themselves; by consulting peers prior to making clinical decisions or in the midst of action; and by attempting to analyse which of our instinctive judgements and readings we should take seriously and which we should hold in abeyance. As a result of this appraisal we take action regarding those procedures and responses that make the most sense in the current situation.

This chapter focuses on the third skill, appraisal, as the phase of clinical reasoning in which thinking is most central. Appraisal entails a detailed critical review of multiple sources, during which we decide to attend to some cues, to discard others, and to reframe interpretations that hold promise but do not entirely explain what we are confronting. In the language of formal research, this involves us in determining the accuracy and validity of assumptions and interpretations that we decide are most appropriate to a situation. In more colloquial terms, we try to judge the fit between what we think is happening and the responses that seem to make most sense.

THE PROCESS OF APPRAISAL: A DEEPER ANALYSIS

As a process, clinical appraisal involves practitioners in recognizing and researching the assumptions that lie behind their clinical practice. Assumptions are the taken-for-granted beliefs about the world and our place within it that seem so obvious to us that they do not need to be stated explicitly. Assumptions give meaning and purpose to who we are and what we do. In many ways we *are* our assumptions. So much of what we think, say and do is based on assumptions about how the world should work, and what we believe counts as clinically appropriate, ethical action within it. Yet frequently these assumptions are not recognized for the provisional understandings that they really are. Ideas and practices that we regard as commonsense conventional wisdom are often based on uncritically accepted assumptions. Some person, institution or authority that we either trust or fear has told us that this is the way things are and we accept their judgement unquestioningly. Clinical appraisal requires that we research these assumptions for the evidence and experiences that inform them. In particular, it involves seeing our assumptions from as many unfamiliar perspectives as we can.

Sometimes we find that assumptions about appropriate clinical responses are justified by our, or others', experiences, in which case we feel a confidence in their accuracy and validity. When we can cite the clinical experiences supporting an assumption, we exhibit an informed commitment to it. At other times, however, we find that our assumptions are flawed, distorted or accurate within a much narrower range of clinical situations than we had originally thought. When this happens we realize that we need to abandon or reframe these assumptions so that they provide more accurate guides to and justifications for our actions.

What makes the process of assumption-hunting particularly complicated is that assumptions are not all of the same character. I find it useful to distinguish between three broad categories of assumption: the paradigmatic, the prescriptive and the causal. *Paradigmatic assumptions* are the hardest of all assumptions to uncover. They are the structuring assumptions we use to order the world into fundamental categories. Usually we do not recognize them as assumptions, even after they have been pointed out to us. Instead we insist that they are objectively valid renderings of reality, the facts as we know them to be true. Some paradigmatic assumptions I have held at different stages of my life as a teacher are that adults are self-directed learners, that critical thinking is an intellectual function characteristic of adult life, that good adult educational processes are inherently democratic, and that education always has a political dimension.

Paradigmatic assumptions are examined critically only after a great deal of resistance, and it takes a considerable amount of contrary evidence and disconfirming experience to change them. But when they are challenged and changed, the consequences for our lives are explosive. I think of them as the foundational building blocks that give structure to the architecture of our worldviews. Paradigmatic assumptions are like load-bearing lintels in the houses of our assumptive clusters – remove them and the whole structure comes crashing down. It is because practitioners sense the potentially traumatic implications of questioning paradigmatic assumptions that they are so reluctant to do this.

Prescriptive assumptions are assumptions about what we think ought to be happening in a particular situation. They are the assumptions that come to the surface as we examine how we think teachers should behave, what good educational processes should look like, and what obligations students and teachers owe to each other. Inevitably they are grounded in, and are extensions of, our paradigmatic assumptions. For example, if you believe that adults are self-directed learners then you assume that the best teaching is that which encourages students to take control over designing, conducting and evaluating their own learning. Prescriptive assumptions are a little easier to discover. They tend to be expressed in institutional mission statements or clearly acknowledged as central to our philosophy of practice. However, although prescriptive assumptions may be espoused passionately they may play a relatively small role in determining our actions. It is not at all uncommon for practitioners to act in ways that bear little relation to their espoused assumptions regarding professional behaviour.

Causal assumptions are assumptions about how different parts of the world work and about the conditions under which these arrangements can be changed. They are usually stated in predictive terms. An example of a causal assumption would be that the use of learning contracts will increase students' self-directedness. Another would be the assumption that if we make mistakes in front of students it creates a trustful environment for learning, in which students feel free to make errors with no fear of censure or embarrassment. Of all the assumptions we hold, causal ones are the easiest to uncover and are the ones most frequently unearthed in workshops and professional conversations. But discovering and investigating these is only the beginning of clinical reasoning. We must then try to find a way to work back to the more deeply embedded prescriptive and paradigmatic assumptions we hold.

CRITICAL APPRAISAL OF CLINICAL REASONING: A CONTEXT-BOUND AND SOCIAL PROCESS

One of the most salient features of clinical appraisal is that it is irrevocably context-bound. The same person can be highly open to re-examining one set of clinical practices, but completely closed to critically reappraising another situation or idea. Nor is a facility for clinical appraisal learned developmentally. There is plenty of evidence to show that after a breakthrough in clinical reasoning people can quite easily revert to an earlier, more naive, way of thinking and being. So clinical reasoning can only be understood, and its development gauged, within a specific context.

Clinical reasoning is also an irreducibly social process. It happens best when we enlist others – clients, patients, supervisors, peers and colleagues – to help us see our ideas and actions in new ways. Very few of us can get very far probing our assumptions on our own. No matter how much we may think we have an accurate sense of our practice, we are stymied by the fact that we are using our own interpretive filters to become aware of our own interpretive filters! This is the pedagogic equivalent of a dog trying to catch its own tail, or of trying to see the back of your head while looking in the bathroom mirror. To some extent we are all prisoners trapped within the perceptual frameworks that determine how we view our experiences. A self-confirming cycle often develops whereby our uncritically accepted assumptions shape clinical actions which then serve only to confirm the truth of those assumptions. It is very difficult to stand outside ourselves and see how some of our most deeply held values and beliefs lead us into distorted and constrained ways of thinking and practising. Our most influential assumptions are too close to us to be seen clearly by an act of self-will.

If clinical reasoning, and especially the process of appraisal, is conceived of as a social learning process then our peers (and teachers) become important critical mirrors. To become critically reflective we need to find some lenses that reflect back to us a stark and differently highlighted picture of who we are and what we do. When our peers listen to our stories and then reflect back to us what they see and hear in them we are often presented with an unexpected version of ourselves and our actions. Hearing colleagues' perceptions helps us gain a clearer perspective on the dimensions to our thoughts and actions that need closer critical scrutiny. It also helps us to understand the commonality of our individual clinical experiences. Although no one person lives practice in exactly the same way as another, there is often much more that unites us than we realize. Talking to colleagues helps us see how much we take for granted in our own practice. Sometimes it confirms the correctness of instincts that we have felt privately but doubted because we thought they contradicted conventional wisdom or accepted clinical protocols. Peer conversation can also help break down the isolation many of us feel. Talking to other practitioners can open up unfamiliar avenues for inquiry and allow us to receive advice on how to deal with the problems we are facing.

THE PRAXIS OF CLINICAL APPRAISAL

Appraisal involves a well-documented praxis of action, reflection on action, further action, reflection on the further action, new, more informed action, and so on, in a continuous cyclical loop. But these alternating phases need not be separated by extensive periods of time. Action can be mindful, thoughtful and informed. At any point in clinical practice we are engaged in a complex series of operations, some of which involve scrutinizing past assumptions, some of which involve exploring new meaning schemes, some of which require us to try on new identities, and so on.

In learning clinical appraisal we can posit the following pattern: initial reflection is usually prompted by some unexpected occurrence – something is happening which does not feel right, which does not fit. This disorienting dilemma (to use Mezirow's (1991) term) occasions reflection on the discrepancy between the assumptions, rules and criteria informing our practice and our experiences of clinical reality. Triggers to clinical reasoning are usually presented as traumatic or troublesome in some way, as cognitive dissonances, or perceptions of anomalies, disjunctions and contradictions between our expectations of clinical practice and its actuality. Practically every theorist of critical thinking emphasizes how trauma triggers appraisal through life-shaking incidents such as divorce, bereavement, unemployment, disability, conscription, forced change of job or geographical location (McMahon 2005). Critical theory – a major intellectual tradition informing critical thinking – explains how such trigger events often cause people to question dominant ideology (Brookfield 2005). After all, if you play by the rules of the dominant culture you are not supposed to have bad things happen to you, so when they do, some of your paradigmatic assumptions are bound to be challenged.

Following the trigger event, periods of denial and depression alternate with attempts to understand the nature of the contradiction or dilemma experienced. During this period clinicians seek desperately for others who are confronting similar anomalies. In formal or informal peer reflection groups, practitioners make an active effort to come to terms with the tension they feel. They reinterpret their experiences to create new meanings as they try to reduce feelings of discomfort or alienation. They may flirt with new identities or new concepts of what it means to be a clinician. They make a deliberate effort to draw on others' experiences and to see the situation from their point of view, so that it can be interpreted from multiple perspectives.

Arising out of this process of exploring and testing new assumptions and beliefs about practice is the development of a changed way of thinking and acting which 'makes sense' or 'fits' the clinical situation. This new perspective on practice is liable, initially at least, to be partial, tentative and fragile. Indeed, there is often a series of incremental confirmations of the validity of this new perspective as clinical experience gradually confirms its accuracy. Having decided that new assumptions and practices make sense in the context of our clinical experiences, we look for ways to integrate these permanently into our practice.

EXPERIENTIAL LENSES OF CLINICAL APPRAISAL

Exploring the discrepancy between what is and what should be is at the heart of clinical appraisal. When we embark on this process we have three experiential lenses through which we can view our clinical practice:

1. our autobiographies as practitioners, teachers and clients
2. our patients' eyes
3. our colleagues' experiences.

Viewing what we do through these different lenses alerts us to distorted or incomplete aspects of our assumptions that need further investigation.

LENS 1: OUR AUTOBIOGRAPHIES AS PRACTITIONERS, TEACHERS AND CLIENTS

Our autobiographies as practitioners, teachers and clients represent some of the most important sources of insight into practice to which we have access. Yet, in much talk and writing about practice, personal experience is dismissed and demeaned as 'merely anecdotal'; in other words, as hopelessly subjective and impressionistic. It is true, of course, that at one level all experience is inherently idiosyncratic. For example, each person experiences the death of a patient in a slightly different way, with a different mix of memories, regrets, affirmations and pain. Yet at the same time, bereavement as a process of recognizing and accepting loss contains a number of patterns and rhythms that could be described as generic (Kubler-Ross 1997).

The fact that people recognize aspects of their individual experiences in the stories others tell is one reason for the success of peer support groups for those in crisis or transition. As I hear you talk about going through a divorce, struggling with illness or addiction, or dealing with the death of partners, friends and parents I am likely to hear echoes of, and direct parallels to, my own experience of these events. The same dynamic holds true in practitioner reflection groups. As we talk to each other about critical events in our practice we start to realize that individual clinical crises are usually collectively experienced dilemmas. The details and characters may differ, but the tensions are essentially the same.

LENS 2: OUR PATIENTS' EYES

Seeing oneself through our patients' eyes constitutes one of the most consistently surprising elements in any clinician's career. Each time we do this we learn something. Sometimes what we find out is reassuring. We discover that patients are interpreting our actions in the way that we mean them. They are hearing what we wanted them to hear and seeing what we wanted them to see. But often we are profoundly surprised by the diversity of meanings patients read into our words and actions. Comments we made incidentally that had no particular significance to us are heard as imperatives. Answers we gave off the cuff to what seemed like inconsequential questions return to haunt them (and us). Long after we have forgotten them they are quoted back at us by patients to prove that what we are saying now is contradicting our earlier advice. What we think is reassuring behaviour on our part is sometimes interpreted as over-protective coddling. A humorous aside, appreciated by some, leaves others feeling insulted.

LENS 3: OUR COLLEAGUES' EXPERIENCES

Talking to colleagues about what we do unravels the shroud of silence in which our clinical practice is wrapped. Participating in critical conversation with peers opens us up to their versions of events we have experienced. Our colleagues serve as critical mirrors, reflecting back to us images of our actions that often take us by surprise. As they describe their experiences dealing with the same crises and dilemmas that we face, we are able to check, reframe and broaden our own theories of practice. Talking to colleagues about problems we have in common, and gaining their perspectives on them, increases our chances of stumbling across a new interpretation that fits what is happening in a particular situation. A colleague's experiences may suggest dynamics and causes that make much more sense than the explanations we have evolved. If this happens we are helped enormously in our effort to work out just what we should be doing to deal with the problem.

Without an accurate reading of the causes of a problem – are they embedded in our actions, in our patients' past histories, in the wider political or professional constraints placed on our clinical practice, or in a particular intersection of all of these? – we are crippled in our attempts to work through it.

Checking our readings of problems, responses, assumptions and justifications against the readings offered by colleagues is crucial if we are to claw a path to critical clarity. It also provides us with a great deal of emotional sustenance. We start to see that what we thought were unique problems and idiosyncratic failings are shared by many others who work in situations like ours. Just knowing that we are not alone in our struggles can be a life-saving realization. Although clinical appraisal often begins alone, it is ultimately a collective endeavour.

CLINICAL REASONING AND THE STRUGGLE AGAINST 'IMPOSTORSHIP'

Thinking in the way that clinical reasoning involves is not without risks. Perhaps the chief of these is the risk of admitting one's own 'impostorship'. Clinical practitioners often feel like impostors. They have a hidden sense that they do not really deserve to be taken seriously as competent professionals because in their heart of hearts they know that they do not really know what they are doing. All they are certain of is that unless they are very careful they will be found out to be practising under false pretences. Such feelings are made worse because of the privacy ethic that prevails in many professional settings. There is no safe place to air uncertainties and request help. Clinicians struck by impostorship have the conviction that they do not really merit any professional recognition or acclaim that comes their way. De Vries (1993, p. 129) summarized these feelings:

> These people have an abiding feeling that they have fooled everyone and are not as competent and intelligent as others think they are. They attribute their success to good luck, compensatory hard work, or superficial factors such as physical attractiveness and likeability. Some are incredibly

hardworking, always over-prepared. However, they are unable to accept that they have intellectual gifts and ability. They live in constant fear that their imposturous existence will be exposed – that they will not be able to measure up to others' expectations and that catastrophe will follow.

The presentation of the false face that impostorship entails is usually done for reasons of survival. We believe that if we do not look as though we know what we're doing then our patients, colleagues and superiors will eat us alive. We think that admitting frailty will be interpreted as a sign of failure. Impostorship also means that many of us go through our professional lives fearing that at some unspecified point in the future we will undergo a humiliating public unveiling. We wear an external mask of control but beneath it we know that really we are frail figures, struggling to make it through to the end of each day. There is the sense that around the corner is an unforseen but cataclysmic clinical event that will reveal us as frauds. When this event happens we imagine that our colleagues' jaws will drop in synchrony. With their collective mouths agape they will wonder out loud, 'How could we possibly have been so stupid as to hire this obvious incompetent in the first place?'

Viewing our practice through any of the experiential lenses of clinical reasoning heightens considerably the chances of our feeling like impostors. For people who are desperately trying to avoid being found out, the last thing they want to endure is a systematic scrutiny of their practice by colleagues. There is always the fear that once their impostorship has been discovered they will be punished. So one of the most important aids to clinical appraisal – having one's practice observed by peers – is also one of the most common triggers to impostorship.

Feelings of impostorship also accompany most attempts at clinical experimentation that spring from our reflection. Any time we depart from comfortable ways of acting or thinking to experiment with a new way of practice we are almost bound to be taken by surprise. The further we travel from our habitual practices the more we run the risk of looking incompetent. The moments of failure that inevitably accompany change and experimentation increase the sense of impostorship by emphasizing how little we can predict and control the consequences of our actions. In the midst of experimentation it is not uncommon for practitioners to resolve never again to put themselves through the experience of looking foolish in front of colleagues and trying desperately to conceal the fact that they do not really know what they are doing.

How can this feeling of impostorship be kept under control? The key, I think, is to make the phenomenon public. Once impostorship is named as an everyday experience it loses much of its power. It becomes commonplace and quotidian rather than a shameful, malevolent secret. To hear colleagues you admire talking graphically and convincingly about their own regular moments of impostorship is enormously reassuring. If they feel exactly the way we do, then perhaps we are not so bad after all. In public forums and private conversations, clinicians who are acclaimed as successful can do a great deal to defuse the worst effects of impostorship by admitting to its reality in their lives.

Being involved in team practice also makes us less prone to being overcome by impostorship. In clinical situations where teaming is required, built-in reflective mirrors are available. As you walk to the cafeteria after what you think is a bad clinical experience and you start to engage in your usual enthusiastic bout of self-flagellation, your colleagues are likely to point out the things that went well. They may tell you about the situations you handled confidently and how impressed they were with your abilities. They may provide you with immediate multiple perspectives on events that you have seen in only one way, and suggest readings of patients' actions that would never have occurred to you.

Clinical conversation groups invariably bring up the theme of impostorship. Once one person has revealed feelings and experiences of this, a ripple or domino effect occurs. One after the other, the members of the group give their own illustrations of the phenomenon. The tricky part is to get someone to admit to it in the first place. This is where experienced practitioners and preceptors can be particularly helpful. By admitting to their feelings of impostorship, experienced practitioners can ease the way for junior colleagues to speak. So joining or forming a reflection group is an important strategy to keep impostorship in its proper place.

TEACHING CLINICAL REASONING THROUGH TEAM MODELLING

How can the phases of clinical reasoning – scanning, gathering and appraisal – be taught? In interviews with practitioners, the factor emphasized more strongly than anything else is their seeing it publicly modelled by figures of authority and power (Brookfield 1995). When clinicians see preceptors and allied health professionals expressing out loud the reasons for their decisions, or disclosing the cues they take seriously and how these help them construct ladders of inference, it becomes clear to novices how experts do clinical reasoning in field settings. Modelling can, of course, be done alone or in teams. For many clinicians the necessities of practice mean it will happen in isolation, where one professional will attempt to model for students or novices her own engagement in clinical reasoning. But, because the clinical appraisal process described in the previous section depends so much on colleagues serving as critical mirrors, one of the most powerful forms of modelling is that undertaken in teams. If those perceived as credible experts demonstrate publicly how they rely on team colleagues to be their critically reflective mirrors it sends a message to newly engaged practitioners that enlisting the help of colleagues is crucial to accurate clinical appraisal. In my view it is impossible to overemphasize the importance of the clinical education faculty undertaking public modelling of their commitment to team learning in their own teaching and writing. The more that faculty members are publicly engaged in team teaching, team research, team writing and team reflection on common problems, the more they convey to practitioners an atmosphere that supports this. One reason it is important that faculty do this is that people often assume that good team behaviour means taking the reins and assiduously demonstrating 'leadership' by speaking frequently, being the author and deliverer of team progress reports, and so on. It is important that

practitioners learn early that effective participation in teams does not boil down to talking a lot and being the person who writes, posts and publicly reports the conversations a group is having. For example, in a doctoral programme I helped design at National Louis University in Chicago, faculty hold a weekend admissions workshop in which applicants are asked to work with each other in small groups accomplishing various team tasks. If someone tries to impress the faculty by immediately dominating a group in the mistaken belief that this demonstrates the exercise of effective team leadership, it is a warning signal that the person may not be suitable for a cohort programme in which participatory learning and team projects are stressed.

When modelling team behaviours for students it is important that faculty members show that effective team participation involves such things as listening carefully, elucidating connections and links between different participants' contributions, showing appreciation for others' contributions, drawing others out through skillful questioning, calling for occasional periods of reflective silence, and being ready to change one's mind in the face of new arguments or information. This is very close to the conditions of Habermas's (1996) ideal speech situation. Effective team participation sometimes also involves people arguing against the conventional wisdom and commonsense explanations a group immediately adheres to, and insisting that certain ignored or discredited ideas and traditions be included. This is what Marcuse (1965) called the practice of liberating tolerance in discussion. For example, critical debate or 'methodological belief' exercises ask participants to spend a limited time seeing a clinical situation from a viewpoint they may never have inhabited before – that of a patient, a patient's family member, or another specialist member of the medical team (anaesthetist, nutritionist, and so on).

If faculty can demonstrate how clinical reasoning happens in their own team-teaching it can help create a greater willingness on the part of students to engage in this same behaviour. Additionally, when a faculty team is dealing with a multi-racial group of learners it is helpful if the faculty group itself is also drawn from a range of racial backgrounds.

The faculty can then talk in front of the students about the contradictions, tensions and pleasures they experienced working as a teaching team, particularly how they negotiated the process of decision making. This helps enormously in readying students to deal with similar tensions in their own multi-racial teams.

EFFECTIVE TEAM PARTICIPATION

It is also helpful if faculty in management education programmes can prescribe indicators of effective team participation that include behaviours that are quieter, more reflective, even silent. For example, in my syllabuses I outline the indicators of effective participation by including specific behaviours such as: 'Ask a question or make a comment that encourages another person to elaborate on something they have already said'; 'Bring in a resource (a reading, Web link, video) not covered in the syllabus but that adds new information or perspectives to our learning'; 'Make a comment that underscores the link between two people's contributions and make this link explicit in your comment'; 'Use body language (in only a slightly exaggerated way) to show interest in what different speakers are saying'; 'Post a comment on the course chat room that summarizes our conversations so far and/or suggests new directions and questions to be explored in the future'; 'Contribute something that builds on, or springs from, what someone else has said and be explicit about the way you are building on the other person's thoughts'; 'When you think it is appropriate, ask the group for a moment's silence to slow the pace of conversation to give you and others time to think'.

MANAGING DYSFUNCTIONAL BEHAVIOURS

One particular issue that is always raised around team learning concerns dysfunctional behaviours, usually defined as one person unfairly dominating the activities of the group. I think we need to be wary of moving too quickly to label certain behaviour as dysfunctional. For example, a group member who insists on others paying attention to a viewpoint, perspective or intellectual tradition that the majority do not see as relevant, may (as I have already argued) be practising liberating tolerance as Marcuse defines it. The others may see this group member as behaving in a dysfunctional way because he or she is preventing the group from coming to a speedy decision on what to accomplish and how to accomplish it. Yet without such a member, groups may never challenge dominant ideology, never explore alternative political or racial perspectives. Stopping a premature rush to consensus may be just what the group will benefit from most in the long run. Clearly, though, there are times when egomaniacs or the extremely needy are taking up far too much of the available air time. What do we do then?

In addressing this problem I think we are helped if some obvious preparatory steps are followed. First, the team has to spend some time developing ground rules for itself. My preference, which I have outlined in *Discussion as a Way of Teaching* (Brookfield & Preskill 2005), is for teams to reflect on their previous experiences of good and bad team learning and to use these to develop commonly agreed ground rules for their activities. If the team has agreed on ground rules they will follow, then their repeated contravention by a particular member becomes a matter for the whole team and not a dispute between a few members of the team. Second, the faculty group should have spent some time modelling team participation in the manner already described. Third, any indicators of effective team participation that are specified in a syllabus can be as made behaviourally specific as possible, to reduce misunderstanding to a reasonable minimum. Of course, you can take all these preparatory steps and a truly disruptive individual can seem to agree to them but in reality be completely oblivious in his or her actual behaviour.

It can be helpful to institute a process through which team members anonymously provide data on how they feel the team is working. The team leader (or faculty member if we are talking about a formal university programme) then summarizes the data and reports back to the team. If opportunities are created for anonymously given data to be supplied by team members then they will immediately identify dysfunctional behaviour – such as a team member taking up 90% of the available air-time and forcing his or her agenda on others – on their anonymous commentary sheets. When feedback sheets on the team's functioning are received in which a majority of team members identify a particular person's behaviour as getting in the way of the team's working well together, two things are possible. First, it can be reported back to the whole team that comments were made about certain behaviours getting in the way of the team's functioning. The problem can be framed as a general problem that the team needs to address, and leaders can then suggest ways members can bring their ground rules to the attention of anyone seen to be flouting them.

Second, the individual identified as dysfunctional can be taken aside and given a summary of the comments made by other team members. Although this is never an easy conversation to have, the team members' comments serve as a body of unequivocal data that the dominating person must take seriously. When a person is presented with data showing that others in a team note his or her behaviour as stifling their own contributions, the talkative member finds it much harder to dismiss the problem or rationalize it away. This helps avoid the dynamic whereby the authority figure is perceived by the domineering team member as trying to control his or her challenge to the leader's power. Instead, the leader becomes the conduit of other people's concerns. Talkative students can deny that they are trying to cut others off, and can maintain that their frequency of speech is just a sign of their enthusiasm and commitment to the class. But they find it difficult to ignore the fact that their peers perceive their behaviour a certain way, no matter how unfair or erroneous they feel these perceptions might be.

When presenting domineering students with comments that refer unflatteringly to their actions, it is important that these students know the conversation is confidential. When I have these conversations I tell the student concerned that there will be no reference to the conversation in class, and that other students will not know their comments have been passed on. I do not want to shame the dominant student in front of his or her peers, nor do I want team members to think of weekly reflection sheets as a way to 'get' students they do not like. So the conversation remains private, a matter of me sharing privately with another student some information about how their peers perceive their behaviour.

This does not mean, of course, that it is easy for me, or the student concerned, to have this conversation. Students often feel that the teacher or other class members are trying to 'get' them. Students react with a complex mixture of anger, embarrassment and humiliation. Sometimes this resentment can be eased by my suggesting specific things the student can do to remedy the situation. I might ask that after making a contribution the student wait until at least three other people have spoken before speaking again, or silently to count to 15 before answering a question another team member has raised. This focus on future actions gives the student a project to work at and helps save some shreds of self-respect.

I can report that these conversations have often had dramatic and positive effects. Students who consistently interrupted other students to correct what they saw as lamentably erroneous comments have become more responsive group members who have struggled to monitor their contributions judiciously. Of course, this does not always happen. There are some students who remain more or less untouched by group ground rules, other students' complaints, data from peers and conversations with teachers. But the frequency of dysfunctional, egomaniacal behaviour has sometimes been reduced when I have followed the procedure I have just described.

CONCLUSION

Clinical appraisal allows us to stand outside situations and see what we do from wider perspectives. It helps us develop a well-grounded rationale for our actions that we call on to help us make difficult decisions in unpredictable situations. This rationale, a set of critically examined core assumptions about why we do what we do in the way that we do it, is a survival necessity. It gives us an organizing vision of what we are trying to accomplish in our practice.

References

Brookfield S D 1995 Becoming a critically reflective teacher. Jossey-Bass, San Francisco

Brookfield S D 2005 The power of critical theory: liberating adult learning and teaching. Jossey-Bass, San Francisco

Brookfield S D, Preskill S 2005 Discussion as a way of teaching: tools and techniques for democratic classrooms, 2nd edn. Jossey-Bass, San Francisco

De Vries M F R K 1993 Leaders, fools, and impostors: essays on the psychology of leadership. Jossey-Bass, San Francisco

Habermas J 1996 Between facts and norms: contributions to a discourse theory of democracy. MIT Press, Cambridge

Kubler-Ross E 1997 On death and dying. Scribner, New York

McMahon C M (ed) 2005 Critical thinking: unfinished business. Jossey-Bass, San Francisco

Marcuse H 1965 Repressive tolerance. In: Wolff R P, Moore B, Marcuse H (eds) A critique of pure tolerance. Beacon Press, Boston, p 81–123

Mezirow J 1991 Transformative dimensions of adult learning. Jossey-Bass, San Francisco

Chapter 7

Clinical reasoning and patient-centred care

Sue Atkins and Steven J. Ersser

Developing effective patient care requires making improvements to the way health professionals relate both to patients and to each other, in an effort to make better healthcare decisions. Clinical reasoning refers to the 'thinking and decision making processes which are integral to clinical practice' (Higgs & Jones, 1995, p. xiv). Fundamental questions may be asked about the part the patient should or can play in these processes and how this may be achieved. It is widely assumed that many patients want and benefit from an active role. Concepts of patient choice, autonomy, empowerment and partnership are being widely examined, advocated and challenged within consumer and professional literature as a means of enhancing patient-centred care (Coulter 2002, Edwards & Elwyn 2001, Mead & Bower 2000). Patient-centred decision making is being promoted by government policy initiatives such as the UK government's National Health Service (NHS) plan (Department of Health 2000) and 'expert patient' initiatives in the UK (Department of Health 2000, 2004). Evidence suggests that a level of participation in clinical reasoning appropriate for the individual contributes to the patient's sense of control. This may positively affect psychological well-being, physical recovery and satisfaction and lead to patients accepting greater responsibility for their health (Michie et al 2003).

It may appear self-evident that clinical decision making would always be formulated in the best interests of the patient. However, there are times when organizational or professional objectives can take precedence over effective decisions that take sufficient account of patients' interests, in terms of both objective clinical facts and patients' experiences and values. Professionals' varying levels of skill when relating to patients may also lead to insufficient account being taken of their concerns and preferences. This in turn can have adverse consequences, such as patient anxiety and dissatisfaction, or sub-optimal clinical outcomes.

This chapter reviews the significance of a patient-centred approach to clinical reasoning. Relevant concepts and theories are introduced to orient the reader to a range of different sociocultural, psychological, ethical and professional perspectives on patient-centred care. Practical strategies that contribute to patient-centred decision making are examined. Finally, a case is made for the promotion of clinical reasoning that is patient-centred to achieve more clinically effective, ethical and humane health care.

PATIENT–CENTRED CARE

Patient-centred care is a complex and difficult concept to define. However, there is an emerging consensus about its key features, particularly in the primary care and general practice literature (Fulford 1996, Mead & Bower 2000, Stewart et al 2003). In a review of the conceptual and empirical literature, Mead & Bower identified five dimensions of patient-centredness which distinguish it from the conventional biomedical model of practice:

- It is crucial to understand a patient's illness within a broader biopsychosocial framework that acknowledges the importance of health promotion.
- There is a concern with understanding the personal meaning of illness for patients, including patients' expectations, feelings and fears where relevant.
- A central feature of patient-centred care is the sharing of power and responsibility between patients and professionals, enabling patients actively to participate in clinical reasoning and to determine treatment and care plans as their condition and motivation allow.

- Patient-centred care also places more emphasis on the personal/professional, therapeutic relationship between health professional and patient, as described in the psychological literature (Rogers 1965).
- The influence of the health professional's personal qualities and subjectivity on the patient–professional relationship is recognized, as is the importance of self-awareness for both parties (Stewart et al 2003).

It has been argued that the health outcomes associated with greater patient involvement in decision making need to be evaluated (Entwistle et al 1998). However, we contend that patient-centredness is fundamentally about the process of care. When patients are enabled to participate in clinical reasoning, the views of professional and patient may be at variance and a decision taken may not necessarily lead to the best clinical outcome. An example would be a patient with cancer or severe chronic psoriasis who expresses reluctance to engage in cytotoxic therapy due to awareness of the risks of major side-effects with such treatment, despite the prospect of therapeutic gain.

RELEVANT CONCEPTS AND THEORIES

Theoretical perspectives drawn from sociology, psychology, ethics and professional literature can contribute to an understanding of the rationale for advocating more patient-centred decision making.

SOCIOCULTURAL PERSPECTIVES

Concepts of health and illness behaviour and professional and patient roles are fundamental to understanding the way in which social factors may shape the way professionals adopt a patient-centred approach to decision making. In particular, a number of different theoretical approaches have been used to analyse the role and function of power relations in doctor–patient relationships (Lupton 2003). These approaches acknowledge that a power differential and 'competence gap' exist between patients and professionals, which may influence or limit patients' involvement in clinical decision making.

Functionalist theory has classically portrayed the patient as a passive recipient of medical expertise. Parsons' (1951) concept of the *sick role* considers patients as exempt from normal social obligations and from accepting responsibility for the management of their illness. Patients are viewed as having a psychological need to leave decision making to the doctor, but with the requirement to cooperate with treatment. There is duty upon the doctor to take control and to be solely guided by the patient's welfare, applying the highest standards of professional competence and scientific knowledge. The sick role may be circumscribed by patients who are unable to fulfil the obligations and expectations that it entails; this applies to the chronically ill. However, it may still be the case that some patients, especially those with life-threatening conditions, prefer to hand over responsibility for managing their illness to professionals.

Political economy theory highlights how professions control knowledge and expertise to secure a position of power in society (Freidson 1970). Whether intentional or not, there is a risk of professionals withholding information from patients about their condition and treatment, thereby limiting patients' scope for participation in decision making. From this perspective, it is argued that the imbalance of power between professionals and patients leads to inequalities in health care, with people from poorer or ethnic minority backgrounds being disadvantaged. A more patient-centred approach therefore requires a review of the professional role and of the impact of professionalization on power use. Self-help and community-led healthcare initiatives are also advocated to improve power balance.

Contemporary approaches to examining social aspects of medical practice, for example social constructionism, have been influenced by the writings of the French philosopher Michel Foucault. Medical knowledge is regarded as a series of relative constructions that are dependent on the sociohistorical settings in which they occur (Lupton 2003). Power relations are viewed as subtle and dynamic. They are constantly negotiated and renegotiated between patient and professional in medical consultations, with patients sometimes taking more control. Medical dominance is considered potentially positive and at times necessary to fulfil patients' expectations and needs for health professionals to exercise medical expertise. Patients who choose to relinquish decision making to health professionals may be regarded positively as engaging in a practice they consider essential to their emotional and physical well-being.

Overall, these sociological perspectives acknowledge that some imbalance of knowledge and power between patients and professionals may be necessary to achieve patient-centred care, and that there are limits to the extent to which patients may participate in clinical reasoning.

HUMANISTIC AND SOCIAL PSYCHOLOGY

Patient-centred decision making requires an understanding of patient–professional relationships. Patient-centredness is influenced by the health professional's beliefs, values and attitudes toward patients in the planning and delivery of care. The whole orientation and comportment of practitioners, in terms of how they view and respond to patients, may have a fundamental bearing on the therapeutic consequences of their interactions (Ersser 1997). Skills are also required, such as the recognition of decisions to be made and the process of facilitating active patient involvement. A patient-centred approach encompasses beliefs about the rights of people and their potential to help themselves, with support. The relationship with the health professional provides the basis for that support. The psychology literature suggests that all therapeutic or helping relationships require qualities of self-awareness, authenticity and empathy (Egan 2002). These ideas have been influenced by humanistic psychology (Schneider et al 2001) and are directly reflected in professional–patient relationships and their effect on decision making.

ETHICAL THEORY

A process of ethical reasoning underpins the decision making of healthcare professionals. Ethical theory can provide a framework to inform and guide clinical reasoning. The bioethical principles of autonomy, beneficence, non-maleficence and justice are widely used in working through ethical problems and dilemmas and in justifying decisions made (Beauchamp & Childress 2001). Patient-centred decisions require professionals to achieve an appropriate balance between respecting the autonomy of 'competent' patients to make their own decisions and meeting the duty of benefi-cence. Beneficence is the primary obligation of all health professionals to 'do good' and act in patients' best interests. Traditionally, health pro-fessionals have been criticized for adopting a paternalistic approach, relying almost exclusively on their own professional knowledge and judge-ment about patients' needs, without due regard for patients' concerns and knowledge (Coulter 2002). Professionals facilitating patient involve-ment and evidence-based patient choice are required to give a higher priority to patient auton-omy. However, it is argued here that beneficence should be reconciled with, and not compete with, respect for patient autonomy. For example, Ashcroft et al (2001) suggested that there may be situations where the professional should challenge a patient's decision if it appears to conflict with the patient's own values. While respecting patients' autonomy and choices, professionals are also obliged to be fair to all patients and uphold the principle of justice when health resources are lim-ited. Despite the value of ethical theory in guiding decision making, clinical reasoning involves more than the application of principles and rules. When conflicts occur between *prima facie* obligations, it rests with the integrity of the professional to make a judgement in a particular situation.

PROFESSIONAL MODELS

Models of professional practice convey different views about the respective roles of professional and patient, the goals of specific types of health care, and the beliefs and values that should under-pin practice. They may also provide pointers to the desirability of patient involvement in clinical reasoning.

In their classic paper, Szasz and Hollender (1956) examined the way in which different models of the doctor–patient relationship related to the patient's degree of participation in care, along a continuum from the passive patient to active

participation. More recently, Charles et al (1999) discussed a shared-decision-making model, which they saw as the middle ground between the con-ventional 'paternalistic' model at one end of the continuum and an 'informed choice' model at the opposite end. Key features of shared decision making are that both professionals and patients share information, build consensus and reach an agreement about the treatment and care to be implemented. The model was developed in rela-tion to cancer care, where there may be several treatment options with different possible side-effects and uncertain outcomes. It emphasizes the importance of professional guidance and support in enabling patients to participate in difficult deci-sion making. In contrast, the informed choice model emphasizes information giving about risks and benefits as the key responsibility of the profes-sional, and that ultimately it is for the patient to take the decision (Charles et al 1999). An example of where this model is likely to be used is in family-planning clinics.

Stewart et al (2003), a group of health and social care professionals working in family medicine in Canada, developed a patient-centred clinical model as a central feature of clinical practice and education. The model identifies six essential and interacting components, encompassing the clinical reasoning process between professional and patient as well as emphasizing the context within which they interact. Steps include exploring both the disease and the illness experience, under-standing the whole person, and finding common ground in terms of problems and goals. Attention is also given to incorporating prevention and health promotion measures, enhancing the profes-sional–patient relationship and being realistic about time and resources. The strengths of this model include its comprehensiveness and rele-vance to different professional and patient con-texts, and its practical detail for teaching purposes.

FACTORS INFLUENCING PATIENT INVOLVEMENT IN CLINICAL REASONING

Clearly, a number of factors influence the extent to which patients are involved in clinical reasoning.

The attitudes and communication skills of health professionals and the extent to which patients are informed and knowledgeable about their illness are crucial factors. Additionally, there is the issue of patients' role preferences and how they are assessed. There is evidence that while the majority of patients want to be well informed about their treatment and care, this does not necessarily mean that they desire an active role in clinical decision making (Guadagnoli & Ward 1998).

PATIENTS' ROLE PREFERENCES

Surveys of patients' preferred roles in clinical decision making have been conducted across Western societies and in relation to a range of illnesses, including cancers and chronic diseases. A systematic review by Benbassat et al (1998) indicated a number of significant demographic patterns. Better educated, younger and female patients were more likely to prefer an active role. People from ethnic minority groups were more likely to prefer a passive role. The severity of the illness may also be an issue, with patients facing acute or life-threatening conditions being more likely to prefer a more passive role than patients with chronic illnesses. Nevertheless, demographic and situational factors explained only 20% of the variability and therefore cannot be used as predictors of an individual's role preferences. Also, some patients' role preferences may change during the course of their illness. Therefore it is apparent that the only way for health professionals to determine patients' role preferences is through direct inquiry.

Several tools have been developed to measure patients' role preferences in clinical consultations and in research studies. The Control Preferences Scale of Degner et al (1997) consists of five cards, each portraying a different role in treatment decision making, using a statement and cartoon. This has been used successfully in busy clinics. However, other authors recommend a more subtle approach. For example, Elwyn et al (2000) considered establishing and reviewing the patient's role preferences to be a fundamental skill of the medical consultation.

STRATEGIES FOR PROMOTING PATIENT–CENTRED CLINICAL REASONING

Specific strategies to promote patient-centred clinical reasoning are advocated in current professional literature. For example, Marshall et al (2005) reviewed a range of approaches to enhancing patient involvement and collaboration within the context of chronic illness, including coaching for patients and communication skills training for professionals. Muir Gray (2002), in his vision of the 'resourceful patient', advocated a range of skills that patients might develop, as well as human and technological resources to support greater patient control and responsibility. Some of these key strategies are now examined.

DEVELOPING PROFESSIONALS' COMMUNICATION SKILLS AND ENHANCING THE PATIENT–PROFESSIONAL RELATIONSHIP

It is clear that the way in which professionals relate to patients directly influences the degree of involvement of patients in decision making about their treatment and care. Increasingly it is expected that professionals will enter into a more complex negotiated relationship, with patients being assisted to take more responsibility and play an active part in clinical reasoning. A clinical illustration may be given from the care of patients with chronic skin conditions, where the professional–patient relationship needs to promote ongoing support, education and discussion, while being open to the fact that some patients will have built up considerable knowledge and experience regarding their condition and treatment. There is likely to be a need to explore patients' understanding of their health beliefs and preferences for treatment, such as their choice of topical treatments that have to fit with their lifestyle if adherence is to be maintained and therapeutic outcomes achieved. Openness and the building of trust will also assist involvement of patients when managing more complex treatment decisions that have serious consequences.

Contemporary models of professional practice emphasize the need to enhance professionals' communication skills to enable them to facilitate effective relationships with patients and engage in patient-centred clinical reasoning. The Cochrane Review by Lewin et al (2002) analysed trials of interventions for health care providers that promoted patient-centred clinical consultations, including training that focused on consultation styles, developing empathy, and identifying and handling emotional problems. It is evident that such training may improve communication with patients, enable clarification of patients' concerns in consultations and improve satisfaction with care, although no link with healthcare outcomes has been demonstrated. In a qualitative study of general practitioner consultations in the UK, Elwyn et al (2000) identified a set of generic competencies and steps for involving patients in decision making within consultations. There would appear to be great potential for this set of competencies to be tested and used as a framework for training health professionals in communication skills.

INFORMATION GIVING AND PATIENT EDUCATION

A key strategy for involving patients in clinical decision making is to provide suitable information about their situation, or provide support to access information sources. Equally important is the need to help patients to acquire the skills to appraise the information available to them (Entwistle 2000, Muir Gray 2002). This is a necessity in this era of wide internet access and sensationalized heathcare reporting and documentaries in the popular media. An important consequence of the informed choice and shared approaches in the current context of evidence-based health care is the need to help patients to understand the inherent uncertainties of clinical decision making where there is limited or unclear information available (Coulter 2002).

Patient education is widely recognized as one of the most effective strategies for empowering patients, especially for those with chronic illness who have to integrate their illness with their lifestyle and manage their own condition (Department of Health 2001, Miller 1992, Panja et al 2005). An important illustration is the help patients require (e.g. pre-discharge self-medication training; Lowe

et al 1995) to engage in effective management of medicines, given the widespread problems of poor treatment adherence and polypharmacy, which commonly leads to increased adverse drug reactions. Health professionals can also support patients indirectly by creating the conditions by which patients learn effectively from each other within social groups. Self-efficacy research suggests that people are more likely to engage in certain health-related behaviours when they believe they are capable of executing those behaviours successfully (Bandura 1997). A practical example of the use of such educational strategies to enhance self-efficacy includes the UK Department of Health (2001) 'Expert Patient' programme, in which patients with chronic conditions help each other to self-manage aspects of their condition effectively.

Effective patient teaching has significant resource implications. Support is needed for the development and dissemination of appropriate materials, the time taken for patients and professionals to discuss the various options and the cost implications of the preferences expressed (Entwistle et al 1997). More recently, there is recognition of the need for quality standards of information resources and the provision of out-of-hours information and advice services (Entwistle 2000). Indeed, in some countries such as the UK, a major policy development has been the establishment of NHS walk-in centres that are designed to meet such needs and to support appropriate patient involvement in self-management (Salisbury et al 2002).

PATIENT DECISION AIDS

Patient decision aids (PtDAs) provide evidence-based information, guidance and support in clarifying values for patients when there are specific and sometimes difficult choices to be made between treatment and health-screening options. Many PtDAs are based on the principles of decision analysis. They have been developed in a variety of different formats, including pamphlets, videos, 'decision boards' and interactive computer or internet packages (O'Connor et al 2003, Whelan et al 2000). A Cochrane systematic review of randomized controlled trials indicates that decision aids can improve patients' knowledge and understanding of the options, help them to consider the personal importance of possible benefits and harms, and participate more actively in the decision-making process (O'Connor et al 2003). However, the development of PtDAs is resource-intensive, and many PtDAs have not been evaluated. There is a need for further evaluative research in relation to professional–patient communication, cost-effectiveness and use in diverse sociocultural settings. O'Connor et al (2005) have also identified the need to set standards for the development and evaluation of PtDAs as more become available from commercial organizations and via the internet.

PATIENT ADVOCACY AND REPRESENTATION

Some health professionals, for example nurses, express aspirations to act as patient advocates (Nursing and Midwifery Council 2004). Porter (1988) argued that nurses' attempts to act as patient advocates are impractical because of their tendency to exercise social control as they professionalize. Indeed, there has been recognition by some that nurses may exacerbate the problem by making patients more passive in their involvement in health care (Fagin & Diers 1983). Current clinical examples continue to highlight the way in which the nature of professional interaction may disempower patients, as illustrated across a wide range of clinical settings (McKain et al 2005, Sainio et al 2001).

Examples can be seen in developments in health policy and infrastructure for patient advocacy and representation in countries such as the USA and more recently the UK. Significant developments have taken place in the USA in the patient advocate movement by employing patient representatives who do not belong to any specific healthcare profession. Ravich and Schmolka (1996) tracked the development of patient representation with reference to pioneering work undertaken at the Mount Sinai Hospital in New York. This strategy developed in response to concerns about the depersonalization of medical care, the variable provision of comprehensive information to patients and the increasing differentiation and technical specialization of health professionals. Patient representatives

play a key role in discussing issues of 'advance directives' with patients. For example, at St Vincent's Hospital in New York, patients are issued with a State booklet specifying their rights. A representative discusses with relevant patients advance directives on issues such as 'do not resuscitate' instructions, healthcare proxies and living wills (New York State 1998).

Although slower to develop, an infrastructure for patient advocacy has developed recently within the NHS in the UK through the establishment of a 'Patient Advice and Liaison Service' (PALS). PALS is part of the NHS modernization programme and arose as a response to the Bristol inquiry (Department of Health 2002) which recommended representation of patient interests at every level of the NHS. The service provides information, advice and support to patients, families and carers and promotes patient involvement in their local health service. The service also acts on behalf of service users when handling patient and family concerns with staff and managers. Another part of the infrastructure is the 'Commission for Patient and Public Involvement in Health' whose role is to ensure the public are involved in decision making about health and health services, largely through 'Patient and Public Involvement Forums' operating within each NHS Trust in England. Evaluations of the PAL service are underway, although it is too early to know the outcome.

TECHNOLOGICAL STRATEGIES

Technology can have a significant role in assisting patients to play a more active role in clinical decision making. Chronically ill patients can be helped to manage their condition through assisting them to monitor their health (e.g. diabetics accurately monitoring their blood glucose levels using a glucometer) and, where appropriate, act on the data obtained. Research evidence can be found in this area, as illustrated by Thomas's (1996) study of patient-controlled analgesia using analgesic pumps. Computer-assisted devices can enable those with disabilities to communicate their views as a basis for involvement in decision making (Thorton 1993). With the dramatic expansion of information through the internet there remains a significant challenge in helping patients and health professionals to use quality-assured information sources for accessing and evaluating health resources (Entwistle & O'Donnell 2001).

Strategic approaches are being taken in some health services, such as the UK NHS, to promote more effective self-management through the use of generic online decision support tools (NHS Direct on-line 2005). Such systems guide patients through algorithms to gauge the level of risk involved and the type of intervention that may be required, whether self-care or emergency services. Electronic tools are also available on this site to aid awareness of an individual's health status, such as assistance with calculating any risks associated with alcohol intake or body weight. Appraisal is needed of the use of these tools and which ones the public find most helpful.

CREATING A HUMANE PATIENT–CENTRED HEALTHCARE ENVIRONMENT

Hospital environments may be experienced by patients as dehumanizing, owing to the attitudes of staff, the ward organization, the presence of technology or the ward atmosphere (Ersser 1997). These factors may stifle patient involvement in decision making, or simply their willingness to express their needs. They can lead to patients experiencing uncertainty and anxiety and losing their ability to cope effectively.

The Planetree Alliance, a US non-profit organization seeking to develop models of health care that focus on healing and nurturing mind, body and spirit, remains a prominent exemplar of patient-centred environments (Frampton et al 2003). Horowitz (1996) illustrated the importance of creating a patient-centred hospital environment at the Beth Israel Medical Centre in New York, which aimed to create a more humanistic environment responsive to patients' emotional and educational needs. Efforts were made to create a less institutional interior in the ward. Attention was given to the aesthetic quality of the setting through use of lighting and art. Modifications were made to key features of the ward, such as the accessibility of the nursing desk for patients. These developments took place in an acute setting. The West Dorset Hospital NHS Trust was one of the first 'patient focus' hospitals to be designed in

the UK (Martin 1996). Prominent but low-cost initiatives to create a more therapeutic environment for patients within an old hospital setting were undertaken by nurses working at the Oxford Nursing Development Unit (Ersser 1988), although few examples are highlighted in more recent literature. However, investigations are taking place seeking patient perceptions of their healthcare environments and how patient-centred indicators may be used to appraise future designs (e.g. Douglas & Douglas 2005).

Attention also needs to be given to key organizational factors, such as the organization of care by nurses, and how this may favourably or adversely affect interaction between staff and patients. The established system of primary nursing employed in some settings is argued to have the potential to achieve a high level of continuity of care, thereby helping to create improved conditions for effective nurse–patient communication (Ersser & Tutton 1991). Its continuing relevance is highlighted in Koloroutis's (2004) recent examination of relationship-based care, which is seen as providing a model to transform practice in a more patient-centred direction. Some researchers have attempted to study the direct clinical impact of changing from task- to client-centred approach to organizing care for vulnerable groups. This is illustrated by Matthews et al (1996), who found such a change can significantly reduce agitation and improve sleep among nursing home residents with dementia.

Re-examination of entrenched practices is required in other aspects of care organization in hospitals such as ward rounds and case conferences. The limited evidence available indicates that patients may continue to feel intimidated and alienated from decision-making processes, even in areas such as acute mental health settings (Wagstaff & Solts 2003). The operation of constraining bureaucratic factors on patients and professionals is also revealed in a study of attempts to involve patients in their discharge planning (Efraimsson et al 2004). The prevailing culture and power structure in healthcare organizations is an important factor that may operate to stifle practical efforts to achieve a client-centred ethos. For instance, O'Cathain et al (2002) found that the culture within which leaflets were designed to improve informed choice in maternity care for women supported the existing normative patterns of care, which led to more informed compliance rather than choice.

LIMITATIONS AND BOUNDARIES OF PATIENT-CENTRED DECISION MAKING

The foregoing analysis emphasizes that patient-centred reasoning is largely dependent upon the attitudes, skills and knowledge of individual patients and professionals and upon the social and physical context within which they interact. There are limits to the extent that healthcare professionals can set aside their values and perspectives and achieve the level of empathy necessary to reach a full understanding of patients' perspectives. Health professionals must also develop the ability to recognize and acknowledge the influence of their own beliefs and values and their level of interpersonal skill on patient involvement; these areas of competence need to be addressed within educational curricula.

Facets of the organizational culture, such as the scope for continuity of care and the prominence of hierarchies, will influence the opportunities for patients and professionals to relate to each other and exchange information. Consideration is also needed of the extent to which organizational and professional practices are directly focused on patient needs and concerns, rather than simply on professional convenience and adherence to tradition. Furthermore, promoting patient-centred reasoning has resource implications. It is likely to be more time-consuming for professionals, and therefore investment is needed in effective training and in evaluation of the most effective patient consultation practices.

CONCLUSION

The development of patient-centred clinical reasoning is a complex issue. It requires an understanding of the range of factors that influence how individuals, professional groups and organizations create or block opportunities for patient involvement. Careful account needs to be taken of the range of factors that impinge on the readiness and ability of patients to benefit from any opportunity created. Patient-centred clinical reasoning is a broader concept than simply encouraging patients to participate in decision making. Wider perspectives are needed to understand the complexities of the issues, to develop a collective understanding and vision of what a patient-centred health service might be and to discover how different theoretical positions can provide explanations and pointers to effective action.

Among the strategies to help promote more active patient involvement in decision making, attention to the professional–patient relationship is of fundamental importance. It provides an anchor for the patient to take more responsibility for decision making, for the building of trust, and for discovery of the patient's and family's capacities. Such collaborative relationships can be cultivated only within an appropriate environment and an organizational system that values patient involvement and a different style of professional practice, and recognizes the alienating aspects of some healthcare structures for patients and their families.

Much emphasis has been given to the necessity for the process of care delivery to be patient-centred and the fact that such initiatives may not necessarily lead to effective clinical outcomes. It is clearly a research priority to ascertain any demonstrable benefits of patient involvement in clinical decision making, and the consultation processes that most effectively lead to such outcomes.

The key factors influencing a patient-centred approach to clinical reasoning have major implications for the education of health professionals. Health service development will take place only when health professionals have the necessary level of awareness and preparation to relate effectively to patients and to influence the organizational changes necessary to bring about change in practice. There remains considerable scope to reform health services and to radically shift care practices from an organizational and professional-centred stance to one that is patient-centred, characterized by widespread and planned patient involvement in clinical decision making.

References

Ashcroft R, Hope T, Parker M 2001 Ethical issues and evidence-based patient choice. In: Edwards A, Elwyn G (eds) Evidence-based patient choice: inevitable or impossible? Oxford University Press, Oxford, p 53–65

Bandura A 1997 Self-efficacy: the exercise of control. W H Freeman, New York

Beauchamp T, Childress J 2001 Principles of biomedical ethics, 5th edn. Oxford University Press, Oxford

Benbassat J, Pipel D, Tidhar M 1998 Patients' preferences for participation in clinical decision making: a review of published surveys. Behavioural Medicine 24(2):81–88

Charles C, Gafni A, Whelan T 1999 Decision-making in the physician-patient encounter: revisiting the shared treatment decision-making model. Social Science and Medicine 49:651–661

Coulter A 2002 The autonomous patient: ending paternalism in medical care. Nuffield Trust, London

Degner L F, Sloan J A, Venkatesh P 1997 The Control Preferences Scale. Canadian Journal of Nursing Research 29(3):31–43

Department of Health 2000 The NHS plan. HMSO, London

Department of Health 2001 The expert patient: a new approach to chronic disease management for the 21st century. HMSO, London

Department of Health 2002 Learning from Bristol: the report of the public inquiry into children's heart surgery at the Bristol Royal Infirmary 1984–1995. HMSO, London

Department of Health 2004 Improving chronic disease management. HMSO, London

Douglas C H, Douglas M R 2005 Patient-centred improvements in health care built environments: perspectives and design indicators. Health Expectations 8(3):264–276

Edwards A, Elwyn G (eds) 2001 Evidence-based patient choice: inevitable or impossible? Oxford University Press, Oxford

Efraimsson E, Sandman P, Hyden L-C et al 2004 Discharge planning: 'fooling ourselves?' – patient participation in conferences. Journal of Clinical Nursing 13:562–570

Egan G 2002 The skilled helper. Brooks/Cole, Australia

Elwyn G, Edwards A, Kinnersley P et al 2000 Shared decision making and the concept of equipoise: the competencies of involving patients in healthcare choices. British Journal of General Practice 50:892–897

Entwistle V A 2000 Supporting and resourcing treatment decision-making: some policy considerations. Health Expectations 3:77–85

Entwistle V, O'Donnell M 2001 Evidence-based health care: what roles for patients? In: Edwards A, Elwyn G (eds) Evidence-based patient choice. Oxford University Press, Oxford, p 34–49

Entwistle V A, Watt I, Sowden A 1997 Information to facilitate patient involvement in decision making: some issues. Journal of Clinical Effectiveness 2(3):69–72

Entwistle V A, Sowden A J, Watt I S 1998 Evaluating interventions to promote patient involvement in decision

making: by what criteria should effectiveness be judged? Journal of Health Service Research and Policy 3(2): 100–107

Ersser S J 1988 Nursing beds and nursing therapy. In: Pearson A (ed) Primary nursing: nursing in the Burford and Oxford Nursing Development Units. Chapman Hall, London, p 60–88

Ersser S J 1997 Nursing as a therapeutic activity: an ethnography. Avebury, Aldershot

Ersser S J, Tutton E (eds) 1991 Primary nursing in perspective. Scutari, London

Fagin C, Diers D 1983 Nursing as a metaphor. New England Journal of Medicine 309:116–117

Frampton S, Gilpin L, Carmel P (eds) 2003 Putting patients first: designing and practicing patient-centred care. Carmel AHA Press, Jossey Bass, San Francisco

Freidson E 1970 Profession of medicine: a study of the sociology of applied knowledge. Dodd, Mead, New York

Fulford K 1996 Concepts of disease and the meaning of patient-centred care. In: Fulford K, Ersser S, Hope T (eds) Essential practice in patient-centred care. Blackwell Science, Oxford, p 1–16

Guadagnoli E, Ward P 1998 Patient participation in decision-making. Social Science and Medicine 47(3):329–339

Higgs J, Jones M 1995 Introduction. In: Higgs J, Jones M (eds) Clinical reasoning in the health professions. Butterworth-Heinemann, Oxford, p xiii–xvi

Horowitz S F 1996 The Planetree model hospital project. In: Fulford K, Ersser S, Hope T (eds) Essential practice in patient-centred care. Blackwell Science, Oxford, p 155–161

Koloroutis M (ed) 2004 Relationship-based care: a model for transforming practice. Springer Publishing, New York

Lewin S, Skea Z, Entwistle V et al 2002 Interventions for providers to promote a patient-centred approach in clinical consultation (Cochrane Review). In: Cochrane Library issue 3, Oxford

Lowe C J, Raynor D K, Courtney E A et al 1995 Effects of self-medication programme on knowledge of drugs and compliance with treatment in elderly patients. British Medical Journal 310:1229–1231

Lupton D 2003 Medicine as culture: illness, disease and the body in western societies. 2nd edn. Sage, London

McKain S, Henderson A, Kuys S et al 2005 Exploration of patients' needs for information on arrival at geriatric and rehabilitation unit. Journal of Clinical Nursing 14(6): 704–710

Marshall S, Haywood K, Fitzpatrick R 2005 Patient involvement and collaboration in shared decision-making: a structured review to inform chronic disease management. Report from the Patient-assessed Health Instruments Group to the Department of Health

Martin T 1996 Commentary on chapter 10. In: Fulford K, Ersser S, Hope T (eds) Essential practice in patient-centred care. Blackwell Science, Oxford, p 162–165

Matthews E A, Farrell G A, Blackmore A M 1996 Effects of an environmental manipulation emphasizing client-centred care on agitation and sleep in dementia sufferers in a nursing home. Journal of Advanced Nursing 24(3): 439–447

Mead N, Bower P 2000 Patient-centredness: a conceptual framework and review of the empirical literature. Social Science and Medicine 51:1087–1110

Michie S, Miles J, Weinman J 2003 Patient-centredness in chronic illness: what is it and does it matter? Patient Education and Counselling 51:197–206

Miller J F 1992 Coping with chronic illness: overcoming powerlessness. F A Davis, Philadelphia

Muir Gray J A 2002 The resourceful patient. eRosetta Press, Oxford

New York State 1998 Your rights as a hospital patient in New York State. New York State

NHS Direct online 2005 Available: www.nhsdirect.nhs.uk 30 Oct 2005

Nursing and Midwifery Council (NMC) 2004 The NMC Code of Professional Conduct: standards for conduct, performance and ethics 07.04. NMC, London

O'Cathain A, Walters S J, Nicholl J P et al 2002 Use of evidence-based leaflets to promote informed choice in maternity care: randomised controlled trial in everyday practice. British Medical Journal 324:643–646

O'Connor A M, Stacey D, Entwistle V et al 2003 Decision aids for people facing health treatment or screening decisions. Cochrane Review. Update Software, Oxford

O'Connor A M, Graham I D, Visser A 2005 Implementing shared decision making in diverse health care systems: the role of patient decision aids. Patient Education and Counselling 57:247–249

Panja S, Starr B, Colleran K M 2005 Patient knowledge improves glycemic control: is it time to go back to the classroom? Journal of Medical Investigation 53(5): 264–266

Parsons T 1951 The social system. Free Press, New York

Porter S 1988 Siding with the system. Nursing Times 84(41): 30–31

Ravich R, Schmolka L 1996 Patient representation: a patient-centred approach to the provision of health services. In: Fulford K, Ersser S, Hope T (eds) Essential practice in patient-centred care. Blackwell Science, Oxford, p 64–84

Rogers C R 1965 The therapeutic relationship: recent theory and research. Australian Journal of Psychology 17:95–108

Sainio C, Lauri S, Eriksson E 2001 Cancer patients' views and experiences of participation in care and decision making. Nursing Ethics 8(2):97–113

Salisbury C, Chalder M, Scoot T M et al 2002 What is the role of walk-in centres in the NHS? British Medical Journal 324:399–402

Schneider K J, Bugental J F, Pierson F (eds) 2001 The handbook of humanistic psychology: leading edges in theory, research and practice. Sage, Thousand Oaks, CA

Stewart M, Brown J, Weston W et al 2003 Patient-centred medicine: transforming the clinical method, 2nd edn. Radcliffe Medical Press, Abingdon, Oxfordshire

Szasz T S, Hollender M H 1956 A contribution to the philosophy of medicine: the basic models of the doctor–patient relationship. Archives of Internal Medicine 97:585–592

Thomas V 1996 Patient controlled analgesia and the concept of patient-centred care. In: Fulford K, Ersser S, Hope T (eds) Essential practice in patient-centred care. Blackwell Science, Oxford, p 103–115

Thorton P 1993 Communications technology: empowerment or disempowerment? Disability, Handicap and Society 8(4):339–349

Wagstaff K, Solts B (2003) Inpatient experiences of ward rounds in acute psychiatric settings. Nursing Times 99(5):34–36

Whelan T, Gafni A, Charles C et al 2000 Lessons learned from the decision board: a unique and evolving decision aid. Health Expectations 3:69–76

Chapter 8

Factors influencing clinical decision making

Megan Smith, Joy Higgs and Elizabeth Ellis

CHAPTER CONTENTS

Research in clinical reasoning has focused strongly on the cognitive aspects of the processes involved. This chapter reports on research that examined the context of and factors influencing clinical decision making. Clinical decision making is both an outcome and a component of clinical reasoning. Given its pivotal place in the practice of health professionals, it is imperative to identify and understand factors that positively or negatively influence decision making. Of particular interest, when considering the quality of health care, are situations when factors influencing decision making contribute to errors or mistakes, with potential adverse outcomes for receivers of health care, or when factors influencing decision making can enhance healthcare experiences or outcomes.

CLINICAL DECISION MAKING

Decision making is a broad term that applies to the process of making a choice between options as to a course of action (Thomas et al 1991). Clinical decision making by health professionals is a more complex process, requiring more of individuals than making defined choices between limited options. Health professionals are required to make decisions with multiple foci (e.g. diagnosis, intervention, interaction and evaluation), in dynamic contexts, using a diverse knowledge base (including an increasing body of evidence-based literature), with multiple variables and individuals involved. In addition, clinical decisions are characterized by situations of uncertainty where not all the information needed to make them is, or can be, known. In this context of clinical decision making there are seldom single decisions made from fixed choices where one decision can be isolated from others. Rather, decisions are embedded in decision–action cycles where situations evolve and where decisions and actions influence each other. Orasanu & Connolly (1993) described the characteristics of decision making in dynamic settings (e.g. healthcare settings) in the following way:

- Problems are ill-structured and made ambiguous by the presence of incomplete dynamic information and multiple interacting goals.
- The decision-making environment is uncertain and may change while decisions are being made.
- Goals may be shifting, ill-defined or competing.
- Decision making occurs in the form of action–feedback loops, where actions result in effects and generate further information that decision makers have to react to and use in order to make further decisions.
- Decisions contain elements of time pressure, personal stress and highly significant outcomes for the participants.
- Multiple players act together with different roles.
- Organizational goals and norms influence decision making.

Clinical decision making has traditionally involved a process of individual healthcare practitioners making decisions on behalf of patients. Chapman (2004) termed this *surrogate decision making*. More recently, emphasis has been placed on clinical decision making as a collaborative process, involving shared and parallel decision making with patients and teams of health professionals (Edwards et al 2004, Patel et al 1996). The collaborative nature of decision making means that any consideration of factors influencing practitioners' clinical decision making could also consider factors influencing team decision making and patient decision making.

Given the multidimensional and complex nature of clinical decision making, factors influencing it may arise from multiple sources, resulting in differing effects for different individuals. In this chapter we describe factors influencing decisions in terms of three key areas: the attributes of and the nature of the task, features of the decision maker, and the context in which the decision takes place.

A RESEARCH PROJECT INVESTIGATING FACTORS INFLUENCING DECISION MAKING

Doctoral research (Smith 2006) was undertaken by Smith in collaboration with Higgs and Ellis to explore factors influencing clinical decision making by physiotherapists practising in acute care settings (hospitals). The emphasis of this research was on seeking an understanding of factors that influenced the decisions and actions of the physiotherapists as they made decisions in the real context of practice. A hermeneutic strategy was adopted, as the emphasis was to seek an understanding of decision making with the context of practice preserved. Physiotherapists from three experience categories (less experienced, intermediate and more experienced) were observed in their everyday practice and interviewed about their decision making with specific discussion of the factors that influenced it. Data analysis involved hermeneutic analysis of the texts constructed from these interviews and observations.

OVERVIEW OF FINDINGS: A MODEL OF FACTORS INFLUENCING CLINICAL DECISION MAKING

The findings of this research revealed that decision making about individual patient care is a complex and contextually dependent process (see Figure 8.1) in which:

- decision making consists of a core process (where decisions are made about patients' healthcare problems, appropriate therapeutic interventions, optimal modes of interaction and methods of evaluation) that is dependent upon attributes of the task such as difficulty, complexity and uncertainty
- decision making involves a dynamic, reciprocal process of engaging with situational factors

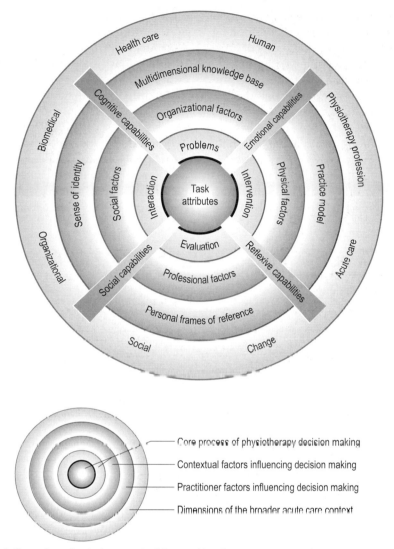

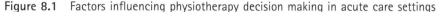

Figure 8.1   Factors influencing physiotherapy decision making in acute care settings

in the immediate context surrounding the decision to identify and use these factors in making decisions and carrying out an optimal course of action, and, at the same time, managing the influence of these factors on decision making to facilitate achievement of an optimal course of action

- practitioner factors (such as their frames of reference, individual capabilities and experience of physiotherapy decision making in the relevant work contexts) influence the decisions they make

- decision making is situated within a broader contextual ethos, with dimensions particular to the practice in the specific workplace
- traversing all of these factors, to manage and make sense of them requires four key capabilities: cognitive, emotional, social and reflexive.

TASK ATTRIBUTES

The task of decision making is to make action-related choices (including, if necessary, not acting). The research revealed that, in the decisions made by physiotherapists in acute care settings, a number of attributes influenced the decision-making process. Decisions can be defined in terms of attributes such as stability, certainty, familiarity, urgency, congruence, risk, and relevance and number of variables (Table 8.1) (Connolly et al 2000, Eraut 2004, Lewis 1997, May 1996, Whitney 2003). In each clinical practice situation decisions are characterized by a unique combination of these attributes.

Our research showed that individual decision attributes have poles of difficulty (e.g. stable versus unstable, familiar versus unfamiliar), with further difficulty and complexity arising from the summation and interplay between attributes (Smith 2006). Attributes that made a decision relatively simple were familiarity, certainty, limited variables, stability, congruence, and low risk. Decisions were more difficult if there was uncertainty, conflict, unfamiliarity, changing conditions, multiple relevant variables, and high risk. Difficult decisions had an ethical and emotional dimension that the participants found challenging. These findings are consistent with the wider body of decision-making research that has identified that individuals adopt different decision-making processes

Table 8.1   Definition of decision attributes

Attributes	Definition	Authors
Uniqueness	The extent to which the features of this decision are unlike other decisions. For example, uniqueness in making decisions about problems relates to the unique features of this patient and their condition in this specific setting	Schön (1988)
Certainty	The amount of information and clear guidelines that exist as to the interpretation of data and to guide a course of action	Lewis (1997), May (1996), Whitney (2003)
Importance/ criticalness/value conflict	The significance of the decision in relation to outcome and effects of negative consequences. Criticalness is used synonymously here to relate to the extent to which the outcome of the decision is of high importance with respect to outcome or where there is the high potential for a negative outcome	Schön (1988), Whitney (2003)
Stability	The extent and rate at which the environment surrounding the decision is changing or evolving. For example an unstable decision environment is where the patient's medical condition is changing at the time the decision is changing such that new data are being received and interpreted requiring a dynamic decision making process	Lewis (1997)
Urgency	The extent to which an immediate decision needs to be made or whether it can be delayed	Smith (2006)
Familiarity	The extent to which the decision being made is similar to decisions made in the past	May (1996)
Congruence/conflict	The extent to which elements of the decision such as the inputs, goals, and environment of the decision fit, match and correspond with each other	Lewis (1997)
Number of variables	The amount of data that need to be considered and interpreted in order to make a decision	Lewis (1997)
Relevance of variables	The extent to which the data available contain information relevant to the decision being made that needs to be sorted from irrelevant material	Lewis (1997)
Risk	The estimation of the chance of an adverse or negative outcome occurring as a result of the decision	Smith (2006)

according to decision attributes (Corcoran 1986, Eraut 2004, Fish & Coles 1998, Hamm 1988, Payne et al 1992). Such differences in decision making are expressed in the types of reasoning approach used in decision making and the speed of decision making. With less time, more rapid responses and less analytical approaches are adopted (Eraut 2004).

Cognitive continuum theory (CCT) is a theory of judgement and decision making that links modes of cognition to features of the task (Hamm 1988, Hammond 1996). Hamm (1988) linked the theory to medical decision making, using a continuum of cognition from intuition to analysis, with modes of cognition occurring in between that use a combination of both approaches. Tasks that induce (slower) analytical approaches are well structured, capable of being broken down into sections, and present with complete information. On the other hand, when tasks are poorly structured and are high in level of uncertainty there is little to analyse and therefore the best approach is one that draws on intuition to integrate material. We argue that professional judgement that is grounded in clinical experience is a preferred term to intuition (see Paterson & Higgs 2001).

These theoretical perspectives are reflected in other research undertaken in clinical settings, with features of decision making such as lack of familiarity and uncertainty slowing nurses' decision-making processes (Bucknall 2003). We also found that, when making decisions in acute care settings, participants responded to simple decisions by choosing a usual mode of practice, choosing an intervention that they found usually worked, and modifying their choice to fit the unique situation by adopting more creative and novel approaches to intervention. In contrast, when decisions were difficult, participants were more likely to experiment, draw upon the knowledge of other people, weigh up the competing aspects of the decision and follow protocols or rules, seeking less opportunity for creativity. Similarly, Corcoran (1986) found that nurses faced with complex tasks used opportunistic planning as opposed to a systematic approach. She noted that they adopted an approach consistent with an intuitive approach, where they pursued

'whatever seem[ed] opportune or promising at the time' (p. 107).

THE NATURE OF THE DECISION TASK

Decision making is influenced by how individuals conceptualize the decision to be made and the outcome they seek to achieve. An assumption in clinical practice is that individuals make decisions with the aim of making the best choice, this being to choose the right diagnosis, or to optimize patient outcomes if the decision is choosing an intervention. This assumption may be a generalization, with healthcare professionals potentially framing the desired outcomes of their decision making in alternative ways. Different factors will be considered to be important, depending on a decision maker's mental representation of the situation (Soman 2004). Schön (1988, p. 66) used the notion of *problem setting* to describe the 'process in which, interactively, we *name* the things to which we will attend and *frame* the context in which we will attend to them'. Framing affects the size of what can be seen, and affects the perspective and what is seen to be the problem. We identified that physiotherapists practising in acute care settings made intervention choices that were directed at improving patient outcome; however, they also aimed to be safe and to ensure that workloads were completed, and wanted their decisions to be justifiable and serving to assure their emotional comfort. The framing of desired outcomes in these different ways has important implications for decision making. Whereas one individual might see the goal of decision making as achieving a desired outcome and is prepared to take a risk to do so, another might see the preferred goal as safety and be much less likely to take a risk.

Tversky & Kahneman (1981, p. 453) used the term *decision frame* to refer to 'the decision-maker's conception of the acts, outcomes, and contingencies associated with a particular choice'. They proposed that the 'frame a decision-maker adopts is controlled partly by the formulation of the problem and partly by the norms, habits, and personal characteristics of the decision maker'. Given this perspective, clinical decision making will be affected by the norms and habits which decision makers have acquired through their experience of clinical practice.

ATTRIBUTES OF DECISION MAKERS

The physiotherapists in our study had a number of frames of reference that guided their decision making. These were:

- a multi-dimensional professional knowledge base
- a conceptual framework for acute care physiotherapy practice
- individual practice models
- personal frames of reference that included their values, beliefs and attitudes.

Decision-making research in the field of psychology has established that attributes of individuals influence decision making, with particular reference to decision-making biases. We found that attributes of decision makers, such as their capabilities, confidence, self-efficacy, emotions, frames of reference, and degree of expertise, also influenced their decision making. Decision makers have been found to make a number of systematic deviations from normative models of decision making. These deviations are referred to as biases in decision making (Keren & Teigen 2004). Some examples of reasoning biases include misinterpreting findings as confirming a hypothesis when they indicate that an alternate finding should be considered (Elstein & Schwarz 2000), overemphasizing the likelihood of rare conditions (Dowie & Elstein 1988), and making different decisions for individuals than for groups of people, even though they have the same condition (Chapman 2004).

We found that physiotherapists in acute care settings had a number of personal qualities or capabilities in decision making that enabled them to make effective decisions in relation to the task, and also in consideration of the context of practice. Bandura (1986) defined capabilities as the cognitive means by which individuals can influence and control their behaviour. He noted that: 'given the same environmental conditions, persons who have the capabilities for exercising many options and are adept at regulating their own behaviour will have greater freedom than will those who have limited means of personal agency' (Bandura 1986, p. 39).

The capabilities of the physiotherapists in our study are shown in Box 8.1. We categorized these as cognitive, metacognitive/reflexive, social and emotional capabilities. The social and emotional capabilities are drawn from the notion of social and emotional intelligence that has been described in the literature (Stephenson 1998). Social and emotional intelligence is concerned with understanding and relating to people (McQueen 2004), and includes self-awareness, self-regulation, self-motivation, social awareness and social skills (Freshman & Rubino 2002). Metacognitive/reflexive capability refers to the self-reflective capability to critically evaluate one's own experience of decision making with a view to informing future practice with similar conditions.

In defining the notion of capabilities, Bandura (1986, p. 391) also used the notion of self-efficacy, that is, 'people's judgements of their capabilities to organize and execute courses of action required to attain designated types of performances'. Self-efficacy has parallels with the notion of confidence in decision making. Our study revealed that in clinical decision making by acute care physiotherapists, self-efficacy and confidence in decision making were important determinants of the decisions that were made. Physiotherapists' feelings and levels of self-efficacy resulted from: (a) evaluating their level of knowledge, particularly in comparison to the knowledge levels of other health professionals with whom they were working; (b) having experienced success and failure; and (c) knowing the likely responses to interventions and the likelihood of adverse events occurring. When self-efficacy was higher there was a greater willingness to take risks and greater confidence in decision making, as opposed to relying on others or deferring decision making. Consistent with previous research (Ewing & Smith 2001) we noted that self-efficacy was linked with experience, with more experience being associated with higher levels of self-efficacy.

Decision makers' emotions and feelings of confidence and controllability influenced our participants' decision making as they sought to control negative outcomes and emotions, particularly under conditions of risk and uncertainty. Feeling confident in decision making can be linked to

Box 8.1 Decision-making capabilities of physiotherapists in acute care settings

Cognitive capabilities

- Capability to identify and collect relevant information (task and contextual) and process these data in order to make decisions in the focal areas of problems, intervention, interaction and evaluation
- Capability to form relevant mental representations of decision-making situations
- Capability to predict the consequences of decisions
- Capability to process and interpret a multitude of decision inputs (task and contextual) to make ethical and justified decisions
- Capability to make pragmatic decisions in the face of uncertainty and/or under-resourcing
- Capability to adapt practice decisions to new and changing circumstances

Metacognitive/reflexive capabilities

- Awareness of the process of decision making and factors that influence one's decision making
- Capability to monitor and evaluate decision making throughout the process of making decisions
- Capability to self-critique experience of and effectiveness of decision making and use this critique in the development of knowledge structures to inform future decision making

Emotional capabilities

- Awareness of emotions and when they are impacting on decision making, particularly awareness of self-efficacy
- Capability to deal with problematic emotions in order to make difficult decisions required for patient management
- Motivation to learn and improve quality of decision making in the face of potentially conflicting emotions that impact on decision making
- Capability to identify and deal with patients' and care-givers' emotions that are impacting on CRP management
- Capability to establish and maintain effective relationships in the workplace with patients, care-givers and work colleagues by managing the emotions of others

Social capabilities

- Capability to interact effectively with others in the decision-making context
- Capability to critically learn from others
- Capability to manage relationships where differentials in power exist and to achieve effective decision making autonomy
- Capability to involve others meaningfully and appropriately in collaborative decision making (including team members and at times patients and carers)

experiencing positive emotions, in contrast to experiencing fear and anxiety in decision making. Individuals have been found to make decisions based on a desire to minimize the experience of negative emotions and maximize the ease of justification of a decision (Payne & Bettman 2004). Decision making may be affected using a process of rule-following which involves the application of rules to situations in an effort to 'find efficient, adaptive, satisfying decisions' (Mellers et al 1998, p. 469). Payne & Bettman (2004) suggested that decision makers can be motivated to solve a problem as well as possible in order to avoid negative emotions, or alternatively to change the amount

of thought involved by avoiding making a decision, letting others make the decision, maintaining the status quo, choosing another option that is easy to justify to others, and avoiding specific aspects of the decision that they find distressing.

A final important attribute that influences decision making is the decision maker's level of expertise, with experts considered superior decision makers making decisions that are faster and more accurate. A distinction is typically made between the extremes of novice and expert. In reality, individual practitioners are more appropriately viewed as being in varying degrees of transition between more and less experienced and expert. As such, they will demonstrate characteristics consistent with their own variable pathways towards expertise, dependent upon their unique experiences.

The more experienced physiotherapists in our study adopted an approach to decision making that was more specific, creative and refined towards the individual needs of patients and the unique contextual dimensions. They used more interpretation and critique in their decision making, being increasingly more confident and self-reliant. They handled uncertainty in decision making more effectively by adopting a practical certainty, being better able to engage in wise risk-taking and possessing a greater knowledge base that decreased the relative uncertainty of decision making. Their knowledge base was broader than that of the novices and contained a higher level of experience-based knowledge. Their knowledge base was personalized, multidimensional, and included a better awareness of the limits of their knowledge with respect to what could be known. More experienced physiotherapists also had more advanced cognitive capabilities for decision making, being more flexible, adaptive and capable of predicting outcomes, as well as having higher levels of emotional capability, being able to separate emotion from task, having a higher awareness of patients' experiences of illness, and knowing how to use their own personality and its effects in their decision making.

The frames of reference of more experienced practitioners are different from those of novices. Experts represent and frame decision-making situations differently from novices, seeing situations more broadly (Corcoran 1986, Phillips et al 2004). Expert decision makers critically apply norms and criteria of decision making. Where novices choose simply to follow rules, experts understand the bases for the rules and thus apply them more wisely (Benner 1984). The more experienced physiotherapists in our study had more developed personal theories of practice consisting of their own set of criteria for practice as opposed to using rules and guidelines for practice derived from their university-based teaching or work-based protocols. Whereas less experienced practitioners framed decision making as needing to make the right decision, more experienced

practitioners sought optimal decisions given the circumstances.

More experienced practitioners were also more capable of managing the context, being more aware of the influences and better able to pragmatically interact with and manipulate contextual factors to achieve optimal decision outcomes. The knowledge base of experts has been found to extend beyond direct patient care, to include knowledge of their work context in terms of the physical environment and organizational structures (Ebright et al 2004).

ATTRIBUTES OF THE EXTERNAL CONTEXT

A key focus of our research was to explore the influence of the external context of practice on decision making. Our research showed that our participants' decision making could not be separated from the context in which it occurred. The physiotherapists accounted for context in their decision making by changing or modifying decisions that they would have otherwise made in response to contextual factors, but also developing strategies to manage and control the context of their practice. This is consistent with other findings such as those of Ebright et al (2003, p. 631), who noted that 'to prevent things from going wrong, practitioners anticipate, react, accommodate, adapt, and cope to manage complexity in the midst of a changing environment.'

We found that the interaction between context and decision making was reciprocal, complex and dynamic. The influence of specific contextual factors upon decision making was dependent upon the unique features of the decision being undertaken at the time. Context was not a fixed entity but was found to be dynamic and variable. A key finding of our research was that contextual factors influencing practitioners' decision making could not be consistently ranked according to their prevalence or importance. Rather, different contextual factors assumed different importance according to the unique circumstances at a given time.

To understand the interaction between context and decision making, Bandura (1986) offered a theory explaining human behaviour in which context (or the environment) acts in a dynamic reciprocal way with the cognition and personal attributes of individual decision makers. He suggested that 'human functioning is explained in terms of a model of triadic reciprocality in which behaviour, cognitive, and other personal factors, and environmental events all operate as interacting determinants of each other' (p. 18).

Bandura (1986) proposed that the effect of behaviour on the environment, and the environment on behaviour, is not always equal. He offered examples where asymmetries exist, such as 'disparities in social power, competencies, and self-regulatory skills' (p. 29), in which environmental influences may take a more dominant role. He argued (p. 39):

> Judgements regarding environmental factors enter into the choice of particular courses of action from among possible alternatives. Choices are not completely and involuntarily determined by environmental events. Rather making choices is aided by reflective cognitive activity, through which self-influence is largely exercised. People exert some influence over what they do by the alternatives they consider, how they foresee and weight the consequences, and how they appraise their capabilities to execute the possibilities they are entertaining.

The broader context of clinical decision making can be seen to consist of different types of factors that become relevant to particular decisions; these include social, professional, organizational, and physical and environmental dimensions. The literature contains a number of examples that illustrate how decisions are influenced by these contextual factors. The social context in particular has been shown to have a large influence on clinical decision making (Chapparo 1997, Denig et al 1993, Greenwood et al 2000). We found that practitioners referred aspects of their decision making to others in the context, particularly when a decision was difficult to make, used chatting with others to check their decision making, used others to generate novel perspectives, and anchored their decision making to decisions others had made in the past. Larrick (2004) indicated that the effects of the social context on decision making can be both positive and negative. Positive influences include using other individuals to check for errors, utilizing positive synergies arising from the combination of team members' knowledge, and recognizing that there is an increased likelihood of generating novel solutions and diverse perspectives when more people are consulted in decision making. Conversely, the social context can have negative effects when individuals choose to do what others do to avoid social rejection or to take advantage of others' decision making rather than being responsible for their own decision making. When 'under conditions of uncertainty, people are susceptible to anchoring on the judgements of others in forming their own judgements' (Larrick 2004, p. 326), and when all members of a group share similar training or dominant workplace norms, people can be inhibited from offering or adopting different perspectives.

Social influences on decision making have also been described in multidisciplinary settings, such as intensive care units. Patel et al (1996) reported that where multiple players were involved in decision making, the process and outcomes were influenced by the urgency of the situation and the hierarchy and social structure of the organization. Similarly, Varcoe et al (2003), investigating moral judgements and decision making by nurses, found that decisions and actions were highly relational and contextual, with decisions of the individual being related to the decisions of others in the organization. Bucknall (2003) found that hierarchical systems existed that provided decision making support for less experienced staff, who passed information and provisional decisions on to more experienced staff until someone made a decision. Beyond direct influences, Ebright et al (2004, p. 531) also noted that nurses 'learn and refine their clinical and caring knowledge from socially determined aspects of their work environment, including the expertise of co-workers, social climate and team functioning, and shared experiences'. Consistent with the literature, we found that social factors directly modified and changed decisions for novices, whereas more experienced practitioners adapted to, controlled and manipulated these factors (Ebright et al 2003, Smith 2006).

In addition to social influences on decision making, we found that organizational systems such as workloads, interruptions, and organizational policies and procedures also influenced decision making. Organizational system factors such as amount and distribution of workload influenced decision making by affecting the time available to make decisions and provide intervention. The acute care physiotherapists responded to high workloads by adapting and incorporating a sense of their workload and their capacity to manage it into their decision making. Where workload resulted in limited time availability, compromises were made in the decisions that could be made. Participants reported prioritizing some patients over others, prioritizing which problems would be addressed, reducing the numbers of times they would see a patient and discharging patients more readily. They also reported effects such as less thinking time, less effective interventions, streamlining assessment, choosing less creative options for treatment, less time for offering patients choice in decision making, and choosing interventions that would be adequate rather than optimal. Bucknall (2003) found that experienced nurses working with more inexperienced staff projected ahead to identify potential increases in their workload and the availability of medical staff. Organizational factors such as time have also been found to influence decision making by affecting the capacity of decision makers to develop rapport with patients. The capacity to get to know patients and their condition was recognized as an important component of decision making by the physiotherapists in our study, consistent with findings in studies of nurses and radiographers (Brown 2004, Jenks 1993).

Hedberg & Sätterlund Larsson (2004) found that the continuity of nurses' decision making was disrupted by organizational matters such as interruptions from others asking questions or asking for assistance, phone calls, and others wanting to exchange information. These authors suggested that such interruptions add to the complexity of the decision-making process, increasing the demands on cognitive capacity to recall information and make decisions. They suggested that interruptions to interactions can positively influence nurse decision making by providing them with additional information, but can also disrupt the flow of ideas causing them to forget as they try to manage different threads of decision making.

Other aspects of organizations that affected the participants' decision making were the systems in place to guide decision making, such as clinical pathways, policies, protocols, and also system definitions of acceptable practice that were represented in the norms, criteria and standards to which individuals working in a centre should adhere (Smith 2006).

Finally the physical environment influenced decision making by affecting the resources available. The participants had to reason and make decisions about the location and supply of equipment, room layout, and which piece of equipment they would use, considering the constraints of the resources they had available. Ebright et al (2003) found that nursing staff needed to develop specific knowledge of the geography of the unit and location of resources. With increased experience of working in the same context nurses developed familiarity with equipment that improved their efficiency and decision making.

CONCLUSION

Quality decision making is an essential component of good clinical practice. If we are to understand, critique and improve clinical decision making, it is imperative that, in addition to understanding the elements of the immediate clinical problem, we make explicit the contextual factors that are taken into account when making decisions. When seeking to improve decision-making, a broad perspective needs to be adopted that considers factors such as the individual's decision-making attributes and the influence of the external context on decision making.

Evidence-based practice is consistently advocated as a means for improving the quality of clinical practice. A broader perspective of factors influencing decision making illustrates how evidence-based practice needs to be integrated with many other influences on practice. Consideration of social and organizational dimensions of context is critical in optimizing the quality of clinical decision making. If we are to promote effective decision making, we need to understand how we can best teach decision making that considers and manages the multiplicity of factors that influence it, rather than focusing only on the immediate clinical decision-making tasks of diagnosis and intervention.

Acknowledgements

The doctoral research project described in this chapter investigating factors influencing decision making was undertaken by Megan Smith. Joy Higgs and Elizabeth Ellis were supervisors and co-researchers in the project.

References

Bandura A 1986 Social foundations of thought and action: a social cognitive theory. Prentice Hall, Englewood Cliffs, NJ

Benner P 1984 From novice to expert: excellence and power in clinical nursing practice. Addison-Wesley, Menlo Park, CA

Brown A 2004 Professionals under pressure: contextual influences on learning and development of radiographers in England. Learning in Health and Social Care 3 (4):213–222

Bucknall T 2003 The clinical landscape of critical care: nurses' decision making. Journal of Advanced Nursing 43 (3):310–319

Chapman G B 2004 The psychology of medical decision making. In: Koehler D J, Harvey N (eds) Blackwell handbook of judgment and decision making. Blackwell Publishing, Malden, MA, p 585–604

Chapparo C 1997 Influences on clinical reasoning in occupational therapy. Unpublished doctoral thesis, Macquarie University, Sydney

Connolly T, Arkes H, Hammond K 2000 Judgement and decision making: an interdisciplinary reader, 2nd edn. Cambridge University Press, Cambridge

Corcoran S A 1986 Task complexity and nursing expertise as factors in decision making. Nursing Research 35 (2):107–112

Denig P, Haauer-Ruskamp F M, Wesseling H et al 1993 Towards understanding treatment preferences of hospital physicians. Social Science Medicine 36 (7):915–924

Dowie J, Elstein A (eds) 1988 Professional judgment: a reader in clinical decision making. Cambridge University Press, Cambridge

Ebright P R, Patterson E S, Chalko B A et al 2003 Understanding the complexity of registered nurse work in acute care settings. Journal of Nursing Administration 33(12):630–638

Ebright P R, Urden L, Patterson E et al 2004 Themes surrounding novice nurse near-miss and adverse-event situations. Journal of Nursing Administration 34 (11):531–538

Edwards I, Jones M, Higgs J et al G 2004 What is collaborative reasoning? Advances in Physiotherapy 6:70–83

Elstein A S, Schwartz A 2000 Clinical reasoning in medicine. In: Higgs J, Jones M (eds) Clinical reasoning in the health professions, 2nd edn. Butterworth-Heinemann, Oxford, p 95–106

Eraut M 2004 Informal learning in the workplace. Studies in Continuing Education 26(2):247–273

Ewing R, Smith D 2001 Doing, knowing, being and becoming: the nature of professional practice. In: Higgs J, Titchen A (eds) Professional practice in health, education, and the creative arts. Blackwell Science, Oxford, p 16–28

Fish D, Coles C (eds) 1998 Developing professional judgement in health care: learning through the critical appreciation of practice. Butterworth-Heinemann, Oxford

Freshman B, Rubino L 2002 Emotional intelligence: a core competency for health care administrators. Health Care Manager 20(4):1–9

Greenwood J, Sullivan J, Spence K et al 2000 Nursing scripts and the organizational influences on critical thinking: report of a study of neonatal nurses' clinical reasoning. Journal of Allied Health 31(5):1106–1114

Hamm R M 1988 Clinical intuition and clinical analysis: expertise and the cognitive continuum. In: Dowie J, Elstein A S (eds) Professional judgement: a reader in clinical decision making. Cambridge University Press, Cambridge, p 78–105

Hammond K R 1996 Human judgement and social policy: irreducible uncertainty, inevitable error. Oxford University Press, New York

Hedberg B, Sätterlund Larsson U 2004 Environmental elements affecting the decision-making process in nursing practice. Journal of Clinical Nursing 13:316–324

Jenks J 1993 The pattern of personal knowing in nurse clinical decision making. Journal of Nursing Education 32 (9):399–405

Keren G, Teigen K H 2004 Yet another look at the heuristics and biases approach. In: Koehler D J, Harvey N (eds) Blackwell handbook of judgment and decision making. Blackwell Publishing, Malden, MA, p 89–109

Larrick R P 2004 Debiasing. In: Koehler D J, Harvey N (eds) Blackwell handbook of judgment and decision making. Blackwell Publishing, Malden, MA, p 316–337

Lewis M L 1997 Decision making task complexity: model development and initial testing. Journal of Nursing Education 36(3):114–120

McQueen A 2004 Emotional intelligence in nursing work. Journal of Advanced Nursing 47(1):101–108

May B 1996 On decision making. Physical Therapy 76(11): 1232–1240

Mellers B A, Schwartz A, Cooke A D J 1998 Judgment and decision making. Annual Review of Psychology 49:447–477

Orasanu J, Connolly T 1993 The reinvention of decision making. In: Klein G A, Orasanu J, Calderwood R et al (eds) Decision making in action: models and methods. Ablex, Norwood, NJ, p 3–20

Patel V L, Kaufman D R, Magder S A 1996 The acquisition of medical expertise in complex dynamic environments. In: Ericsson K A (ed) The road to excellence: the acquisition of expert performance in the arts and sciences, sports, and games. Lawrence Erlbaum, Hillsdale, NJ, p 127–165

Paterson M, Higgs J 2001 Professional practice judgement artistry. CPEA Occasional Paper 3. Centre for Professional Education Advancement, University of Sydney, Australia

Payne J W, Bettman J R 2004 Walking with the scarecrow: the information-processing approach to decision research. In: Koehler D J, Harvey N (eds) Blackwell handbook of judgment and decision making. Blackwell Publishing, Malden, MA, p 110–132

Payne J W, Bettman J R, Johnson E J 1992 Behavioural decision research: a constructive processing perspective. Annual Reviews in Psychology 43:87–131

Phillips J K, Klein G, Sieck W R 2004 Expertise in judgment and decision making: a case for training intuitive decision skills. In: Koehler D J, Harvey N (eds) Blackwell handbook of judgment and decision making. Blackwell Publishing, Malden, MA, p 297–315

Schön D A 1988 From technical rationality to reflection-in-action. In: Downie J, Elstein A (eds) Professional judgement: a reader in clinical decision making. Cambridge University Press, Cambridge, p 60–77

Smith M C L 2006 Clinical decision making in acute care cardiopulmonary physiotherapy. Unpublished doctoral thesis, University of Sydney, Sydney

Soman D 2004 Framing, loss aversion, and mental accounting. In: Koehler D J, Harvey N (eds) Blackwell handbook of judgment and decision making. Blackwell Publishing, Malden, MA, p 379–398

Stephenson J 1998 The concept of capability and its importance in higher education. In: Stephenson J, Yorke M (eds) Capability and quality in higher education. Kogan Page, London, p 1–13

Thomas S A, Wearing A J, Bennett M J 1991 Clinical decision making for nurses and health professionals. W B Saunders/Ballière Tindall, Sydney

Tversky A, Kahneman D 1981 The framing of decisions and the psychology of choice. Science 211(4481):453–458

Varcoe C, Rodney P, McCormick J 2003 Health care relationships in context: an analysis of three ethnographies. Qualitative Health Research 13(7):957–973

Whitney S N 2003 A new model of medical decisions: exploring the limits of shared decision making. Medical Decision Making 23:275–280

Chapter **9**

Dimensions of clinical reasoning capability

Nicole Christensen, Mark A. Jones, Joy Higgs and Ian Edwards

In the context of our complex healthcare environment, most clinical situations are characterized by varying levels of certainty and agreement as to the appropriate or 'right' decision to be made and course of action to be undertaken. This uncertain and at times unpredictable practice environment presents many clinical reasoning challenges, even for experienced clinicians. When we consider the array and magnitude of potential challenges this same practice context poses for less experienced or new clinicians, the need is clear for a focus on the development of capability in clinical reasoning during professional entry educational programmes.

This chapter draws from findings of a doctoral research project undertaken by Christensen, in collaboration with Jones, Edwards and Higgs, which explored how the development of capability in clinical reasoning can be facilitated in the context of professional entry physical therapist education (Christensen 2007). This research employed a hermeneutic approach to the interpretation of texts constructed from previously published literature and transcribed records of interaction with research participants. The research involved focus group and individual interviews with student physical therapists who were nearing the completion of their respective professional education programmes at four different physical therapy schools in California. Here, we introduce and discuss the concept of clinical reasoning capability, one of the main outcomes of this research. Ways in which students can be guided towards development of that capability during the professional entry education process are discussed in Chapter 36.

CAPABILITY

In our explorations we adopted the term *capability* from the higher education literature. Capability was defined by John Stephenson (1992, 1998) as the justified confidence and ability to interact effectively with other people and tasks in unknown contexts of the future as well as known contexts of today. Stephenson (1998, p. 2) explained that 'to be "justified", such confidence needs to be based on real experience'. Specifically, capability is observed in confident, effective decision making and associated actions in practice; confidence in the development of a rationale for decisions made; confidence in working effectively with others; and confidence in the ability to navigate unfamiliar circumstances and learn from the experience (Stephenson 1998).

In their phenomenological study of professional doctoral students in a work-based learning programme, Doncaster & Lester (2002) sought to understand what is involved in being and becoming capable. They concluded that capability may best be conceptualized as 'an "envelope" or complex bundle of abilities and attributes which is personal to individual practitioners, and which is exercised in equally personal ways in relevant contexts' (p. 98). Participants' descriptions of 'being capable' included both 'outer' and 'inner' dimensions. The outer dimension of capability was linked with action; capable action involved initiating or managing change, especially in difficult or complex contexts. Closely related to this was the ability to work effectively with others to effect change through collaboration and consensus. The inner dimensions of capability varied considerably among participants, but Doncaster & Lester identified several commonly recognized qualities and skills that contributed to effectiveness. Specific examples were the ability to get things done, leadership ability and ability to inspire others into action in support of ideas and goals. All of these abilities required skills in communication, listening, facilitation, tact, persuasion and the ability to work with others. Other key elements of capability included intellectual or thinking abilities, such as critical thinking, reflection, synthesis, creativity, evaluation and intuition. Closely related to these were breadth and depth of understanding in action, involving the ability to see the big picture, understand the wider context and wider implications (of policies or actions) and engage in systems thinking.

Capability, then, cannot be precisely defined and therefore cannot be tied to a list of profession-specific technical skills and abilities, characteristic of 'capable practice'. Rather, high-level capability results when practitioners have opportunities and resources for professional growth, encounter events or circumstances that spur them to action in this regard and are motivated to succeed or change in their practice (Doncaster & Lester 2002). In other words, capable individuals are skilled experiential learners. Capable individuals are motivated to develop their knowledge intentionally, through application and processing of their knowledge via reflective learning from practice.

CLINICAL REASONING CAPABILITY

Clinical reasoning is a process that links and integrates all elements of practice (such as philosophy of practice, generation and use of practice knowledge, profession-specific technical skills, communication and collaboration, ethics and identity). Within clinical reasoning, these integrated elements are brought to life and developed. Capability in clinical reasoning involves integration and effective application of thinking and learning skills to make sense of, learn collaboratively from and generate knowledge within familiar and unfamiliar clinical experiences.

Our recent research has identified that key elements of capability are directly applicable and recognizable in the clinical reasoning of skilled and experienced physiotherapists, and that capability in clinical practice is best observed through the clinical reasoning of skilled clinicians (Christensen 2007). Descriptions of characteristics of the clinical reasoning and practice of expert physiotherapists (Edwards et al 2004, Jensen et al 1999) show deep similarities to descriptions of performance of capable individuals: for example confidence and effectiveness in decision making, in providing contextual justification for actions and decisions, in motivating self and others, in communicating and collaborating with others to effect change and in critical, reflective thinking.

There are also similarities between capability and the Aristotelian notions of practical knowledge and reasoning, and obvious links to descriptions of the application and generation of practice knowledge in the clinical reasoning of skilled practitioners (Higgs et al 2004). Practical reasoning involves the application of both theoretical knowledge and, most significantly, experiential knowledge. A key feature of practical reasoning is that this experiential knowledge is both applied to and arises from practical activity, and is open to revision or expansion by processing new experiences in light of past experiences (Gadamer 1989). Practical reasoning is highly contextualized in that it is applied to concrete situations and results in particular actions relevant to the specific situation(s).

Another key feature of practical reasoning is that it is inherently ethical in nature. This is because it requires subsequent decisions for action, decisions that are determined by close consideration of the broader moral and ethical issues at play in the context of a particular situation (Dunne 1993). This action is oriented towards 'doing the right thing' based on taking all situational variables and constraints into account (Gadamer 1989, Schwandt 2001). Recently authors have described the practice of expert physiotherapists as profoundly influenced by their context, ethics, values and virtues (Edwards et al 2005, Jensen & Paschal 2000). Likewise, capability is observed when we see people 'taking effective and appropriate action within unfamiliar and changing circumstances', which 'involves ethics, judgements, the self-confidence to take risks and a commitment to learn from the experience' (Stephenson 1998, p. 3).

The clinical reasoning process is the 'navigation system' upon which skilled clinicians can confidently rely for direction in decision making and action, in both familiar and unfamiliar clinical situations. 'Justified confidence' in thinking, learning and associated actions is the hallmark of capability and is developed through successful experience in living out, or putting into action, what one knows (Stephenson 1998). Capability is characterized by the confidence to take risks, to try new things in practice and to make mistakes.

Clinical reasoning provides a firm foundation for practice, not only for making decisions in uncertain situations and trialling new procedures but also for prompting reflection and learning from practice experiences both familiar and innovative.

LINKING CLINICAL REASONING CAPABILITY AND EXPERIENTIAL LEARNING

Clinical reasoning is the vehicle for experiential learning from practice; it is well accepted that the process of thinking about one's own thinking and the factors that limit it facilitates learning from clinical practice experience (Eraut 1994, Higgs & Jones 2000, Schön 1987). Thus, clinical reasoning serves to develop as well as to demonstrate practice capability.

Experiential learning is a goal of capable action and results from translating knowledge and reason into action in the context of living and working with others (Stephenson 1998). A key element in any individual embodiment of capability is the motivation and skill to learn through experiences in any (known or unknown) situation. Christensen (2007) found that capability in clinical reasoning was observed in clinicians who were confident in their skills and motivated to continually learn from collaborative work with patients in practice. We propose that clinical reasoning capability develops from, and contributes to, skill in collaborative clinical reasoning and experiential learning from reasoning experiences. Capable practitioners have been described in the literature as skilled and motivated experiential learners (Doncaster & Lester 2002, Stephenson 1998). Capable clinical reasoners, then, are skilled and motivated to learn from experience through intentional reflective processing of their reasoning in practice (Christensen 2007).

INVESTIGATING THE THINKING AND LEARNING SKILLS INHERENT IN CLINICAL REASONING CAPABILITY

The research reported in this chapter (Christensen 2007) showed that capable clinical reasoners demonstrated sound thinking *and* learning skills. Dimensions of clinical reasoning capability, as discussed below, can be interpreted as being congruent with the descriptions of clinical reasoning of expert physiotherapists in recent research-based literature (Edwards et al 2004, Jensen et al 1999). These dimensions were often underdeveloped, disconnected, or absent in the conceptions of and reflections on clinical reasoning of the student physical therapist research participants studied by Christensen. The limited connection between these thinking and learning skills in the understandings of, and reflections on, clinical reasoning of most of the student physical therapists participating in the study served to highlight the lack of adequate attention to the learning of clinical reasoning in their professional educational journeys and clearly indicated the importance of developing the clinical reasoning skills of capable practitioners.

Given that capability has been described as a complex and multifaceted construct, not amenable to descriptions of specific technical skills or qualities, we suggest that the dimensions of clinical reasoning capability discussed here are not a comprehensive set of dimensions. Nor can they completely comprise the capable individual clinical reasoner's 'envelope' or bundle of abilities and qualities. They have been chosen for their pivotal role in the reasoning of skilled practitioners and for the type of thinking in clinical reasoning that facilitates experiential learning. Learning from clinical practice requires thinking and learning skills to be integrated and applied to both the *doing* of the clinical reasoning (for example dialectical thinking, complexity thinking) and the *processing* of the experience of clinical reasoning (for example reflective thinking, critical thinking, complexity thinking). The four dimensions of clinical reasoning capability described here are *reflective thinking, critical thinking, dialectical thinking*, and *complexity thinking*.

Reflective thinking

The process of reflection relates to clinical reasoning of a practitioner, both when engaged with a patient over a period of time, considering and evaluating performance in past experience, and also in an immediate sense, reflecting in the moment while working with a patient. Schön (1987) described

two types of reflection in practice that illustrate this distinction as *reflection-on-action* and *reflection-in-action*.

Reflection-on-action refers to thinking back on experiences 'to discover how our knowing-in-action may have contributed to an unexpected outcome' (Schön 1987, p. 26). In this sense, reflection becomes a way of cognitively organizing experience through construction of a sense of coherence, and facilitating planning for future action (Forneris 2004).

Reflection-in-action, as described by Schön (1987, p. 26), is reflection that occurs in the midst of action, without interruption of the action upon which the practitioner is reflecting. He described this type of reflection as thinking that modifies what is being done while it is being done, and which can thus impact on the situation at hand while it is still being experienced. Some scholars, however, have expressed concern about identifying as reflection this phenomenon that is characterized by the rapidity and relative superficiality with which someone can truly reflect on a situation while engaged in action (Eraut 1994, Van Manen 1995). Eraut (p. 149) suggested that this sort of reflection is more accurately viewed as a metacognitive activity than a reflective one. On the one hand this disagreement is about terminology; on the other it relates to the nature of reflection and metacognition as phenomena. In this chapter we propose that a heightened level of awareness involving critique of one's thinking and other actions (which we have previously called 'metacognition'; see Higgs & Jones 2000) is an essential element of sound clinical reasoning. This behaviour broadens the 'bigger picture' focus of experiential learning engendered by (after the event) reflection-on-action to also include the potential to learn from the smaller decisions and critiques within practice. Such reflective self-awareness (metacognition) facilitates concurrent learning within the details and patterns of response to individual decisions, actions and procedures in practice.

It is important to differentiate the process of reflection, as discussed above, from the process of critical reflection. The following section details critical thinking and describes the role of reflection in critical thinking in practice.

Critical thinking

Critical thinking in professional practice is intimately linked to the process of reflection. However, 'reflection is not, by definition, critical' (Brookfield 2000, p. 126). Scriven & Paul (2004, p. 1) defined critical thinking as 'the intellectually disciplined process of actively and skilfully conceptualising, applying, analysing, synthesising and/or evaluating information gathered from, or generated by, observation, experience, reflection, reasoning or communication, as a guide to belief and action'. It is a skill that can be applied when developing an understanding of a particular situation or context, and also can be applied to the examination of thinking (one's own or that of others) in the context of particular situations.

Forneris (2004, p. 1) argued that, 'the outcome of thinking critically in practice is the achievement of a *coherence of understanding*. This can be defined as an awareness of assumptions, and how these assumptions connect to the reasoning used within the context of a situation to create new knowledge and generate an appropriate new action'. With grounding in an extensive comparative analysis of the work of the educational theorists Freire, Schön, Argyris, Mezirow, Brookfield and Tennyson, Forneris (2004) identified four core attributes of critical thinking: reflection, context, dialogue and time. When applied to clinical reasoning, these four attributes of critical thinking are a useful framework within which to conceptualize all the different elements of practice and the factors influencing collaborative clinical reasoning that are linked to critical thinking.

Reflection attaches meaning to information, and 'illuminates the *why* and the *reason for* what we do and how we critically discriminate what is relevant' (Forneris 2004, p. 4). As Mezirow (2000) explained, reflection allows for interpretation of experience; as part of reflection the thinker comes to know the 'why' of a situation by subjectively and objectively reframing the context to bring to light the underlying assumptions used to justify beliefs. New knowledge may then be produced if a new perspective on experience is achieved. 'Reflection, as an attribute, is a means of engaging critical thinking processes in practice' (Forneris 2004, p. 5).

Context refers to the 'nature of the world in a given moment' (Forneris 2004, p. 8). Through experience of living amongst the realities of a situation, understanding of that situation is achieved. Critical thinking in practice implies achievement of understanding in the context of that moment in practice. 'Context encompasses culture, values, facts, ideals, and assumptions. All of these shape how we construct knowledge in practice' (p. 9).

Dialogue is an 'interactive process of evaluating perspectives and assumptions within context, in order to develop an understanding' (Forneris 2004, p. 10). Brookfield (2000) contended that a critical dialogue requires an ongoing, evolving exploration of how the context of a situation influences the way that situation is understood. This interaction in critical conversation 'involves participation in constructive discourse to use the experience of others to assess reasons justifying these assumptions, and making an action decision based on the resulting insight' (Mezirow 2000, pp. 7–8). Critical conversation can occur with oneself, with patients/clients, peers, and mentors; any of these potential partners in constructive discourse related to any of the many facets of clinical reasoning in practice can serve to provide the clinician with an opportunity to self-examine more clearly from another perspective, and can facilitate experiential learning.

Time as an attribute of critical thinking connotes that past learning may be recalled in the present context and may also inform future action. Time also influences understanding, in that time taken to reflect on experience is necessary to the development and understanding of patterns and meaning (Forneris 2004). This is a key element that must be considered when working toward the facilitation of experiential learning through clinical reasoning.

Extending the idea and role of critical thinking to focus on thinking about thinking, Paul & Elder (2006, p. 4) defined critical thinking as 'the art of analyzing and evaluating thinking with a view to improving it'. In effect, critical thinking about thinking promotes learning from and about thinking. Skilled critical thinkers, when applying their critical thinking to any situation, have been characterized as employing self-direction, self-monitoring and self-correction in the development of their thinking (Scriven & Paul 2004). In action, critical thinking is characterized by a consistent commitment to raise well-formulated and clear questions; to gather and assess relevant information; to think open-mindedly within alternative systems of thought; to recognize and assess assumptions, implications and the associated practical consequences; to communicate effectively with others in engaging with and finding solutions to complex problems (Paul & Elder 2006).

There are clear links between the above description of critical thinking as applied to one's own thinking and the process of metacognition. *Metacognition* has been described as the integrative link between knowledge and cognition in the clinical reasoning process (Higgs et al 2004), and as the self-monitoring employed by the therapist in order to detect links or inconsistencies between the current situation and expectations based on learning from past clinical experience (Higgs & Jones 2000). Metacognition may involve reflecting on and critiquing data collection processes and results, considering different strategies of reasoning and reviewing personal biases or limitations in knowledge depth, breadth or organization.

Examining the writings of certain theorists about critical thinking, Forneris (2004) perceived that the meaning implied by their use of the word *critical* was overtly political (Argyris 1992, Brookfield 2000, Freire 1970). For example, Brookfield (2000, p. 126) explained that the word involves 'some sort of power analysis of the situation or context in which the learning is happening'. Critical thinkers and learners must 'try to identify assumptions they hold dear that are actually destroying their sense of well-being and serving the interests of others: that is, hegemonic assumptions' (p. 126). This focus then promotes social action towards change when 'people learn to recognize how uncritically accepted and unjust dominant ideologies are embedded in everyday situations and practices' (p. 128). This interpretation of critical thinking relates directly to the role of critical thinking in recent discussions of the emancipatory nature of collaborative clinical reasoning (Trede et al 2003) and is relevant to improving one's thinking and to fostering recognition of habits of thought and unfounded beliefs in the thinking of others.

Dialectical thinking

The clinical reasoning of expert physiotherapists has been described as dialectical reasoning (Edwards & Jones 2007). In the context of their model, *dialectic* refers to movement between two fundamentally different (and potentially opposing) ways of thinking. Through this dialectic process of engagement in various reasoning strategies (some aligned with empirico-analytical thinking and others aligned with interpretive thinking, for example), physiotherapists collaborate with their patients to achieve a holistic understanding of both the biomedical aspects and the lived experience aspects of the patients' worlds (Edwards & Jones 2007, Edwards et al 2004). A number of scholars (e.g. Basseches 1984, Kramer & Melchior 1990, Riegel 1973) have discussed the development of dialectical thinking in adults as an advanced skill level, or stage of cognitive development, which allows adults to cope with the inherent contradictions and complexity of life (Merriam & Caffarella 1999).

Basseches (1984) situated dialectical thinking as a middle course between what he described as universalistic formal thinking and relativistic thinking. Universalistic formal thinking assumes that there are fixed universal truths and a universal order to things (a perspective that can be aligned with an empirico-analytical research paradigm). Relativistic thinking assumes there is no one universal order to things, and that 'order in the universe is entirely relative to the people doing the ordering' (p. 10) (a perspective that can be broadly aligned with the interpretive research paradigm). Dialectical thinking moves along a continuum between the poles of universalistic formal thinking and relativistic thinking, drawing upon each as needed to promote appropriate interpretation of the many different facets of a particular phenomenon or situation, and to facilitate development of understanding in complex circumstances.

There are strong arguments for this sort of thinking, considering the perspective that a clinician is a complex human being, working with other complex human beings within a complex environment – the 'swampy lowland', where 'messy, confusing problems defy technical solution' (Schön 1987, p. 3). Dialectical thinking 'considers both the deductive and inductive aspects of a situation in terms of an open system subject to feedback and change' (Pesut 2004, p. 157). Dialectical thinking has also been discussed as an integral component of thinking within a complexity perspective.

Complexity thinking

Current literature and models of clinical reasoning (e.g. Higgs & Jones 2000, Pesut 2004) have characterized the thinking involved in the clinical reasoning process as non-linear, and not truly represented by the stepwise single-dimensional process found in early models of diagnostic reasoning in medicine. Current conceptions of clinical reasoning portray a type of thinking in practice where practitioners are 'required to weave multiple threads together into a fabric of care' (Pesut 2004, p. 152).

Increasingly, authors have advocated the adoption of the metaphors contained within complexity science as a way to understand and cope with the escalating complexity in health care (e.g. Plsek 2001, Sweeney & Griffiths 2002, Zimmerman et al 2001). It is argued that 'we must abandon linear models, accept unpredictability, respect (and utilize) autonomy and creativity, and respond flexibly to emerging patterns and opportunities' (Plsek & Greenhalgh 2001, p. 323). Suggestions (explicit or implicit) for the application of the concepts of complexity theory to ways of thinking in practice have also begun to appear in recent nursing and allied health literature (Forneris 2004; Pesut 2004; Stephenson 2002, 2004). These metaphors, derived from complexity science, include the foundational concept of complex adaptive systems. 'A complex adaptive system is a collection of individual agents with freedom to act in ways that are not always totally predictable, and whose actions change the context for other agents' (Plsek & Greenhalgh 2001, p. 625). Examples of complex adaptive systems encountered in the practice of health care include the human behaviour of patients, the whole of the healthcare system, the immune system, the patient and his or her family, the musculoskeletal system and healthcare teams within healthcare centres.

Description of the systems involved in health care (social, political, professional, human) as complex adaptive systems is contrasted with the more historical, traditional medical view of systems as

mechanical in nature (for example the body as a machine metaphor, derived from Newtonian scientific principles) (Plsek 2001, Sweeny & Kernick 2002, Zimmerman et al 2001). Mechanical systems are characterized by linearity and predictability, and as such it is possible to know and predict in great detail what each of the parts will do in response to a given stimulus in a variety of circumstances, as they rarely if ever demonstrate surprising or emergent behaviour (Plsek 2001).

Proponents of the adoption of a complexity view of health care argue that, in today's world, there are growing numbers of situations in which the traditional medical paradigm, and even early interpretations of the biopsychosocial model, are insufficient to frame and explain situations and provide guidance for action (Borrell-Carrió et al 2004, Holt 2002, Plsek 2001, Zimmerman et al 2001). In his discussion of the limitations to our understanding that arise as a result of the continued dominance of an inadequate traditional scientific model, Holt described linear thinking as 'a sort of "mischief" which creeps into much of the way we conceptualize the world' (p. 36).

We contend that current models of expert physiotherapist practice and of the clinical reasoning of expert physiotherapists (Edwards & Jones 2007, Edwards et al 2004, Jensen et al 1999), when viewed within a complexity perspective, also demonstrate characteristics of complex adaptive systems. Arguments for the inclusion of 'systems thinking' as a key skill in clinical reasoning have been presented by several authors (Pesut 2004, Stephenson 2004). Contemporary systems thinking, as described by these authors, reflects the complexity perspective and implies recognition of the dynamic relationships between the many elements and players in a given situation. This thinking incorporates induction (forward reasoning, reasoning from specific cues toward a general judgement), deduction (reasoning from a general premise toward a specific conclusion), and dialectical thinking (Pesut 2004, Stephenson 2004).

Richard Stephenson (2004) also discussed the thinking required for individualized consideration of the weighting of all relevant factors acting within the person acting as a system as essential to the reasoning process. In discussing clinical reasoning in the context of a complexity view of human behaviour, Stephenson (2004) described the need for consideration of each agent or component within the system (for example motor skills, thoughts and beliefs, communication, emotional arousal responses) as variable in degree of influence on and from the behaviour of the system as a whole. The degree to which a particular agent influences or 'drives' the behaviour of a system depends on both the internal (within the person) and external (the context within which the person is functioning) conditions acting in the system at the time (Stephenson 2002). Stephenson (2004) referred to this degree of influence of a particular component or agent within a system as its 'weight', explaining that due to the ability of complex adaptive systems to self-organize through feedback, this weighting of agents results from past history of activity which either positively or negatively impacts upon the system, and thus increases or decreases the amount of influence an individual agent holds over the system at present.

Stephenson (2004, p. 171) portrayed clinical reasoning (including the dialectical thinking processes involved) as a 'tool through which the potential weight of each influence can be explored, requiring knowledge of all potential influences'. He stressed that as a whole system, no one component or agent acting in the human system has assumed priority or dominant influence on emerging behaviour. In addition, when considering which influences are driving the system in particularly adaptive or non-adaptive ways, different health professions cannot consider specific components in isolation from the whole of the system of influences (for example physical health as distinct from environmental and psychosocial influences on disability). Thus it can be argued that complexity thinking is required for the sort of holistic clinical reasoning required to make wise decisions in such complex situations involving complex human beings.

IMPLICATIONS OF VIEWING CLINICAL REASONING AS CAPABILITY IN A COMPLEX ENVIRONMENT

The argument has been put forth in recent medical literature that education of new practitioners for capability, as opposed to competence, is essential when preparing new professionals to practise in today's complex healthcare environment (Fraser & Greenhalgh 2001, Rees & Richards 2004). Capability extends beyond the notion of competence to include the capacity of individuals to realize their potential in unknown future circumstances; this is related to the ability to adapt to change, generate new knowledge, manage one's own continual professional development and contribute to shaping the future (Fraser & Greenhalgh 2001, Stephenson 1998).

For allied health professions this focus on capability meets the call for education that focuses on preparation for practice in the complex healthcare environment of today and tomorrow. In particular, professional education curricula need to focus on the development of generic thinking and learning skills (in addition to technical, profession-specific content). Development of thinking, learning, and clinical reasoning skills are critical when considering that new healthcare practitioners must not only be qualified to practise as individuals, but also need to be able to work in teams and be ready to contribute to the development of the profession (Higgs et al 1999, Jensen & Paschal 2000).

We suggest that development of students' thinking and learning skills that contribute to capability in clinical reasoning should be a priority, not just for academic and clinical educators but for all practitioners. There is widespread agreement that expertise evolves over time as clinical practice experience is accumulated. However, it is also well recognized that any number of years of experience will not automatically result in expert clinical performance. It can be argued, then, that experts are clinicians who are more successful than non-experts in learning from their practice (Cervero 1992, Higgs et al 2004). We have proposed that skilled practitioners must be capable clinical reasoners. Facilitating the development of capability in clinical reasoning in professional education programmes is one step towards facilitating movement of all clinicians towards more expert practice, and thereby facilitating the generation of high quality practice knowledge for development of the profession itself.

Stephenson (1998) argued that the outcome of any higher education process should be judged by the extent to which it: (a) graduates students who are confident and able to take responsibility for their continued personal and professional development; (b) prepares students to interact effectively within their life and work contexts; and (c) promotes and motivates students to continue to pursue excellence in the generation and use of knowledge and skills in practice. Capability implies both fitness for purpose (working and adapting to change within an existing system) and fitness of purpose (envisioning and working for change to the system itself) (Doncaster & Lester 2002). Similarly, capability in clinical reasoning implies a motivation to learn from and improve personal practice – effective work within a system – but also a motivation to learn about and work to change for better professional practice itself – effective work on a system.

References

Argyris C 1992 Reasoning, learning and action: individual and organizational. Jossey-Bass, San Francisco

Basseches M 1984 Dialectical thinking and adult development. Ablex Publishing Corporation, Norwood, NJ

Borrell-Carrió F, Suchman A L, Epstein R M 2004 The biopsychosocial model 25 years later: principles, practice, and scientific inquiry. Annals of Family Medicine 2(6): 576–582

Brookfield S D 2000 Transformative learning as ideology critique. In: Mezirow J (ed) Learning as transformation: critical perspectives on a theory in progress. Jossey-Bass, San Francisco, p 125–148

Cervero R 1992 Professional practice, learning, and continuing education: an integrated perspective. International Journal of Lifelong Education 10:91–101

Christensen N 2007 Development of clinical reasoning capability in student physical therapists. Unpublished PhD thesis, University of South Australia

Doncaster K, Lester S 2002 Capability and its development: experiences from a work-based doctorate. Studies in Higher Education 27(1):91–101

Dunne J 1993 Back to the rough ground: 'phronesis' and 'techne' in modern philosophy and in Aristotle. University of Notre Dame Press, London

Edwards I, Jones M 2007 Clinical reasoning and expertise. In: Jensen G M, Gwyer J, Hack L M, Shepard K F (eds) Expertise in physical therapy practice, 2nd edn. Elsevier, Boston, p 192–213

Edwards I, Jones M, Carr J et al 2004 Clinical reasoning strategies in physical therapy. Physical Therapy 84(4): 312–335

Edwards I, Braunack-Mayer A, Jones M 2005 Ethical reasoning as a clinical-reasoning strategy in physiotherapy. Physiotherapy 91:229–236

Epstein R M, Hundert E M 2002 Defining and assessing professional competence. JAMA 287(2):226–235

Eraut M 1994 Developing professional knowledge and competence. Falmer Press, London

Forneris S G 2004 Exploring the attributes of critical thinking: a conceptual basis. International Journal of Nursing Scholarship 1(1) Article 9. Online. Available:http://www.bepress.com/ijnes/vol1/iss1/art9 28 December 2006

Fraser S W, Greenhalgh T 2001 Complexity science: coping with complexity: educating for capability. British Medical Journal 323:799–803

Freire P 1970 Pedagogy of the oppressed, 30th anniversary edn. Continuum International Publishing Group, New York

Gadamer H-G 1989 Truth and method, 2nd revised edn. Continuum, New York

Higgs J, Jones M, Refshauge K 1999 Helping students learn clinical reasoning skills. In: Higgs J, Edwards H (eds) Educating beginning practitioners: challenges for health professional education. Butterworth-Heinemann, Oxford, p 197–203

Higgs J, Jones M 2000 Clinical reasoning in the health professions. In: Higgs J, Jones M (eds) Clinical reasoning in the health professions, 2nd edn. Butterworth Heinemann, Oxford, p 3–14

Higgs J, Jones M, Edwards I et al 2004 Clinical reasoning and practice knowledge. In: Higgs J, Richardson B, Abrandt Dahlgren M (eds) Developing practice knowledge for health professionals. Butterworth-Heinemann, Edinburgh, p 181–199

Holt T 2002 Clinical knowledge, chaos and complexity. In: Sweeney K, Griffiths F (eds) Complexity and healthcare: an introduction. Radcliffe Medical Press, Oxford, p 35–57

Jensen G M, Paschal K A 2000 Habits of mind: student transition toward virtuous practice. Journal of Physical Therapy Education 14(3):42–47

Jensen G M, Gwyer J, Hack L M et al 1999 Expertise in physical therapy practice. Butterworth-Heinemann, Boston

Kramer D, Melchior J 1990 Gender, role conflict, and the development of relativistic and dialectical thinking. Sex Roles 23(9):553–575

Merriam S B, Caffarella R S 1999 Learning in adulthood: a comprehensive guide, 2nd edn. Jossey-Bass, San Francisco

Mezirow J 2000 Learning to think like an adult: core concepts of transformation theory. In: Mezirow J (ed) Learning as transformation: critical perspectives on a theory in progress. Jossey-Bass, San Francisco, p 3–33

Paul R, Elder L 2006 The miniature guide to critical thinking: concepts and tools, 4th edn. Foundation for Critical Thinking, Dillon Beach, CA

Pesut D J 2004 Reflective clinical reasoning. In: Haynes L C, Butcher H K, Boese T A (eds) Nursing in contemporary society: issues, trends, and transition to practice. Pearson Prentice Hall, Upper Saddle River, NJ, p 146–162

Plsek P E 2001 Redesigning health care with insights from the science of complex adaptive systems. In: Institute of Medicine Committee on Quality of Healthcare in America (ed) Crossing the quality chasm: a new health system for the 21st century. National Academies Press, Washington, DC, p 309–322, Appendix B

Plsek P E, Greenhalgh T 2001 Complexity science: the challenge of complexity in health care. British Medical Journal 323:625–628

Rees C, Richards L 2004 Outcomes-based education versus coping with complexity: should we be educating for capability? Letter to the editor, Medical Education 38:1203–1205

Riegel K 1973 Dialectic operations: the final period of cognitive development. Human Development 16346–370

Schön D 1987 Educating the reflective practitioner: toward a new design for teaching and learning in the professions. Jossey-Bass, San Francisco

Schwandt T A 2001 Dictionary of qualitative inquiry, 2nd edn. Sage Publications, Thousand Oaks, CA

Scriven M, Paul R 2004 Defining critical thinking. Foundation for Critical Thinking. Online. Available: http://www.criticalthinking.org/aboutCT/definingCT.shtml 28 July 2006

Stephenson J 1992 Capability and quality in higher education. In: Stephenson J, Weil S (eds) Quality in learning: a capability approach to higher education Kogan Page, London

Stephenson J 1998 The concept of capability and its importance in higher education. In: Stephenson J, Yorke M (eds) Capability and quality in higher education. Kogan Page, London, p 1–13

Stephenson R 2002 The complexity of human behaviour: a new paradigm for physiotherapy? Physical Therapy Reviews 7:243–258

Stephenson R C 2004 Using a complexity model of human behaviour to help interprofessional clinical reasoning. International Journal of Therapy and Rehabilitation 11(4):168–175

Sweeney K, Griffiths F 2002 Complexity and healthcare: an introduction. Radcliffe Medical Press, Oxford

Sweeney K, Kernick D 2002 Clinical evaluation: constructing a new model for post-normal medicine. Journal of Evaluation in Clinical Practice 8(2):131–138

Trede F, Higgs J, Jones M et al 2003 Emancipatory practice: a model for physiotherapy practice? Focus on Health Professional Education: A Multidisciplinary Journal 5(2): 1–13

Van Manen M 1995 On the epistemology of reflective practice. Teachers and Teaching: Theory and Practice 1(1):33–50

Zimmerman B J, Lindberg C, Plsek P E 2001 Edgeware: insights from complexity science for health care leaders, 2nd edn, VHA, Irving, TX

SECTION 2

Reasoning, expertise and knowledge

SECTION CONTENTS

Chapter 10

The development of clinical reasoning expertise

Henny P.A. Boshuizen and Henk G. Schmidt

CHAPTER CONTENTS

The main objective of medical schools is to turn relative novices into knowledgeable and skilled professionals. Despite all the efforts of teachers and students, clinical teachers are not always content with the outcomes. One complaint is that students might have knowledge about subjects X or Y but do not demonstrate that knowledge in contexts where it has to be applied. Another complaint is that students are not able to solve clinical problems, especially in practical settings. Over the years, these observations have been made by many teachers, inspiring a great deal of research (e.g. Barrows et al 1978, Elstein et al 1978) and the introduction of new approaches to teaching medicine, such as problem-based learning (Norman & Schmidt 1992) aiming at the improvement of clinical reasoning in medicine.

In this chapter we seek to answer the question of whether clinical reasoning can be taught to medical students. We start by describing the development from novice in medicine to expert, providing a theoretical framework. Several approaches to clinical reasoning skills training are then described, and the implications are considered of this theory for the way medical education can improve students' clinical reasoning.

A THEORY OF THE DEVELOPMENT OF MEDICAL EXPERTISE

For a long time it has been thought that the human mind can be trained in logical thinking, problem-solving or creativity. For that purpose children are encouraged to play chess, or to learn Latin in school. Polya's (1957) problem-solving training programme also cherishes this general idea about the human mind. In the same vein, it was thought that experts in an arbitrary domain had trained their minds and had developed general problem-solving and thinking skills. This opinion has, however, been superseded, since research outcomes have shown that experts in a specific domain have not developed separate problem-solving skills that can be applied across domains. Instead, domain knowledge and the associated skills to use this knowledge in problem solving develop simultaneously and interdependently.

In medicine, research has shown that clinical reasoning is not a separate skill acquired independently of medical knowledge and other diagnostic skills. Instead, it suggests a stage theory of the development of medical expertise, in which knowledge acquisition and clinical reasoning go hand in hand (Boshuizen & Schmidt 1992, Schmidt & Boshuizen 1992, Schmidt et al 1990, Schmidt et al 1992). This theory of medical diagnosis is essentially a theory of the acquisition and development of knowledge structures upon which a student or a physician operates when diagnosing a case. Dramatic changes in problem solving or clinical reasoning are the result of structural changes in knowledge.

During the first stage, medical students acquire large amounts of knowledge about the biomedical basic sciences. They acquire concepts linked together in a knowledge network. Gradually, more concepts are added and refined and more and better connections are made. Knowledge accretion and validation are the students' main concerns in this period of their study. This process takes much more time than teachers might expect. In particular, the integration and integrated use of knowledge from different domains (such as the clinical sciences, biochemistry, pathophysiology and microanatomy) is not self-evident (Boshuizen & Van de Wiel 1998, Groothuis et al 1998). During this stage the clinical reasoning process is characterized by lines of reasoning consisting of chains of small steps commonly based on detailed, biomedical concepts. An example of detailed reasoning is given in Table 10.1. It has been taken from a longer protocol in which a fourth year medical student is dealing with a case of pancreatitis. His initial hypothesis set contained gallbladder and pancreas disease. Apparently, this student is entertaining the hypothesis of biliary tract obstruction. First, he reasons whether the new

Table 10.1 Lines of reasoning by a fourth year medical student*

Case item (number and text)	Think–aloud protocol
31. (History) Defecation: paler and more malodorous stools according to the patient	. . . not so much undermines that idea . . . er . their frequency . and their pattern compared with colour and the like . their smell er . . . yes . . . no problems with defecation, that means in any case no constipation, which you wouldn't expect with an obstruction of the biliary tract . . . well yes
32. (History) Last bowel movement was yesterday	. . .
32. (History) Temperature: 37°C at 6 p.m.	so no temperature
33. (Physical examination) Pulse rate: regular, 72/min	. . . er . yes . . . the past two . . . together . means that there's er no inflammation . . . and that would eliminate an er . . . an er . cholecystitis . . . and would rather mean an . . . er . . . obstruction of the biliary tract . . . caused by a stone, for instance . . . or, what may be the case too, by a carcinoma, but I wouldn't . . . although, it might be possible, lost 5 kilograms in weight . . .

*Protocol fragment obtained from a 4th year medical student working on a pancreatitis case showing detailed reasoning steps. See Boshuizen and Schmidt (1992) for a detailed description of the experiment.

finding about the patient's stools affects this hypothesis and decides that this is not the case. Next, three items later, he combines the information acquired and concludes that there is no inflammation (causing this obstruction) (step 1), hence, no cholecystitis (step 2), hence the biliary tract must be obstructed by something else, a stone for instance (step 3), or a carcinoma (step 4), which might be the case because the patient has lost weight (step 5).

By the end of the first stage of knowledge acquisition students have a knowledge network that allows them to make direct lines of reasoning between different concepts within that network. The more often these direct lines are activated the more these concepts cluster together, and students become able to make direct links between the first and last concept in such a line of reasoning, skipping intermediate concepts. We have labelled this process 'knowledge encapsulation', a term that refers to the clustering aspect of the process and can account for the automatization involved (e.g. Boshuizen & Schmidt 1992, Schmidt & Boshuizen 1993). Many of these concept clusters have (semi-) clinical names, such as microembolism, aorta insufficiency, forward failure or extrahepatic icterus, providing a powerful reasoning tool. Encapsulation of biomedical knowledge results in the next stage of development of clinical reasoning skills, in which biomedical knowledge has been integrated into clinical knowledge. At this stage, students' clinical reasoning processes no longer involve many biomedical concepts. Students tend to make direct links between patient findings and clinical concepts that have the status of hypotheses or diagnoses in their reasoning process. However, if needed, this encapsulated biomedical knowledge can be unfolded again, for instance when dealing with a very complicated problem. Van de Wiel et al (2000) showed that experts' clinical knowledge structures subsumed biomedical knowledge. Rikers et al (2005) demonstrated that in expert clinical reasoning, biomedical knowledge is also activated, operating in a sort of stand-by mode.

At the same time, a transition takes place from a network type of knowledge organization to another type of structure, which we refer to as 'illness scripts'. Illness scripts have three components. The first component refers to *enabling conditions* of disease; that is, the conditions or constraints under which a disease occurs. These are the personal, social, medical, hereditary and environmental factors that affect health in a positive or a negative way, or which affect the course of a specific disease. The second component is the *fault* – that is, the pathophysiological process that is taking place in a specific disease, represented in encapsulated form. The third component consists of the *consequences of the fault* – that is, the signs and symptoms of a specific disease (also see Feltovich & Barrows, 1984, who introduced this theoretical notion). Contrary to (advanced) novice knowledge networks, illness scripts are activated as a whole. After an illness script has been activated, no active, small-step search within that script is required; the other elements of the script are activated immediately and automatically. Therefore, people whose knowledge is organized in illness scripts have an advantage over those who have only semantic networks at their disposal. While solving a problem, a physician activates one or a few illness scripts. Subsequently the illness script elements (enabling conditions and consequences) are matched to the information provided by the patient. Illness scripts not only incorporate matching information volunteered by the patient, they also generate expectations about other signs and symptoms the patient might have. Activated illness scripts provide a list of phenomena to seek in history taking and in physical examination. In the course of this verification process the script is instantiated; expected values are substituted by real findings, while scripts that fail in this respect will deactivate. The instantiated script yields a diagnosis or a differential diagnosis when a few competing scripts remain active. An example of script activation by an experienced physician, dealing with the same clinical case as the student in Table 10.1, is given in Table 10.2. The information he heard about the patient's medical past and psychosocial circumstances (summarized in the protocol) was combined with the presenting complaint and activated a few competing illness scripts: pancreatic disease, liver disease and abdominal malignancy (which he considers implausible because of the patient's age) and stomach perforation. In addition, he thought of cardiomyopathy as an effect of excessive drinking. In the course of the think-aloud protocol he seemed to monitor the level of instantiation of every illness script. Except for gallbladder disease, no new scripts were activated.

Table 10.2   Illness script activation by a family physician**

Case item (number and text)	Think–aloud protocol
8. Complaint Continuous pain in the upper part of the abdomen, radiating to the back	. . . well, when I am visiting someone who is suffering an acute . . . continuous – since when? – pain in his upper abdomen, radiating to the back, who had pancreatitis a year before . . . of whom I don't know for sure if he still drinks or not after that course of Refusal®, but of whom I do know that he still has mental problems, so still receives a disability benefit, then I think that the first thing to cross my mind will be: well, what about that pancreas, . . . how's his liver . . . and also that – considering his age – eh it is not very likely that there will be other things wrong in his abdomen . . . eh . . . of a malign thing er nature . . . of course eh if he's taking huge amounts of alcohol there's always the additional possibility of a stomach eh problem, a stomach perforation . . . excessive drinking can also cause eh serious cardiomyopathy, which eh may cause heart defects mm I can't er judge the word continuous very well yet in this context

**Protocol fragment obtained from an experienced family physician working on a pancreatitis case. Earlier, he had received information about enabling conditions such as mental problems and alcohol abuse. See Boshuizen & Schmidt (1992).

So far we have seen that expert and novice knowledge structures differ in many respects. As a consequence, their clinical reasoning differs as well. Medical experts, who have large numbers of ready-made illness scripts that organize many enabling conditions and consequences associated with a specific disease, will activate one or more of these illness scripts when dealing with a case. Activation will be triggered by information concerning enabling conditions and/or consequences. Expert hypothesis activation and testing can be seen as an epiphenomenon of illness script activation and instantiation. These are generally automatic and 'unconscious' processes. As long as new information matches an active illness script, no active reasoning is required. Only in cases of severe mismatch or conflict does the expert engage in active clinical reasoning. During this process either illness-script based expectations are adjusted based on specific features of the patient, or the expert reverts to pure biomedical reasoning, drawing on de-encapsulated biomedical knowledge. An example of the first process is given by Lesgold et al (1988) who described expert radiologists' interpretations of an enlarged heart shadow on an X-ray screen. These experts took into consideration the marked scoliosis of the patient's thoracic spine affecting the position of his heart relative to the slide. Hence, they concluded that the heart was not actually enlarged.

Students, on the other hand, can rely only on knowledge networks which are less rich and less easily activated than experts' illness scripts. For that reason they require more information before a specific hypothesis will be generated, only because the disease labels in the network are linked to a very limited number of enabling conditions or consequences. Semantic networks must be reasoned through, step by step. This is a time-consuming process and often requires active monitoring. Hence, contrary to illness scripts, the knowledge structures which students activate do not automatically generate a list of signs and symptoms that are expected. Active searching through their networks is needed in order to generate a list of symptoms that might verify or falsify the hypotheses entertained. In general, students' clinical reasoning is less orderly, less goal-oriented and more time-consuming, but most importantly, it is based on less plausible hypotheses resulting in less accurate diagnoses than those of experts.

The differences described thus far were all investigated in the context of solving cases that did not require further data collection. This rather artificial task has the advantage that participants can devote all their attention and all the time they need to the cognitive processing of the information given. However, authentic clinical reasoning takes place during the action of data gathering and evaluation. A recent study by Wagenaar et al (submitted) has shown that third year students have great difficulty combining data collection and clinical reasoning. They are very dependent on the information the client volunteers and seem unable to reason in action. Instead, they try to collect as much information as possible and only after they have completed the interview do they review the information collected to formulate a diagnosis. Experts, on the other hand, think on their feet, adapting their data collection to the level of verification or falsification of their hypotheses and to the time available. Table 10.3 summarizes these differences between novices, intermediates and experts. The picture that emerges here is that novices and intermediates are handicapped in two ways: their knowledge is insufficient and it requires extra cognitive capacity when solving problems. Both aspects negatively influence clinical problem solving; they also hinder learning. Teaching should be organized in such a way that both aspects, knowledge structure and demand on cognitive capacity, improve.

TEACHING CLINICAL REASONING

Until this moment we have avoided definition of the concepts of clinical reasoning and clinical reasoning skills, first giving attention to the knowledge structures upon which these reasoning processes operate. Nor have we addressed the question of whether clinical reasoning can be taught. Yet there is huge pressure on the profession to improve the quality of diagnosis and treatment. Generally, clinical reasoning equals the thinking process occurring while dealing with a clinical case. Most researchers differentiate between different stages in the clinical reasoning process: beginning with hypothesis generation, inquiry strategy, data analysis, problem synthesis or diagnosis and finally ending with diagnostic and treatment decision making. Most often these different stages are thought to require different skills: hypothesis generation skills, inquiry skills, data analysis skills, etc.

Traditional approaches to enhancing clinical reasoning in students are based on the assumption that clinical reasoning or problem solving is a skill, separate from content knowledge. A typical

Table 10.3   Knowledge restructuring, clinical reasoning and levels of expertise level

Expertise level	Knowledge representation	Knowledge acquisition and (re)structuring	Clinical reasoning	Control required in clinical reasoning	Demand on cognitve capacity	Clinical reasoning in action
Novice	Networks	Knowledge accretion and validation	Long chains of detailed reasoning steps through pre-encapsulated networks	Active monitoring of each reasoning step	High	Difficulty to combine data collection and evaluation and clinical reasoning
Intermediate	Networks	Encapsulation	Reasoning through encapsulated network	Active monitoring of each reasoning step	Medium	. . .
Expert	Illness scripts	Illness script formation	Illness script activation and instantiation	Monitoring of the level of script instantiation	Low	Adjust data collection to time available and to verification/ falsification level of hypotheses

example is described by Elstein et al (1978). In that training programme, students were taught a few heuristics that had been derived from analysis of the reported and observed errors of diagnostic reasoning committed by medical students. For instance, as the planning heuristic, students were taught that each piece of information they requested should be related to a plan for solving the problem. They were also taught that they should have at least two or three competing hypotheses under consideration, and that each piece of information should be evaluated with respect to all hypotheses presently considered. It was found, however, that this training programme had no significant effects on the students' diagnostic accuracy and cost. Furthermore, it was found that students varied widely in their ability to apply the heuristics recommended in different cases. This finding and the outcomes of comparisons of experts and weaker problem solvers suggested to the investigators that differences were more to be found in the repertory of individuals' experiences organized in long-term memory than in differences in the planning and problem-solving heuristics employed. In terms of our theory: knowledge differences seem to play a larger role than differences in problem-solving skill.

Barrows & Pickell (1991) took the position that experts, performing better, are supposed to have better skills than novices and intermediates. They assumed that the clinical reasoning process itself could be improved. From the description of our theory it will be evident that we take a different position. Despite these differences, there are many correspondences as well. Therefore, in order to picture our position most clearly, we will compare our approach with and differentiate it from that of Barrows & Pickell. In their book *Developing Clinical Problem Solving Skills: A Guide to More Effective Diagnosis and Treatment*, Barrows & Pickell (1991, pp. xii–xiii) emphasized:

There are two components of expert clinical problem-solving that need to be considered separately, even though they cannot be separated in practice. One is content, the rich, extensive knowledge base about medicine that resides in the long-term memory of the expert. The other is process, the method of knowledge manipulation the expert uses to apply that knowledge

to the patient's problem. In expert performance these components are inexorably intertwined. Both are required; a well developed reasoning process appropriately bringing accurate knowledge to bear on a problem in a most effective manner . . . . This book should help you *perfect the process of clinical reasoning* [italics added] to best deliver the knowledge that you now have (and will acquire in the future) to the care of your patients . . . . To develop these skills you must practice, analyse, and repractice them until they are automatic. More important, if you associate your medical-school learning with this regime, your knowledge will be organised for effective recollection in your clinical work.

Their advice focuses on the different stages of clinical reasoning and associated skills, such as hypothesis generation and testing. For instance, they suggested that students should practise their scientific clinical reasoning skills at every opportunity. They provided the following advice (Barrows & Pickell 1991, pp. 215–216; in the first sentence, the term 'initial concept' refers to the first interpretation and representation of a patient's problem constructed by the doctor or student):

To develop an accurate initial concept, look carefully for important initial information as the patient encounter begins.

Generate a complete set of hypotheses in every patient encounter, carefully watching their degree of specificity and their complementarity. Be sure to watch out for hidden biases.

Use your creativity, and your inductive skills, to develop these hypotheses.

Use your critical deductive skills to inquire in a manner that will establish the more likely hypothesis.

Generate new hypotheses whenever your inquiries become unproductive or new data make your present hypotheses less likely.

In both your hypothesis generation and in inquiry strategy, be guided by an awareness of the basic pathophysiologic mechanism that may be operative in your patient's problem.

Superficially, the advice given suggests many correspondences with our theory. For instance, the authors' suggestion to look for important initial information as the patient encounter begins agrees with our emphasis on the role of enabling conditions in script activation. But what if a student does not have any scripts? Furthermore, their proposition to be aware of the basic 'pathophysiologic mechanism' that might play a role corresponds with our conceptions of *fault*. In our theory, applying biomedical knowledge would be helpful if a diagnostician cannot activate a matching illness script. However, the difference between our approach and that of Barrows & Pickell is that these authors suggest that every student and physician, independent of level of expertise, should always apply these skills. Our theory suggests that undertaking these activities is only fruitful when it affects the knowledge structure acted upon, while the quality and extent of the knowledge structure determine whether an exercise such as applying information about enabling conditions or activating basic science knowledge will help. More importantly, as long as the student does not have the relevant knowledge, many of the suggestions given may only be counterproductive.

This analysis brings us back to the question of whether clinical reasoning skills can be taught and trained as such, or whether other educational measures will be needed in order to improve students' clinical reasoning. It might be evident that our theory and previous experiences with direct training programmes suggest that other measures are needed, as far as the reasoning component of the diagnostic process is concerned. What is more important, our theory suggests that in order to improve clinical reasoning, education must focus on the development of adequate knowledge structures. Hence, teaching, training, coaching, modelling or supervising should adapt to the actual knowledge organization of the student. During the first stage in which knowledge accretion and validation take place, students should be given ample opportunity to test the knowledge they have acquired for its consistency and connectedness, to correct concepts and their connections and to fill the gaps they have detected. Students will do many of these things by themselves if they are provided with stimuli for thinking and with appropriate feedback. This stuff for thinking does not necessarily have to consist of patient problems. One could

also think of short descriptions of physiological phenomena (e.g. jet lag) that have to be explained. During the following stage of knowledge encapsulation, students should deal with more elaborate patient problems. As students go through the process of diagnosing a patient and afterwards explaining the diagnosis to a peer or a supervisor, biomedical knowledge will become encapsulated into higher level concepts. For instance, diagnosing a patient with acute bacterial endocarditis will first require detailed reasoning about infection, fever reaction, temperature regulation, circulation, haemodynamics, and so on. Later, a similar case will be explained in terms of bacterial infection, sepsis, microembolisms and aortic insufficiency (Boshuizen 1989). These problems are not necessarily presented by real patients in real settings. Paper cases and simulated patients will serve the same goal, sometimes even better. Especially during the earlier stage of knowledge encapsulation, when students have to do a great deal of reasoning, it might be more helpful to work with paper cases that present all relevant information. Reasoning through their knowledge networks in order to build a coherent explanation of the information available, students need not be concerned whether the information on which they work is complete and valid. Later in this stage, when knowledge has been restructured into a more tightly connected format, greater uncertainty can be allowed. Finally, the stage of illness script acquisition requires experience with real patients in real settings. Research by Custers et al (1993) suggests that at this stage, practical experience with typical patients (i.e. patients whose disease manifestations resemble the textbooks) should be preferred over experiences with atypical patients. There are no empirical data that can help to answer the question of whether illness script formation requires active dealing with the patient, or whether observing a doctor–patient contact could serve the same goal. On the other hand, since encapsulation and script formation go hand in hand, especially earlier in this stage, it is probable that 'hands on' experience is to be preferred. Having to reason about the patient would result in further knowledge encapsulation, while direct interaction with the patient provides the opportunity for perceptual learning, adding 'reality' to the symbolic concepts learned from textbooks. During this phase students might initially be overwhelmed by the information available in reality. They can easily overlook information when they do not know its relevance. This will especially affect their perception of *enabling conditions*. Therefore, it might be helpful to draw the student's attention to the enabling conditions operating in specific patients, to make sure that their illness scripts are completed with this kind of information. Boshuizen et al (1992) emphasize that in this stage of training a mix of practical experience and theoretical education is needed. They have found that during clinical rotations students tend to shift towards the application of clinical knowledge although it is not yet fully integrated into their knowledge base. A combination of the two ways of learning can help students to build a robust and flexible knowledge base.

Thus we see that working on problems and diagnosing and explaining patient cases, applying biomedical knowledge and providing feedback on students' thinking, might help them to form a knowledge system that enables efficient and accurate clinical reasoning that does not require all control capacity available (monitoring of reasoning on encapsulated concepts in a network requires less control than monitoring of reasoning on pre-encapsulated, detailed concepts; see Table 10.3). However, in practice, clinical reasoning must be performed in a context of real patients. In the end students should be able to collect information through history-taking, physical examination and laboratory, guided by their clinical reasoning process, and to find a (preliminary) diagnosis in the time available. Again there are indications that students have problems with collecting information in real settings (Wagenaar et al, submitted). A well-organized knowledge base is a first requirement, along with well-trained social, perceptual and psychomotor skills, though these skills also have a knowledge component, which makes it quite difficult to train them in isolation, separate from knowledge acquisition. Students must therefore learn to do their clinical reasoning and to perform these skills in a coordinated way. This again necessitates training and practice on whole training tasks that stimulate the integration of knowledge and skill into a further integrated knowledge base (Patrick

1992). The same discussion as occurred earlier in this chapter concerning the possibility of separating knowledge acquisition and the acquisition of clinical reasoning can be repeated regarding the question of whether a well-organized knowledge base and well-trained social, perceptual and psychomotor skills could be acquired independently. Van Merriënboer et al (2003) have shown that good planning and design of the learning process, such that integration and automatization are fostered, are very important. A good combination of learning environments, such as part-task practice, timely presentation of information, whole-task practice and elaboration and understanding, adjusted to the student's mastery and knowledge and the cognitive demand of the task, might be the key to success.

The reader might have observed a similarity between what has been proposed in this chapter and problem-based curricula. This similarity is not incidental. However, our suggestions for learning with cases and from practical experience do not necessarily require a problem-based curriculum. They can be applied in traditional course-based curricula as well. On the other hand, not every problem-based curriculum is structured in the way we have proposed. For example, a programme that uses problems as a starting point for learning may neglect the encapsulation function of working with cases. In our opinion it is essential that students do not work with problems and cases only. They also need an educational programme, based on an insight into the different obstacles that students experience at successive stages of development toward expertise. Studies by Prince (2006) and Dornan (2006) have shown that on the one hand, not observing these development issues results in a practice shock even in problem-based learning (PBL), and on the other hand, developing a curriculum with a combination of PBL and practical experience requires a complete rethinking of the role of the clinical teacher.

Acknowledgements

Preparation of this chapter was enabled by a grant to Henny P. A. Boshuizen by the Spencer Foundation, National Academy of Education, USA.

References

Barrows H S, Pickell G C 1991 Developing clinical problem-solving skills: a guide to more effective diagnosis and treatment. Norton, New York

Barrows H S, Feightner J W, Neufeld V R et al 1978 An analysis of the clinical method of medical students and physicians. Report to the Province of Ontario Department of Health, McMaster University, Hamilton, ONT

Boshuizen H P A 1989 De ontwikkeling van medische expertise; een cognitief-psychologische benadering [The development of medical expertise; a cognitive-psychological approach]. PhD thesis, University of Limburg, Maastricht

Boshuizen H P A, Schmidt H G 1992 On the role of biomedical knowledge in clinical reasoning by experts, intermediates and novices. Cognitive Science 16:153–184

Boshuizen H P A, Van de Wiel M W J 1998 Multiple representations in medicine: how students struggle with it. In: Van Someren M W, Reimann P, Boshuizen H P A, de Jong T (eds) Learning with multiple representations. Elsevier, Amsterdam, p 237–262

Boshuizen H P A, Hobus P P M, Custers E J F M et al 1992 Cognitive effects of practical experience. In: Evans A E, Patel V L (eds) Advanced models of cognition for medical training and practice. Springer Verlag, New York, p 337–348

Custers E J F M, Boshuizen H P A, Schmidt H G 1993 The influence of typicality of case descriptions on subjective disease probability estimations. Paper presented at the Annual Meeting of the American Educational Research Association, Atlanta, GA

Dornan T 2006 Experienced based learning; learning clinical medicine in workplaces. PhD thesis Maastricht University

Elstein A S, Shulman L S, Sprafka S A 1978 Medical problem solving: an analysis of clinical reasoning. Harvard University Press, Cambridge, MA

Feltovich P J, Barrows H S 1984 Issues of generality in medical problem solving. In: Schmidt H G, De Volder M L (eds) Tutorials in problem-based learning: a new direction in teaching the health professions. Van Gorcum, Assen, p 128–142

Groothuis S, Boshuizen H P A, Talmon J L 1998 Analysis of the conceptual difficulties of the endocrinology domain and an empirical analysis of student and expert understanding of that domain. Teaching and Learning in Medicine 10(4):207–216

Lesgold A M, Rubinson H, Feltovich P J et al 1988 Expertise in a complex skill: diagnosing X-ray pictures. In: Chi M T H, Glaser R, Farr M J (eds) The nature of expertise. Lawrence Erlbaum, Hillsdale, NJ, p 311–342

Norman G R, Schmidt H G 1992 The psychological basis of problem-based learning: a review of the evidence. Academic Medicine 67:557–565

Patrick J 1992 Training: theory and practice. Academic Press, London

Polya G 1957 How to solve it. Doubleday, Garden City, NY

Prince K 2006 Problem-based learning as a preparation for professional practice. Unpublished PhD thesis, Maastricht University

Rikers R M J P, Schmidt H G, Moulaert V 2005 Biomedical knowledge: encapsulated or two worlds apart? Applied Cognitive Psychology 19(2):223–231

Schmidt H G, Boshuizen H P A 1992 Encapsulation of biomedical knowledge. In: Evans A E, Patel V L (eds) Advanced models of cognition for medical training and practice. Springer Verlag, New York, p 265–282

Schmidt H G, Boshuizen H P A 1993 On acquiring expertise in medicine. Educational Psychology Review 5:205–221

Schmidt H G, Norman G R, Boshuizen H P A 1990 A cognitive perspective on medical expertise: theory and implications. Academic Medicine 65:611–621

Schmidt H G, Boshuizen H P A, Norman G R 1992 Reflections on the nature of expertise in medicine. In: Keravnou E (ed) Deep models for medical knowledge engineering. Elsevier, Amsterdam, p 231–248

Van de Wiel M W J, Boshuizen H P A, Schmidt H G 2000 Knowledge restructuring in expertise development: evidence from pathophysiological representations of clinical cases by students and physicians. European Journal of Cognitive Psychology 12(3):323–355

Van Merriënboer J J G, Kirschner P A, Kester L 2003 Taking the load off the learner's mind: instructional design for complex learning. Educational Psychologist 38:5–13

Wagenaar A, Boshuizen H P A, Muijtjens A et al (submitted) Cognitive processes of beginning and experienced counsellors: differences in diagnostic reasoning during a diagnostic interview.

Chapter **11**

Expertise and clinical reasoning

Gail Jensen, Linda Resnik and Amy Haddad

In all professions, there are individuals who perform exceptionally well and who are held in high
regard by their colleagues and their patients – in
other words, experts. The simple definition of an
expert is someone 'capable of doing the right thing
at the right time' (Holyoak 1991). In research on
expertise there are several variations on this definition. An expert can be defined as someone who *performs* at the level of an experienced professional
such as a master or grandmaster in chess or a clinical specialist in medicine (Ericsson & Smith 1991,
Rikers & Paas 2005). Experts can also be defined
as top performers who excel in a particular field,
for example elite athletes or musicians, or those
clinicians who achieve the best clinical outcomes
(Rothstein 1999). Experts can also be seen as those
who achieve at least a moderate degree of success
in their occupation (Boshuizen et al 2004).

Knowing more about the development of expertise, components of expertise and expert practice
are all critical elements in expertise research. Ideally, an enhanced understanding of what distinguishes novices from experts should facilitate
learning strategies for more effective education.
Novice development in pursuit of expertise is an
area of great interest in professional education as
it lays the foundation for entry into practice
(Boshuizen et al 2004). Expertise is much more of
a process or continuum of development than a
static state resulting from a cluster of attributes
such as knowledge and problem-solving skills or
high level performance (Bereiter & Scardamalia
1993). This does not mean that the process of
moving toward expertise is based merely on

the gathering of years of experience. Without learning mechanisms or reflection used to mediate improvement from experience there will be little acquisition of expertise (Tsui 2003).

One of the most critical and complex dimensions of expertise is clinical reasoning and decision making. A core assumption we make in this chapter is that we must not separate the critical analysis of clinical reasoning from the deliberate action that results as part of the reasoning and decision-making process. This is an interactive relationship where analysis and action each influence the other (Kennedy 1987). Clinical reasoning, then, is a process in which the healthcare professional, through interacting with the patient, family or care givers and other members of the healthcare team, structures meaning, goals and health management strategies based on clinical data, client preferences and values, knowledge and professional judgement (Higgs & Jones 2000). We begin this chapter with a 'deconstruction of the concept of expertise' achieved through a brief, analytical overview of key elements in traditional expertise theory and research. Next we explore the essential role of clinical reasoning and expertise in the context of everyday practice. Here we draw on predominantly qualitative research that has been carried out with practitioners in the context of practice. From this review, we generate a working list of attributes that we believe need to be considered when talking about clinical reasoning and decision making. In the final section of the chapter we engage in a discussion of strategies for facilitating learning and novice development in clinical reasoning. The goal of understanding expertise and clinical reasoning is the translation to more effective teaching and student learning and ultimately the delivery of the highest quality care.

DECONSTRUCTING THE CONCEPT OF EXPERTISE

EXPERTISE AS MENTAL PROCESSING AND PROBLEM SOLVING

Expertise is a complex multidimensional concept that has captured the interest of researchers over 50 years (Rikers & Paas 2005). Early work was in the field of cognitive psychology and accepted a tradition of basic information-processing capabilities of humans. Initial work in expertise concentrated on mental processing or, more simply, the conceptualization of problem solving. In deGroot's well known work with chess players he began to look at differences between chess players with varying levels of expertise (deGroot 1966). He found that chess masters were able to recognize and reproduce chess patterns more quickly and accurately than novice players. Newell & Simon (1972) suggested that reasoning brought progressive expansion of knowledge of a problematic situation that continued until the problem was solved. They proposed that general methods or heuristics could be used for problem solving or information processing in all fields. An *expert* was someone who was particularly skilled at carrying out this heuristic search (Chase & Simon 1973, Ericsson & Smith 1991, Holyoak 1991). Investigative work required experts and novices to think aloud, or verbalize, as a way to explore thought processes and assess problem-solving skills. Subsequent studies in areas such as chess (Chase & Simon 1973) and physics (Chi et al 1981) revealed that expertise depended not only on the method of problem solving but also on the expert's detailed knowledge in a specific area, ability to memorize, and ability to make inferences.

The well-known research by Elstein et al (1978, 1990) in medical problem solving was based on elements from early cognitive work in clinical reasoning and problem solving. They used various methods to analyse subjects' reasoning processes, including the use of simulated patients, recall tasks and verbalization. Several major findings from this work have had a strong influence on education in medicine and other health professions (Elstein & Schwartz 2000; Elstein et al 1978, 1990; Rothstein & Echternach 1986). The hypothetico-deductive method that they identified continues to be incorporated into models that represent the clinical reasoning process in health professional education (Barrows & Pickell 1991, Elstein & Schwartz 2000, Elstein et al 1990, Jones 1992, Jones & Rivett 2004, Rothstein & Echternach 1986). In hypothetico-deductive reasoning the focus is on a process that includes cue acquisition, hypothesis generation, cue interpretation and hypothesis evaluation. The process of collecting data or cues from the patient and generating hypotheses is considered a technique for transforming an unstructured problem (e.g. a patient presenting with several complications) into a structured problem by generating a small possible set of solutions.

One of the most fundamental differences between experts and novices is that experts will bring more and better organized knowledge to bear on a problem. In medicine, the ability to determine the proper patient diagnosis was discovered to be highly dependent on the physician's knowledge in a particular clinical specialty area, called *case specificity* (Elstein & Schwartz 2000, Rikers & Paas 2005). Case specificity implies that a successful reasoning strategy in one situation may not apply in a second case, because the practitioner may not know enough about the area of the patient's problem. Identification of case specificity focused attention on the role of knowledge in expertise. Both clinician experience and the features of the case are factors that affect the problem-solving strategy that is used. Experts appear to have not only methods of problem solving but also the ability to combine these methods with knowledge and an understanding of how the knowledge necessary to solve the problem should be organized (Boshuizen et al 2004, Brandsford et al 2000, Chi et al 1988, Ericsson 1996). In a test of diagnostic reasoning, both successful and unsuccessful diagnosticians used a hypothesis-testing strategy (Rikers & Paas 2005). Research on the clinical reasoning of expert physicians demonstrated that in familiar situations experts did not display hypothesis testing but instead used rapid, automatic and often nonverbal strategies. This showed that expert reasoning in non-problematic situations is similar to pattern recognition or retrieval of a well-structured network of knowledge (Elstein & Schwartz 2000, Norman et al 1994). Experts can make connections or inferences from the data by recognizing the pattern and links between clinical findings and a highly structured knowledge base. This explains why experts tend to ask fewer, more relevant questions and perform examinations more quickly and accurately than novices. Novices and intermediate subjects tend to use hypothetico-deductive processes that involve setting up hypotheses and gathering clinical data to prove or disprove them (Elstein & Schwartz 2000). Thus, less experienced clinicians tend to ask patients more questions than do experts, and in the same order, regardless of their relevance to the case (Rivett & Higgs 1995).

EXPERTISE AS SKILL ACQUISITION

For health professions where diagnosis is not the predominant decision point, there has been perhaps no more influential work in expertise than that done by Benner (Benner 1984; Benner et al 1996, 1999). In her original work Benner applied a model of skill acquisition developed by Hubert Dreyfus, a philosopher, and Stuart Dreyfus, a mathematician and system analyst (Dreyfus & Dreyfus 1980). Their work came out of a reaction to the cognitive psychology tradition that intelligent practice is not just the application of knowledge and rules for instrumental decision making. A central premise in this work is that human understanding is a skill akin to knowing how to find one's way about the world, rather than knowing a lot of facts and rules for relating them. 'Our basic understanding was thus a knowing how rather than a knowing that' (Dreyfus & Dreyfus 1980, 1996). From their research on chess players and airline pilots they put forward a five stage model for the acquisition and development of skill (novice, advanced beginner, competent, proficient and expert) (Table 11.1).

The Dreyfus & Dreyfus conception of expertise is much more focused on the context of actual practice. Several critical elements emerged from their model (Dreyfus & Dreyfus 1980, 1996): (1) expertise is more about 'knowing how' (procedural knowledge, knowing how to do things) rather than 'knowing what' (declarative knowledge, knowing information and facts); (2) expert knowledge is embedded in the action of the expert rather than from propositional knowledge; (3) experience is a critical factor in the development of expertise; (4) much of expert performance is automatic and non-reflective (but when a situation is novel, experts engage in deliberation before action); (5) intuition of experts or the knowing how to do things is both experiential and tacit.

In her analysis of nursing practice Benner found that much of expert performance in nursing emphasizes individual perceptions and decision-making abilities rather than just the performance

Table 11.1   The Dreyfus & Dreyfus (1980) model of skill acquisition (adapted from Benner 1984)

Stage	Knowledge use	Action	Orientation	Decision making
Novice	Factual	Given rules for actions	Cannot see whole situation	Rule-governed, relies on others
Advanced beginner	Objective facts	Begin use of intuition in concrete situations	Limited situational perception	Less rule-governed, more sophisticated rules, relies on others
Competent	Hierarchical perspective	Devise new rules based on situation	Conscious of situation	Makes decisions, feels responsible
Proficient	Situational	Intuitive behaviours replace reasoned responses	Perceives whole situation	Decision making is less labored, can discriminate
Expert	Knows what needs to be done based on practiced situational discrimination	Intuitive and deliberate rationality; where intuition not developed, reasoning is applied	Can discriminate among situations and know when action is required	Know how to achieve goals

of the skill. Skill is identified as an overall approach to professional action that includes both perception and decision making, not just what we would think of as technical skill or technique (Benner 1984; Benner et al 1996, 1999). The knowledge necessary to perform the skill is *practical knowledge* (i.e. knowing how to perform a skill in its real setting). Practical knowledge contrasts with knowing material in a textbook or theoretical knowledge that is learned in the classroom (Eraut 1994, Ryle 1949).

The Dreyfus model captured the complexity of nursing expertise that is acquired from deep, intuitive and holistic understanding of a situation. Benner argued that skilled know-how or practical knowledge is a form of knowledge, not just application of it. Furthermore, knowledge is not possessed by an individual in isolation, but rather is based upon the 'shared life of a work group', whereby clinicians learn from watching and interacting with others in collaborative and cooperative teamwork (Benner et al 1997).

Gruppen & Frohna (2002, p. 221), reviewing clinical reasoning research in medical education, wrote about the importance of context in research on clinical reasoning:

> Too often studies of clinical reasoning take place in a vacuum. A case or scenario is presented to subjects ... stripped of any 'irrelevant' noise that

stems from the physician's prior relationship with the patient .... The traditional methodology of providing clinical cases that are decontextualized and 'clean' may not be particularly valid means of assessing the full range of processes and behaviors present in clinical reasoning in natural settings.

KEY ELEMENTS IN EXPERTISE RESEARCH

Although there has been prolonged debate and controversy in expertise research on the acquisition of expert characteristics, there continues to be strong agreement on the characteristics of experts. In fact, that consistency is seen here in the characteristics of experts identified by Glaser & Chi (1988):

- Experts mainly excel in their domain of expertise.
- Experts are faster than novices in performing skills.
- Experts can solve problems more quickly and with little error.
- Experts have superior short-term and long-term memory.
- Experts can see the problem in their domain at a deeper, more principled level than novices, who have a more superficial representation of the problem.

- Experts spend more time trying to understand the problem and experts have strong self-monitoring skills.

Another way to look at the key elements of expertise is to cluster them into categories. Sternberg & Horvath (1995) described three such clusters of categories for thinking about expertise in real-world settings:

- Domain knowledge. Experts bring knowledge to bear more effectively on problems within their domain.
- Efficiency of problem solving. Experts can solve problems within their domain more efficiently through self-regulation and use of metacognitive strategies.
- Insight. Experts are more likely to arrive at creative solutions to problems. They often redefine the problem to reach an insightful solution that would not occur to others.

In summary, experts are knowledgeable because they have extensive, accessible, well-organized knowledge. Experts continue to build their practical knowledge base through a repertoire of examples, images, illness scripts, and understanding learned through experience (Eraut 1994, Schön 1983). Experts learn from experience by using reflective inquiry or metacognitive strategies to think about what they are doing, what worked and what did not work. Although much of the expertise research has been done contrasting the performance of novices and experts, it is investigations of actual practice that provide an opportunity to explore more fully the knowledge, experience and complex human decision making embedded in expertise (Schön 1983, 1991).

EXPERTISE AND CLINICAL REASONING IN EVERYDAY PRACTICE

Qualitative research methods have been central tools in investigative work and theoretical writing done in several applied professions such as nursing (Benner 1984; Benner et al 1996, 1999), teaching (Berliner 1986, Sternberg 1998, Tsui 2003), occupational therapy (Fleming & Mattingly 2000, Mattingly & Fleming 1994), and physical therapy

(Edwards et al 2004; Gwyer et al 2004; Jensen et al 1999, 2000, 2007; Resnik & Hart 2003; Shepard et al 1999). These are all professions where human interactions and care are central aspects of the work. In these studies we find that the clinical reasoning process is not as analytical, deductive or rational because the focus of care is a much larger process that extends beyond the identification of a diagnosis. The clinical reasoning process is iterative and ongoing. Knowing a patient, understanding his or her story, fitting the patient's story with clinical knowledge and collaborating with the patient to problem-solve are the kinds of integral components of clinical reasoning that emerge from these studies. Here we discuss and compare in greater detail key findings from conceptual and theoretical work in clinical reasoning and expertise in occupational therapy, physical therapy and nursing. Each of these investigations represents important and provocative theory development for these professions, that led to sustained work exploring the context of everyday practice.

In their ethnographic study of clinical reasoning in occupational therapy, Mattingly & Fleming (1994) originally proposed three types of reasoning in their 'theory of the three-track' mind.

1. Procedural reasoning. This type of reasoning is similar to hypothetical-propositional reasoning in medicine, but in the case of occupational therapy the focus is on identifying the patient's functional problem and selecting procedures to reduce the effects of the problem.
2. Interactive reasoning. This is the reasoning that takes place during face-to-face interactions between therapist and patient. Active interaction and collaboration with the patient are used to understand the patient's perspective.
3. Conditional reasoning. This form of reasoning is based on social and cultural processes of understanding and is used to help the patient in the difficult process of reconstructing a life that is now changed by injury or disease.

A fourth form of reasoning, narrative reasoning (Fleming & Mattingly 2000, Mattingly & Fleming 1994), is used to describe the story-telling aspect of patient cases. Often therapists use narrative thinking and telling of a kind of 'short story' in coming to understand or make sense of the human experience. This making sense of the illness experience is shifting the thinking and dialogue from a physiological event to a personally meaningful one for the patient. Reflecting on ethnographic research work done in occupational therapy since their original work, Mattingly & Fleming (1994) highlighted two key concepts in clinical reasoning: active judgement and narrative. Working together, these two streams of reasoning are core processes for occupational therapists.

In physical therapy, Jensen and colleagues developed a grounded theory of expert practice in physical therapy (Jensen et al 1999, 2000; Shepard et al 1999). It is proposed in this model that expertise in physical therapy is some combination of multidimensional knowledge, clinical reasoning skills, skilled movement and virtue (Figure 11.1). All four of these dimensions (knowledge, reasoning, movement and virtue) contribute to the therapist's philosophy of practice. For novices, each of these core dimensions of expertise may exist but they do not appear to be as well integrated (Figure 11.2) (Jensen et al 2007). As novices continue to develop, each of the dimensions may become stronger, yet they may not be well integrated for proficient practice. When the expert therapist has fully integrated these dimensions of expertise, that in turn leads to an explicit philosophy of practice (Figure 11.2) (Jensen et al 2007). In this model of expertise it is difficult to highlight only one dimension such as clinical reasoning, as all dimensions could be seen as contributing to thinking and actions of expert practitioners. For example, experts' knowledge is

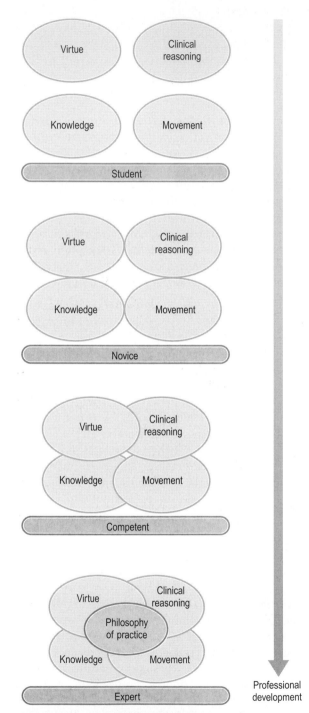

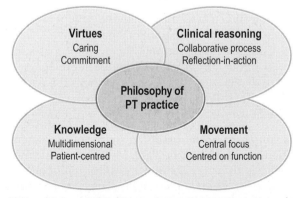

Figure 11.1   Model of expert practice in physical therapy

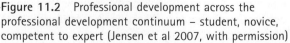

Figure 11.2   Professional development across the professional development continuum – student, novice, competent to expert (Jensen et al 2007, with permission)

multidimensional and patient-centred. Therapists draw from several sources such as specialty knowledge, clinical knowledge gained through reflection on practice and listening carefully to their patients. Experts trust their tacit or craft knowledge and use it in making intuitive decisions about patient care.

The clinical reasoning dimension of the model has two core components: (1) it is a collaborative process between therapist and patient in which the patient is seen as an important source of knowledge; and (2) therapists demonstrate evidence of strong self-monitoring reflection skills in this collaborative process. Function, as defined by the patient, forms the core of a framework used in establishing patient care goals. Skilful facilitation of movement focused on function, done through data gathering, hands-on skills, assessment palpation and touch, is the central aim of therapists. One final element of the expert model is virtuous practice, seen in behaviours such as care and compassion for patients, non-judgemental approaches to patients, admitting mistakes and taking deliberate actions such as reporting unethical behaviour of colleagues or advocating for patients.

Subsequent work by Resnik & Jensen (2003) corroborated the presence of a patient-centred approach to care seen in collaborative clinical reasoning and promotion of patient empowerment. At the foundation of the patient-centred approach they identified an ethic of caring and a respect for individuality, a passion for clinical care and a desire to continually learn and improve. The primary goals of empowering patients, increasing self-efficacy beliefs and involving patients in the care process are facilitated by patient–therapist collaborative problem solving and enhanced through attentive listening, trust building and observation. The patient-centred approach is exemplified by the therapist's emphasis on patient education and by strong beliefs about the power of education. This approach alters the therapeutic relationship and enhances patients' abilities to make autonomous choices. Resnik & Jensen reported that these efforts not only promoted patient empowerment and self-efficacy, but also resulted in greater continuity of services, more skilful care, and more individualized plans of care and ultimately better outcomes.

Although experts in that study possessed a broad, multidimensional knowledge base, Resnik & Jensen (2003) discovered that years of clinical experience and specialty certification did not appear to be mandatory in achieving expertise. This seemed to challenge a basic assertion of the Dreyfus model, that experience is a critical factor in development of expertise. In Resnik & Jensen's study this was not observed, and in fact, some therapists classified as experts were relatively new physical therapists. In these instances, they theorized, knowledge acquisition was facilitated by work and life experience prior to attending physical therapy school, by being in a work environment that offered access to pooled collegial knowledge, and by practitioners' values and virtues of inquisitiveness and humility which drove their use of reflection. This combination of factors helped accelerate the acquisition and integration of knowledge. Furthermore, expert therapists used the rich knowledge base of colleagues and sought out knowledgeable mentors to assist them in challenging cases. Thus, in their theoretical model, expert therapists' knowledge base comprised knowledge gained from personal experience and movement and rehabilitation, colleagues, patients, clinical experience, teaching experience, specialty work and entry-level education, as well as continuing education.

In-depth ethnographic work by Edwards and colleagues (2004) on expert physical therapists' clinical reasoning strategies further revealed an interplay of different reasoning strategies in every task of clinical practice (for example interactive reasoning, diagnostic reasoning, narrative reasoning, ethical reasoning, reasoning about teaching). Rather than contrasting the cognitively-based rational models of reasoning and interactive models of reasoning, Edwards et al proposed a dialectic model of clinical reasoning that moves between the cognitive and decision-making processes required to diagnose and manage patients' physical disabilities and the narrative or communicative reasoning and action required to understand and engage patients and caregivers. Critical reflection is required with either process.

The work of Benner and colleagues in *Expertise in Nursing Practice: Caring, Clinical Judgment and Ethics* (Benner et al 1996) and *Clinical Wisdom and Interventions in Critical Care: A Thinking-in-action Approach* (Benner et al 1999) represents the richness and the relevance of 'learning from practice' in order to improve understanding of expert practice. They used observations and narrative accounts of actual clinical examples as primary tools for understanding the everyday clinical and caring knowledge and practical reasoning that were used in nursing practice. Important findings from this work include these aspects of clinical judgement and skilful comportment of experienced nurses (Benner et al 1999):

1. Reasoning-in-transition. This refers to practical reasoning in an evolving or open-ended clinical situation. The clinician is always interpreting the present clinical situation in terms of the immediate past condition of the particular patient.

2. Skilled know-how. This is the skilful performance of interventions done by practitioners that is visible through observation. For example, one would see differences between novices and experienced nurses in where they locate themselves when monitoring a patient. Expert nurses position themselves where they can use all their senses while they are engaged in completing non-direct aspects of patient care.

3. Response-based practice. Excellent clinicians are able to read a situation and engage in proactive, response-based actions. For example, skilled nurses have learned that the hypertension may be triggered by emotion and anxiety, and will attempt to talk the patient down before using a pharmacological intervention.

4. Agency. This refers to the moral agency seen through the practitioner's ability to act upon or influence a situation. It is not enough just to go through routine clinical actions based on objective findings. The practitioner must be engaged in the clinical situation demonstrated through action, reasoning and the relationship with the patient and family. Here one would see the nurse or practitioner taking a stand in promoting what he or she considered to be in the patient's best interests as she does not see herself as ever standing outside of the situation. Agency is seen as a critical component of expertise.

5. Perceptual acuity and skill of involvement. Perceptual acuity requires skilful engagement with both the problem and the person. Emotions play a key role in the perception of the problem. Benner (1984) suggested that they may even act as a moral compass in learning a practice. The interpersonal skill of engaging with the clinical and human situation is called the skill of involvement.

What do these examples of investigative work centred on everyday practice tell us about clinical reasoning and expertise? As we look across the three health professions, we see striking similarities that emerge from understanding the context of practice (Table 11.2). It is the human or relationship side of practice that emerges as a central component of clinical reasoning and expertise. The critical analysis that is fundamental to clinical reasoning is not just a matter of matching the signs and symptoms to the practitioner's existing knowledge base. It is a complex process where critical analysis must take place within the context of the action and interaction with the patient. That analysis and thinking must lead to wise judgement and action. It is these key attributes or habits of mind that are the focus of our discussion in the final section of this chapter.

CLINICAL REASONING AND NOVICE DEVELOPMENT: DEVELOPING HABITS OF MIND ACROSS THE PROFESSIONAL DEVELOPMENT CONTINUUM

Understanding the context in which practice occurs is critical in the clinical reasoning and decision-making process of experts, yet challenging for novices who are often focused on technical skills. Experts do much more than 'make a diagnosis'; they engage in a process of reasoning and decision making that includes patients as a partners in their care. Although we use patient-centred language in professional association documents and professional journals, we spend little time focusing on the development of patient-centred skills in our novices.

The university setting does well in training analytic 'habits of mind' but it does far less in developing practical skills and capacity for professional

Table 11.2   Learning from everyday practice: comparisons across professions

Health profession theoretical elements	Key themes	Common themes shared by two or more professions
Occupational therapy		
Procedural reasoning Interactive reasoning Conditional reasoning Narrative reasoning	Use of hypothetico-deductive reasoning for identifying functional problems Collaboration with patient to understand patient's perspective Integration of social and cultural processes for understanding Narrative as important tool for making sense of the illness experience	Hypothetico-deductive reasoning used for specific procedural issues The patient is a respected and central aspect of the work Collaboration with the patient is a critical strategy in clinical reasoning and decision making Metacognitive skill (reflection) is an integral aspect of patient care
Physical therapy		Narrative is a critical tool for understanding the clinical situation including patient, caregivers as well as the clinical knowledge that is part of the story Moral agency and deliberate actions are essential elements of what it means to be 'good' at one's work (it is difficult to separate clinical and ethical reasoning)
Multidimensional knowledge base Clinical reasoning is collaborative and patient centred; reflection; self-monitoring Function central to movement Virtuous practice; deliberate action Dialectic reasoning Instrumental reasoning (hypothetico-deductive for diagnosis and management) Communicative/narrative for understanding	Use of hypothetico-deductive reasoning for identifying diagnosis, patient management Collaboration with the patient is an important aspect of clinical reasoning Knowledge comes from many sources including the patient Reflection, self-monitoring is a critical skill Non-judgemental approach, deliberate actions Narrative/communicative reasoning and action for understanding patient or caregiver experience	

judgement. Sullivan (2005) argued that in professional education, the strong emphasis on formal analytic reasoning and knowledge creation leaves out perhaps one of the most important elements, the act of inquiry in the context of the relationship. 'The clearest way to grasp the insufficiency of the positivist model of professional expertise is to notice what the positivist account of knowledge leaves out and must take for granted' (Sullivan 2005, p. 242). While expert practitioners bring scientific evidence, analysis and problem-solving skills to the clinical situation, they also bring the skills of practical reasoning as they listen to patients, reflect on and make meaning of what they hear. It is this narrative understanding and practical reasoning that is informed by scientific knowledge but guided by concern for human well-being that is central to

expertise. The challenge for professional education is how to teach this complex ensemble of analytic thinking, skilful practice and wise judgement that is required in the professions. How do we go about developing habits of mind in our students? We, along with many others (Benner et al 1996, 1999; Dewey 1910; Epstein 1999; Higgs & Tichen 2001; Kennedy 1987; Schön 1987), argue that the relationship between patient and practitioner is a critical element of skilful ethical comportment, and that it is foundational in expert work and therefore an essential foundation for novice development.

The choice of the metaphor of *foundation* is important in that it emphasizes the supportive nature of ethical comportment. A foundation allows something, in this case expert work, to stand on a solid base. If something is lacking in a foundation, or is shakily built, then it will not be strong enough to withstand the stresses encountered in clinical practice. Skilful ethical comportment draws on at least three basic approaches to ethics: principled reasoning, virtue and a care orientation. A solid moral foundation includes all these approaches because an expert needs to understand moral norms and theories and the use of such tools to examine moral problems and practices. However, 'theories and principles are only starting points and general guides for the development of norms of appropriate conduct' (Beauchamp & Childress 2001, p. 2). An expert must also possess the virtues or character to do the right thing. If a clinician knows the correct moral action but lacks the courage or compassion to act, then the knowledge is of little significance. Lastly, a solid foundation in ethics includes the ability to discern what is worth caring about in healthcare practice. A care orientation considers what values should be pursued, nurtured or sustained and, conversely, what should be disvalued. Approaches that include only abstract principles or duties often lead to conclusions that minimize the particulars of individual circumstances that are considered morally relevant to care orientation. An orientation to care allows health professionals and patients to interact on the basis of 'receptivity, relatedness, and responsiveness' (Noddings 1984, p. 35).

Ethical comportment requires balancing all of these approaches as well as translating a judgement into action. Moral judgements can be about abstract, distant issues or they can be about up-close and personal issues involving 'identified lives': 'The more personally involved we feel, the more emotive and aesthetic elements play a role; the farther the situation is from us, the less the force of emotion or aesthetics will be' (Loewy 2000, p. 222). Within the realm of expert practice, the emotions of compassion, sympathy and empathy have a central place in our understanding of humane and ethical treatment of patients. Beyond these basic expressions of care, patients expect a range of emotional responsiveness appropriate to context. For example, in an emergency situation most patients would prefer quick and competent action to save their lives rather than heartfelt empathy. However, it is clear that in certain cases the emotional tone matters deeply. It is the life

work of health professionals to recognize those situations and adapt their emotional response to the particular needs of the patient at that time.

In addition to these central emotions that are a part of care, other emotions are evoked through interactions with patients that are not always positive. It is important that students develop emotional sensitivity and realize that emotions or felt affect are distinct from thought or action: 'Thus, to grieve, pity, show empathy or love is to focus on an aspect of self or other and to grasp information to which purer cognition or thought may not have access' (Sherman 1995, p. 664). One way to attend to emotions is to encourage novices to reflect on the emotional content of interactions with patients or peers as this is an often overlooked component of ethical decision making. Reflection on emotions emphasizes the relationship between behaviours or words that begin or trigger an emotional response. By openly acknowledging that different emotions are evoked in different circumstances, novices have an opportunity to reflect on their emotional repertoire in a way that is encouraging and safe.

The processes of self-reflection, reflecting together between novice and expert at the moment of a clinical encounter, or small group discussion on the identification and understanding of emotions are steps in strengthening novices' capacity to hold on to and name their emotional experiences. Rather than novices being told what they should feel or should have felt (such as empathy and compassion) when interacting with patients or others, opportunities should be provided to let novices interact with simulated patients or real patients in clinically complex situations and then reflect on their experiences in their own words.

Although emotions are sometimes seen as a somewhat fragile platform upon which to build such heavy obligations as moral duty or care, by attending to emotions we can see that they highlight certain aspects of a situation, serve as a mode of communication, lead to deeper self-knowledge and provide insight into motivation. Grounding and naming emotions in specific examples from novices' and experts' experiences in clinical practice begins to create a framework that legitimizes this component of the self in one's professional role. Novices can then examine, question and develop their skills in emotional sensitivity – an important part of ethical comportment and caring for others.

In health professional education we have certainly heard and embraced the concepts of reflection and helping students develop their skills of reflective inquiry (Harris 1993; Schön 1983, 1991). Our understanding of reflection as an important metacognitive skill is often just that, a skill to be taught and a process to be applied by the student. Yet we know from experts that there is much more to reflection than writing down or discussing insights from one's experience. Expert clinicians have the capacity to engage in critical self-reflection. Expert clinicians are more sensitive to contextual cues, as they are aware of their own mental processes, listen more attentively, are flexible, recognise bias and judgements and therefore act with compassion based on insight (Benner et al 1999, Epstein 1999, Gwyer et al 2004, Jensen et al 1999, Shepard et al 1999).

It is essential that novices have multiple opportunities to act on ethical judgements in a safe environment and reflect not only on the reasons for a particular action or set of actions but also on the thinking and responses that led up to the action. Novices need to hear experts 'think out loud' after a particularly difficult exchange with a patient or colleague, so that the process of arriving at a sound decision becomes more transparent. The habit of reflecting on what is going on ethically in a situation, what should be done about it, and the meaning for the broader professional and public community can be fostered throughout professional education.

CONCLUSION

In this chapter we have argued that expertise is not a static state, congruent with a list of specific attributes or obtained through years of experience. It is much more a continuum of development and a dynamic process where critical reflection and deliberate action are central components. Experts continue to learn and build extensive, well organized practical knowledge through the use of reflective inquiry and metacognitive strategies. Clinical reasoning is a complex process where critical analysis and reflection take place in the context of the action and interaction with the patient. Experts demonstrate their patient-centred focus through a consistent commitment to knowing the patient, intense listening that leads to a rich understanding of the patient's perspective, and character to do the right thing. It is the ability of experts to engage in reflective analysis in patient care that leads to deliberate action to do the right thing with their patients. The challenge in professional education is to teach the complex ensemble of analytic thinking, skilful practice and wise judgement that is required in the health professions. This skilful ethical comportment based on principled reasoning, virtue and a care orientation is the foundation of expertise.

References

Barrows H S, Pickell G C 1991 Developing clinical problem-solving skills: a guide to more effective diagnosis and treatment. Norton, New York

Beauchamp T, Childress J 2001 Principles of biomedical ethics, 5th edn. Oxford University Press, Oxford

Benner P 1984 From novice to expert: excellence and power in clinical nursing practice. Addison-Wesley, Menlo Park, CA

Benner P, Tanner C A, Chesla C A 1996 Expertise in nursing practice. Springer, New York

Benner P, Tanner C A, Chesla C A 1997 The social fabric of nursing knowledge. American Journal of Nursing 97(6): 16BBB–16DDD

Benner P, Hooper-Kyriakidis P, Stannard D 1999 Clinical wisdom and interventions in critical care. W B Saunders, Philadelphia

Bereiter C, Scardamalia M 1993 Surpassing ourselves: an inquiry into the nature and implications of expertise. Open Court Press, Chicago

Berliner D 1986 In pursuit of the expert pedagogue. Educational Researcher 15(7):5–13

Boshuizen H, Bromme R, Gruber H 2004 Professional learning: gaps and transitions on the way from novice to expert. Kluwer Academic, Norwell, MA

Brandsford J, Brown A, Cocking R 2000 How people learn: brain, mind, experience and school. National Academy Press, Washington, DC, p 31–50

Chase W G, Simon H A 1973 Perception in chess. Cognitive Psychology 4:55–81

Chi M T, Feltovich P J, Glaser R 1981 Categorization and representation of physics problems by experts and novices. Cognitive Science 5:121–152

Chi M T, Glaser R, Farr M 1988 The nature of expertise. Lawrence Erlbaum, Hillsdale, NJ

DeGroot A D 1966 Perception and memory versus thought. In: Kleinmuntz B (ed) Problem solving research, methods, and theory. Wiley, New York, p 19–50

Dewey J 1910 How we think. University of Chicago, Chicago

Dreyfus H L, Dreyfus S L 1980 A five stage model of the mental activities involved in directed skill acquisition. Unpublished report supported by the Air Force of Scientific Research (AFSC), USAF (Contract F49620-79-C—63), University of California, Berkeley

Dreyfus H L, Dreyfus S E 1996 The relationship of theory and practice in the acquisition of skill. In: Benner P, Tanner C A, Chesla C A (eds) Expertise in nursing practice. Springer, New York, p 29–48

Edwards I, Jones M, Carr J et al 2004 Clinical reasoning strategies in physical therapy. Physical Therapy 84(4): 312–335

Elstein A S, Schwartz A 2000 Clinical reasoning in medicine. In: Higgs J, Jones M (eds) Clinical reasoning in the health professions, 2nd edn. Butterworth-Heinemann, Oxford, p 95–106

Elstein A S, Shulman L S, Sprafka S A 1978 Medical problem solving: an analysis of clinical reasoning. Harvard University Press, Cambridge, MA

Elstein A S, Shulman L S, Sprafka S A 1990 Medical problem solving: a ten year retrospective. Evaluation and the Health Professions 13:5–36

Epstein R M 1999 Mindful practice. Journal of the American Medical Association 282:833–839

Eraut M 1994 Developing professional knowledge and competence. Falmer Press, London

Ericsson K A (ed) 1996 The road to excellence. Lawrence Erlbaum, Mahwah, NJ

Ericsson K A, Smith J (eds) 1991 Toward a general theory of expertise. Cambridge University Press, New York

Fleming M H, Mattingly C 2000 Action and narrative: two dynamics of clinical reasoning. In: Higgs J, Jones M (eds) Clinical reasoning in the health professions, 2nd edn. Butterworth-Heinemann, Oxford, p 54–61

Glaser R, Chi M TH 1988 Overview. In: Chi M TH, Glaser R, Farr M J (eds) The nature of expertise. Lawrence Erlbaum, Hillsdale, NJ, p xv–xxviii

Gruppen L D, Frohna A Z 2002 Clinical reasoning. In: Norman G R, van der Vleuten C PM, Newble D I (eds) International handbook of research in medical education. Kluwer Academic, Dordrecht, p 205–230

Gwyer J, Jensen G M, Hack L et al 2004 Using a multiple case-study research design to develop an understanding of clinical expertise in physical therapy. In: Hammell K W, Carpenter C (eds) Qualitative research in evidence-based rehabilitation. Churchill-Livingstone, New York, p 103–115

Harris I B 1993 New expectations for professional competence. In: Curry L, Wergin J F et al (eds) Educating professionals: responding to new expectations for competence and accountability. Jossey-Bass, San Francisco, p 17–52

Higgs J, Jones M 2000 Clinical reasoning in the health professions, 2nd edn. Butterworth-Heinemann, Oxford

Higgs J, Titchen A 2001 Practice knowledge and expertise in the health professions. Butterworth-Heinemann, Oxford

Holyoak K J 1991 Symbolic connectionism: toward third-generation theories of expertise. In: Ericsson K A, Smith J (eds) Toward a general theory of expertise. Cambridge University Press, New York, p 301–336

Jensen G M, Gwyer J, Hack L M et al 1999 Expertise in physical therapy practice. Butterworth-Heinemann, Boston

Jensen G M, Gwyer J, Shepard K F et al 2000 Expert practice in physical therapy. Physical Therapy 80(1):28–43

Jensen G M, Gwyer J, Hack L M et al 2007 Expertise in physical therapy practice. 2nd edn. Saunders-Elsevier, St Louis

Jones M A 1992 Clinical reasoning in manual therapy. Physical Therapy 72:875–884

Jones M A, Rivett D A 2004 Clinical reasoning for manual therapists. Butterworth-Heinemann, Edinburgh

Kennedy M 1987 Inexact sciences: professional education and the development of expertise. Review of Research in Education 14:133–168

Loewy E H 2000 The role of reason, emotion, and aesthetics in making ethical judgments. In: Thomasma D, Kissell J (eds) The health care professional as friend and healer. Georgetown University Press, Washington, DC, p 210–226

Mattingly C, Fleming M H 1994 Clinical reasoning: forms of inquiry in a therapeutic practice. F A Davis, Philadelphia

Newell A, Simon H A 1972 Human problem solving. Prentice-Hall, Englewood Cliffs, NJ

Noddings N 1984 Caring: a feminine approach to ethics and moral education. University of California Press, Berkeley

Norman G R, Trott A L, Brooks L R et al 1994 Cognitive differences in clinical reasoning related to postgraduate training. Teaching and Learning in Medicine 6:114–120

Resnik L, Hart D 2003 Using clinical outcomes to identify expert physical therapists. Physical Therapy 83:990–1002

Resnik L, Jensen G M 2003 Using clinical outcomes to explore the theory of expert practice in physical therapy. Physical Therapy 83(12):1090–1106

Rikers R, Paas F 2005 Recent advances in expertise research. Applied Cognitive Psychology 19:145–149

Rivett D, Higgs J 1995 Experience and expertise in clinical reasoning. New Zealand Journal of Physiotherapy 23(1): 16–21

Rothstein J 1999 Foreword II. In: Jensen G, Gwyer J, Hack L et al (eds) Expertise in physical therapy practice. Butterworth-Heinemann, Boston, p xviii

Rothstein J M, Echternach J L 1986 Hypothesis-oriented algorithm for clinicians: a method for evaluation and treatment planning. Physical Therapy 66:1388–1394

Ryle G 1949 The concept of the mind. University of Chicago Press, Chicago

Schön D A 1983 The reflective practitioner: how professionals think in action. Basic Books, New York

Schön D 1987 Educating the reflective practitioner. Jossey-Bass, San Francisco

Schön D A (ed) 1991 The reflective turn: case studies in and on educational practice. Teachers College Press, New York

Shepard K, Hack L, Gwyer J et al 1999 Describing expert practice. Qualitative Health Research 9:746–758

Sherman N 1995 Emotions. In: Reich W (ed) The encyclopedia of bioethics, 2nd edn. Macmillan, New York, p 664

Sternberg R 1998 Abilities are forms of developing expertise. Educational Researcher 28:11–20

Sternberg R J, Horvath J A 1995 A prototype view of expert teaching. Educational Researcher 24:9–17

Sullivan W 2005 Work and integrity: the crisis and promise of professionalism in America. Jossey-Bass, San Francisco, p 221–256

Tsui A 2003 Understanding expertise in teaching. Cambridge University Press, New York

Chapter 12

Clinical reasoning and biomedical knowledge: implications for teaching

David R. Kaufman, Nicole A. Yoskowitz and Vimla L. Patel

Health science curricula worldwide are undergoing significant structural changes that are likely to shape the practice of the health sciences for decades to come. The role of biomedical knowledge in clinical medicine is one of the focal issues in this transformation. Basic science knowledge reflects a subset of biomedical knowledge, although the two terms are often used interchangeably. There are many competing views and assumptions concerning the role of biomedical knowledge and its proper place in a health science curriculum. In this chapter we consider some of these arguments in the context of empirical evidence from cognitive studies in medicine. The role of basic science knowledge is a subject of considerable debate in medical education. It is generally accepted that basic science or biomedical knowledge provides a foundation upon which clinical knowledge can be built. However, its precise role in medical reasoning is controversial (Norman 2000). Biomedical knowledge has undergone a dramatic transformation over the past 30 years, presenting unique and formidable challenges to medical education (Association of American Medical Colleges (AAMC) 2004). There is considerable uncertainty concerning the relationship between basic science conceptual knowledge and the clinical practice of physicians (e.g. Woods et al 2005). There continues to be a dramatic increase in the volume of medical knowledge, especially in cellular and molecular biology (Shaywitz et al 2000). In the past, medical schools have typically responded by adding the new content to existing courses, increasing the number of lectures and textbook readings (D'eon

& Crawford 2005). This has changed somewhat as clinical courses have become more routine in the first two years of medical school (AAMC 2004). In addition, basic science courses are increasingly competing with new curricular demands and objectives, for example to improve professionalism and patient-centred care (AAMC 2006).

THE FUTURE ROLE OF BASIC SCIENCE KNOWLEDGE

There have been increasing expressions of dissatisfaction with basic science teaching in medicine. It has been argued that substantial parts of the basic science in medical schools are irrelevant to the future needs of practitioners (Neame 1984). Furthermore, the method of presenting information in a didactic lecture format and with text readings that do not usually include clinical reasoning exercises encourages passivity and rote learning, which inhibits the development of understanding (Patel et al 2004). This has been increasingly recognized by medical educators, and medical schools have taken steps to make basic science teaching more clinically relevant (Benbassat et al 2005).

In the past 20 years, information technology has had a profound effect on the practice of medicine (Shortliffe & Blois 2006). However, the ways in which these changes should affect clinical training is the subject of ongoing debate in medical informatics (Patel & Kaufman 2006). Information technology can provide access to a wealth of information and has the potential to improve patient care substantially. Serious concerns have been raised about whether future health science practitioners will continue to require the kinds of scientific training that their predecessors received. According to Prokop (1992), there are clear historical trends that are likely to continue. New discoveries in science will continue to provide physicians with increasingly powerful investigative tools with which to see the workings of the human body and through which to prevent disease. When we consider the historical precedents, it seems likely that the best clinical judgement will require a broader understanding of both biology and medicine than ever before (Prokop 1992). A relatively recent report by the AAMC (2001, p. 5) proposed:

> Medical practice should be based on a sound understanding of the scientific basis of contemporary approaches to the diagnosis and management of disease. Therefore, knowledge and understanding of the scientific principles that govern human biology provide doctors not only with a rationale for the contemporary practice of medicine, but also with a framework for incorporating new knowledge into their practices in the future.

It is likely that advances in genomics, proteomics (defined as 'the study of the set of proteins produced (expressed) by an organism, tissue or cell, and the changes in protein expression patterns in different environments and conditions'; University of Indiana 2007) and bioinformatics will influence clinical medicine in the near future and it will therefore need to be incorporated into medical curricula. In addition, an increased risk for infectious diseases such as SARS and bird flu, as well as the potential dangers of agents of bio-terrorism are new risks that physicians must be prepared to grapple with (Debas 2000, Fauci 2005). Given that treatment guidelines are unlikely to cover the spectrum of emerging illnesses, it may be necessary for clinicians to have a deeper understanding of dangerous pathogens and how they may affect human disease.

CURRICULAR AND EPISTEMOLOGICAL ISSUES

Clinical knowledge includes knowledge of disease entities and associated findings, and basic science knowledge incorporates subject matter such as biochemistry, anatomy and physiology. Basic science or biomedical knowledge provides a scientific foundation for clinical reasoning. It had been widely accepted that biomedical and clinical knowledge can be seamlessly integrated into a coherent knowledge structure that supports all cognitive aspects of medical practice, such as diagnostic and therapeutic reasoning (Feinstein 1973). From this perspective, clinical and biomedical knowledge become intricately intertwined, providing medical practice with a sound scientific basis. Since the Flexner report (1910), medical schools have made a strong commitment to this epistemological framework. The report recommended the partitioning of the medical curriculum into a basic science component and an applied component. Medical educators and researchers have argued over how to best promote clinical skill as well as foster robust conceptual change (Boshuizen & Schmidt 1992, Clough et al 2004, Patel & Groen 1986).

Traditionally, the curricula of most medical schools during the first and second years involve preclinical courses which predominantly teach the basic sciences. The remaining two years of medical school and further postgraduate training consist of clinical courses and practica. This has begun to change in recent years, in part as a result of the growing popularity of problem-based learning (PBL). In PBL programmes, instruction involving clinically meaningful problems is introduced at the beginning of the curriculum. This practice is guided by the assumption that scientific knowledge taught abstractly does not help students to integrate it with clinical practice (Norman & Schmidt 2000). Recently, conventional or traditional clinical schools have embraced the idea of emphasizing a more clinically relevant basic science curriculum. Following PBL, they have also incorporated small group teaching and have focused more on fostering clinical skills. The renewed emphasis on skills and competency has been partly in response to reports indicating that patient care is sub-optimal. In particular, reports by the Institute of Medicine (e.g. 2001) characterized a state of affairs in which medical errors have caused an alarming number of deaths in the USA and the quality of care has been found to be deficient in significant respects. Studies have also indicated that physicians are not very effective in communicating with patients (Debas 2000) or in conducting physical examinations (Benbassat et al 2005), deficiencies which are likely to contribute to the problems associated with quality of care.

The AAMC issued reports (e.g. 2004, 2006) outlining a vision for undergraduate, graduate and continuing medical education. The reports advocate a series of strategies for reforming medical education to promote a more patient-centred approach and a more rigorous approach for ensuring that students and residents are acquiring the knowledge, skills, attitudes and values deemed necessary to provide high-quality patient care. It

is hard to quarrel with the objectives set forth in the AAMC reports. However, the renewed focus on clinical skills and competencies introduces additional demands on an already crowded undergraduate curriculum. The first two years of medical school were largely devoted to basic science content, but now there is a need to shift towards a more clinically-centred model.

Medical problem solving can be characterized as ill-structured, in the sense that the initial states, the definite goal state and the necessary constraints are unknown at the beginning of the problem-solving process. In a diagnostic situation, the problem space of potential findings and associated diagnoses is enormous. The problem space becomes defined through the imposition of a set of plausible constraints that facilitate the application of specific decision strategies (Pople 1982). For example, when faced with a multi-system problem such as hypokalemic periodic paralysis associated with hyperthyroidism, a physician may need to confirm the more common disorder of hyperthyroidism before solving the more vexing problem of hypokalemia. Once this is confirmed, there is a set of constraints in place such that there are classes of disorders that co-occur with hyperthyroidism and there is a set of symptoms that have not yet been accounted for by this disorder and are consistent with hypokalemic periodic paralysis. As expertise develops, the disease knowledge of a clinician becomes more dependent on clinical experience, and clinical problem solving is increasingly guided by the use of exemplars, becoming less dependent on a functional understanding of the system in question. Biomedical knowledge, by comparison, is of a qualitatively different nature, embodying elements of causal mechanisms and characterizing patterns of perturbation in function and structure.

The focus of the instructional approach for the biomedical curriculum is necessarily on the extensive coverage of a broad corpus of knowledge as opposed to in-depth conceptual understanding. The volume of information in any one of the basic science disciplines is now so large that it cannot be completely mastered even by a full-time graduate student pursuing doctoral studies for 5 years (Prokop 1992). It is unreasonable to expect that medical students can master five or more fields in the first 24 months of medical school. In our view it is not tenable, given a finite time frame and finite psychological resources, to coordinate these multiple sources of knowledge and harmonize all biomedical knowledge with a clinical body of knowledge of disease entities and associated findings.

Feltovich and colleagues (1993) proposed that medicine can be construed as a domain of advanced knowledge acquisition. These domains necessitate learning that takes place beyond the initial or introductory stages. For example, medical students are expected to have a substantial background in the biological sciences. Much of the basic science subject matter in medical schools is predicated on the fact that students have a basic mastery of the introductory materials, so that instructors can focus on more advanced topics. The goal of introductory learning is to provide exposure to large areas of content with the goal of providing a basic literacy or familiarity with the domain. There is not much emphasis on conceptual mastery of knowledge. Advanced knowledge acquisition carries the expectation of students attaining a deeper understanding of the content material and the ability to use it flexibly and productively in diverse contexts. Although we view many of the curricular changes as a substantive improvement, there are lingering questions as to the effect on mastery of basic science knowledge.

RESEARCH IN CLINICAL REASONING

In this section we review some of the pertinent research in medical reasoning, particularly research that addresses the role of basic science knowledge in clinical medicine. Studies in medical clinical reasoning encompass different domains of knowledge (e.g. cardiology and radiology), a wide range of performance tasks, and various theoretical approaches (e.g. expert reasoning as a process, as memory, and as knowledge representations).

CLINICAL REASONING STRATEGIES AND EXPERTISE

Lesgold et al (1988) investigated the abilities of radiologists at different levels of training and expertise to interpret chest X-ray pictures and provide a diagnosis. Experts were able to initially detect a general pattern of disease with a gross anatomical localization, serving to constrain the possible interpretations. Novices had greater difficulty focusing on the important structures, being more likely to maintain inappropriate interpretations despite discrepant findings in the patient history. The authors concluded that the knowledge that underlies expertise in radiology includes the mental representation of anatomy, a theory of anatomical perturbation, and the constructive capacity to transform the visual image into a three-dimensional representation. The less expert subjects had greater difficulty in building and maintaining a rich anatomical representation of the patient.

Norman et al (1989) compared dermatologists' performance at various levels of expertise in tasks that required them to diagnose and sort dermatological slides according to the type of skin lesion evident. Expert dermatologists were more accurate in their diagnoses and took significantly less time to respond than novices. The sorting task revealed that each group sorted the slides according to different category types. Experts grouped the slides into superordinate categories such as viral infections, which reflected the underlying pathophysiological structure. Novices tended to classify lesions according to surface features such as scaly lesions. The implication is that expert knowledge is organized around domain principles which facilitate the rapid recognition of significant problem features. It supports the idea that experts employ a qualitatively different kind of knowledge to solve problems based on a deeper understanding of domain principles.

The picture that emerges from research on expertise across domains is that experts use a quite different pattern of reasoning from that used by novices or intermediates, and organize their knowledge differently. Three important aspects are that experts: (a) have a greater ability to organize information into semantically meaningful, interrelated chunks; (b) do not process irrelevant information; and (c) in routine situations, tend to use highly specific knowledge-based problem-solving strategies (Ericsson & Smith 1991). The use of knowledge-based strategies has given rise to an important distinction between a data-driven strategy (forward reasoning) in which hypotheses are generated from data, and a hypothesis-driven strategy (backward reasoning) in which one reasons backward from a hypothesis and attempts to find data that elucidate it. Forward reasoning is based on domain knowledge and is thus highly error-prone in the absence of adequate domain knowledge. Backward reasoning is slower and may make heavy demands on working memory (because one has to keep track of goals and hypotheses), and is most likely to be used when domain knowledge is inadequate. Backward reasoning is characteristic of non-experts and experts solving non-routine problems (Patel et al 2005).

In experiments with expert physicians in cardiology, endocrinology and respiratory medicine, clinicians showed little tendency to use basic science in explaining cases, whereas medical researchers showed preference for detailed, basic scientific explanations, without developing clinical descriptions (Patel et al 1989). In medicine, the pathophysiological explanation task has been used to examine clinical reasoning (Feltovich & Barrows 1984). This task requires subjects to explain the causal pattern underlying a set of clinical symptoms. Protocols from this task can be used to investigate the ability of clinicians to apply basic science concepts in diagnosing a clinical problem. In one study (Patel & Groen 1986), expert practitioners (cardiologists) were asked to solve problems within their domain of expertise. Their explanations of the underlying pathophysiology of the cases, whether correctly or incorrectly diagnosed, made virtually no use of basic science knowledge. In a similar study (Patel et al 1990), cardiologists and endocrinologists solved problems both within and outside their domains of expertise. The clinicians did not appeal to principles from basic biomedical science, even when they were working outside their own domain of expertise; rather, they relied on clinical associations and classifications to formulate solutions. The results suggest that basic science does not contribute directly to reasoning in clinical problem solving for experienced clinicians. However, biomedical information was used by practitioners when the task was difficult or when they were uncertain about their diagnosis. In these cases, biomedical information was used in a backward-directed manner, providing coherence to the explanation of clinical cues that could

not be easily accounted for by the primary diagnostic hypothesis that was being considered.

There have been many other studies highlighting the difficulty of integrating basic and clinical knowledge (e.g. Boshuizen & Schmidt 1992, Patel et al 1993, Woods et al 2005). Pathophysiological information is used by physicians and senior medical students either when the problem-solving process breaks down (i.e. no obvious solution) or to explain loose ends (i.e. leftover findings) that cannot be accounted for by the diagnostic hypothesis(es). In general, there is evidence to suggest that unprompted use of biomedical concepts in clinical reasoning decreases as a function of expertise. In addition, students have difficulty in applying basic science concepts in contexts that differ from the initial conditions of learning (Patel et al 1993). The first three studies described in this section focus on expertise in visual diagnosis and suggest a more transparent role for basic science knowledge than does the work on expertise in the domains of cardiology and endocrinology. Although pattern recognition is an important aspect of all diagnostic expertise, certain domains necessitate a greater use of core biomedical concepts in understanding even basic problems.

BASIC SCIENCE IN STUDENTS' EXPLANATIONS OF CLINICAL CASES

We conducted a series of experiments to elucidate the precise role of basic science in clinical reasoning and to determine to what extent the two areas are complementary (Patel et al 1990, 1991). Subjects were McGill University medical students who were either first year students, second year students who had completed all basic medical sciences but had not begun any clinical work, or final year students 3 months before graduation. Students were presented with three basic science tests (e.g. microcirculation) immediately prior to a clinical case of acute bacterial endocarditis (Patel et al 1989). This procedure was designed to maximize the likelihood that subjects would use related information from separate knowledge sources. Subjects read the four texts, recalled in writing what they had read, and then explained the clinical problem in terms of the basic science texts.

In general, subjects' recall of the basic science texts was poor, indicating a lack of well-developed knowledge structures in which to organize this information. Recall of the clinical text appeared to be a function of clinical experience, but there was no similar correlation between basic science and experience. In the explanation of the problem, second year students made extensive use of basic science knowledge. Fourth year students gave explanations that resembled those of expert physicians outside their domain of specialization, except that the students made more extensive use of basic science information than found in experts' explanations. It was interesting to note that their greater use of basic science actually resulted in more consistent inferences. Our results indicate that basic science knowledge was used differently by the three groups of subjects.

In a second experiment, students recalled and explained cases when basic science information was provided after the clinical problem (Patel et al 1990). We can characterize reasoning as a two-stage process: diagnostic reasoning is characterized by inference from observation to hypothesis; and predictive reasoning is characterized by inference from hypothesis to observations. Fourth year students were able to use the basic science information in a highly effective manner, facilitating both diagnostic and predictive reasoning. Second year students were also able to use this information effectively, but diagnostic reasoning was not facilitated. First year students were not able to use basic science information any more effectively when it was given after the clinical problem than when it was given before the clinical problem. These results suggest that reasoning toward a diagnosis from the facts of a case was frustrated by attempting to use basic science knowledge unless the student had already developed a strong diagnostic hypothesis. Thus, the addition of basic science knowledge seemed to improve the accuracy of diagnoses offered by final year medical students, but did not improve the accuracy of diagnoses by first and second year students. It is likely that final year students, who had had some clinical experience, relied on clinically relevant features in a case to (broadly) classify the diagnosis and make selective predictions of

features that were susceptible to analysis in terms of the basic science facts they had read (Patel et al 1989). This tendency of clinical solutions to subordinate basic scientific ones, and for basic science not to support the clinical organization of facts in a case, was evident among expert physicians as discussed earlier. These results were also consistent with other findings suggesting that unprompted use of biomedical concepts in clinical reasoning decreases as a function of expertise (Boshuizen & Schmidt 1992).

REASONING AND BIOMEDICAL KNOWLEDGE IN DIFFERENT MEDICAL CURRICULA

As discussed previously, in problem-based learning (PBL) programmes, instruction involves the introduction of clinically meaningful problems introduced at the beginning of the curriculum, based on the assumption that scientific knowledge taught abstractly does not help students to integrate it with clinical practice (Norman & Schmidt 2000). In general, research evaluating the performance of PBL and conventional curricula (CC) programmes has found negligible differences in terms of clinical skills (Jolly 2006). Nevertheless, the different curricula are predicated on different assumptions about how best to foster conceptual change. PBL programmes are based on the necessity of connecting scientific concepts to the conditions of application, whereas CC programmes emphasize the importance of fostering a foundation of general scientific knowledge that is broadly applicable. The CC runs the risk of imparting inert knowledge, much of which is not retained beyond medical school and is not readily applicable to clinical contexts. On the other hand, PBL curricula may promote knowledge that is so tightly coupled to context (e.g. a featured clinical case of hypothyroidism) as to have minimum generality beyond the immediate set of problems.

Patel et al (1993) attempted to replicate the above studies in an established PBL medical school at McMaster University. Results showed that when basic science information was provided before the clinical problem, there was again a lack of integration of basic science into the clinical context. This resulted in a lack of global coherence in knowledge structures, errors of scientific fact and disruption of the diagnostic reasoning process. When basic science was given after the clinical problem, there was again integration of basic science into the clinical context. It is concluded that clinical problems cannot be easily embedded into a basic science context, but basic science can be more naturally embedded within a clinical context. It is our belief that when one is attempting to learn two unknown domains, it is better to learn one well so that it can be used as an 'anchor' for the new domain. Basic science knowledge may serve as a better anchor than clinical knowledge. It may be useful to introduce some core basic science at the beginning of the curriculum, followed by an early introduction of clinical problems that are thematically connected to the specific scientific concepts.

The findings of these studies suggest that in the conventional curriculum: (a) basic science and clinical knowledge are generally kept separate; (b) clinical reasoning may not require basic science knowledge; (c) basic science is spontaneously used only when students get into difficulty with the patient problem; and (d) basic science serves to generate globally coherent explanations of the patient problem with connections between various components of the clinical problem. It is proposed that in a conventional curriculum, the clinical aspect of the problem is viewed as separate from the biomedical science aspect, the two having different functions. In the PBL curriculum, basic science and clinical knowledge are spontaneously integrated. However, this integration results in students' inability to decontextualize the problem, in that the basic science is so tightly tied to the clinical context that students appear unable to detach it even when the clinical situation demands it. In addition, a greater number of elaborations are made when students think about problem features using basic science and clinical information. However, these greater elaborations result in fragmentation of knowledge structures, resulting in the lack of global coherence (various parts of the problem are not connected). Finally, within PBL such elaborations result in factual errors that persist from first year students' responses to the final year. There are multiple competencies involved in the

practice of medicine, some of which are best fostered in the context of real-world practice and others best acquired through a process of formal learning. It has become more apparent that the extent to which aspects of a domain are best learned in context is determined jointly by the nature of domain knowledge and the kinds of tasks that are performed by practitioners (Patel & Kaufman 2006).

Recently, Patel et al (2001) compared the problem-solving performance of house staff with undergraduate medical training in CC or PBL schools. As in the previous studies, house staff were given two clinical cases to read, after which they provided differential diagnoses and explanations of the pathophysiology of the problem. Results showed that CC house staff focused on clinical information from the given case rather than biomedical information and used more forward reasoning, whereas the PBL house staff generated more biomedical inferences and used more backward reasoning. These findings are consistent with the performance of medical students in PBL schools (Patel et al 1993), suggesting that the effects of medical training endure well into residency.

Small group teaching (SGT) is one of the characteristics of PBL, though many conventional curricula have begun to incorporate it as well. Patel et al (2004) investigated the relationship between SGT and lecture teaching and how biomedical and clinical knowledge is integrated across these teaching formats. Whereas the lecture served as a means to cover core biomedical material broadly, the small groups allowed for further discussion and integration of the biomedical and clinical knowledge in an interactive and intimate environment. Thus the use of both lectures and SGT supported the objective of providing students with a strong foundation in biomedical knowledge, which could be integrated and used in clinical practice. This point has been supported by another study (Patel et al 2005), where the effects of introducing problem-based small group tutorials into a conventional medical curriculum were evaluated among students at various levels of expertise. Findings suggested that a hybrid medical curriculum may be effective at promoting integration of biomedical and clinical knowledge. Valuable insights can be gained by investigating the ways in which learning activities employed in the different systems differentially contribute to clinical competencies and knowledge.

PROGRESSIONS IN UNDERSTANDING OF BIOMEDICAL CONCEPTS

In the preceding studies we examined the role of basic science knowledge in a clinical context. In this section, we focus on a study related to students' understanding of important biomedical concepts. Patel et al (1991) examined medical students' understanding of complex biomedical concepts in cardiopulmonary physiology. They found that students at the end of their first year of medical school exhibited significant misconceptions in reasoning about ventilation–perfusion matching in the context of a clinical problem, and that they were not able to map clinical findings onto pathophysiological manifestations. The findings of this study are consistent with other research (cf. Patel et al 1989) that indicates that students' oversimplified representations of biomedical phenomena fail to support clinical reasoning. The research of Feltovich et al (1993) in the related domain of congestive heart failure documented widespread misconceptions in students' and in some medical practitioners' understanding of the structure and function of the cardiovascular system.

We conducted a study (Kaufman et al 1996, Kaufman & Patel 1998) to characterize students' and physicians' understanding of biomedical concepts in cardiovascular physiology. Subjects were presented with questions and problems pertaining to the concepts of cardiac output, venous return and the mechanical properties of the cardiovascular and circulatory system. The stimulus material covered basic physiology (e.g. the effects of an increase in preload on stroke volume); applied physiology (e.g. extreme exercise); pathophysiology (e.g. the haemodynamic effects of haemorrhage); medical disorders (e.g. congestive heart failure); and brief clinical problems. This afforded us an opportunity to investigate subjects' reasoning within and across levels in the hierarchical chain of biomedicine.

In general, we observed a progression of mental models as a function of expertise, as evidenced in predictive accuracy which increased with expertise and in the quality of explanations (Kaufman & Patel 1998). Progression was also noted in the quality of explanations in response to individual questions and problems and in terms of the overall coherence of subjects' representations of the cardiovascular and circulatory system (see Patel et al 2000). The study documented a wide range of conceptual errors in subjects at different levels of expertise. There were particular misconceptions that would appear to be a function of formal learning. For example, a misconception was manifested in the responses of six subjects, including two fourth year students and two cardiology residents. It was related to a confounding of venous resistance and venous compliance. The notion is that since an increase in venous resistance is associated with a decrease in compliance, then the net effect of resistance would be to increase venous return. If one considers the meaning of resistance, which all of these subjects clearly understood, then it appears quite counterintuitive that resistance can facilitate (as opposed to impede) blood flow. This would suggest that this misconception is a function of formal learning rather than acquired through experience.

The more advanced subjects in our study, including the senior students and physicians, experienced more difficulty in responding to the basic physiology than they did applying the same concepts in more clinically oriented problems. On several occasions, the physicians would use clinical analogies to explain physiological processes. More often than not, the analogies did not successfully result in correct explanations. However, when provided with pathophysiological conditions or medical disorders requiring pathophysiological explanations (e.g. congestive heart failure), the physicians drew on their clinical knowledge to great effect. The distance in the hierarchy (e.g. from physical science to pathophysiology) had a considerable effect on the likelihood of successful transfer of knowledge. Understanding of these basic science concepts could have implications for particular therapeutic practices such as fluid management.

This section serves to highlight the complexity of basic science knowledge in medicine. As in other domains, novices as well as more experienced subjects exhibited misconceptions that led to faulty patterns of reasoning. Mental models, even in expert subjects, tended to be imperfect and at times imprecise. Experienced physicians who were less than experts showed evidence of significant faults in their understanding of biomedical knowledge. However, these faults did not necessarily impair their ability to engage in clinical reasoning except under circumstances where such knowledge is necessary (e.g. a very complex case).

THE WORLDS OF BIOMEDICAL KNOWLEDGE AND CLINICAL SCIENCE

We have considered epistemological and curricular issues related to the role of basic science knowledge in clinical medicine, discussed empirical studies related to the use of biomedical knowledge in clinical reasoning contexts, and considered studies that examined students' and physicians' understanding of biomedical concepts. What inferences can we make concerning the role of basic science knowledge in clinical reasoning? We will consider two theoretical hypotheses.

Patel & Groen (1991) proposed that clinical and basic science knowledge bases constitute 'two worlds' connected at discrete points. Schmidt and Boshuizen offered a more integrative perspective. The basis of their theory is a learning mechanism, *knowledge encapsulation*, which explains how biomedical knowledge becomes subsumed under clinical knowledge in the development of expertise (Boshuizen & Schmidt 1992, Schmidt & Boshuizen 1993). The process of knowledge encapsulation involves the subsumption of biomedical propositions and associative relations under a small number of higher level clinical propositions with the same explanatory power. These authors argued that through repeated application of knowledge in medical training and practice, networks of causal biomedical knowledge become incorporated into a comprehensive clinical concept (Van de Wiel 1997). Basic science knowledge is not typically used in routine circumstances by experts, but is readily available. The knowledge encapsulation thesis has spawned an impressive body of research. In this section we consider both hypotheses, starting with the two worlds hypothesis.

The crux of the two worlds hypothesis is that these two bodies of knowledge differ in important respects, including the nature of constituent knowledge elements and the kinds of reasoning they support. Clinical reasoning involves the coordination of diagnostic hypotheses with clinical evidence. Biomedical reasoning involves the use of causal models at varying levels of abstraction (e.g. organ and cellular levels). The evidence from medical problem-solving studies suggests that routine diagnostic reasoning is largely a classification process in which groups of findings become associated with hypotheses. Basic science knowledge is not typically evident in expert think-aloud protocols in these circumstances.

Under conditions of uncertainty, physicians resort to scientific explanations which are coherent, even when they are not completely accurate. The role of basic science, aside from providing the concepts and vocabulary required to formulate clinical problems, is to create a basis for establishing and assessing coherence in the explanation of biomedical phenomena. Basic science does not provide the axioms, analogies or abstractions required to support clinical problem solving. Rather, it provides the principles that make it possible to organize observations that defy ready clinical classification and analysis. Biomedical knowledge also provides a means for explaining, justifying and communicating medical decisions. It also facilitates retention and retrieval (Woods et al 2005). In the absence of basic science, the relationships between symptoms and diagnoses seem arbitrary.

The two worlds hypothesis is consistent with a model of conceptual change in which clinical knowledge and basic science knowledge undergo both joint and separate processes of reorganization. This is partly a function of the kinds of learning experience that students undergo. The premedical years are focused primarily on the acquisition of biomedical knowledge. As students become increasingly involved in clinical activities, the prioritization of knowledge also shifts to concepts that support the process of clinical reasoning. Schmidt & Boshuizen (1993) proposed a developmental process in which students early in their training acquire 'rich elaborated causal networks explaining the causes and consequences of disease' in terms of biomedical knowledge (p. 207). Through repeated exposure to patient problems, the basic science knowledge becomes encapsulated into high-level simplified causal models explaining signs and symptoms. The knowledge structures acquired through different developmental phases remain available when clinical knowledge is not adequate to explain a clinical problem.

Intermediates require additional processing time to accomplish a task as compared to experts and at times, even novices. For example, in pathophysiological explanations, intermediates generate lengthy lines of reasoning that employ numerous biomedical concepts. On the other hand, experts use shortcuts in their line of reasoning, skipping intervening steps (Kuipers & Kassirer 1984). A common finding is that intermediates (typically senior medical students or residents early in their training) recall more information from a clinical case than either novices or experts. Novices lack the knowledge to integrate the information, whereas experts selectively attend to and recall only the relevant information. Similarly, in pathophysiological explanation tasks, intermediates tend to use more biomedical knowledge and more elaborations than either novices or experts. The extra processing is due to the fact that these subjects have accumulated a great deal of conceptual knowledge, but have not fully assimilated it or tuned it to the performance of clinical tasks.

Schmidt and colleagues (Schmidt & Boshuizen 1993, Van de Wiel et al 2000) conducted several studies in which they varied the amount of time that an individual was exposed to stimulus materials. They demonstrated that intermediates were negatively affected by having less time to process the stimulus material, whereas experts were largely unaffected by a reduction in time. The argument is that the immediate activation of a small number of highly relevant encapsulating concepts enables experts to rapidly formulate an adequate representation of a patient problem. On the other hand, students have yet to develop knowledge in an encapsulated form, relying more on biomedical knowledge and requiring more time to construct a coherent case representation. In other studies, Schmidt and colleagues demonstrated that expert clinicians could unfold their abbreviated lines of reasoning into longer chains of inferences that evoked more elaborate

causal models when the situation warranted it (Rikers et al 2002). This was seen as further evidence to support the knowledge encapsulation theory.

The knowledge encapsulation theory may on the one hand overstate the capabilities of experts to rapidly activate elaborated biomedical models when circumstances warrant it. On the other hand, by its focus on lines of reasoning, the theory may undermine the generative nature of expert knowledge. Lines of reasoning would suggest that experts have access to limited patterns of inference resulting from repeated exposure to similar cases. There is evidence to suggest that they do have access to a repertoire of such patterns and use it as circumstances warrant it (Van de Wiel et al 2000). It is apparent that people learn to circumvent long chains of reasoning and chunk or compile knowledge across intermediate states of inference. This results in shorter, more direct inferences which are stored in long-term memory and are directly available to be retrieved in the appropriate contexts. We agree that repeated exposure to recurrent patterns of symptoms is likely to result in the chunking of causal inferences that will subsequently be available for reuse (Kaufman & Patel 1998).

However, experts are also capable of solving novel and complex problems which necessitate the generation of new causal models based on a deep understanding of the system. This enables them to work out the consequences of a pathophysiological process that is anomalous or one not previously encountered (Kaufman & Patel 1998). This is necessary when encapsulated knowledge is not available. Mastery of biomedical knowledge may be characterized as a progression of mental models which reflect increasingly sophisticated and robust understandings of pathophysiological processes. Given the vast quantities of knowledge that need to be assimilated in four-year medical curricula, it is not likely that one can develop robust understanding of the pathophysiology of disease. Clinical practice offers selective exposure to certain kinds of clinical cases. Even experts' mental models can be somewhat brittle when stretched to the limits of their understanding (Kaufman & Patel 1998). Knowledge encapsulation may partially account for the process of conceptual change in biomedicine. Clearly, the diversity of biomedical knowledge and clinical reasoning tasks requires multiple mechanisms of learning.

In our view, the notion of knowledge encapsulation represents an idealized perspective of the integration of basic science in clinical knowledge. The reasons for our scepticism lie in several sources. Basic science knowledge plays a different role in different clinical domains. For example, clinical expertise in perceptual domains such as dermatology and radiology requires a relatively robust model of anatomical structures, which is the primary source of knowledge for diagnostic classification (Norman 2000). In other domains, such as cardiology and endocrinology, basic science knowledge has a more distant relationship with clinical knowledge. Furthermore, the misconceptions evident in physicians' biomedical explanations would argue against well-developed encapsulated knowledge structures where basic science knowledge can easily be retrieved and applied when necessary. Our contention is that neither conventional nor problem-based curricula can foster the kind of learning suggested by the encapsulation process.

It is our view that the results of research into medical clinical reasoning are consistent with the idea that clinical medicine and biomedical sciences constitute two distinct worlds, with distinct modes of reasoning and quite different ways of structuring knowledge (Patel et al 1989). Learning to explain how a set of symptoms is consistent with a diagnosis may be very different from learning to explain what causes a disease. The challenge for medical schools is to strike the right balance between presenting information in applied contexts and allowing students to derive the appropriate abstractions and generalizations to further develop their models of conceptual understanding.

We have proposed that basic science knowledge is valuable in the development of coherence in the explanation of clinical phenomena. In response to the proposal that the teaching of basic science and clinical knowledge should be completely merged, Trelstad (1991, p. 1186) argued that 'basic science is a unique and special activity that when melded into a clinical environment, will only be diluted in focus and quality'. This suggestion echoes the concerns and issues raised in this chapter. We believe that although teaching basic science in context is important, it is not sufficient for promoting the robust transfer of usable knowledge. The 'two worlds' hypothesis implies that each body of knowledge be given special status in the medical curriculum and that the correspondences between the two worlds need to be developed. As discussed previously, medical curricular reform is faced with competing pressures. A recent report by the AAMC (2001) articulates a concern that the amount of time devoted to basic science in medical curricula is decreasing. The concern is made more acute by the fact that new knowledge in the biological sciences is increasing rapidly and by the emergence of new scientific domains (e.g. bioinformatics) 'that promise paradigm shifts in clinical thinking'.

References

Association of American Medical Colleges 2001 Report IV. Contemporary issues in medicine: basic science and clinical research. Medical School Objectives Project, Washington, DC

Association of American Medical Colleges 2004 Educating doctors to provide high quality medical care: a vision for medical education in the United States. Report of the Ad Hoc Committee of Deans, Washington, DC

Association of American Medical Colleges 2006 Implementing the vision: group on educational affairs responds to the IIME Dean's Committee report. Washington, DC

Benbassat J, Baumal R, Heyman S N et al 2005 Suggestions for a shift in teaching clinical skills to medical students: the reflective clinical examination. Academic Medicine 80:1121–1126

Boshuizen H P A, Schmidt H G 1992 On the role of biomedical knowledge in clinical reasoning by experts, intermediates and novices. Cognitive Science 16:153–184

Clough R W, Shea S L, Hamilton W R 2004 Weaving basic science and social sciences into a case-based, clinically oriented medical curriculum: one school's approach. Academic Medicine 79:1073–1083

D'eon M, Crawford R 2005 The elusive content of the medical-school curriculum: a method to the madness. Medical Teacher 27:699–703

Debas H T 2000 Medical education and practice: end of century reflections. Archives of Surgery 135:1096–1100

Ericsson K A, Smith J (eds) 1991 Toward a general theory of expertise. Cambridge University Press, New York

Fauci A S 2005 Emerging and reemerging infectious diseases: the perpetual challenge. Academic Medicine 80:1079–1085

Feinstein A R 1973 An analysis of diagnostic reasoning: the domain and disorders of clinical macrobiology. Yale Journal of Biology and Medicine 46:264–283

Feltovich P J, Barrows H S 1984 Issues of generality in medical problem solving. In: Schmidt H G, De Volder M L (eds) Tutorials in problem-based learning: a new direction in teaching the health professions. Van Gorcum, Assen, p 128–142

Feltovich P J, Spiro R, Coulson R L 1993 Learning, teaching and testing for complex conceptual understanding. In: Frederiksen N, Mislevy R, Bejar I (eds) Test theory for a new generation of tests. Erlbaum, Hillsdale, NJ, p 181–217

Flexner A 1910 Medical education in the United States and Canada, Bulletin number four. Carnegie Foundation for the Advancement of Teaching, New York

Institute of Medicine 2001 Crossing the quality chasm: a new health system for the 21st century. National Academy Press, Washington, DC

Jolly B 2006 Problem-based learning. Medical Education 40:494–495

Kaufman D R, Patel V L 1998 Progressions of mental models in understanding circulatory physiology. In: Singh I, Parasuraman R (eds) Human cognition: a multidisciplinary perspective. Sage Publications, New Delhi, p 300–326

Kaufman D R, Patel V L, Magder S A 1996 The explanatory role of spontaneously generated analogies in reasoning about physiological concepts. International Journal of Science Education 18:369–386

Kuipers B J, Kassirer J P 1984 Causal reasoning in medicine: analysis of a protocol. Cognitive Science 8(4):363–385

Lesgold A M, Rubinson H, Feltovich P J et al 1988 Expertise in a complex skill: diagnosing X-ray pictures. In: Chi M T H, Glaser R, Farr M J (eds) The nature of expertise. Lawrence Erlbaum, Hillsdale, NJ, p 311–342

Neame R L B 1984 The preclinical course of study: help or hindrance. Journal of Medical Education 59:699–707

Norman G R 2000 The essential role of basic science in medical education: the perspective from psychology. Clinical Investigative Medicine 23:47–51

Norman G R, Schmidt H G 2000 Effectiveness of problem-based learning curricula: theory, practice and paper darts. Medical Education 34:721–728

Norman G, Brooks L R, Rosenthal D et al 1989 The development of expertise in dermatology. Archives of Dermatology 125:1063–1068

Patel V L, Groen G J 1986 Knowledge-based solution strategies in medical reasoning. Cognitive Science 10:91–116

Patel V L, Groen G J 1991 The general and specific nature of medical expertise: a critical look. In: Ericsson A, Smith J (eds) Toward a general theory of expertise: prospects and limits. Cambridge University Press, New York, p 93–125

Patel V L, Kaufman D R 2006 Cognitive science and biomedical informatics. In: Shortliffe E H, Cimino J J (eds) Biomedical informatics: computer applications in health care and biomedicine. Springer-Verlag, New York, p 133–185

Patel V L, Evans D A, Groen G 1989 Biomedical knowledge and clinical reasoning. In: Evans D A, Patel V L (eds) Cognitive science in medicine: biomedical modelling. MIT Press, Cambridge, p 49–108

Patel V L, Evans D A, Kaufman D R 1990 Reasoning strategies and use of biomedical knowledge by students. Medical Education 24:129–136

Patel V L, Kaufman D R, Magder S 1991 Causal reasoning about complex physiological concepts by medical students. International Journal of Science Education 13:171–185

Patel V L, Groen G J, Norman G R 1993 Reasoning and instruction in medical curricula. Cognition and Instruction 10:335–378

Patel V L, Kaufman D R, Arocha J F 2000 Conceptual change in the biomedical and health sciences. In: Glaser R (ed) Advances in instructional psychology, vol 5. Lawrence Erlbaum, Hillsdale, NJ, p 329–392

Patel V L, Arocha J F, Leccisi M S 2001 Impact of undergraduate medical training on housestaff problem-solving performance: implications for problem-based curricula. Journal of Dental Education 65:1199–1218

Patel V L, Arocha J F, Branch T et al 2004 Relationships between small group problem-solving activity and lectures in health science curricula. Journal of Dental Education 68(10):1058–1080

Patel V L, Arocha J F, Chaudhari S et al 2005 Knowledge integration and reasoning as a function of instruction in a hybrid medical curriculum. Journal of Dental Education 69:186–211

Pople H E 1982 Heuristic methods for imposing structure on ill-structured problems: the structuring of medical diagnostics. In: Szolovitz P (ed) Artificial intelligence in medicine. Westview Press, Boulder, CO, p 119–190

Prokop D J 1992 Basic science and clinical practice: how much will a physician need to know? In: Marston R Q, Jones R M (eds) Medical education in transition. Robert Wood Johnson Foundation, Princeton, p 51–57

Rikers R M J P, Schmidt H G, Boshuizen H PA et al 2002 The robustness of medical expertise: clinical case processing by medical experts and subexperts. American Journal of Psychology 114:609–629

Schmidt H G, Boshuizen H PA 1993 On acquiring expertise in medicine. Educational Psychology Review 5:205–221

Shaywitz D A, Martin J B, Ausiello D A 2000 Patient-oriented research: principles and new approaches to training. American Journal of Medicine 109(2):136–140

Shortliffe E H, Blois M S 2006 The computer meets medicine and biology: emergence of a discipline. In: Shortliffe E H, Cimino J J (eds) Biomedical informatics: computer applications in health care and biomedicine. Springer-Verlag, New York, p 133–185

Trelstad R L 1991 The nation's medical curriculum in transition: progression or retrogression? Reactions to the Robert Wood Johnson Foundation Commission on Medical Education. Human Pathology 22:1183–1186

University of Indiana 2007 Online genomics glossary. Available: http://www.homepages.indiana.edu/120800/text/glossary.html 09 Jan 2007

Van de Wiel M 1997 Knowledge encapsulation: studies on the development of medical expertise. Dissertation, Ponsen and Looijen

Van de Wiel M W J, Boshuizen H P A, Schmidt H G 2000 Knowledge restructuring in expertise development: evidence from pathophysiological representations of clinical cases by students and physicians. European Journal of Cognitive Psychology 12(3):323–355

Woods N N, Brooks L R, Norman G R 2005 The value of basic science in clinical diagnosis: creating coherence among signs and symptoms. Medical Education 39:107–112

Chapter 13

Knowledge, reasoning and evidence for practice

Joy Higgs, Mark A. Jones and Angie Titchen

CHAPTER CONTENTS

In this chapter we examine knowledge and its place in clinical reasoning and decision making, and the relationship between knowledge and evidence for practice. The context of this paper is the current tension between three often conflicting influences on professional healthcare practice: the evidence-based practice movement, the push towards patient-centred care that incorporates patient input into clinical decision making, and management-oriented approaches to the operation of healthcare systems. We argue that one form of knowledge will not satisfy all of these demands and that understanding the nature of knowledge, its derivations and use is necessary to effectively use professional knowledge in clinical reasoning and clinical practice.

KNOWLEDGE

What counts as knowledge is a matter of definition. The traditional definition of knowledge as a description of the world's structure and functions states that knowledge emerges from what we believe or hold to be true. This definition is related to the Platonic concept of *episteme*, from which the term epistemology derives (Gustavsson 2004). For something to be held to be true and to be accepted as a justified, true belief it must be supported by sound arguments. The concept of knowledge became much broader as a result of the contribution of Aristotle in the fourth century BC. Aristotle, in his *Nicomachean Ethics* (see Table 13.1), added to *episteme* the concepts of *techne* and *phronesis*.

Table 13.1   Knowledge categorizations

Plato (400 BC) (P) Aristotle (300 BC) (A) (in Gustavsson 2004)	Vico (in Berlin 1979)	Kolb (1984)	Carper (1978) Sarter (1988)*	Reason and Heron (1986)	Higgs and Titchen (1995)
Episteme (P) Objective knowledge, represents scientific knowledge, theoretical knowledge	Deductive knowledge Things that are true either by definition or by deduction from propositions or assumptions which are themselves true purely by definition		Interpretive knowledge (philosophical analysis)	Propositional knowledge Knowledge of things, gained through conversation, reading, etc.	Propositional knowledge Knowledge derived through research and/or scholarship; it is formal, explicit and exists in the public domain. It may be expressed in propositional statements that describe relationships between concepts or cause–effect relationships, thus permitting claims about generalizability. Or it may be presented in descriptive terms which allow for transferability of use
	Scientific knowledge Requires objectively valid, reliable and reproducible evidence. Only evidence gained by the senses, through observation, description and measurement, may be counted. Knowledge remains 'true' only for as long as it is not objectively refuted; when it fails the crucial test it becomes obsolete, to be replaced by a superior formula/ findings		Empirical knowledge		
Techne (A) Knowledge used in the process of producing, manufacturing and creating products	Experiential knowledge Is gained by personal experience. Some crucially important human knowledge	Experiential knowledge • Concrete experience • Reflective observation • Abstract conceptualization	• Aesthetic knowledge (artistic) pattern of knowing, derived from experience	Non propositional (a) Experiential knowledge from direct encounters with	Non-propositional/ experience-based (a) Professional craft knowledge

Phronesis (A)
Practical knowledge or wisdom used in the process of social interaction; incorporates ethical understanding of the values and norms that help people frame their ideas of a good life

exists which is distinct from and not reducible to either scientific or deductive knowledge

- Active experimentation

- Personal pattern of knowing self
- Ethical (moral) pattern of knowing

persons, places/things
(b) Practical knowledge gained through activity and related to skills or competencies

Can be tacit and is embedded in practice; it comprises general professional knowledge gained from health professionals' practice experience and also specific knowledge about a particular client in a particular situation (see Titchen & Ersser 2001)
(b) Personal (individual) knowledge
Includes the collective knowledge held by the community and culture in which the individual lives, and the unique knowledge gained from the individual's life experience

These three forms of knowledge deal with science, production/creativity and practical wisdom/ethics respectively, and form different ways of knowing the physical and human worlds.

Influenced by international technological and economic developments, the 1980s saw, according to Gustavsson (2004), an emerging focus on the content of practical knowledge and its relation to professional competence. Instead of the previous focus on scientific or theoretical knowledge – seen as separate from practical knowledge and as disseminated via experts and then added to practical knowledge – there was a shift to seeing such knowledge as embedded in practical actions and activities. The importance of reflection on practical experience became more clearly recognized, drawing on the philosophical perspectives of Ludwig Wittgenstein (1921), who distinguished between what can be said and that which is beyond words; he contended that we must remain silent about that which is beyond words. Other important perspectives were contributed by Michael Polanyi (1958), who presented knowledge as resting upon tacit background knowledge, and Gilbert Ryle (1949) who distinguished between *knowing that* and *knowing how*.

KNOWLEDGE CATEGORIES

The broad distinctions between 'knowing that' (or propositional knowledge) and 'knowing how' (non-propositional knowledge) (Polanyi 1958, Ryle 1949) reflect the two major categorizations of knowledge recognized in contemporary Western society. Propositional knowledge is generated formally through research and scholarship, and includes scientific knowledge (from the sciences), logic (from philosophy) and aesthetics (from the arts); it represents the 'knowledge of the field'. Non-propositional knowledge is generated primarily through practice experience. The former is commonly regarded in modern society and in professional discourse as having a higher status, in keeping with the hegemony of the physical sciences and the scientific method. In opposing this viewpoint, Ryle (1949) argued that procedural (practical) knowledge has primacy over propositional (theoretical) knowledge, which

follows rather than drives procedural knowledge. He contended that some theory is inside (part of) practice, while other (external) theory is utilized *in* practice. Barnett (1990) has argued that modern society is unreasonably dominated by the cognitive framework of science, with other forms of knowledge being downgraded and not even regarded as real knowledge. He argued that in a world where problems are not discrete nor solutions definite, we need knowledge beyond science.

Table 13.1 presents an overview of various ways people have categorized knowledge. Knowledge in any one category can be (and often is) translated into or subsumed within another category. For instance, knowledge derived from experience can subsequently be transformed into formal, publicly assessable propositional knowledge through theorization and/or rigorous critique and debate among practice communities. Propositional knowledge (of the field) can on the other hand also arise through basic or applied research. It can then be elaborated and particularized through practice experience to become part of the experience of the individual.

Both personally owned and publicly owned knowledge have contributions to make to professional practice. The knowledge base of an individual (Eraut 2000, p. 114) refers to 'the cognitive resource which a person brings to a situation that enables them to think and perform . . . this incorporates codified (i.e. public or propositional) knowledge in its personalized form, together with procedural knowledge and process knowledge, experiential knowledge and impressions in episodic memory . . . [and] personal knowledge [that] may be either explicit or tacit'. Personal knowledge, an important concept in the work of Polanyi (1958), is a recurring theme through all these categorization systems. It 'promotes wholeness and integrity in the personal encounter' (Carper 1978, p. 20), it arises from personal and professional experiences accompanied by reflection, and it provides the individual's frame of reference (Higgs & Titchen 1995). All forms of knowledge have limitations and must therefore be subject to continual critical reflection.

For effective clinical reasoning, we consider that health professionals rely upon the scientific knowledge of human behaviour and body responses in health and illness, the aesthetic perception of significant human experiences, a personal understanding of the uniqueness of the self and others and their interactions, and the ability to make decisions within concrete situations involving particular moral judgements. Each way of knowing, therefore, has a place in the education of health science students and in the practice of clinical reasoning.

RESEARCH KNOWLEDGE

Apart from distinguishing between research- and theory-generated (propositional) knowledge and experience-based (non-propositional) knowledge, it is also useful to consider the different forms of knowledge that are generated through different research paradigms (see Table 13.2).

Research paradigms provide frameworks for generating knowledge. The term *paradigm* is used to describe the model within which a community of scientists generates knowledge. Within a paradigm, assumptions, problems, research strategies, criteria and techniques are shared by the community. Therefore to justify that we are working within a particular research paradigm, we need to understand and be able to articulate to others, for critical review purposes, the principal assumptions and conventions of that paradigm. In particular, researchers (and practitioners in relation to their non-propositional knowledge) should be able to answer the following questions:

What can we know? What is reality?

This question relates to the ontological assumptions underpinning the different research paradigms. Ontology deals with issues of what exists, what is reality, and what is the nature of the world.

How can what exists be known?

Epistemology deals with how what exists may be known, and has been described as 'the philosophical theory of knowledge which seeks to define it, distinguish its principal varieties, identify its sources, and establish its limits' (Bullock & Trombley 1988, p. 279). Adopting Kuhn's (1970) notion of paradigms means acknowledging that a paradigm is a very fundamental orientation that determines such issues as which research is relevant, which questions can be asked and addressed by research, and what constitutes and justifies evidence. Other writers take the stance that the research question determines the type of methodology and paradigm to be adopted (Domholdt 1993, Guba & Lincoln 1994). However, Kuhn would argue that it is not possible to step out of paradigms at will because they do not suit one's questions or interests.

The fundamental issue of epistemology is that the type of knowledge obtained from research is dependent on the paradigm in which the research is conducted. Similarly, the type of knowledge desired is influenced by how the research question is posed.

Table 13.2 presents three broad research paradigms and the types of knowledge associated with these paradigms.

A) THE EMPIRICO–ANALYTICAL PARADIGM

This paradigm, which underlies the medical model, has dominated the philosophy of science from the 1920s to the 1960s (Manley 1991). The scientific paradigm or empiricist model of knowledge creation utilizes the scientific method and relies on observation and experiment in the empirical world, resulting in generalizations about the content and events of the world which can be used to predict future experience (Moore 1982). In many of the health professions it is questioned whether the medical model is a sufficient, or indeed the preferred, model for the health sciences. The medical model is increasingly regarded as inadequate for addressing the breadth of human challenges faced in health care. In some situations (e.g. care of older people or people with chronic conditions, community health, industrial and occupational health) other healthcare models (e.g. biopsychosocial, person-centred, relationship-centred or emancipatory models) are seen as preferable. Such preferences have been identified by some writers in nursing (Holmes 1990, McCormack 2001), physiotherapy (Parry 1997, Shepard 1987), medicine (Borrell-Carrió et al 2004) and occupational therapy (Denshire 2004, Mattingly 1991). Practitioners in these fields identify a dissonance between the philosophical bases for practice and research (Holmes 1990, Manley 1991). There is a greater emphasis,

Table 13.2 Research paradigms and knowledge

Research paradigm	Knowledge in this paradigm (Higgs & Titchen 1995)	Knowledge classification (Habermas 1972)	Description
The empirico-analytical paradigm	• Is discovered, i.e. universal and external truths are grasped and justified • Arises from empirical processes which are reductionist, value–neutral, quantifiable, objective and operationalizable • Contends that statements are valid only if publicly verifiable by sense data	Technical	Predictive knowledge where the emphasis is on a cause–effect relationship
The interpretive paradigm	• Comprises constructions arising from the minds and bodies of knowing, sensate, conscious and feeling beings • Is generated through a search for meaning, beliefs and values, and through looking for wholes and relationships with other wholes	Practical	Knowledge is associated with and embedded in the world of meanings and of human interactions and being
The critical paradigm	• Is emancipatory and developmental for people, organizations and communities • Requires becoming aware of how our thinking is socially, culturally, politically and historically constructed and how this limits our actions • Enables people to challenge learned restrictions, compulsions or dictates of habit • Is not grasped or discovered but is acquired through critical debate and critical empirical inquiry	Emancipatory	Knowledge about how to transform current structures, relationships and conditions which constrain development and reform

in nursing and occupational therapy in particular, on the humanistic movement and on knowledge generated within the interpretive and critical paradigms, while at the same time research conducted in the empirico-analytical paradigm is valued for the different purposes of answering questions about efficacy and effectiveness.

B) THE INTERPRETIVE PARADIGM

The interpretive paradigm is often more suited to the generation of knowledge in the human sciences, in both its philosophical stance and the methods utilized. Ontologically, this paradigm recognizes local, multiple and specific constructed or embodied realities. Researchers within this paradigm seek to generate practical knowledge through describing and/or interpreting phenomena, particularly human phenomena, exploring the whole phenomenon in its context, taking account of the context, the timings, the subjective meanings and intentions within the particular situation (in some types of interpretive research), or embodied, unarticulated, situational meanings (in other types), and seeking to uncover the meanings and significant aspects of the situation from the perspective of the people being studied. Research approaches in the paradigm include hermeneutic inquiry (hermeneutics is concerned with the theory and practice of interpretation), ethnography (which describes a phenomenon from a given societal or cultural focus), and phenomenology (concerned with describing, interpreting and understanding people's lived experiences of the phenomenon being studied).

C) THE CRITICAL PARADIGM

The critical paradigm generates emancipatory knowledge that enhances awareness of how our thinking is socially and historically constructed and how this limits our actions. The critical paradigm is chosen when researchers not only want to create new knowledge but also intend to act to bring about transformation of themselves, other individuals, teams, organizations or communities by using the new knowledge to underpin their transformational actions (Carr & Kemmis 1986). Such researchers are concerned with overcoming obstacles within themselves as well as with changing systems, management strategies, cultures, power relationships and communication channels. Critical researchers may be practitioner–researchers who are investigating their own practices and contexts. They use a variety of research approaches that are collaborative, participative and inclusive, such as cooperative inquiry or action research. They aim to create emancipatory knowledge or critical practice theories about how to overcome the obstacles that get in the way of, for example, person-centred, evidence-based care (Titchen & Manley 2006).

USING KNOWLEDGE FROM ALL THREE PARADIGMS

Just as healthcare practitioner-researchers make decisions based on research from all three paradigms about the kind of services/care they should provide, so do healthcare practitioners when engaging in clinical reasoning in relation to a particular patient/client. As we know, technical/propositional knowledge (from the empirico-analytical paradigm) is useful in predicting the effectiveness of a range of therapeutic interventions which might be helpful for a patient/client. In a complementary way, practical knowledge (from the interpretive paradigm) helps the practitioner to use this technical knowledge in the best interests of the particular patient/client/family member. For example, such knowledge informs the practitioner's understanding of how to create and negotiate partnerships with the patient/client/family member and enable genuine involvement in decision making about the intervention that best suits this particular person, at this particular time, in this particular context. Use of professional craft knowledge and personal knowledge are particularly important in particularizing the technical knowledge for the patient/client/family member and facilitating real partnerships that result in care interventions that are effective and also meet the needs of patients/clients/family members as they see them. Emancipatory knowledge may be useful to the practitioner and patient/client/family member if an obstacle is met in relation to giving or receiving the care intervention that has been chosen because it offers strategies, processes and/or tools for surmounting them.

KNOWLEDGE AS EVIDENCE FOR PRACTICE

In previous writings we have argued:

- The complex context of health science practice requires that health professionals utilize a rich array of knowledge and practice skills that should not be restricted by narrow definitions of what constitutes competence or evidence for practice (Higgs et al 2004, Jones et al 2006, Rycroft-Malone et al 2004).
- The status, definition and operation of professions rely heavily on their knowledge bases; such knowledge is essential for professional reasoning and decision making (Higgs & Titchen 2000).
- A knowledge base that includes propositional, practice and personal knowledge provides a sound foundation for human, ethical, holistic and patient-centred practice (Higgs et al 2001a, Titchen & McGinley 2003).
- The current focus on evidence-based practice has arisen from the climate of increasing demands confronting the health sector for public accountability and the assurance of quality health care in the face of decreasing public funds (Jones & Higgs 2000).
- Best practice which is associated with evidence-based practice needs to be interpreted as being situationally applicable, not absolutely and objectively definable. The practitioner's (and the system's) duty of care is to provide high quality and relevant services, and to provide credible evidence in support of the chosen services; these parameters, rather than a prescribed or predetermined management strategy, constitute the essence of best practice (Jones & Higgs 2000).
- Evidence-based practice requires professional judgement and sound reasoning. It does not dictate the prescriptive use of evidence for cookbook decision-making (Higgs et al 2001b, Jones et al 2006).
- Clinicians need to use professional judgement in providing care which best addresses patients' needs and well-being, in part because of the complexity and variability of professional practice and in part because health care

relies on inexact sciences that can provide only limited 'hard' evidence for the grey areas of practice and knowledge (Higgs et al 2001b).

In professional discourse the higher status of propositional knowledge is particularly prominent when it comes to determining what counts as evidence. This is most apparent in the evidence-based practice movement, where the dominant research paradigm is the empirico-analytical paradigm. The use of randomized controlled trials to investigate the effectiveness of therapeutic interventions is valued as the pre-eminent research approach in this paradigm, as evident in the 'levels of evidence' hierarchies (Sackett et al 2000) for ranking the quality of information available to guide practice. The continued perceived supremacy of the empirico-analytical paradigm, along with the limitations with respect to population homogeneity, diagnostic inclusion criteria, intervention details and outcome measures commonly found within health professions empirico-analytical paradigm research and reporting (Jones et al 2006), has resulted in a dominant body of research that is incomplete to adequately guide practitioners in the management of the multitude of patient problems encountered. Many authors now argue for the place of qualitative, interpretive paradigm research in expanding the scope of evidence available for practice (Barbour 2000, Bithell 2000, Higgs et al 2004, Jones et al 2006, Ritchie 1999). This broader view of evidence is more consistent with the World Health Organization's (2001) biopsychosocial philosophy of health and disability. Psychosocial factors cannot be separated from biomedical factors, and as such psychosocial effects must be considered alongside biomedical outcomes (Borrell-Carrió et al 2004).

Evidence-based practice itself does not constrain decision making. Instead, it emphasizes the role of clinicians in using evidence to answer their own clinical problems (Herbert et al 2001). However, given the continued status of empirico-analytical research above interpretive research, and the methodological limitations with much of the effectiveness research, practising clinicians face the daunting challenge of maintaining best practice based on best evidence when the evidence is still largely not available or is incomplete. For the practitioner this underlines the importance of using skilled clinical reasoning in applying research evidence and managing patients who fall outside the available evidence. The value of clinical expertise has been emphasized by Sackett et al (2000) in the statement 'external clinical evidence can inform, but never replace, individual clinical expertise. [This] expertise will assist the practitioner in deciding whether the external evidence applies to the individual client at all and, if so, how it should be integrated into the clinical decision' (p. 73).

Empirico-analytical research alone is insufficient to understand patients' disability experiences. For health professionals, this realization emphasizes the need both for greater recognition of the strengths and limitations of the two research paradigms and for a breakdown of the political barriers separating the two groups of researchers. Interpretive research is ideal for providing the context currently lacking in the traditional quantitative approach that dominates evidence-based practice, and innovative strategies are needed that link and combine the two paradigms, with clinical questions being the common ground on which to unite them (Miller & Crabtree 2000, Ritchie 1999).

In the context of clinical reasoning within person-centred, evidence-based care, the use of research knowledge does not occur in isolation, as indicated above. Other categories of knowledge are used too. For example, person-centred care is grounded in a particular philosophical tradition and ethical (moral) stance that has been articulated through philosophical and scholarly research. For this tradition and stance to live, the practitioner draws on non-propositional knowledge of various kinds, such as aesthetic and ethical patterns of knowing, professional craft knowledge and the personal knowledge of the patient/client/family member. Practitioners use all these different types of knowledge within clinical reasoning and caregiving: a unique blending of these kinds of knowledge occurs that is particular to this patient, this situation, and so on. This unique knowledge blend is intermingled with the practitioner's qualities, intelligence, practical wisdom, cognitive and metacognitive processes, practical skills and therapeutic use of self. Building on Schön's (1987) ideas, Titchen and Higgs (2001) described this capacity to uniquely blend all these things, in the hot action of practice, as *professional artistry*.

CONCLUSION

Making sound and patient-centred clinical decisions in an era that demands accountability and evidence-based practice requires not only scientific knowledge, but also a deep knowledge of the practice of one's profession and of what it means to be human in the world of combined strength and vulnerability that is health care. Therefore, knowledge from a variety of research paradigms and from practice experience is necessary for clinical decision making. Restricting ourselves to any single paradigm or way of knowing can result in a limitation to the range of knowledge and the depth of understanding that can be applied to a given problem situation.

The accumulated propositional, professional and personal knowledge of the individual constitutes his or her unique knowledge base. Such knowledge bases have contextual influences generated by the societal, professional, paradigmatic and experiential situations in which the individual's knowledge was generated. The relevance of the individual's knowledge base to the task in hand is important (Feltovich et al 1984), and the effective use of this knowledge in the reasoning process is an essential element in quality health care. As part of professional responsibility to contribute to their own and their profession's knowledge base practitioners are expected to undertake knowledge creation and validation, and can facilitate this process in students and novices.

The exploration of knowledge in this chapter has demonstrated the richness of the forms of knowledge that practitioners can bring to the task of clinical decision making. It has also identified the many issues that face those who would use knowledge knowingly: what constitutes knowledge, what forms of knowledge are needed for practice, and how knowledge is shaped and used within different frames of reference (such as paradigms). The critical, informed and meaningful use of knowledge in practice, along with person-centred, evidence-based practice, requires professional artistry which is often tacit, embedded and unarticulated in practice. The next chapter pursues the topic of knowledge further in consideration of practice epistemology.

References

Aristotle (trans. T Irwin) 1985 Nichomachean ethics. Hackett, Indianapolis

Barbour R S 2000 The role of qualitative research in broadening the 'evidence base' for clinical practice. Journal of Evaluation in Clinical Practice 6:155–163

Barnett R 1990 The idea of higher education. Society for Research into Higher Education and Open University Press, Buckingham

Berlin I (ed) 1979 Against the current: essays in the history of ideas. London: Hogarth Press

Bithell C 2000 Evidence-based physiotherapy: some thoughts on 'best evidence'. Physiotherapy 86:58–61

Borrell-Carrió F, Suchman A L, Epstein R M 2004 The biopsychosocial model 25 years later: principles, practice, and scientific inquiry. Annals of Family Medicine 2(6): 576–582

Bullock A, Trombley S 1988 The Fontana dictionary of modern thought. 2nd edn. Fontana, London

Carper B A 1978 Fundamental patterns of knowing. Advances in Nursing Science 1:13–23

Carr W, Kemmis S 1986 Becoming critical: education, knowledge and action research. Falmer Press, London

Denshire S 2004 Imagination, occupation, reflection: an autobiographical model of empathetic understanding. In: Whiteford G (ed) Qualitative research as interpretive practice: proceedings of the RIPPLE (Centre for Research into Professional Practice, Learning and Education) QRIP (Qualitative Research as Interpretive Practice) conference. Albury, Australia, p 21–38

Domholdt E 1993 Physical therapy research: principles and applications. W B Saunders, Philadelphia

Eraut M 2000 Non-formal learning and tacit knowledge in professional work. British Journal of Educational Psychology 70:113–136

Feltovich P J, Johnson P E, Moller J H et al 1984 The role and development of medical knowledge in diagnostic expertise. In: Clancey W J, Shortliffe E H (eds) Readings in medical artificial intelligence: the first decade. Addison-Wesley, Reading, MA, p 275–319

Guba E G, Lincoln Y S 1994 Competing paradigms in qualitative research. In: Denzin N K, Lincoln Y S (eds) Handbook of qualitative research. Sage, London, p 105–117

Gustavsson B 2004 Revisiting the philosophical roots of practical knowledge. In: Higgs J, Richardson B, Abrandt Dahlgren M (eds) Developing practice knowledge for health professionals. Butterworth-Heinemann, Oxford, p 35–50

Habermas J (trans. J J Shapiro) 1972 Knowledge and human interest. Heinemann, London

Herbert R D, Sherrington C, Maher C et al 2001 Evidence-based practice – imperfect but necessary. Physiotherapy Theory and Practice 17:201–211

Higgs J, Titchen A 1995 Propositional, professional and personal knowledge in clinical reasoning. In: Higgs J, Jones M (eds) Clinical reasoning in the health professions. Butterworth-Heinemann, Oxford, p 126–146

Higgs J, Titchen A 2000 Knowledge and reasoning. In: Higgs J, Jones M (eds) Clinical reasoning in the health professions, 2nd edn. Butterworth-Heinemann, Oxford, p 23–32

Higgs J, Titchen A, Neville V 2001a Professional practice and knowledge. In: Higgs J, Titchen A (eds) Practice knowledge and expertise in the health professions. Butterworth-Heinemann, Oxford, p 3–9

Higgs J, Burn A, Jones M 2001b Integrating clinical reasoning and evidence-based practice. AACN Clinical Issues: Advanced Practice in Acute and Critical Care 12 (4):482–490

Higgs J, Andresen L, Fish D 2004 Practice knowledge – its nature, sources and contexts. In: Higgs J, Richardson B, Abrandt Dahlgren M (eds) Developing practice knowledge for health professionals. Butterworth-Heinemann, Oxford, p 51–69

Holmes C A 1990 Alternatives to natural science foundations for nursing. International Journal of Nursing Studies 27:187–198

Jones M, Higgs J 2000 Will evidence-based practice take the reasoning out of practice? In: Higgs J, Jones M (eds) Clinical reasoning in the health professions, 2nd edn. Butterworth-Heinemann, Oxford, p 307–315

Jones M, Grimmer K, Edwards I et al 2006 Challenges in applying best evidence to physiotherapy. Internet Journal of Allied Health Sciences and Practice, 4(3). Online. Available: http://ijahsp.nova.edu/

Kolb D 1984 Experiential learning: experience as the source of learning and development. Prentice-Hall, Englewood Cliffs, NJ

Kuhn T S 1970 The structure of scientific revolutions. 2nd edn. University of Chicago Press, Chicago

McCormack B 2001 Negotiating partnerships with older people: a person-centred approach. Ashgate, Aldershot

Manley K 1991 Knowledge for nursing practice. In: Perry A, Jolley M (eds) Nursing: a knowledge base for practice. Edward Arnold, London, p 1–27

Mattingly C 1991 The narrative nature of clinical reasoning. American Journal of Occupational Therapy 45:998–1005

Miller W L, Crabtree B F 2000 Clinical research. In: Denzin N K, Lincoln Y S (eds) Handbook of qualitative research, 2nd edn. Sage Publications, London, p 607–631

Moore T W 1982 Philosophy of education: an introduction. Routledge and Kegan Paul, London

Parry A 1997 New paradigms for old: musings on the shape of clouds. Physiotherapy 83:423–433

Polanyi M 1958 Personal knowledge: towards a post-critical philosophy. Routledge and Kegan Paul, London

Reason P, Heron J 1986 Research with people: the paradigm of cooperative experiential enquiry. Person-Centred Review 1:457–476

Ritchie J 1999 Using qualitative research to enhance the evidence-based practice of health care providers. Australian Journal of Physiotherapy 45:251–256

Rycroft-Malone J, Seers K, Titchen A et al 2004 What counts as evidence in evidence based practice? Journal of Advanced Nursing 47(1):81–90

Ryle G 1949 The concept of mind. Penguin Books, Harmondsworth

Sackett D L, Straus S E, Richardson W S et al 2000 Evidence-based medicine: how to practice and teach EBM. 2nd edn. Churchill Livingstone, Edinburgh

Sarter B (ed) 1988 Paths to knowledge: innovative research methods for nursing. National League for Nursing, New York

Schön D 1987 Educating the reflective practitioner: toward a new design for teaching and learning in the professions. Jossey-Bass, San Francisco

Shepard K F 1987 Qualitative and quantitative research in clinical practice. Physical Therapy 67:1891–1894

Titchen A, Ersser S J 2001 The nature of professional craft knowledge. In: Higgs J, Titchen A (eds) Practice knowledge and expertise in the health professions. Butterworth-Heinemann, Oxford, p 35–41

Titchen A, Higgs J 2001 Towards professional artistry and creativity in practice. In: Higgs J, Titchen A (eds) Professional practice in health, education and the creative arts. Blackwell Science, Oxford, p 273–290

Titchen A, McGinley M 2003 Facilitating practitioner-research through critical companionship. NTResearch 8(2): 115–131

Titchen A, Manley K 2006 Spiralling towards transformational action research: philosophical and practical journeys. Educational Action Research: An International Journal 14(3):333–356

Wittgenstein L 1921/1963 Tractatus logico-philosphicus. Suhurkamp, Frankfurt

World Health Organization 2001 International classification of functioning, disability and health. World Health Organization, Geneva

Chapter 14

Knowledge generation and clinical reasoning in practice

Joy Higgs, Della Fish and Rodd Rothwell

CHAPTER CONTENTS

Health professionals have a responsibility to contribute to the development of their profession's knowledge base and to continually expand and critique the knowledge used in practice (Higgs & Titchen 2000). Practitioners need to be able to critically appreciate knowledge, generate knowledge from practice and recognize the practice epistemology that underpins their practice.

To commence our own critical appreciation of knowledge, we define it as follows:

Knowledge is a dynamic and context-bound phenomenon that utilizes language to construct meaning. Language serves as a tool for thinking, learning and making meaning (Vygotsky 1986, Wittgenstein 1958) (see Chapter 31). Knowledge is constructed in the framework of sociopolitical, cultural and historical contexts. Practice knowledge evolves within a dynamic 'history of ideas' (see Berlin 1979, Lovejoy 1940) contained in the particular practice domain and within the history of how ideas born in that practice domain have shaped and been shaped by that practice (Higgs et al 2001).

Each of these dimensions and contexts of knowledge has particular relevance to how we use knowledge in reasoning and generate knowledge from within reasoning. During professional socialization, practitioners learn the ways of being, acting, thinking and communicating that characterize their profession.

PRACTICE EPISTEMOLOGY

In Chapter 3 the importance of practitioners knowing and choosing their practice models was argued. In this chapter we extend this argument to the understanding and adoption of a position relating to practice epistemology. To say that 'this is the epistemological position that underpins my practice' is to recognize that my practice is carried out within the context of a certain discursive tradition (a scientific and professional community in this case) of knowledge generation. This tradition, with its rules and norms of practice, determines what constitutes knowledge and what strategies of knowledge generation are valid. Within the biomedical practice framework (or model), for example, with its inherent physical sciences epistemological stance, knowledge is seen as an objective, predictive, empirical, generalizable, explanatory phenomenon that arises from the use of the natural scientific method and theorization in a world of external objective reality. In humanistic, psychosocial practice models, located in the human and social sciences and the arts, knowledge is seen as being interpretive, theoretical, and constructed in social worlds that recognize and seek to interpret multiple constructed realities. In emancipatory practice models, located in the critical social sciences, knowledge is recognized as being historically and culturally constructed, and historical reality is something that, once understood more deeply, can be changed in order to seek positive changes in practice.

We begin our reflections on this topic in acknowledgement of the position that knowledge and practice are inseparable (see Fish & Coles 1998, Higgs et al 2001, Ryle 1949). Indeed professional practice, with clinical reasoning at its core, could be viewed as knowing in practice. And professional knowledge should be considered not as a repository of knowledge of the discipline combined with the individual practitioner's store of knowledge, but rather as a practice of knowing within the broader field of professional practice. Thus the knowing and the doing of practice are concurrent, intertwined journeys of being and becoming in practice.

APPRECIATING PRACTICE AND PRACTICE KNOWLEDGE

To appreciate something involves *sensing, becoming aware of, understanding* and *valuing* it. *Critical appreciation* is a process of examining and seeking to understand an activity or an object by as many means and from as many points of view as possible. This incorporates:

- reflecting upon its creator's or originator's intentions, methods and values
- recognizing the traditions and context within which it was created
- evaluating its achievements and failures
- seeing in it meanings beyond the surface
- recognizing that it is often representative of a set of principles and beliefs beyond itself.

This process can lead the 'appreciator' away from the specific activity or object under review, towards a view of the bigger picture surrounding it (Fish 2001).

Critical appreciation and professional judgement have much in common. Professional judgement can focus on the product of clinical reasoning, that is, the decisions or judgements made in clinical practice; this is comparable to the evaluation made by connoisseurs (Eisner 1985) who use critical appreciation to make judgements about their field of expertise (e.g. art). The processes of clinical reasoning and critical appreciation both involve using discretionary judgement and self-evaluation (Freidson 1994, 2001). This process of self-critique also applies to the continual refinement and updating of practitioners' knowledge bases. They are expected to seek out the best and most salient knowledge available to deal with practice tasks and problems and to recognize when their knowledge is deficient, redundant or irrelevant. In such cases they need to pursue further learning, reflect on practice to generate experience-based knowledge, and seek out other people's knowledge (including that of their clients) as input to professional decision making.

Part of appreciating practice knowledge is recognizing that what counts as knowledge is a matter of perspective. The dominant view of knowledge in Western society and in the health professions is the largely unquestioned view of knowledge from the physical sciences or empirico-analytical paradigm. This is the 'hypothetico-deductive' approach, in which knowledge generation is viewed not as a process of creation of knowledge but as a process of discovery of empirical 'facts' about the (physical) world/universe. Knowledge in this view is an account or a theory of what is 'out there'; it represents or mirrors aspects of the natural world. This is the epistemology of representationalism, the notion that theories (and language) represent nature rather than the notion developed here, that theories are created in the context of human activity. In critique of this positivist epistemology (the idea that scientific propositions are given to the senses by nature itself), the British philosopher Karl Popper (1959, 1970) argued that the discovery of scientific fact begins by a process of theoretical conjecture, not, as the positivists would argue, through objective or empirical observation. From this conjunction arise testable or 'falsifiable' hypotheses. Thus in epistemological terms, science follows a process or method involving disproof, not proof. One cannot speak about truth in the traditional sense, that a hypothesis matches reality precisely or perfectly, but rather that empirical research has not yet proved the hypothesis incorrect. Theories that have withstood the strictures of empirical testing or experimentation give scientists a degree of certainty and confidence about them. While seeking *the truth*, such research actually generates knowledge or *a truth* that is currently undisproved by testing through observation or experimentation.

As scholars, educational practitioners and researchers we support a constructionist interpretation of knowledge according to which all knowledge is a construction of human beings (individuals or groups) who are striving to know about nature and experience. This view of knowledge involves an appreciation of knowledge as a sociohistorical political construct and recognition of the value of different forms of knowledge for different communities and contexts. We are socialized (in life, education and work) to value different forms of knowledge, often unquestioningly accepting the values and expectations of these social groups. Vygotsky (1978) referred to

this process of acquiring knowledge as 'internalization of activity', and Rogoff (1995) used the term 'participatory appropriation' to emphasize the dynamic, relational and mutual nature of learning. This differs from a perspective of learning that implies pieces of knowledge being transferred from the outside to the inside of the individual.

New knowledge can be challenging in that it requires appreciation (evaluating, critique and valuing). This process of appreciation requires us to question previous values and entails a new thematic understanding of previously implicit ways of seeing and understanding. It is a dynamic process, where individuals are placed in the position of critics who do not blindly accept what their professional leaders or experts espouse, but actively question and interpret it in light of their own previous and current experience. They may in fact reject the new or emerging knowledge and suggest alternatives. Given the dynamic nature of contexts, not only can the circumstances that surround knowledge use, creation and acknowledgement change, but the knower's frame of reference (including knowledge needs, values and knowledge abilities) might also change. All these changes impact on professional practice and must be internalized by both new learners and skilled practitioners. Much of this change may well occur around us, even in some instances without our initial explicit awareness, but it can also arise from continuous reflection on our practice.

EMPLOYING, CREATING AND MODIFYING KNOWLEDGE IN PRACTICE

In this section our goal is to explore strategies through which knowledge can come to be appreciated, generated, validated and valued. Employing existing or learned knowledge in practice is not simply a matter of transferring this knowledge to a new setting. This process customarily requires modification, particularly because knowledge generated through research or by theorists is inevitably generalized, and does not always meet the needs of the particular practice in the field. The knowledge generated by others does not always fit the perceived needs of a particular practitioner who may seek to deconstruct and reconstruct formal theory in terms that make it more intelligible and user-friendly. In practice, not only are propositional and non-propositional knowledge modified for and through practice, but they are also combined, extended, converted from one form to another and, most importantly, particularized (see Fish & de Cossart 2007, Montgomery 2006). For example, in designing a healthcare plan for a particular patient the practitioner adapts general research knowledge to suit that patient's unique combination of life and health circumstances, drawing on experience-based knowledge from working with other similar situations.

The practice setting is a vital arena for the construction of new knowledge by practitioners themselves. First, professional judgement is utilized by practitioners in the selection of knowledge to be used *and* the kind of use to which that knowledge is put in the practice setting. Here, practitioners consider what is appropriate knowledge, how it might be used and whether it should be modified to suit the particular case. That modification is itself a version of creating knowledge *in* practice. Second, new knowledge may be created in the practice setting, when practitioners identify the need to develop new procedures or when they face new challenges. Evidence-based practice can exist only insofar as relevant evidence exists and is known by practitioners (Beeston & Simons 1996, Ford & Walsh 1994, Grahame-Smith 1995, Jones & Higgs 2000, White 1997). Further, it is important to recognize that for practitioners to use evidence

in their practice it needs to be appropriated internally by them, an internalization that occurs when the evidence is seen to have relevance for their practice. In practical settings, professionals are continually adapting both formal public knowledge and their own informal knowledge to particular cases, or they are extending existing knowledge in response to the current case. Third, and perhaps most significantly, knowledge is created by practitioners in the practice setting when they theorize about their practice and make explicit and refine the tacit knowledge that lies embedded within and beneath their actions, activities and know-how.

In Figure 14.1 we attempt to illustrate a loosely sequenced series of activities which can be included in the process of making sense of the world of practice in order to produce knowledge. This is not intended to represent an empirical observation or generalization of knowledge generation in a prescriptive or predictive sense; neither is it a set of rules for generating knowledge. Rather, we propose that these interactive, reflexive, cognitive and communicative processes and actions can usefully contribute to knowledge development. The sequence commences with the formulation of ideas and proceeds through a deepening understanding of the phenomenon or reality that the thinker is seeking to appreciate. The next phase involves evaluative and critiquing processes which can result in a level of certainty that can be called conviction or validation of the truth,

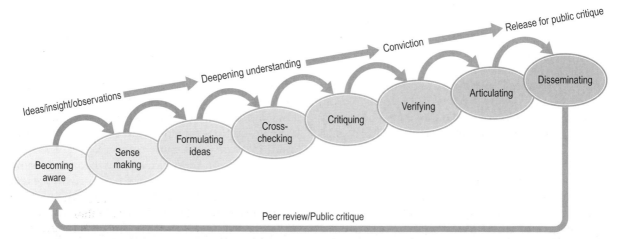

Figure 14.1 Appreciating practice knowledge (from Higgs et al 2004, with permission of Butterworth-Heinemann)

at which point the notion is judged to reflect reality satisfactorily. This allows or prompts the knower to release this knowledge claim for public critique. The cycle then progresses through critique by others and by the field, so that the knowledge claims become part of the accepted knowledge base of the group/profession/society. These phases are detailed below.

FORMULATING IDEAS

Healthcare practitioners are expected to notice things; to become aware of their patients' needs and responses. They are expected to critically appraise their own performance, role and actions. In so doing they can become aware of patterns of behaviour and outcomes in their clinical interventions. For example, they can reflect on the relative effectiveness and patient preference for different modes of treatment and the circumstances surrounding these findings. Fish (1998) has argued that this processing of noticing with heightened awareness and a learned habit requires the development of a 'discerning eye'. For many practitioners, this awareness may be channelled directly into their clinical role, almost without conscious recognition. That is, they may acquire a large store of mainly tacit knowledge and experience.

Tacit knowledge plays an important role in practice. According to Heidegger (1926/1990), craft activity (involving a form of tacit knowledge) must remain tacit to work well and is brought to awareness only when the practitioner makes a mistake. This mistake then focuses the practitioner's attention; the activity becomes explicit; the correction is made consciously (or *thematically*, to use Heidegger's term) and practice knowledge is realized. Heidegger would argue that craft work must operate on a tacit basis, otherwise it ceases to become craft work and is articulated into a set of guidelines.

However, we argue that tacit knowledge can also be made explicit by practitioners deliberately reflecting upon the underlying elements of their practice in order to understand it, communicate it to other practitioners and teach it to students. In the context of healthcare practice, which blends science, art and craft, the wholeness and at times the essence of the artistry or craft of practice cannot be articulated. However, there is much about practice that needs to be further explored and can be made explicit. In particular, experience-based knowledge gained by one practitioner could greatly enhance the practice of others if it were presented to, validated and adopted by the profession. This requires articulation. Thus we distinguish between 'unspeakable' tacit knowledge, which is deeply embedded in the actions of practice, and the vast amount of procedural knowledge that awaits exploration. This exploration can occur when an appropriate exploration tool is identified, when an opportunity or stimulus (such as a critical incident) occurs to prompt reflection, or when health professionals take the time to explore and critique their practice. In their recent book *Developing the Wise Doctor*, Fish & de Cossart (2007) introduce the term 'the invisibles of practice' to refer to key elements of practice which are tacit (but can be made explicit) or are implicit (lying just beneath the surface of human endeavour, but can be easily made explicit when prompted). Their book offers a range of resources for developing clinicians' understanding of these invisible dimensions of practice.

The act of noticing in practice is the first step to making practice epistemology an ingrained practice of practitioners as well as of researchers. The goal is to make paying attention to how knowledge is used in practice and created through practice a living part of practice. Noticing, however, as with the other knowledge generation actions discussed below, should not be just the actions of the isolated practitioner. Each of these actions should become part of professional education and socialization; they are part of working and being in a learning community and of a profession with both a tradition of knowledge-making and a future of knowledge evolution.

Practitioners often explore their existing knowledge base when seeking to make sense of a new idea, an insight, an observed pattern or inconsistency. They look at the compatibility of the new idea with existing knowledge, the value of the new idea, patterns emerging across a number of cases or situations, and whether the new idea is unique to the particular situation. And they challenge their existing knowledge to see what needs to be replaced or updated. Self-questioning and reflection play a major role here in appreciating the subtleties of a situation and developing understandings and explanations.

CROSS-CHECKING AND CRITIQUING

New ideas, variations, techniques and strategies are often explored and tested out in practice. Such active experimentation is part of creating new knowledge and cross-checking emerging knowledge. Checking may also take the form of self-debate, with the new idea or potential intervention strategy being analysed, deconstructed, examined from multiple perspectives to further the process of refining and testing it in terms of credibility, coherence, relevance, etc. The issue of the compatibility of new knowledge with practitioners' existing knowledge is a critical factor in clinical effectiveness and the development of practitioners' knowledge bases. In clinical reasoning, practitioners often need to deal with and make sense of differences between new knowledge and existing propositional and experience-based knowledge. Conflicts between such forms of knowledge could be due to the presence of existing knowledge that is obsolete, inadequate, incomplete, erroneous or irrelevant to the given situation, or there could be a problem with the new knowledge (e.g. lack of relevance or validity). There can also be some aspects of health care that remain irreconcilable, and practitioners need to be able to make professional judgements to deal with such situations rather than developing a clear knowledge position.

In critiquing emerging knowledge claims, practitioners need to address the relevance, credibility and currency of this potential knowledge for their practice. They can perform this critique against internal yardsticks, that is, their existing knowledge base and their capacity to scrutinize knowledge claims against first principles (using scientific knowledge and theory). They can also compare emerging knowledge against the knowledge of their field through literature reviews, systematic reviews and so on. And they can trial the knowledge claims during clinical reasoning in relation to real and hypothetical cases.

In relation to practical knowledge practitioners could ask, for example: Can my knowledge of biomechanics, anatomy or physiology help to explain why a newly invented treatment technique or variation should work? What could be the possible consequences of taking this course of action? How does this new approach sit with the professional knowledge base and the literature pertaining to evidence-based practice? If I use this knowledge or technique in my practice, do my self-knowledge and my knowledge of ethics, culture and professional standards create ease of use or difficulties?

Beyond the immediate questioning of emerging knowledge claims, this process of generating knowledge from practice addresses further questions. On one hand there is a seeking after some truth (or matching with reality), but there is also a critique of the rightness, justification and compatibility with self and others in the use of this knowledge in practice. To critique includes dealing with issues of relevance and appropriateness for the setting (e.g. individual client, culture, professional role). In addition, at a 'meta' level, we advocate an exploration of the nature of knowledge and its generation in the context of the particular practice arena, that is, practice epistemology. Is this knowledge or just an idea or observation? Can I verify it? Does this knowledge claim stand the test of scrutiny against my own and my profession's way of being in our practice world and our way of knowing about this world?

VERIFYING

Verification of claims to knowledge requires rigour and conviction. Rigour in knowledge generation is both an intention (to seek truth or *a* truth) and an approach (including providing transparency of method to facilitate critique, being systematic and thorough in testing truth with open-mindedness in the pursuit of clarity and truthfulness). Yet the nature of the rigour is also dependent upon the knowledge tradition being utilized. In the positivist tradition, the requirement for rigour arises from the goal of the research, to generalize from its findings. Here, rigour is manifest in strict adherence to rules of the scientific method (e.g. objectivity, reliability and validity) and to the protocols of experimental research (e.g. random allocation of subjects, use of blind trials, measurement of statistical significance).

In keeping with the aim of the professional artist to generate meaning, confer significance or offer insight rather than to develop propositional knowledge, the major means of collecting evidence in the connoisseurship model is the practitioner through whom the meaning is developed and expressed (see Eisner 1981). And, just as the piece of art itself is the place from which art critics draw their evidence, so the arena in which practitioners seek evidence is the practice arena. Eisner also emphasized the importance of the connoisseur approach as a way of communicating meaning in a manner that is understandable to the relevant community. If no one but the connoisseur can recognize the description, it will not be regarded as a competent interpretation.

Rigour associated with the expertise of critical appreciation (the processes, language and form) develops within the context of a critical community, as argued by Schön (1983), who proposed that the professional knowledge by which practitioners 'make sense of practice situations, formulate goals and directions for action, and determine what constitutes acceptable professional conduct' is 'embedded within the socially and institutionally constructed context shared by a community of practitioners' (p. 33). Beyond individual critique and metacognitive scrutiny, rigour is achieved by peer critique through validating knowledge by exposing it to the professional community (as discussed below).

To be convinced that a claim to knowledge has been verified, knowers need to have reached a point where they believe that the evidence accumulated is sufficient to judge the claim to be acceptable or true. Thus conviction is a decision and a judgement rather than a point of absolute certainty. Ayer (1956, p. 222) argued that when seeking to verify knowledge claims we should take scepticism of these claims seriously. Such scepticism will enable us to learn 'to distinguish the different levels at which our claims to knowledge stand'. Thus, knowing is a continual process of generating, refining and understanding knowledge.

ARTICULATING

One of the most difficult challenges in knowledge generation is to articulate knowledge clearly, in a form and language meaningful to the people (within and outside the health professions) who use that knowledge. In health care this is likely to include professional practitioners and their clients, and thus different forms of expression are needed to take account of different levels of medical knowledge and different language and cultural backgrounds.

Articulation (oral and written) of new practice knowledge can include definitions, explanations, illustrations, examples and arguments. Writing and dialogue play major roles in shaping, refining and communicating new knowledge. Such processes place the knowledge in the context of the practice community, hold the emerging ideas up against the challenge of existing knowledge and look at the resonance of the language and ideas with existing discourse. Writing is a process of making meaning as well as presenting meaning. Meaning emerges from the writing just as an artefact emerges from the work of the artist. The process of writing (or making meaning) takes the originator beyond what was planned and what was known at the beginning. Writing enables writers to discover what they really think, understand and want to say. And because the evolution of new knowledge emerges through a series of drafts, which seek to capture complex ideas in order to refine them, the oral tradition does not provide a sufficient basis for developing professional practice (see Fish 1998).

DISSEMINATING AND PEER REVIEWING

Practice knowledge varies across different health professions and within individual professions as they work with specific client groups or within specific contexts of care (Beeston & Higgs 2001). In this way knowledge and practice norms and traditions are social entities which emerge from practice and are shared by communities of practitioners. Krefting (1991) argued that the rigour of peer review by professional communities is concerned with credibility and transferability rather than with validity. The credibility of practice knowledge 'requires that others in the community of practice find the meaning that is expressed to be credible in terms of the traditions of practice, and that they find it can be transferred to their own practice and applied in other contexts' (Beeston & Higgs 2001, p. 114).

Many strategies are used to disseminate knowledge in professional communities, including conference presentations, journal articles and other publications, educational programmes and informal communications. As part of presenting the new knowledge to the field to allow for wider consideration and investigation, articulation of the knowledge should also include description of how it was generated and in what context, so that the knowledge claim can be critiqued.

ONGOING DEVELOPMENT

Ongoing development of knowledge is part of the search for truth in a changing world, recognizing that it is a dynamic phenomenon. Kleinig (1982, p. 152), for instance, argued that 'the knowing subject must continually reflect on and test what [knowledge] is presented'. Practitioners need to develop an appreciation of the credibility of their knowledge, to be able to defend their knowledge, but at the same time to acknowledge that much of the range and depth of their knowledge has conditional certainty in terms of contextual relevance and durability.

Thus, knowledge claims developed by individuals or groups need to be critiqued and validated in the field in practice settings. At the simplest level this involves identifying whether the knowledge informs practice and is compatible with practice demands and tasks. However, the empirical improvement in patient outcomes as a result of utilizing this new knowledge is only part of the equation. Another important element of the validation of the new knowledge in the practice setting involves a critical appreciation of the professional practice within which the new knowledge is being activated. Appreciating practice (see Fish 1998, pp. 205–206) involves:

- understanding the context (the history, traditions and physical context) within which the practice is carried out
- discerning beneath professional practice the professional's aims, intentions and, above all, vision
- being clear about the moral ends of the practice and the appropriateness of the means to these ends
- being aware of the worth of the practice as professional practice

- recognizing the professional's skills, capacities and abilities, theories, values, emotions, beliefs and personal qualities
- seeing the artistic nature of the performance and perceiving what the professional has done to achieve this artistry
- discerning within practice the fusion (the balance and harmony, integration and unity) of the visible with the invisible (skills, thoughts, theories, values, abilities, emotions and personal qualities), and thus discerning the value of the practice as a whole
- identifying the employment of imagination within the practice
- distinguishing and distilling out from this picture the observer's own vision.

Understanding and developing practice, from the practitioners' perspective, is a matter not of looking at practice via theory, but of working from within practice itself to enquire into practice (Eraut 1994, Fish 1998, Fish & Coles 1998). This allows new knowledge to be used, critiqued and refined in the practice context and may result in the identification of deeper understanding of professional practice itself.

Generating experience-based knowledge is one way of creating knowledge out of practice. Research is another. We are not talking here of research done out of the context of practice, but rather research that begins with an insight or observation arising from practice, or research that is conducted as part of practice or within the practice setting and, above all, research that serves the goal of enhancing practice.

The starting point of practice-based research can be a recognition that experience-based knowledge does indeed count as knowledge, that it arises from observation and awareness of experience (including professional practice) and that it undergoes a process of testing and verification, as discussed above, that can be just as rigorous as other research (experimental, phenomenological and critical). The second valuable realization is that this knowledge is different in source and process of generation and is different in kind (non-propositional) from research-generated (propositional) knowledge. Thirdly, it is valuable to recognize that both these forms of knowledge can often benefit from translation into the other form. For instance, the starting point of research could be professional craft knowledge of effective treatments; post-research this becomes empirically tested, generalized knowledge with claims of population applicability. Conversely, generalized knowledge for a broad and criterion-referenced population can be translated through the practice application and testing of skilled practitioners to become particularized, context-rich professional craft knowledge suitable for unique individuals or within population complex subgroups.

There is a particular need, whether by generating experience-based knowledge in practice or by researching practice wisdom, to take the professional craft knowledge of experienced practitioners, particularly their implicit and tacit knowledge, and seek to understand, test and share this knowledge for the enhancement of practice, education and patient outcomes. After the identification of dimensions of practice, particularly of expert practice, empirical research may then be used to test the efficacy of that knowledge more

broadly across a range of practitioners and settings. Through this testing process, the professional craft knowledge of individuals can be transformed into propositional knowledge of the profession. It is then ready to be reconsidered by practitioners themselves. In this way the ongoing spiral of the development and use of knowledge in professional practice continues.

CONCLUSION

Practitioners who explore their own practice are an important starting point in the generation of new practice knowledge. They are a vital and primary source of evidence about clinical knowing and thinking, and they provide the key means of sharing and refining new visions of practice. For this reason the professional development of practitioners is vital to the welfare of patients and the progress of the profession. Being part of a professional group requires this attention to expanding one's own as well as the profession's knowledge base.

References

Ayer A J 1956 The problem of knowledge. Penguin, London

Beeston S, Higgs J 2001 Professional practice: artistry and connoisseurship. In: Higgs J, Titchen A (eds) Practice knowledge and expertise in the health professions. Butterworth-Heinemann, Oxford, p 108–117

Beeston S, Simons H 1996 Physiotherapy practice: practitioners' perspectives. Physiotherapy Theory and Practice 12:231–242

Berlin I (ed) 1979 Against the current: essays in the history of ideas. Hogarth Press, London

Eisner E 1981 On the differences between scientific and artistic approaches to qualitative research. Educational Reader, April:5–9

Eisner E W 1985 The art of educational evaluation: a personal view. Falmer Press, London

Eraut M 1994 Developing professional knowledge and competence. Falmer Press, London

Fish D 1998 Appreciating practice in the caring professions: refocusing professional development and practitioner research. Butterworth-Heinemann, Oxford

Fish D 2001 Mentoring and the artistry of professional practice. In: Mentoring in the new millennium: a selection of papers from the Second British Council Regional Mentor Conference, April 2000. Cluj-Napocca, Romania, Editura Napocca Star, p 11–26

Fish D, Coles C (eds) 1998 Developing professional judgement in health care: learning through the critical appreciation of practice. Butterworth-Heinemann, Oxford

Fish D, de Cossart L 2007 Developing the wise doctor. Royal Society of Medicine Press, London

Ford P, Walsh M 1994 New rituals for old: nursing through the looking glass. Butterworth-Heinemann, Oxford

Freidson E 1994 Professionalism reborn: theory, prophesy and policy. Polity Press, Cambridge

Freidson E 2001 Professionalism: the third logic. Polity Press, Cambridge

Grahame-Smith D 1995 Evidence-based medicine: Socratic dissent. British Medical Journal 310:1126–1127

Heidegger M (trans. J Macquarie, E Robinson) 1926/1990 Being and time. Basil Blackwell, Oxford

Higgs J, Titchen A 2000 Knowledge and reasoning. In: Higgs J, Jones M (eds) Clinical reasoning in the health professions, 2nd edn. Butterworth-Heinemann, Oxford, p 23–32

Higgs J, Titchen A, Neville V 2001 Professional practice and knowledge. In: Higgs J, Titchen A (eds) Practice knowledge and expertise in the health professions. Butterworth-Heinemann, Oxford, p 3–9

Higgs J, Fish D, Rothwell R 2004 Practice knowledge – critical appreciation. In: Higgs J, Richardson B, Abrandt Dahlgren M (eds) Developing practice knowledge for health professionals. Butterworth-Heinemann, Oxford, p 89–105

Jones M, Higgs J 2000 Will evidence-based practice take the reasoning out of practice? In: Higgs J, Jones M (eds) Clinical reasoning in the health professions, 2nd edn. Butterworth-Heinemann, Oxford, p 307–315

Kleinig J 1982 Philosophical issues in education. Routledge, London

Krefting L 1991 The culture concept in the everyday practice of occupational and physical therapy. Physical and Occupational Therapy in Pediatrics 11(4):1–16

Lovejoy A O 1940 Reflections on the history of ideas. Journal of the History of Ideas 1(1):3–23

Montgomery K 2006 How doctors think: clinical judgement and the practice of medicine. Oxford University Press, Oxford

Popper K 1959 The logic of scientific discovery. Cambridge University Press, Cambridge

Popper K R 1970 Normal science and its dangers. In: Lakatos I, Musgrave A (eds) Criticism and the growth of knowledge. Cambridge University Press, New York, p 51–58

Rogoff B 1995 Observing socio-cultural activity on three planes: participatory appropriation, guided participation, and apprenticeship. In: Wertsch J V (ed) Socio-cultural studies of mind. Cambridge University Press, Cambridge, p 139–164

Ryle G 1949 The concept of mind. Penguin, Harmondsworth

Schön D A 1983 The reflective practitioner: how professionals think in action. Basic Books, New York

Vygotsky L S 1978 Mind in society: the development of higher psychological processes. Harvard University Press, Cambridge, MA

Vygotsky L S (trans. A Kozulin) 1986 Thought and language. MIT Press, Cambridge, MA [originally published 1962]

White S 1997 Evidence-based practice and nursing: The new panacea? British Journal of Nursing 6:175–178

Wittgenstein L (trans. G E M Anscombe) 1958 Philosophical investigations, 3rd edn. Prentice Hall, Upper Saddle River, NJ [originally published 1953]

Chapter **15**

Understanding knowledge as a sociocultural historical phenomenon

Dale Larsen, Stephen Loftus and Joy Higgs

INTRODUCTION

Knowledge is an essential component of clinical reasoning. In this chapter we take the view that knowledge is both a tool and a sociocultural historical phenomenon. To explore and substantiate this view we locate this argument as follows:

- Health professions emerge and operate within sociocultural, political and historical frames of reference, generating and continually refining the knowledge and language of these professions.
- Knowledge exists and is used in a historical frame of reference. This is examined in the discipline of the history of ideas.
- Cultural communities interact via artefacts or tools, particularly knowledge and language, which are core and defining features of such communities.

This framing of knowledge was recently examined in two research projects. The first investigated the evolution of practice knowledge in a disciplinary context (Larsen 2003, Larsen et al 2003). The second explored the place of sociocultural, historical frameworks and practice communities in developing the ability of practitioners to use practice knowledge in clinical decision making (Loftus 2006, Loftus & Higgs 2006). Both projects identified the importance to professional practice of the way knowledge is construed. Understanding knowledge as a sociocultural historical phenomenon enabled Dale Larsen (2003) to examine in detail the nature, depth and changing patterns of knowledge that practitioners (in manual therapy) have used to support their practice, to produce a rational and rich contextual framework of the knowledge practitioners currently use in this discipline, and to provide a critique of the forms and origins of knowledge used. This, it is argued, is one of the responsibilities of professionals: to understand and critique the knowledge they use in practice. Stephen Loftus (2006) identified the substantial influences of sociocultural factors and the personal history and socialization experiences of individual practitioners and students on the way they understand what knowledge is and how they use and name it in practice. From his work (see also Chapter 31) we can identify the importance of understanding knowledge as a key tool for decision making and practice actions in the changing sociocultural and historical worlds of practice.

LOCATING KNOWLEDGE, REASONING AND PRACTICE WITHIN SOCIOCULTURAL FRAMES OF REFERENCE

Professions are practice communities that evolve in sociocultural, political and historical frames of reference. They are occupations constantly in search of greater professionalization. They are influenced by forces from within, such as a drive towards self-regulation and autonomy. In addition, they are driven by a need for external recognition, the pursuit of ongoing credibility and viability in the marketplace, the desire for recognized status and respect in a competitive practice arena, and an ongoing drive towards continued development of their knowledge base and practice.

Professions face many external influences, including changing demographics, the expectations and demands of society and consumers, perpetually fluctuating economic and political demands of governments and employers, and persistent changes in the resources and demands of their knowledge, physical, technological and human worlds. Practitioners endeavour to locate and pursue their reasoning, knowledge evolution and use, and their practice in these contexts. In turn, it is their knowledge, reasoning and practice

that help more broadly to shape their practice communities, the world of healthcare practice and society. For example, multicultural communities often seek a mixture of healthcare services, blending traditional practices of different cultural groups and mainstream medicine. In the health sector there is a matching trend to provide services which combine (through referrals or integrated practices) mainstream and complementary medicine approaches (Grace et al 2006).

CLINICAL REASONING AND KNOWLEDGE AS ACCULTURATED PHENOMENA

For centuries, Western thought was dominated by the Cartesian notions that reasoning and knowing were essentially activities of individuals operating in isolation. These ideas have been challenged in recent decades by scholars such as Vygotsky (1978, 1986) and Bakhtin (1986). In their view reasoning and knowing begin as activities embedded in social interaction; they are primarily intersubjective processes provided to us by our culture. They become gradually internalized by individuals who can then use such knowledge and reasoning for themselves. We become acculturated into societies that provide us with a cognitive toolkit of knowledge and ways of using such knowledge. Professionalization can be viewed as a specialized form of this acculturation. Professional education and training are primarily about socializing students into particular ways of knowing and thinking about the world of practice.

In Vygotskian terms, professional ways of thinking and knowing are higher mental functions. Vygotsky (1978) distinguished higher mental functions from the lower mental functions which we share with animals. He claimed that higher mental functions, which would include clinical reasoning, are qualitatively different from the lower, and cannot be reduced to them. Higher mental functions need a different conceptual framework, one that takes into account their cultural and historical nature. Unfortunately, the dominant cognitivist and behaviourist paradigms within fields such as professional and clinical reasoning are reductionist, and so have been unable adequately to conceptualize the issues involved in such higher mental functions. Schön (1987) addressed another aspect of this problem when he discussed the way that language, in the form of our terminology, has been used to close off inquiry. He contended that the observation that outstanding practitioners have more wisdom, or talent, or artistry should be the point from which we can open up inquiry into the nature of these concepts. In fact, these terms are often used to bring inquiry to an end, as concepts such as artistry and talent do not fit within the domain of propositional knowledge. The cognitive paradigm is based upon a metaphor of *the mind as a computer*. Concepts such as artistry, talent and wisdom have no place within this metaphor, and therefore become effectively invisible to those who think this way. Cognitivism admits knowledge in one form only, that of technical rationality.

However, there is a growing realization that knowledge and rationality can be conceptualized in different ways. Wells (2000), taking a Vygotskian viewpoint, differentiated five types of knowledge: instrumental, procedural, substantive, aesthetic and theoretical. These are said to form an ascending hierarchy of more and more sophisticated forms of knowledge. From this perspective, these different forms of knowledge have emerged over the course of human history as a result of the development of culture that requires people to engage in various activities. The Western world has been dominated by one model of rationality for several centuries, the model of rationality based upon science. Consequently, the health professions have come to view themselves as sciences when it could be argued they should be seen as scientifically informed practices (Montgomery 2006). A science and a scientifically informed practice are quite different. Lawyers might use forensic science in a courtroom but they are not scientists; they are scientifically informed practitioners. Montgomery (2006) argued that medicine (and by implication all health professions) should be seen in the same way, emphasizing that there are other ways than scientific technical rationality of being rational. She discussed notions such as Geertz's (1983) insights into so-called 'common sense'. Geertz observed that the common sense of a culture might be obvious to people immersed in that culture. However, on closer examination it is quite clear that common sense is a sophisticated body of knowledge. According to Montgomery (2006), health professionals often ascribe their expertise to common sense, forgetting that it is a hard-won common sense, available only to insiders in the profession. It is a form of rationality that is 'culturally engendered' and 'communally reinforced' (p. 165). The *phronesis*, or practical rationality, of Aristotle is a closely related notion. This is the difficult to articulate knowledge acquired only through the experience of doing one's practice. Professional craft knowledge (Higgs & Titchen 1995) is a related concept.

HISTORY OF IDEAS

The knowledge that health professionals possess is embedded in and arises from the context of their practice. As all professions are human practices they can best be understood by appreciating the close interrelationship of knowledge and history. Professional knowledge is located within the wider history of ideas and the broader knowledge of society (Higgs et al 2004). Professional practice knowledge evolves as a consequence of individual and group reflection on the profession's knowledge and practice. The exploration of the history of ideas within a practice can therefore assist practitioners to contextualize their understanding of contemporary practice and enhance their ability to work more effectively on developing it.

The development of practice knowledge of the health professions occurs within a variety of contexts. These contexts include the historical era, and the cultural, social and individual perspectives of practitioners, scholars and researchers engaged in the exploration of practice and practice knowledge. Educators who are informed about the development of knowledge in their discipline can help their students to understand the history of ideas and the evolution of the theories underpinning current practice. Clinicians can gain insight into their clinical reasoning and beliefs through an understanding of the development of knowledge and the strengths and limitations of practice knowledge within their area of practice. A sense of history also assists researchers to focus on important practice themes, to avoid short-lived and questionable fads and fashions in the field, and to identify gaps or problem areas in knowledge which require investigation.

The discipline of the history of ideas was popularized by the American philosopher Arthur Lovejoy (1873–1962) in the 1920s (Burke 1988, Kelley 1990). The term *history of ideas* encompasses study approaches which centre on how the meaning and associations of ideas change according to history (Burke 1988). Lovejoy (1936, p. 20) proposed that the task of the history of ideas is to:

> attempt to understand how *new* beliefs and intellectual fashions are introduced and diffused, to help to elucidate the psychological character of the processes by which changes in the vogue and influence of ideas have come about; to make clear, if possible, how conceptions dominant, or extensively prevalent in one generation lose their hold upon men's minds and give place to others.

Lovejoy's argument was that we understand ourselves better by understanding the ways in which we have evolved, or the manner in which we have come, over time, to hold the ideas that we do. A history of ideas aims at interpretation and unification of ideas, seeking to correlate matters which in a reductionist way of thinking may appear unconnected. According to Lovejoy (1936, p. 15), to understand an idea fully, 'its nature and its historic role [need] . . . to be traced connectedly through all the phases of a man's reflective life in which [the workings of that idea] manifest themselves or through as many of them as the historian's resources permit.' History needs to be concerned with ideas that attain a wide diffusion, and to cross barriers between different disciplines and thinking, recognizing the fact that ideas that emerge at any one time usually manifest themselves in more than one direction (Lovejoy 1936, 1940).

Lovejoy's successors considered the term 'intellectual history' preferable to 'history of ideas' as it more accurately reflects its purpose (i.e. to trace the history of thinking) and the interdisciplinary scope of the enterprise (Kelley 1990, Mandelbaum 1983, Tosh 2000). According to Kelley (1990, p. 19), 'intellectual history can now be seen as an approach or range of approaches to historical interpretation.' In general these approaches begin with the study of cultural and linguistic forms but do not presume the conventions of academia or formal logical discourse.

The subject of intellectual historians is texts, or their cultural analogues, and the intelligible field of study is generally language (Kelley 1990): 'Intellectual history is at least as concerned with the reading as with the writing of texts – the reception and distortion, as well as creation and transmission of ideas and culture' (p. 24). Questions of text, context and in many cases authorial intention are basic to the task of the intellectual historian and the hermeneutical (or interpretive) condition of intellectual history. In this sense Hamilton (1993) proposed that intellectual history can be visualized as multiple sets of concentric circles representing ideas, people, social structures and culture. The researcher must be able to visualize each of the circles and understand their interrelationships if a credible explanation is to be formulated.

Throughout the ages different cultures have had their own visions, sets of values and ideas. Since a history of ideas is a synthesis of intellectual history, it is a powerful tool in identifying important themes in knowledge development (Lovejoy 1983). A history of ideas approach allows the origins of ideas to be known and one's own ideas to be placed in perspective (Adams 1987). 'One of the safest (and most useful) generalizations from a study of the history of ideas is that every age tends to exaggerate the scope or finality of its own discoveries, or rediscoveries, to be so dazzled by them that it fails to discern clearly their limitations' (Lovejoy 1940, p. 17). An understanding of the history of ideas or concepts that have previously been the subject of investigation helps to clarify the knowledge increment contributed by one's own findings (Adams 1987). A history of ideas is therefore 'a program mindful of the extent . . . to which the community in the context of which that author does his thinking includes not only those presently living but those who have gone before' (Oakley 1987, p. 245).

There are three basic commitments that have long been associated with intellectual history, the first of which is thinking itself (in intellectual history, thinking is the event). The second commitment is to the belief in the significance of thinking done by persons whose social function was to produce or disseminate ideas. The third commitment is to the idea that thinking occurs in a social context, that is, a background of socially constructed beliefs, values and symbolic meanings which can either facilitate or restrict what people say and think (Hollinger 1985). Such social contexts have been described as communities of practice.

COMMUNITIES OF PRACTICE

Disciplines and professions are examples of communities of practice (Lave & Wenger 1991). A community of practice is a group of people participating in communal activity, such as the dental profession promoting and supporting the oral health of a population. A shared identity is both created and experienced by participating in the activities of that community. A community of practice is distinguished by the organization of people around particular knowledge and activities that matter to them. Such communities can be informal or highly organized. The concept of communities of practice focuses attention on the social interactions that foster learning rather than the private cognitive processes of individuals.

Wenger (1998) developed the community of practice notion to highlight the dialectical nature of professional knowledge, such as the tension between explicit and tacit knowledge. Explicit knowledge is the official knowledge of the group, such as might be found in a textbook. Tacit knowledge, on the other hand, is difficult to articulate and comes only with the experience of practice. Tacit knowledge is linked to the 'know-how', as opposed to the 'know-what' of explicit knowledge. Both are needed to be a competent professional. Tacit knowledge connects with the notions of *phronesis* and with the highly specialized common sense of a profession. These forms of knowledge can only be acquired and mastered in practice, and they need active communities of practice to sustain and develop them over time. Such forms of knowledge are difficult to document and are dependent on a community of active practitioners implementing the knowledge in their work. It is the practice itself that integrates the tacit and the explicit knowledge and gives them both meaning.

This is why someone cannot become a doctor or a dentist or a physiotherapist (etc.) by reading the profession's textbooks. Practitioners must become immersed in the work before they can begin to grasp how the knowledge and the practice (of their profession) all fit together. When practitioners become immersed in the dialogue between knowledge and practice, then, and only then, are they in a position to understand what it is they are doing.

KNOWLEDGE AND LANGUAGE

Central to all forms of knowledge is language. As Halliday (1993, p. 94) wrote, 'language is the essential condition of knowing, the process by which experience *becomes* knowledge'. Fundamental to the mastery of any knowledge field is the mastery of the appropriate language. Members of a community of practice are expected to use language in certain ways. This means they will use knowledge in ways that fit within the norms laid down by the profession.

For Vygotsky (1978, 1986) the power of language lay in the ways it is embedded or interwoven into the rest of our activities, including professional activities and the knowledge that is required for such activities. Vygotsky asserted that humans can only be understood when pursuing their normal activities within a realistic and relevant context. There is always a sociocultural context, even when working alone. There is a 'situatedness' in people's lives which cannot be divorced from their activities if we wish to understand those activities. He introduced the notion that the mediation of artefacts is central to human activity and its underlying knowledge. This recognition of the centrality of artefacts in human life was one of his most important insights.

An artefact is 'an aspect of the material world that has been modified over the history of its incorporation into goal-directed human action' (Cole 1996, p. 117). Artefacts can be anything that humans use, and they are simultaneously ideal and material. They vary from material tools, such as stethoscopes and other hardware, to intellectual artefacts such as the knowledge base of a profession. The most important artefact by far is language itself, such as the professional terminology of a healthcare profession. The social institutions in which we participate are also artefactual.

An important aspect of artefacts is the way they carry the past into the present. Mastering the use of artefacts and the practices in which they are employed enables people to assimilate the history, knowledge base and culture of their professions and to become proficient practitioners in their own right. Mastering the artefact of language is a particularly crucial aspect by which clinicians become acculturated into their professions. Using language appropriately, in both written and verbal forms, is a key aspect of demonstrating professional competence. Vygotsky maintained that artefacts are not external to human thought, acting upon it. Rather, he proposed that artefacts, particularly language, fundamentally shape thought, and they constitute and transform it. If we wish to understand how people acquire professional knowledge we can use Vygotsky's insights in exploring how clinicians use language as a psychological tool to shape their perceptions and actions and become members of their professional community.

CONCLUSION

Collective and individual practice professional knowledge is generated and refined within socio-cultural, political and historical contexts. Within these contexts practitioners are acculturated into professional communities as they seek to pursue their knowledge, reasoning and practice, which in turn impacts on health care and society more broadly. The development of professional knowledge, therefore, necessitates both individual and collective reflection on what a professional knows and understands within the context of the era in which this evolution occurred. An understanding of the history of ideas underpinning professional practice can assist practitioners to gain greater insight into (and develop) their clinical reasoning and beliefs. Viewing health professions as communities of practice which embody different types of knowledge, and which sustain and develop that knowledge in a dialogical manner, provides a conceptual framework for a better understanding of what being a responsible, effective, decision-making health professional entails.

References

Adams J 1987 Historical review and appraisal of research on learning, retention, and transfer of human motor skills. Psychological Bulletin 10(1):41–74

Aristotle (trans. T Irwin) 1985 Nichomachean ethics. Hackett, Indianapolis

Bakhtin M (trans. V W McGee) 1986 Speech genres and other late essays. University of Texas Press, Austin, TX

Burke P 1988 History of ideas. In: Bullock A, Stallybrass O, Trombley S (eds) The Fontana dictionary of modern thought, 2nd edn. Fontana, London, p 388

Cole M 1996 Cultural psychology: a once and future discipline. Harvard University Press, Boston

Geertz C 1983 Local knowledge: further essays in interpretive anthropology. Basic Books, New York

Grace S, Higgs J, Horsfall D 2006 Integrating mainstream and complementary and alternative medicine: investing in prevention. In: Proceedings of the University of Sydney From Cell to Society 5 Conference, November 9–10, 2006, p 18–25

Halliday M A K 1993 Towards a language-based theory of learning. Linguistics and Education 5:93–116

Hamilton D B 1993 The idea of history and the history of ideas. Image: Journal of Nursing Scholarship 25(1):45–48

Higgs J, Titchen A 1995 The nature, generation and verification of knowledge. Physiotherapy 81:521–530

Higgs J, Andresen L, Fish D 2004 Practice knowledge – its nature, sources and contexts. In: Higgs J, Richardson B, Abrandt Dahlgren M (eds) Developing practice knowledge for health professionals. Butterworth-Heinemann, Edinburgh, p 51–69

Hollinger D 1985 In the American province: studies in the history and historiography of ideas. Johns Hopkins University Press, Baltimore

Kelley D R 1990 What is happening to the history of ideas? Journal of the History of Ideas 51(1):3–25

Larsen D 2003 The development of a conceptual framework spinal manual therapy in physiotherapy. Unpublished PhD Thesis, University of Sydney, Australia

Larsen D, Higgs J, Refshauge K et al 2003 The development of knowledge in spinal manual therapy. Presented at 14th International Congress of the World Confederation for Physical Therapy, 7–12 June, Barcelona

Lave J, Wenger E 1991 Situated learning: legitimate peripheral participation. Cambridge University Press, Cambridge

Loftus S 2006, Language in clinical reasoning: learning and using the language of collective clinical decision making. PhD Thesis. University of Sydney, Australia, Online. Available: http://ses.library.usyd.edu.au/handle/2123/1165

Loftus S, Higgs J 2006, Learning and using the language of collective clinical decision making. In: Proceedings of the ANZAME Conference 'Fill the Gaps', Gold Coast, Australia, 29 June – 2 July, p 56

Lovejoy A D 1936 The great chain of being: a study of the history of an idea. Harvard Press, Cambridge, MA

Lovejoy A O 1940 Reflections on the history of ideas. Journal of the History of Ideas 1(1):3–23

Lovejoy A O 1983 The study of the history of ideas. In: King P (ed) The history of ideas: an introduction to method. Croom Helm, London, p 179–197

Mandelbaum M 1983 On Lovejoy's historiography. In: King P (ed) The history of ideas: an introduction to method. Croom Helm, London, p 198–210

Montgomery K 2006 How doctors think: clinical judgment and the practice of medicine. Oxford University Press, Oxford

Oakley F 1987 Lovejoy's unexplored option. Journal of the History of Ideas 48(2):231–245

Schön D A 1987 Educating the reflective practitioner. Jossey-Bass, San Francisco

Tosh J 2000 The pursuit of history, 3rd edn. Pearson Education, Harlow

Vygotsky L S 1978 Mind in society: the development of higher psychological processes. Harvard University Press, Cambridge, MA

Vygotsky L S (trans. A Kozulin) 1986 Thought and language. MIT Press, Cambridge, MA [originally published 1962]

Wells G 2000 Dialogic inquiry in education: building on the legacy of Vygotsky. In: Lee M C, Smagorinsky P (eds) Vygotskian perspectives on literary research. Cambridge University Press, Cambridge, p 51–85

Wenger E 1998 Communities of practice: learning, meaning, and identity. Cambridge University Press, Cambridge

Chapter 16

Professional practice judgement artistry

Margo Paterson and Joy Higgs

INTRODUCTION

A reflective revolution is occurring in professional practice which requires knowledge beyond science to best provide quality client-centred professional services (Edwards et al 2004; Fulford et al 1996; Higgs & Titchen 2001a, b). In this revolution there is an increasing interest among various professions in challenging the hegemony of biomedical science and the medical model. There is growing support for a wellness orientation in care, and recognition of the unique blend of reasoning approaches which characterize and enrich health care (e.g. Edwards et al 2004, Mattingly & Fleming 1994). If we are to incorporate in practice the breadth of evidence that serves the interests of client/patient-centred care as well as evidence-based practice (which need not be mutually exclusive) then we need to address one of the greatest challenges facing the health professions today; that is, the need to make visible and credible the many invisible, tacit and as yet unexplored aspects of professional practice that are vital to the success of the professions.

This chapter reports on recent research (Paterson 2003, Paterson & Higgs 2001) that addressed this topic by focusing on the fusion of two such invisible and tacit aspects of advanced and expert practice: professional judgement and practice artistry. The construct *professional practice judgement artistry* (PPJA) was developed to name this merged skill.

PROFESSIONAL ARTISTRY IN PRACTICE

In client-centred health care we are seeing a significant trend to explore and embrace emerging literature (Eraut 1994, Fish 1998, Higgs & Titchen 2001c, Scott 1990, Titchen 2000) that acknowledges the value of artistry within professional practice, alongside science and humanism. Professional artistry is a uniquely individual view of practice within a shared tradition involving a blend of practitioner qualities, practice skills and creative imagination processes (Higgs & Titchen 2001c). It is concerned with 'practical knowledge, skilful performance or knowing as doing' (Fish 1998, p. 87) and is developed through the acquisition of a deep and relevant knowledge base and extensive experience (Beeston & Higgs 2001). Importantly, professional artistry does not negate research and theoretical knowledge or scientific evidence for practice; rather the professional artist practitioner uses such knowledge as a significant part of the range of knowledge (including experience-based knowledge) that serves as tools, input and a framework for clinical decision making.

PROFESSIONAL JUDGEMENT

Professional judgement refers to the ways in which practitioners interpret patients' problems and issues and demonstrate saliency and concern in responding to these matters. It involves deliberate, conscious decision making and is associated with professional competence and judgements that reflect holistic discrimination, intuition and responsiveness reflective of proficient and expert performance (Dreyfus & Dreyfus 1986, p. 2). Judgement is both an action, the process of making evaluative decisions, and the product of these decisions. Health professionals constantly make judgements within, about and as a result of practice. We speak of making a judgement in much the same way as making a clinical decision, but with perhaps a greater emphasis, in judgement making, on the importance of higher level awareness, discrimination and evaluation in the face of the greyness (complexity) of professional practice due to its complexity, humanity, uncertainty and

indeterminacy. If decision making in professional practice were entirely procedural and logical it could potentially be reduced to the realm of rules and manuals. However, from the viewpoint of PPJA, to be a professional and to provide professional services means that the client is receiving the benefit of extensive education and the capacity of the professional to make complex, situationally relevant judgements, utilizing a deep and broad store of professional knowledge. Skilled professionals are expected to have both propositional knowledge of the field and also experience-derived knowledge. Clients seek this blend of knowledge in the same way that they want technical competence as well as a depth of experience and artistry in refining these skills to address their unique needs.

OVERVIEW OF THE PPJA RESEARCH

A hermeneutic study (Paterson 2003) was conducted to investigate the question 'How can the term judgement artistry be understood in relation to occupational therapy (OT) practice?' The hermeneutic strategy, derived from the work of Gadamer and colleagues (Gadamer 1976, 1981; Gadamer et al 1988), was implemented as a hermeneutic spiral incorporating three hermeneutic strategies:

- A *dialogue of questions and answers* resulted in the creation of two sets of texts, the first based on existing research and theoretical interpretations of professional judgement, clinical decision making and professional artistry as the substrates of judgement artistry, and the second comprising transcripts of interviews and focus groups with 53 experienced OT educators and practitioners. The dialogue continued as a hermeneutic conversation between the text and the researchers (see Koch 1999).
- The term *hermeneutic circle* is used to describe 'the experience of moving dialectically between the parts and the whole' (Koch 1996, p. 176). This involved the researchers moving repeatedly between interpretations of parts of the text and interpretations of the whole text, the latter

representing an emerging understanding of the phenomenon.

- A *fusion of horizons* involved different researcher and participant interpretations of the phenomenon under investigation (in this case professional practice judgement artistry) being brought together through dialogue to produce shared understanding.

The text interpretation process involved repeated engagement with the texts, using these three strategies in the hermeneutic spiral. The researchers became deeply immersed in the texts, examining the parts or segments of the texts and then spiralling out to answer questions posed and reflect on the emerging whole or bigger picture of the phenomenon of PPJA being interpreted. Further details of the research strategy are presented in Paterson & Higgs (2005).

PPJA RESEARCH FINDINGS

A) PARTICIPANTS' UNDERSTANDING OF JUDGEMENT ARTISTRY

The *artistry of the judgements*, being individually tailored and perceived, is impossible to represent as a single image. However, many of the participants in this research used various metaphors of professional artists at work to portray the special characteristics of judgement artistry. Examples included the artisan (artistry in painters, sculptors and jewellers), the athlete (in dance and sports), the cook/chef and the musician/conductor. In all cases the intention of these metaphors was to illuminate participants' understanding of PPJA from the viewpoint of either an educator or a practitioner, elicited in a focus group or an individual interview. The unattributed quotations in this chapter are from participants in these different contexts.

An example of describing the therapist with PPJA as a cook came from one participant:

> You need proportions of technical skill, philosophy, life experience and you need equal proportions. It is like baking a cake – to be successful you need the right proportions – you've got to get the temperature right, the ingredients right.

An educator said that a practitioner with PPJA is similar to:

> The notion of an artisan ... I think it is like a jeweller: somebody who, for instance, knows the science of the materials they work with, has a vision about what they want to produce, and has some skills and techniques in terms of being able to take the raw materials to the end product ... There's a big difference between a jeweller who has an inert material, which is gold, and working with another human being who is very much not inert. When we look at people who have genius, like Leonardo da Vinci ... what they've actually done if you look carefully, they've actually taken more than one body of knowledge and combined them.

In the tasks of processing and unravelling the highly complex problems that arise in professional practice, PPJA utilizes the unique knowledge base, frame of reference and reasoning capacity of individual practitioners, along with the skilled valuing and inclusion of the client's knowledge, capabilities and frame of reference. Such problems can involve demanding moral and ethical issues, questions of values, beliefs and assumptions, and the intricacies of health issues as they impact on people's lives.

B) DIMENSIONS OF PPJA

Four key dimensions of PPJA were identified: professionalism, multifaceted judgements, practice artistry and reflexivity (Table 16.1). Within these dimensions were a range of generic elements, some relevant across different professions and some specific to OT. In Table 16.1 the generic elements are so called because as researchers we found authenticity in these labels for many professions, in keeping with literature beyond OT that portrays professional artistry and practice wisdom (Scott 1990), and at multidisciplinary workshops and conferences where we received feedback on the applicability of these elements in other disciplines. More research in other disciplinary areas is required to investigate this question further and to develop other discipline-specific elements.

Table 16.1   Key dimensions and generic elements of PPJA

	Professionalism	Multifaceted judgement	Practice artistry	Reflexivity
Generic elements	Having credibility Having a strong professional identity Setting (own) high standards of excellence Practising with artistic efficiency Balancing autonomy and accountability Dealing with ethical and workplace dilemmas	Micro-, macro- and meta-judgements Value judgements 'Thinking outside the box' Risk taking Critique, challenge Professional intuition Articulation of judgements/ reasoning	Embodied knowing Attunement (being in tune with people) Passion Grace and finesse Wise practice	Heightened self-awareness Critical self-evaluation Self-development
OT elements	Client-centred practice	OT practice wisdom Mutual decision making/collaboration	OT identity • Flow • Interactivity • Conscious use of self • Preserving self integrity	Ongoing self-development as an OT

OT = Occupational therapy; PPJA = Professional practice judgement artistry

Professionalism

Professionalism is seen as an integral aspect of PPJA, as well as being the broader context for making high level/artistic professional/clinical judgements. That is, professionalism is a key ingredient of making sound judgements and demonstrating judgement artistry as well as being the overall framework within which professional practice occurs. Professionalism is portrayed by Eraut (1994) as an ideology, characterized by the traits and features of an 'ideal type' profession. Professionals are expected to practise with integrity and personal tolerance, to communicate effectively across language, cultural and situational barriers (Josebury et al 1990) and to demonstrate social responsibility (Prosser 1995), accountability and recognition of their limitations (Sultz et al 1984).

During interviews and focus groups the research participants clearly identified the professional nature of practice judgements. For them, practitioners with judgement artistry constantly go beyond required levels of competence in 'furthering their professional knowledge; keeping up to date with journals; making the theory and practice link; processing and integrating highly complex information'. They blend technical efficiency and evidence with humanity. On an individual client level they weigh 'the evidence versus the everyday, "what's important", the priorities for the person'. The connection with efficiency was identified:

> Sound clinical reasoning [is needed] to confirm why [professionals] were doing what they were doing. They had really fantastic networks, they were using literature . . . they were thinking all the while, it does come into time, it comes into efficiency.

Multifaceted judgement

This is a major feature of PPJA (as opposed to standard decision making), and involves a deep understanding of professional judgement, along with the capacity to artistically, credibly and effectively juggle the many human, technical and contextual facets of judgement at micro, macro and meta levels. Recognition of these different levels and facets of judgement was an important finding of this research (Table 16.2). Judgements can occur at micro (within process), macro (in outcomes

Table 16.2   Types of professional judgement

Type of judgement	Definition	Example
Micro-	Process decisions, or decisions within decisions	Reliability of data, choice of next action/test/question
Macro-	Output decisions or conclusions	Diagnosis, prognosis, management plan, agreement with client on healthcare goals
Meta-	Reflective evaluative decisions	Awareness of change in client's responses to intervention, self-monitoring, recognition of communication difficulties

and conclusions), and meta (monitoring) levels. Micro-judgements are made constantly in clinical practice. They deal with such questions as: Are these data reliable? How does this joint feel? What instruments and equipment do I need for this procedure? References to macro-judgements occur frequently in the extensive literature on clinical reasoning with a particular focus on making decisions about diagnosis, treatment, and prognosis. The meta-judgement level involves employing metacognition within reasoning and decision making, to refine, question and monitor the reasoning process and challenge the decisions being made. This requires a heightened level of awareness of one's actions and thinking, and the capacity critically to reflect upon and modify thinking in response to self-evaluation. Meta-judgement is also employed in coming to understand one's reasoning and learning how to use and choose strategies for making, critiquing and refining judgements.

An example of micro-judgement is recognizing 'a change in response to different cues'. The larger, macro-judgements are 'being able to make the right decision at the right time or [within] the bigger picture, bringing together a whole lot of different things'. Meta-judgements involve metacognition and 'being able to kind of conceive of a big picture and bring a whole lot of pieces together, as distinct from making your actual decision about what your actual intervention's going to be today'.

Different levels and purposes of judgement were described by one participant as follows:

You see there are different sorts of judgements, aren't there? ... If you have a judgement in the sense of a skilled medical clinical judgement, then there is a collection of data [that leads the practitioner] to make a professional judgement that this is going to be this choice rather than that, and therefore the judgement is critical to deciding on the nature of the treatment. ... And then there is the [sort of] judgement that says what should I do now and why; and you make one judgement, and then 30 seconds later you are making another judgement and 30 seconds later you are making another judgement because what you are doing is making decisions about how to handle and support or process this evolving thing that is happening between you and another person or a situation at a particular time. That is a judgement but it is very different from the other two sorts of judgements ... It is about the irretrievability of the decision-making: that moment in time has gone and nobody can say whether your decision was right or wrong. ... So there is something about the ... ephemeral [nature of] professional judgements. ... They vanish. They go. They are not there. They are lost in time. You cannot get them back.

Practice artistry

Practice artistry is the embodiment of knowing in practice whereby practitioners bring all of their knowledge and judgement to realization in their practice acts and being.

Embodied knowing was mentioned by various participants as:

something in the eyes [of the practitioner] – the aliveness, the alertness, the constantly watching to see what is going on ... that way of connecting, spiritual level, subconscious level – you hear patterns;

being able to read body language;

being

very aware of what was going on with people, very insightful;

the ability to

change tack in the way that they're working with people, they can do it and there's no jarring, it just happens in a really sort of smooth, easy manner that's quite comfortable . . . so smooth that you don't even see the wheels turning in their head;

a particular flavour to that integration of all of your experience, your knowledge, your skill, your craft, your science, your systems, your beliefs . . . which you are choosing to use as professional artistry . . . it could be therapeutic excellence.

Reflexivity

Reflexivity is linked both to the outcome of judgement artistry (i.e. growth and enhanced capability of the practitioner) and an inherent process within it. Judgement artistry by its very nature is reflexive. Within the making of judgements, practitioners are constantly reflecting on their judgements, their capacity for judgement and their practice actions, and learning from these reflections. This is a process of self-critique and self-development. As stated by one educator, you need 'to be open to growth and development'. Participants believed that ongoing self-development was an important aspect of judgement artistry. For example:

[in] some areas of my practice I'm probably getting towards the top, but I've always got lots of reading to do and I always find a client who has got a new problem or a different situation. So I don't think I will ever be an expert . . . when you're more experienced you get through faster. You still consider huge amounts of things.

Overlap of dimensions. In looking at the dimensions listed, the overlap evident between attributes of practice as a whole and judgement which is a part

of practice is both remarkable and 'right'. For the practitioner who is a professional artist, there can be no practice without advanced judgement (PPJA), and for judgement to be demonstrated as advanced artistry it must be embedded within and congruent with the overall practice artistry approach. Just as the professional artist practitioner embodies grace and humanity in interpersonal relationships and finesse in implementing the technical skills of his/her profession, so too, PPJA must be the embodiment of such finesse, grace and humanity in thinking and decision making.

C) DEFINING PPJA

In drawing the dimensions together we generated the following definition: PPJA refers to 'the capacity of professional artist practitioners to make highly skilled micro-, macro- and meta-judgements that are optimal for the circumstances of the client and the context' (Paterson & Higgs 2001).

D) A MODEL OF PPJA

The research findings were formulated into a *model of PPJA* (Figure 16.1) which reflects the four dimensions of professional practice judgement artistry (upper section) and PPJA in occupational therapy (lower section). The image created is one of a dynamic whole (PPJA) entering the arena of OT and drawing out elements of PPJA that are consistent with and characteristic of OT. The OT section illustrates the way that PPJA has a deep connection with the philosophical underpinnings of OT in art, science and humanism. In OT the place of occupation is central and the four elements derived from the research participants' words and text interpretation reflect the essence of OT: client-centred practice, OT practice wisdom, OT identity and ongoing self-development. (For further discussion of PPJA in OT see: Paterson 2003; Paterson et al 2005, 2006.)

WHAT DOES IT MEAN TO PRACTISE USING PPJA?

Firstly, it means understanding professionalism as a means of engaging with people rather than

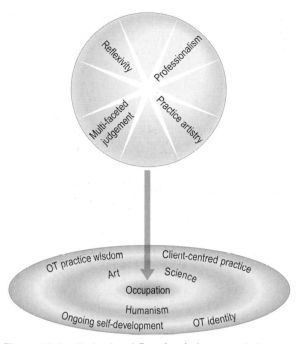

Figure 16.1 Professional Practice Judgement Artistry model in occupational therapy

distancing oneself from them. It means knowing one's professional identity and engaging in self critique, being able to set high standards for one's practice and learning to blend artistry and efficiency.

In clinical reasoning education and literature, much attention is given to knowledge and practical skills, with a growing emphasis on clinical decision making. However, even in the latter the focus is on making decisions, the reasoning processes, decision outcomes, novice–expert differences and reasoning in relation to evidence-based practice. This is the approach of science and education; it gives little attention to the subtleties of judgement. Advanced skills and capacity for judgement were identified by the participants in this study as moving beyond mere accuracy and defensibility. Instead, this PPJA mode of making judgements was highly reflexive, requiring heightened levels of self-awareness and critique and resulting in continual self-development. Practitioners evidencing PPJA continued to learn and deepen their professional craft knowledge and understanding of self and others.

In addition, PPJA was recognized in this study as being multifaceted. For such practitioners, judgements were made at multiple levels about multiple aspects of practice, ranging from the evaluation of a single piece of data to being aware of their own values and the values of others and seeking to accommodate diversity in cultural, personal and system values. Judgement involves risk taking rather than rule following. It is the key tool and challenge of the skilled practitioner and is used in making difficult decisions in the majority of clinical situations where the clarity and comfort of black and white decisions are absent and complexity, variability and 'shades of greyness' are the order of the day. Making these judgements requires practitioners to draw heavily on all their professional learning, their professional craft knowledge and their professional intuition (that is, a heightened level of awareness and perceptiveness with a greater capacity to make insightful judgments relevant to the unique situation). Articulating the judgements made and the judgements within judgements (why and how the judgement was made) requires practitioners to understand and bring to awareness, through reflection and dialogue, the nature of judgements and judgement making. One participant described a practitioner with PPJA as:

> a very good trainer, she's a very good supervisor and she's a very good manager; and she's very adaptable, she's very reflective in her practice. She was very open to change and was constantly re-evaluating her practice and the practice of the service. [Especially when she is] compared with other colleagues, who might be very resistant to change, be resistant to evaluation. And she wasn't evangelical to me, but you wouldn't really know that she was striving to improve things. She did this quite quietly really, but it was in her nature to be a good practitioner. And being a reflective practitioner, you can learn an awful lot more from those people, because they include you in that question, they include you in that problem-solving.

To practise using PPJA demands more than producing legally-, professionally- or evidence-based decisions and outcomes. Those issues and reasoning strategies are not negated by practitioners engaging in PPJA but are subsumed into a holistic approach that places the patient firmly at the centre of practice and recognizes that practice artistry requires more. It demands of the practitioner passion for wise implementation of practice, caring for others, and an understanding and embodiment of all that practice can be beyond technology and efficiency, to achieve an artistry of practice characterized by grace, attunement and finesse. As stated by an educator:

> I was talking about grace ... something outside ourselves even that allows us to become master clinicians or experts in the area. Some of it is environmental that I went from job to job, always a different area and then [I was] able to put those pieces together, and some people might not be able to do that, but I do think about [it] and I suppose I use grace instead of luck because I think of it some way more deliberate or more thoughtful a word than luck that allows some of us to be able to have that [grace]. ... John Dewey talks about intellectual grace. He talks about the idea that there is a moment when the teacher and the learner are transformed to the experience, which to me is the same thing as what I would call the therapeutic grace. There is the moment (and I mean it goes on to be a lifelong moment for some of the clients) where the client and I are transformed or transcend or whatever, so I really like that idea of his [Dewey]. ... There is something in the interaction that becomes bigger than all of us.

Some participants spoke about the difference between expertise and judgement artistry. For example:

> You can have someone who is technically expert. For instance if you have a hand therapist, who is marvellous at what she does, or he does, and gets the [client's] hands back and is absolutely wonderful, but doesn't have the humanism and the ability to nurture the whole person within that injury. The trauma of the injury, the hand injury. ... they are an expert, they are marvellous, but they haven't got that judgment artistry.

WHY IS PPJA RELEVANT TO HEALTH PROFESSIONAL PRACTICE AND HEALTH CARE TODAY?

Within the context of the growing dissatisfaction with the biomedical model as a complete framework for practice today, and the concurrent support for models of wellness and patient-centred care, a common element in healthcare rhetoric is the recognition of the importance of the human world and personal relevance of health care. In part, this is being addressed by a greater valuing and focus on the human sciences in concert with the physical and biomedical sciences. Such an argument is built around the recognition that the value of scientific study is not limited to the physical world, and the status that science accords and receives in the public arena can be shared across both the human and physical worlds.

Secondly, there is the recent trend towards models of collaborative reasoning (Edwards et al 2004). This collaborative trend is a reflection of an increasing societal movement toward greater self-management and prevention (Higgs & Hunt 1999, Richardson 1999), a higher level of accessibility of web-based healthcare information, changing views of health care as empowerment (Mattsson et al 2000, Trede et al 2003), changing healthcare funding strategies with increasing expectations of 'user pays' and community care (Lorig et al 1999), and demographic changes (including population ageing, increase in numbers of chronically ill people).

Thirdly, there is recognition of the value of interpretive and critical paradigm research (often jointly called qualitative research) for investigating human and social aspects of health and health care, alongside quantitative or empirico-analytical research with its emphasis on empirical measurement for description, testing and prediction.

Next there is an ongoing debate about what constitutes evidence (Higgs et al 2001). And finally, there is a need to look beyond science to the world of artistry in an endeavour to explore those aspects of care that are reflected in artistry, embodied knowing and the more ephemeral, person-centred and situationally-relevant aspects of caring.

References

Beeston S, Higgs J 2001 Professional practice: artistry and connoisseurship. In: Higgs J, Titchen A (eds) Practice knowledge and expertise in the health professions. Butterworth-Heinemann, Oxford, p 108–117

Dreyfus H L, Dreyfus S E 1986 Mind over machine: the power of human intuition and expertise in the era of the computer. The Free Press, New York

Edwards I, Jones M, Higgs J et al 2004 What is collaborative reasoning? Advances in Physiotherapy 6:70–83

Eraut M 1994 Developing professional knowledge and competence. Falmer Press, London

Fish D 1998 Appreciating practice in the caring professions: refocusing professional development and practitioner research. Butterworth-Heinemann, Oxford

Fulford K W M, Ersser S, Hope T 1996 Essential practice in patient-centred care. Blackwell Science, Oxford

Gadamer H G 1976 Philosophical hermeneutics (trans & ed Lange D E). University of California Press, Berkeley, CA

Gadamer H 1981 Reason in the age of science. MIT Press, Cambridge, MA

Gadamer H G, Specht E K, Stegmuller W 1988 Hermeneutics vs. science. University of Notre Dame Press, Notre Dame, IN

Higgs J, Hunt A 1999 rethinking the beginning practitioner: introducing the 'interactional professional'. In: Higgs J, Edwards H (eds) Educating beginning practitioners: challenges for health professional education. Butterworth-Heinemann, Oxford, p 10–18

Higgs J, Titchen A (eds) 2001a Practice knowledge and expertise. Butterworth-Heinemann, Oxford

Higgs J, Titchen A (eds) 2001b Professional practice in health, education and the creative arts. Blackwell Science, Oxford

Higgs J, Titchen A 2001c Rethinking the practice-knowledge interface in an uncertain world: a model for practice development. British Journal of Occupational Therapy 64(11):526–533

Higgs J, Burn A, Jones M 2001 Integrating clinical reasoning and evidence-based practice. AACN Clinical Issues: Advanced Practice in Acute and Critical Care 12(4): 482–490

Josebury H E, Bax N D S, Hannay D R 1990 Communication skills and clinical methods: a new introductory course. Medical Education 24:433–437

Koch T 1996 Implementation of a hermeneutic inquiry in nursing: philosophy, rigour and representation. Journal of Advanced Nursing 24:174–184

Koch T 1999 An interpretive research process: revisiting phenomenological and hermeneutical approaches. Nurse Researcher 6(3):20–34

Lorig K R, Sobel D S, Stewart A L et al 1999 Evidence suggesting that a chronic disease self-management program can improve health status while reducing utilization and costs: a randomized trial. Medical Care 37:5–14

Mattingly C, Fleming M H 1994 Clinical reasoning: forms of inquiry in a therapeutic practice. F A Davis, Philadelphia

Mattsson M, Wikman M, Dahlgren L et al 2000 Physiotherapy as empowerment – treating women with chronic pelvic pain. Advances in Physiotherapy 2: 125–143

Paterson M 2003 Professional practice judgement artistry in occupational therapy practice. Unpublished PhD thesis, The University of Sydney, Australia

Paterson M, Higgs J 2001 Professional practice judgement artistry. CPEA Occasional paper 3, Centre for Professional Education Advancement, The University of Sydney, Australia

Paterson M, Higgs J 2005 Using hermeneutics as a qualitative research approach in professional practice. Qualitative Report 10(2):339–357. Online. Available: http://www.nova.edu/ssss/QR/QR10-2/paterson.pdf 20 Jul 2006

Paterson M, Higgs J, Wilcox S 2005 The artistry of judgement: a model for occupational therapy practice. British Journal of Occupational Therapy 68(9):409–417

Paterson M, Higgs J, Wilcox S 2006 Developing expertise in judgement artistry in OT practice. The British Journal of Occupational Therapy 69(3):115–123

Prosser A 1995 Teaching and learning social responsibility. Higher Education Research and Development Society of Australasia, Canberra

Richardson B 1999 Professional development: 2. professional knowledge and situated learning in the workplace. Physiotherapy 85(9):467–474

Scott D 1990 Practice wisdom: the neglected source of practice research. Social Work 35:564–568

Sultz H A, Sawner K A, Sherwin F S 1984 Determining and maintaining competence: An obligation of allied health education. Journal of Allied Health 13(4):272–279

Titchen A 2000 Professional craft knowledge in patient centred nursing and the facilitation of its development. Ashdale Press, Oxford

Trede F, Higgs J, Jones M et al 2003 Emancipatory practice: a model for physiotherapy practice? Focus on Health Professional Education: A Multidisciplinary Journal 5(2):1–13

SECTION **3**

Clinical reasoning research trends

SECTION CONTENTS

Chapter 17

Methods in the study of clinical reasoning

José F. Arocha and Vimla L. Patel

This chapter presents an overview of some of the methods used in the study of clinical reasoning. It does not constitute an exhaustive overview. Rather, it presents major features of the most common approaches used in the study of clinical reasoning. In addition, we include a range of new and promising research methodologies used in clinical reasoning research and elsewhere.

From purely behaviouristic and psychometric roots, the study of clinical reasoning (see Patel et al 2005 for a review) has diversified to include different methodological commitments and techniques, developing a multiplicity of methods, and continues to do so. We have found it useful to categorize such methods along different dimensions (see Figure 17.1). One is the individual–group dimension, or the extent to which a study focuses on the individual or the group as units of analysis. A second dimension is the quantitative–qualitative dimension, or the extent to which the study makes of use quantitative or qualitative methods of data gathering and analysis. Specific studies can, of course, vary along these dimensions and may use quantitative methods to identify average differences between groups together with verbal protocol methods to characterize individual performance (Hashem et al 2003, Patel et al 2001) or use of verbal protocols in combination with interpretive methods (Ritter 2003).

QUANTITATIVE METHODS

Quantitative methodologies for investigating medical reasoning have been used in various clinical

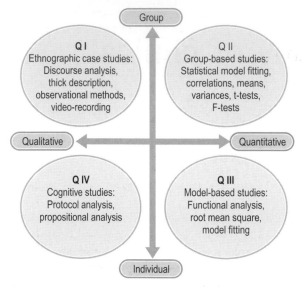

Figure 17.1 Dimensions along which research methods in clinical reasoning can be categorized

tasks. One aspect of clinical reasoning that has been investigated using group-based quantitative methods is the study of diagnosis in perceptual tasks such as X-ray or dermatological slide interpretation (Crowley et al 2003; Lesgold et al 1988; Norman et al 1989a, b). In such studies, subjects are presented with a series of X-rays or slides and then, after a period, are asked to interpret or recall the information in them. The goal is to show how variations in the subjects' interpretations (e.g. assessed through verbal recall) relate to the variations on the experimental conditions (e.g. types of slide). These data are then quantified using descriptive statistics and subjected to standard statistical analysis (e.g. null-hypothesis testing). The same methods have been employed by others (e.g. Patel & Frederiksen 1984, Schmidt & Boshuizen 1993) to compare clinical performance by groups with different levels of expertise using verbal materials such as the clinical case as independent variable and various dependent measures such as recall (Patel & Frederiksen 1984), diagnostic accuracy (Patel & Groen 1986), probability assignments (e.g. Hasham et al 2003), or decision times (Rikers et al 2005).

Although quantitative methods are most commonly used to investigate average group differences (e.g. between experimental and control

groups or between expertise levels), there is a fundamental reason for also investigating individual subjects quantitatively, namely the search for behavioural or cognitive invariants across all individuals (Runkel 1990, 2003; Simon 1990). If the overall goal of research is to understand the functioning of human beings, how they are organized such that they are capable of producing what we observe them producing, then that organization must be the same for everyone. Although unfortunately little use has been made of such methods, their addition to the methodological toolbox of the clinical reasoning researcher is welcome.

Theoretical approaches underlying individual subject research are varied, including behaviouristic, information processing, control theoretic or system dynamic approaches. Some stress the changes in overt behaviour across time while others stress the process of thinking and reasoning, the role of goals and intentions as part of people's attempts to engage in interaction with the external environment, or the perceived consequences of such engagement (Runkel 2003). The basic idea is that humans operate according to a set of principles described by the model, which must be known in order to give an accurate account of human performance in detail.

One strategy for conducting individual subject research developed from the behaviouristic research is to look at changes across condition for each individual, where the individual serves as his or her own control, by comparing multiple measures of behaviour at baseline and after experimental intervention (Sterling & McNally 1992, Weiner & Eisen 1985). Another strategy consists of generating models of individual organization, such as a computational model, and then testing the fit of the model to individual data, using quantitative fitting measures, such as the root-mean square or correlations. Research consistent with this strategy has been associated mostly with research in artificial intelligence (e.g. Clancey 1997).

A quantitative model-based methodology that sheds light on the study of reasoning is exemplified by the decision-making approach, originating from the study of economic decisions, although widely applied to other fields, including medical decisions. Typically, researchers in decision making start with a formal model of decision making and then collect data which are compared to the model. The models can be of various types, such as simple regression models, Bayesian estimation models and decision-theoretic models. The latter are the most mathematically sophisticated (Christensen et al 1991).

Decision theory has its roots in the work of Von Neumann & Morgenstern (1944) on game theory. The theory deals with making decisions in situations of uncertainty. The basic principle of the theory is that a rational person should maximize his or her expected utility, which is defined as the product of probability by utility. Hammond (1967) gave the following example: a businessman faces the decision of either winning $500,000 or losing $100,000, both of which have the same probability, 0.5. The expected utility in this case would be of $200,000 [0.5 (500,000) − 0.5 (100,000)]. Decision theory has been used mostly as a model for rational decision making. Previously, the theory was thought to describe actual human decision making, but empirical research on the psychological bases of decision making has falsified its claims as a descriptive theory (Tversky & Kahneman 1974). The theory also has been used as a normative theory under the assumption that the maximization of the expected utilities is rational. Under this assumption, to be rational, people's decisions must mirror those derived from the model. If people's decisions depart from those specified by the model, it is taken as evidence that they are not behaving rationally. This assumption, and therefore the normative character of the theory, has also been severely questioned (Allais & Hagen 1979, Bunge 1985, Hammond 1967). In short, critics argue that it is not always rational to maximize one's expected utility and therefore the theory cannot be taken as a prescription for action.

Whatever its merits either as a descriptive or a prescriptive theory, decision theory has stimulated a great deal of research in medicine (Weinstein et al 1980) and various other domains (Carroll & Johnson 1990, Dawes 1988). The research on decision theory uses a model that serves as comparison for the empirical studies. Consistent with its assumptions, most utility models are assumed to be models of rationality such that lack of agreement between the subject's responses and the model is taken as evidence that the subject does not make decisions rationally.

Decision theory also makes use of other explicit numerical models for the evaluation of human decisions. The most used models, beside the expected utility model, are the regression and the Bayesian models. These are called weighted additive models because of the assumption that the decision process has the form of an additive function, $Y_i = (X_{ij})$, in which i represents the alternative, j represents the number of attributes, and f is the function that relates the decision to the set of weighted attributes.

Typically, in a decision-making study, the subject is asked to generate a series of attributes that are of most importance for a given situation (e.g. a clinical case) and to rank them in order of importance or preference. Once this is done, a set of weights is gathered for each of the attributes. The data are then combined into a decision formula (i.e. the decision model) and a decision is generated from the model. This is then used either to help the human decision maker arrive at a good decision or as a description of the decision maker's behaviour.

These models – also called input/output models – do not take into account any mediating process between the attributes and the decision. Most of them also assume that the decision function is linear. The methods used within these approaches consist of collecting a series of responses to a limited set of choices. The models assume that all the alternatives and their consequences are known. The subject's task is to choose among these alternatives.

It is important to note that for such models to apply, all the information has to be available to the subject (and to the model). Also note that only the selection of alternatives (e.g. diagnoses) is illustrated by these models. Such observations have provoked some researchers (Fox 1988) to argue for an expansion in the study of decision making to include also the intermediate processes between the selection of attributes and the reaching of the decision. The argument supports the developing of knowledge-based decision methods based on the techniques of artificial intelligence, which calls for the inclusion of heuristics (e.g. means–ends analysis) and knowledge structures in the decision model. Although decision models have been used to describe human behaviour, psychological research (Tversky & Kahneman 1974) has shown that subjects do not behave according to the models. People show various kinds of biases that depart systematically from the models' predictions.

In summary, quantitative methods as they are used in the study of clinical reasoning cover a large variety of theoretical approaches and techniques. Some involve the collection of easily scoreable responses to investigate input/output connections with no direct examination of the processes mediating these connections, whereas others involve the development of mathematical models or computational models that serve to investigate underlying cognitive processes or reasoning strategies.

QUALITATIVE METHODS

This section deals with what are considered to be, overall, qualitative methods – those in quadrants I and IV of Figure 17.1. The methods described in this section vary widely in terms of their origins and applications and cover think-aloud protocols, discourse analysis and ethnographic methods. The first originates in the study of problem solving and the computer simulation of thought processes (Elstein et al 1990, Newell & Simon 1972), the second in the analysis of text comprehension (Frederiksen 1975) and conversation (Schiffrin et al 2001) and the third in the analysis of complex, mostly social, situations (Suchman 1987).

A common theme in all these methods is that they deal with real-life or close to real-life situations. Another common aspect is that they have become accepted as methods of scientific study by scientists, often to complement other methods. A third common feature is that they are applied to unique situations. By this we mean that each case, consisting, for example, of a physician solving a case or a pair of nurses discussing a patient problem, is taken as a unit. In contrast to the quantitative methods discussed above, qualitative researchers attempt to describe single episodes in detail rather than obtaining gross average measures of many situations.

VERBAL REPORTS

There are two kinds of verbal report. One kind is the 'think-aloud' method used in clinical reasoning and expertise research (Kassirer et al 1982). The second is the retrospective protocol, such as stimulated recall (Elstein et al 1978) and the explanation protocol (Arocha et al 2005, Patel & Arocha 1995, Patel & Groen 1986). In both cases, the researcher uses verbalizations as data, without involving introspection. That is, subjects are asked to verbalize their thoughts without 'theorizing' about their cognitive processes. Any theorizing is the responsibility of the experimenter and not of the subject (Ericsson & Simon 1984, Newell & Simon 1972). Analysis methods can be found in Ericsson & Simon (1984).

Think–aloud protocols

In typical think-aloud research, subjects are presented with a clinical case, most frequently in written form, which may contain anything from a single sentence to a whole patient record including the clinical interview, the physical examination results and the laboratory results (e.g. Hashem et al 2003). The subject is asked to read the information and verbalize whatever thoughts come to mind. If the subject pauses for a few seconds, the experimenter intervenes with questions such as 'What are you thinking about?' or, more appropriately, with demands such as 'Please, continue', which encourage the subject to carry on talking without introspecting.

Once the protocol has been collected, it is subjected to an analysis aimed at uncovering the cognitive processes and the information that were used. The analysis of the protocol is then compared to a reference or domain model of the task to be solved. This model is frequently taken either from an expert collaborator in the study or from printed information about the topic, such as textbooks or scholarly expositions. For instance, Kuipers & Kassirer (1984), in their study of causal reasoning, used a model of the Starling equilibrium mechanism which was compared to the protocols from subjects at different levels of expertise: medical students, residents, and expert physicians. In the same vein, Patel and her colleagues (Joseph

& Patel 1990, Patel & Groen 1986) used a reference model of the clinical cases, which served as a standard for comparison with subjects' protocols.

For think-aloud reports to be valid, it is necessary that some conditions be met. The conditions pertain to the type of task that should be used, the kinds of instruction given to the subject, and the familiarity of the subject with the task. Ericsson & Simon (1984) developed an extensive description of these conditions, and there is also independent research that has shown the validity of the methods (White 1988). The theory of protocol analysis is based on the assumption that verbalizations reflect a subject's search through a problem space of hypotheses and data.

Retrospective protocols

Retrospective protocols are collected after the situation described has already happened. In most situations they are collected and analysed in the same manner as think-aloud protocols, but with different goals in mind. They differ in that in think-aloud protocols subjects are asked to report whatever comes to mind without making any evaluation of their thinking. In this sense the verbalizations at time t are hypothesized to be the contents of short-term memory at time t_1. In retrospective protocols, verbalizations do not refer to the contents in short-term memory alone but are probably a mixing of short- and long-term memory information (Newell & Simon 1972). Therefore, whereas think-aloud protocols can be reliably used to characterize clinical reasoning, retrospective protocols can be used to characterize processes that are not dependent on the concurrent presentation of the stimulus materials. They may be used as a complement to think-aloud protocols or to investigate other cognitive aspects associated with reasoning such as comprehension, metacognitive activities and the use of knowledge. These methods have been used by Patel & Groen (1986), Schmidt et al (1988) and Norman et al (1989a, b) to investigate clinical tasks.

Explanation protocols

Explanation protocols are a form of retrospective protocol. Patel & Groen (1986) used such protocols with the aim of investigating expert/novice differences in medical reasoning. Influenced by the research on text comprehension (Frederiksen 1975; Kintsch 1974, 1998), they used the concept of the proposition (i.e. an idea unit) as a cognitive unit of thought. The explanation protocol is based on a number of assumptions (Arocha et al 2005). First, information, such as a clinical case description, is processed serially. That is, the information generated from a clinical problem passes through working memory first, and then linked later to information in long-term memory, which provides context for interpretation. Second, the temporal sequence in an explanation protocol follows that of the underlying reasoning, in the sense that ideas that are verbalized first are processed first. Third, although the clinical problem may be the same, the reasoning strategies and the final response (e.g. final diagnosis) vary because people process clinical information at several levels of generality, from the very specific symptom level to the general diagnostic level. Research shows that the critical factor in determining generality is the expertise of the clinician. Finally, both reasoning strategies and inferences used during clinical reasoning are a function of domain-specific prior knowledge of the clinician.

The explanation protocol method consists of asking research subjects to explain the pathophysiology of a case. The explanation is then represented in the form of a propositional structure (see Table 17.1). Analysis consists of several steps: (1) segment the subject protocol (the explanation of the case) into clauses according to the clause analysis method of Winograd (1972); (2) determine the propositions in each clause, by taking each idea unit separately as a proposition; (3) relate the propositions in a semantic network in which the relations between propositions are labelled following the propositional grammar developed by Frederiksen (1975). A semantic network is a structure of concepts and relations among concepts. Concepts are represented as nodes and relations are represented as links between nodes, according to graph theoretic notions (Sowa 1984). The relations in the semantic networks contain mostly conditional and causal links. Thus a semantic network is a connected graph in which the connections among concepts as well as the direction of reasoning are represented. A graph is connected

Table 17.1 Example of propositional analysis. Sentence: Painless recurrent haematuria suggests a possible tumour of the urinary tract

	Propositional analysis	
Proposition number	Predicate	Arguments
1.0	COND:	[1.1], [1.2]
1.1	HAEMATURIA	ATT:painless; ASPECT::ITER(recurrent)
1.2	SUGGEST	THM:1.3
1.3	TUMOUR	LOC:tract, MOD:QUAL:(possible)
1.4	TRACT	ATT:urinary

Propositions are numbered within segments and consist of a predicate and labelled arguments. A predicate may be an action (e.g. examine), an object (e.g. tumour) or a relation connecting propositions (COND). For instance, proposition 1.1 expresses the idea that haematuria is painless and recurrent. COND (condition), ATT (attribute), THM (theme), LOC (location), MOD:QUAL (modal qualifier) are semantic tags that serve to categorize the types of ideas expressed.

if there exists a path, directed or undirected, between any two nodes. The types of nodes correspond either to data given in the problem or to hypothesized information.

Reasoning is characterized in the following form. When the direction of the relations is from the given data in the problem to the hypothesized node, it is coded as forward or data-driven reasoning. When the link is from the hypothesized node to explain the data in the problem, it is coded as backward reasoning, or hypothesis-driven reasoning. A series of inferences between the two is coded as an elaboration. With this methodology it has been possible to investigate some aspects of expert and novice reasoning in diagnostic tasks. More specifically, the method has been used to uncover the kinds of reasoning pattern used by expert physicians, which has served to identify several kinds of expertise, such as general and specific expertise (Groen & Patel 1988).

INTERPRETIVE METHODS

Philosophers (e.g. Taylor 1971) and social sciences researchers (e.g. Suchman 1987) have argued that the traditional scientific approach to research is inadequate for investigating human issues, preferring instead methods that take into account the 'social construction of shared meaning' in analogy with the reading of texts. That is, just as a word in a text obtains its meaning from the context provided

by other words, situations involving human actions are comprehensible only in the context where they occur. In both cases, the reader/observer's task is to *interpret* the meaning of the text/actions. Interpretive research has had a long history in educational research (Glaser & Strauss 1967, Lincoln & Guba 1985).

In this line of thinking, ethnographic researchers aim to describe 'whole real-life situations' in order to grasp their meaning (Benner 1984, Ramsden et al 1989) and argue for the need of collecting rich descriptive information, including the context of behaviour and the interaction among members of a group. Furthermore, rather than investigating behaviour in an objective manner and minimizing interaction, the researcher becomes a participant of the 'community' he or she is studying, which better informs the researcher about the phenomenon under investigation. Typically, data are collected by asking clinicians to study patient records, taking as much time as they need. They are then asked questions in a non-directive way with the aim of eliciting information about their understanding of the problem and their ways of solving it. The analysis consists of generating categories that can meaningfully characterize what subjects are doing from their own perspective.

In a study by Benner (1984) on nursing expertise, paired interviews were conducted with novice and expert nurses about a situation that was common to both. Benner's research was based on the models of skill acquisition and expertise developed by Dreyfus & Dreyfus (1986), whose work was, in turn, inspired by the phenomenological philosophy of Martin Heidegger (1962). Benner's method consisted of interpreting each situation by independent observers/interpreters and then comparing their interpretations and reaching a consensus about the meaning of the situations. The idea behind this method is to capture subjects' experiences in terms of their interpretations of the problem. Other studies in the interpretive tradition (e.g. Roberts & Sarangi 2005) have focused on how meaning is negotiated and decisions are reached during interaction among people in their naturalistic settings. For instance, theme-oriented discourse analysis uses combined ethnographic observation with interviews with the goal of understanding all aspects involved in their complexity (both the local as well as the wider context, in all their complexity). This methodology has been applied to research on genetic counselling (Sarangi et al 2003) and primary care (Roberts et al 2004).

Situated cognition methods

Reasoning in naturalistic settings, such as organizations and institutions, is an increasingly important topic of research (Patel et al 1996). The transition from studying individual subjects to investigations of group interaction in naturalistic environments requires an expanded methodological framework that captures cognition and action in complex settings. These settings are characterized (Orasanu & Connolly 1993) as dynamic and ill-structured, where ambiguous and incomplete information is the rule and where unpredictable changes may occur resulting in high stress and sometimes high risk situations. Such situations involve multiple players, where decisions are distributed over a set of cooperating individuals who try to coordinate their activities. In such settings, verbal protocols must be complemented by other techniques of data collection such as note-taking, interviews and video recording in order to capture the whole event that is occurring.

Although indirectly related to the interpretive approach, situated cognition developed independently of qualitative research (Greeno 1989). In common with the interpretive approach, the situated

approach proposes the collection and analysis of rich ethnographic descriptions of persons acting in their environment, because reasoning is conceived of as taking place in interaction with situations, rather than inside someone's mind (e.g. as a set of knowledge structures and operations on them). The shift proposed by the situated cognition approach involves a new consideration of the environmental aspect in theories of cognition. Since proponents of the situated approach view thinking as occurring in a situation, they record not only verbal protocols, but also the actions and tasks people perform and the interactions among people. To these ends, data collection commonly relies on the use of videotaping to capture the situated character of reasoning and thinking.

Video coding and analysis

Videotaping and video analysis are essential methodological tools in interpretive approaches (Greeno 1989, Jordan & Henderson 1995). The selection of such tools is in keeping with the emphasis on analysing the context of action as part of the subject/environment, where reasoning is treated as a relation between persons and the environment where they act. In fact, the method allows better characterization of cognitive processing, by providing extra nonverbal information, such as gestures, movements and gazes, which complements the information obtained from the subjects' verbal protocols. In this way, video data (e.g. behavioural data from the subject, the environmental situation, visible aspect of the task) can be used to support hypotheses made from verbal data or can suggest new hypotheses. Furthermore, video data are helpful in analysing tasks designed to externalize subjects' thought processes. In such tasks, both verbalizations and physical actions (e.g. pointing, gazing) can be analysed in a more complete fashion. An interesting variation of the use of videotaping method (Unsworth 2005) consists of using a camera on the subject's head so that the video generated focuses on what the subject is perceiving at the time of performance. The assumption is that focusing on what the subject perceived at the moment of performance will facilitate the recall of his or her explanation. Methods of analysis often involve the classification of streams of behaviour into a coding scheme that is developed beforehand, based typically on a theoretical understanding of the phenomenon under consideration (e.g. Frederiksen et al 1992, Roberts & Sarangi 2005).

CONCLUSION: ISSUES FOR THE FUTURE

In their 1990 article reviewing the progress of the field of medical cognition, Elstein et al foresaw several possible orientations adopted in the study of clinical reasoning in the health sciences. Despite their earlier optimism regarding the unification of the decision-making and information-processing approaches (see also Berner 1984, Elstein et al 1978), the field has moved in different directions. This has generated a multiplicity of methodologies ranging from the more traditional quantitative methods still in much use to interpretive methods (Benner 1984, Ramsden et al 1989).

Methodological pluralism is healthy as long as it is accompanied by the development of a theory of expertise, of which a theory of reasoning would be a major component. Pluralism brings also a needed awareness of what the methods are designed for, what questions they should answer, and what their limitations are. It may be that such proliferation of methods has contributed to the fragmentation of research approaches with little integration, but we hope that such diversity of methods also contributes to an overarching view of clinical reasoning.

Among the issues that are being clarified is the goal that a particular methodological approach is supposed to meet. It is common to criticize an investigation for failing to give answers that are not relevant to that study. An objection frequently made about qualitative research concerns the generalizability of its research results. However, this criticism misses the point of qualitative research, which aims at characterizing a given phenomenon to provide evidence for its existence rather than determining its generality. This should, in turn, help develop theories that include what Simon (1990) has called 'laws of qualitative structure'. Questions about generalizability of results can be meaningfully asked of studies that are based on statistical comparisons, because they invariably are designed to answer such questions. The interest in carrying out such studies is not in determining whether or not a phenomenon exists but how general it is.

A second issue concerns the external validity of the research. Some critics argue that the artificiality of research conditions places serious doubts on the quality of research studies. This artificiality would severely distort what actually happens in real-life situations, enough to make this kind of research meaningless. However, maybe because of the extreme empiricist biases of many behavioural scientists, these critics fail to see the point of artificiality. The claim is that it is the results of an experiment that should be judged as valid or invalid. But conducting research in artificial environments implies a different view of what is valid or not. It is not the results of the study per se but the theoretical conclusions that are logically tied to such results. Let us present an example. In a study carried out by Coughlin (1985; see also Vicente & Wang 1998) in which a clinical text describing a patient was presented with the sentences scrambled, it was found that expert physicians were able to reorganize the text in a way that novices were unable to do. Of course, this study could be criticized for failing to approximate the conditions where expert physicians work; after all, they are unlikely to read patient reports in which the information has been scrambled. But criticizing the study for this reason would totally miss its point. The conclusion of this study was not that expert physicians were better at unscrambling clinical cases, but rather that their memory for clinical information was organized differently from that of novices. Only this theoretical conclusion can be meaningfully made.

A major goal of science is to generate laws that account for the phenomena under consideration. Some researchers believe that laws of behaviour and cognition are impossible to achieve; others, that these laws are not universal as in the case of the mature sciences (Simon 1990). Others hold the belief that it is by inductive generalizations that laws are obtained. Empirical generalizations, if strongly confirmed, then become laws of the discipline. Although there is some truth to the last position, most laws in the hard sciences are much more than empirical generalizations. They are theoretical propositions that possess referential universality and that have no counterpart in empirical terms. That is, they explain but are not empirical regularities themselves. Rather, they refer to the unobservable underlying processes that produce the empirical regularities. The solution is to acknowledge that science admits several kinds of laws. We mentioned the laws of qualitative structure (Simon 1990), which can be uncovered by proposing models and then testing them by comparing them with human performance. The advantage of laws of this kind is that they not only describe a phenomenon, but also account for it.

Different methodologies serve different purposes. Early research into reasoning was too monolithic, giving primacy to the standard methods typically studied in research design courses. As research becomes more sophisticated, new methods and techniques become increasingly used and new approaches to research are tried out. To be effective, methodological pluralism needs to be accompanied by a real effort to develop rigorous theories of reasoning. Theorizing about such a complex field as clinical reasoning is a challenging task, but one that can not be postponed.

Despite promises of unification, the study of clinical reasoning has branched into diverse methodological and substantial areas. This diversity has been welcomed to the extent that it has encouraged investigators to study reasoning more freely. It has also obviously resulted in some lack of communication among researchers involved in different research programmes. There is, however, the hope of providing some unification to the field, as witnessed by attempts outside the area of clinical reasoning (Clancey 1997, Greeno 1998, Patel et al 1995). This unification involves a plethora of methodologies, each serving the purpose of investigating all aspects of cognition, including mental heuristics, knowledge generation and utilization, the process of discovery and interpretation of evidence, and collaborative reasoning. It is time for clinical reasoning researchers to take steps in this direction. This requires that researchers of clinical reasoning with diverse backgrounds, from artificial intelligence to psychology and education, help promote the development of a unified theory of clinical reasoning and decision making.

Acknowledgments

The updating of this chapter was supported by grants from the Social Sciences and Humanities Research Council of Canada (41095206 and 410951208).

References

Allais M, Hagen O 1979 Expected utility hypothesis and the Allais paradox. D Reidel, Dordrecht

Arocha J F, Wang D, Patel V L 2005 Identifying reasoning strategies in medical decision making: a methodological guide. Journal of Biomedical Informatics 38:154–171

Benner P 1984 From novice to expert: excellence and power in clinical nursing practice. Addison-Wesley, Menlo Park, CA

Berner E 1984 Paradigms and problem solving: a literature review. Journal of Medical Education 59:625–633

Bunge M 1985 Philosophy of social sciences and technology, treatise on basic philosophy, vol 7. D Reidel, Dordrecht

Carroll J S, Johnson E S 1990 Decision research. Sage, Newbury Park, CA

Christensen C, Elstein A S, Bernstein L M et al 1991 Formal decision support in medical practice and education. Teaching and Learning in Medicine 3:62–70

Clancey W J 1997 Situated cognition: on human knowledge and computer representations. Cambridge University Press, Cambridge

Coughlin L D J 1985 The effects of randomization on the free recall of medical information by experts and novices. Department of Educational Psychology, McGill University, Montreal, Quebec

Crowley R S, Naus G J, Stewart J et al 2003 Development of visual diagnostic expertise in pathology – an information-processing study. Journal of the American Medical Informatics Association 10:39–51

Dawes R M 1988 Rational choice in an uncertain world. Harcourt Brace Jovanovich, New York

Dreyfus H L, Dreyfus S E 1986 Mind over machine: the power of human intuition and expertise in the era of the computer. Free Press, New York

Elstein A S, Shulman L S, Sprafka S A 1978 Medical problem solving: an analysis of clinical reasoning. Harvard University Press, Cambridge, MA

Elstein A S, Shulman L S, Sprafka S A 1990 Medical problem solving: a ten year retrospective. Evaluation and the Health Professions 13:5–36

Ericsson K A, Simon H A 1984 Protocol analysis: verbal reports as data. MIT Press, Cambridge, MA

Fox J 1988 Formal and knowledge-based methods in decision technology. In: Dowie J, Elstein A (eds) Professional judgment: a reader in clinical decision making. Cambridge University Press, Cambridge, p 226–252

Frederiksen C H 1975 Representing logical and semantic structure of knowledge acquired from discourse. Cognitive Psychology 7:371–458

Frederiksen J R, Sipusic M, Gamoran M et al 1992 Video portfolio assessment: a study for the national board for professional teaching standards. Educational Testing Service, Princeton, NJ

Glaser B, Strauss A 1967 The discovery of grounded theory. Aldine, Chicago

Greeno J 1989 A perspective on thinking. American Psychologist 44:134–141

Greeno J 1998 The situativity of knowing, learning, and research. American Psychologist 53:5–26

Groen G J, Patel V L 1988 The relationship between comprehension and reasoning in medical expertise. In: Chi M, Glaser R, Farr M (eds) The nature of expertise. Erlbaum, Hillsdale, NJ, p 287–310

Hammond J S 1967 Better decision with preference theory. Harvard Business Review 45:123–141

Hashem A, Chi M T, Friedman C P 2003 Medical errors as a result of specialization. Journal of Biomedical Informatics 36:61–69

Heidegger M 1962 Being and time. Harper and Row, New York

Jordan B, Henderson A 1995 Interaction analysis: foundations for practice. Journal of the Learning Sciences 4:39–103

Joseph G M, Patel V L 1990 Domain knowledge and hypothesis generation in diagnostic reasoning. Medical Decision Making 10(1):31–46

Kassirer J P, Kuipers B J, Gorry G A 1982 Toward a theory of clinical expertise. American Journal of Medicine 73:251–259

Kintsch W 1974 The representation of meaning in memory. Erlbaum, Hillsdale, NJ

Kintsch W 1998 Comprehension: a paradigm for cognition. Cambridge University Press, Cambridge

Kuipers B J, Kassirer J P 1984 Causal reasoning in medicine: analysis of a protocol. Cognitive Science 8(4):363–385

Lesgold A M, Rubinson H, Feltovich P J et al 1988 Expertise in a complex skill: diagnosing X-ray pictures. In: Chi M T H, Glaser R, Farr M J (eds) The nature of expertise. Lawrence Erlbaum, Hillsdale, NJ, p 311–342

Lincoln Y S, Guba E G 1985 Naturalistic inquiry. Sage, Beverly Hills, CA

Newell A, Simon H A 1972 Human problem solving. Prentice-Hall, Englewood Cliffs, NJ

Norman G, Brooks L R, Allen S W 1989a Recall by expert medical practitioners and novices as a record of processing attention. Journal of Experimental Psychology: Learning, Memory, and Cognition 15:1116–1174

Norman G, Brooks L R, Rosenthal D et al 1989b The development of expertise in dermatology. Archives of Dermatology 125:1063–1068

Orasanu J, Connolly T 1993 The reinvention of decision making. In: Klein G A, Orasanu J, Calderwood R et al (eds) Decision making in action: models and methods. Ablex, Norwood, NJ, p 3–20

Patel V L, Arocha J F 1995 Cognitive models of clinical reasoning and conceptual representation. Methods of Information in Medicine 34:47–56

Patel V L, Frederiksen C H 1984 Cognitive processes in comprehension and knowledge acquisition by medical students and physicians. In: Schmidt H G, De Volder M L (eds) Tutorials in problem-based learning. Assen, van Gorcum, Holland, p 143–157

Patel V L, Groen G J 1986 Knowledge-based solution strategies in medical reasoning. Cognitive Science 10:91–116

Patel V L, Kaufman D R, Arocha J F 1995 Steering through the murky waters of a scientific conflict: situated and symbolic models of clinical cognition. Artificial Intelligence in Medicine 7:413–438

Patel V L, Kaufman D R, Magder S A 1996 The acquisition of medical expertise in complex dynamic environments. In: Ericsson K A (ed) The road to excellence: the acquisition of expert performance in the arts and sciences, sports, and games. Lawrence Erlbaum, Hillsdale, NJ, p 127–165

Patel V L, Arocha J F, Leccisi M S 2001 Impact of undergraduate medical training on housestaff problem-solving performance: implications for problem-based curricula. Journal of Dental Education 65:1199–1218

Patel V L, Arocha J F, Zhang J 2005 Reasoning in medicine. In: Holyoak K J (ed) Cambridge handbook of thinking and reasoning. Cambridge University Press: Cambridge, p 727–750

Ramsden P, Whelan G, Cooper D 1989 Some phenomena of medical students' diagnostic problem solving. Medical Education 23:108–117

Rikers R M, Loyens S, Winkel W et al 2005 The role of biomedical knowledge in clinical reasoning: a lexical decision study. Academic Medicine 80:945–949

Ritter B J 2003 An analysis of expert nurse practitioners' diagnostic reasoning. Journal of the American Academy of Nurse Practitioners 15:137–141

Roberts C, Sarangi S 2005 Theme-oriented discourse analysis of medical encounters. Medical Education 39:632–640

Roberts C, Sarangi S, Moss B 2004 Presentation of self and symptom in primary care consultations involving patients from non-English speaking backgrounds. Communication and Medicine 12:159–169

Runkel P J 1990 Casting nets and testing specimens: two grand methods of psychology. Praeger, New York

Runkel P J 2003 People as living things: the psychology of perceptual control. Hayward, Living Control Systems, CA

Sarangi S, Bennert K, Howell L et al 2003 'Relatively speaking': relativisation of genetic risk in counselling for predictive testing. Health, Risk and Society 5:155–170

Schiffrin D, Tannen D, Hamilton H E 2001 The handbook of discourse analysis. Blackwell, Oxford

Schmidt H G, Boshuizen H P 1993 On the origin of intermediate effects in clinical case recall. Memory and Cognition 21:338–351

Schmidt H, Boshuizen H P A, Hobus P P M 1988 Transitory stages in the development of medical expertise: the 'intermediate effect' in clinical case representation studies. Proceedings of the Tenth Annual Conference of the Cognitive Science Society, Erlbaum, Hillsdale, NJ, p 139–145

Simon H A 1990 Invariants of human behavior. Annual Review of Psychology 41:1–19

Sowa J F 1984 Conceptual structures: information processes in mind and machine. Addison-Wesley, Reading, MA

Sterling Y M, McNally J A 1992 Single-subject research for nursing practice. Clinical Nurse Specialist 6:21–26

Suchman L 1987 Plans and situated action: the problem of human/machine communication. Cambridge University Press, Cambridge, MA

Taylor C 1971 Interpretation and the sciences of man. Review of Metaphysics 25:3–51

Tversky A, Kahneman D 1974 Judgment under uncertainty: heuristics and biases. Science 185:1124–1131

Unsworth C A 2005 Using a head-mounted video camera to explore current conceptualizations of clinical reasoning in occupational therapy. American Journal of Occupational Therapy 59(1):31–40

Vicente K J, Wang J H 1998 An ecological theory of expertise effects in memory recall. Psychological Review 105:33–57

Von Neumann J, Morgenstern O 1944 Theory of games and economic behavior. Princeton University Press, Princeton

Weiner I S, Eisen R G 1985 Clinical research: the case study and single-subject designs. Journal of Allied Health 14:191–201

Weinstein M C, Fineberg H V, Elstein A S et al 1980 Clinical decision analysis. W B Saunders, Philadelphia, PA

White P 1988 Knowing more about what we can tell: 'introspective access' and causal report accuracy 10 years later. British Journal of Psychology 79:13–45

Winograd T 1972 Understanding natural language. Cognitive Psychology 3:1–191

Chapter 18

A history of clinical reasoning research

Stephen Loftus and Megan Smith

INTRODUCTION

Clinical reasoning has been a topic of research for several decades. The history of this research is important as it provides insights into the various ways in which both cognition and clinical reasoning have been conceptualized over the years and provides a context for current understanding of clinical reasoning and the ways in which it is taught to novice health professionals. In this chapter we draw on two recent research studies which have investigated clinical reasoning as used by different health professionals. These studies (Loftus 2006, Smith 2006) were situated within an understanding of clinical reasoning derived from the variety of research approaches that have been used to study clinical reasoning.

Early research into clinical reasoning was based predominantly within the empirico-analytical paradigm. The first studies came from behavioural psychology, and were followed by studies based on cognitive psychology. A separate but related body of research, generally referred to as medical decision theory, adopted a more probabilistic and statistical approach to conceptualizing clinical reasoning. Research into novice/expert differences has also constituted a distinct topic throughout the history of research into clinical reasoning. In more recent years, research situated in the interpretive and critical paradigms has appeared and grown in volume, especially in healthcare professions other than medicine.

BEHAVIOURISM

The oldest research tradition in clinical reasoning is behaviourism. Behaviourism is the view that mental phenomena like clinical reasoning can be understood only by analysing behaviour. Behaviour such as clinical reasoning is taken to be a dependent variable, and the independent variables that produce it are the stimuli that might lawfully cause that behaviour. The behavioural laws that link stimuli to behaviour are assumed to be similar in kind to the laws of physics and chemistry. Internal states of consciousness are excluded from this view of psychology as being beyond scientific study. Some research into clinical reasoning has been conducted within the behaviourist paradigm. For example, Rimoldi (1988) tested diagnostic skills of medical practitioners and students in the 1950s and 1960s, showing that as expertise increased so the numbers of questions asked and the time taken to solve diagnostic problems decreased.

Behaviourism has affected the teaching of clinical reasoning and other skills. For example, the notion that students should receive immediate corrective feedback on their performance comes from behaviourism, as does the precept of providing explicit aims and objectives that are related to measurable outcomes (Custers & Boshuizen 2002, Greeno et al 1996, Smith & Irby 1997).

Many features of modern medical curricula that have a direct bearing on the way that clinical reasoning is taught and practised can be traced to influences from behaviourist principles. These features include frequent and progressive testing, and close monitoring of students (Custers & Boshuizen 2002). Behaviourism may have many weaknesses but it has been of some benefit when intelligently applied. However, as an explanation of all learning, behaviourism is conceptually weak and does not go far enough. It ignores context, sociocultural interaction and intersubjectivity. In the endeavour to address some of these weaknesses cognitivism emerged as a more powerful conceptual model for thinking about mental phenomena such as clinical reasoning (Patel & Arocha 2000).

COGNITIVISM

Cognitive science seeks to account for intelligent activity as exhibited by living organisms or machines. Cognitivism replaced the behaviourist metaphor of cognition, as a black box having environmental inputs and behavioural outputs, with the metaphor of cognition as a form of computation and information processing, similar in kind to that carried out by computers.

Cognitivism allows for 'mental' structures and processes, whereas behaviourism does not. Information processing, memory representation and problem solving are three core concepts (Case & Bereiter 1984). There have been a number of attempts to characterize knowledge structures according to a cognitive view, and these feature prominently in much clinical reasoning research within the cognitive paradigm. The mental structures which purportedly play such a prominent role have included successively: categories, prototypes, instances, schemas, scripts and networks (Gruppen & Frohna 2002). Each concept was introduced in turn as a response to the perceived weaknesses of its predecessors. For example, according to the theory of instances, knowledge organization occurs around an individual instance rather than as an abstract based on several cases. This idea was proposed in response to the weaknesses perceived in the construct of prototypes (Brooks et al 1991, Homa et al 1981).

This preoccupation with mental structures and access to them is typical of cognitivism and is symptomatic of the underlying conceptual model of cognition as a form of computation. Along with the concern for cognitive structures is an interest in the cognitive processes by which individuals make use of such structures. The most popular process for utilizing these cognitive structures in clinical reasoning is held to be hypothetico-deductive reasoning.

HYPOTHETICO-DEDUCTIVE REASONING

Research investigating the hypothetico-deductive method as a foundation in clinical reasoning was divided by Bradley (1993) into two groups.

Researchers in the first group used think-aloud protocols with patients or simulated patients (e.g. Elstein et al 1978). Those in the second group used case vignettes (e.g. Eddy & Clanton 1982). There were weaknesses with both kinds of study, such as the artificial nature of the think-aloud protocols that tended to be used. However, the concept of hypothetico-deductive reasoning is generally considered to be a robust element of the cognitive paradigm, and one that could be adopted in different models that may reject many of the assumptions of cognitivism. The cognitivist body of research also highlighted the differences between experts and novices in clinical reasoning.

EXPERT/NOVICE RESEARCH

Much of the effort in cognitivist research into clinical reasoning has consisted of attempts to delineate differences between novices and experts, which is therefore sometimes called the contrastive method. Most of this research has been experimental. A problem-solving approach is generally used, in which cognitive processes are studied in tasks that attempt to represent medical thinking. Typically, protocol analysis has been used, as in the work of Ericsson & Simon (1993), who claimed that experts' use of forward-directed reasoning was 'one of the most robust findings' (p. 132) of research in this field. Forward reasoning is supposed to occur when someone gathers data and, with the aid of a great deal of pattern recognition invoking 'if-then' production rules, eventually reaches a conclusion (Patel & Groen 1986). Backward reasoning is supposed to occur when someone selects a hypothesis early and then proceeds to test it by gathering data that will confirm or refute it. This is believed to work well if the hypothesis is correct, but means that the problem-solver may need to start again if it becomes clear that the data being gathered tend to refute the hypothesis. This view of expert–novice difference is widespread in the clinical reasoning literature. It began about 1980 when researchers claimed that these differences existed between experts and novices in physics (Larkin et al 1980). These studies influenced the research of Elstein et al (1978)

into clinical reasoning, seeking the same phenomenon of forward and backward reasoning.

The finding that forward and backward reasoning distinguish experts and novices has now been extensively investigated and 'confirmed' within medicine (Patel et al 1990), and is now widely accepted. However, the relevant studies were experimental and can be criticized as being highly artificial. In general they used written protocols, with all the relevant information presented simultaneously on a single page. The researchers asked individuals to read the case and verbalize or write down their thoughts. Analysis of these verbalizations produced the apparent distinction between forward and backward reasoning.

Variations on the research into novice–expert differences in reasoning have continued to recent times. For example, Norman & Schmidt (2000) also devised experiments to test forward and backward reasoning strategies among novices and experts. Their findings showed clearly that novices did better when using backward reasoning. This kind of finding has been used to provide a theory of what happens during problem-based learning, and this is why the hypothetico-deductive model is still an important theory in the teaching of clinical reasoning (Barrows & Feltovich 1987).

However, as Norman et al (1999) have observed, the concept of forward and backward reasoning is problematic owing to the artificial nature of the decontextualized settings in which it was established. In other words, these findings may be a laboratory artefact. Lemieux & Bordage (1992) discussed the issue of research into forward versus backward clinical reasoning at length. They concluded that laboratory-based studies were far too limiting, and that the results were often more a reflection on the method of investigation than the actual reasoning of the clinician. This criticism is supported by the work of Laufer & Glick (1996), who investigated novice–expert differences in real-world work settings, using an ethnographic approach informed by ideas from the cultural psychology of Vygotsky (1978, 1986).

Cognitivism entails an essentially individualistic view of expert–novice differences. Even as early as 1980, some researchers were dissatisfied with cognitivism as an explanatory model. For example, Norman (1980) complained that cognitivism was inadequate for conceptualizing the influence of interaction with others and the ways in which an individual's personal life history and cultural background could affect reasoning skills. If cognition is in fact not a computational process then the search for the purported cognitive structures and processes may be misguided and doomed to failure. It can be argued that the similarities between cognition and computation are trivial, such as the ability to do simple mental arithmetic in one's head. Much of the research referred to above, which sets out to establish the nature of the cognitive structures in clinical reasoning and other forms of cognition, assumes what it sets out to prove. The underlying metaphor of cognition being a form of computation is open to challenge. Humans undertake procedures such as mathematical calculations differently from computers, and the way they do them varies depending on the circumstances (Dreyfus 1992). Cognitivism has an essentially individualistic view that expertise in skills such as clinical reasoning is a collection of behaviours and thoughts which are unique personal constructions. This directly contrasts with the sociocultural view that expertise is fundamentally best viewed as a social phenomenon. From this perspective expertise would, in large part, be selective assimilations of prevalent social practices and values. There is limited research into clinical reasoning from a sociocultural perspective. Engeström (1995) used a sociocultural approach to study medical expertise in clinical consultations with real patients, and was able to richly describe and articulate his findings in a manner that would have been precluded by a purely cognitivist framework.

THE COGNITIVE CONTINUUM

There are other models for understanding clinical reasoning. There is wide acceptance of the notion that experts use intuition and pattern recognition. Intuition and pattern recognition are not well understood. The cognitive continuum is a construct that some have used in an attempt to accommodate all these different types of thinking within one model (Hamm 1988). The proposal is that different modes of thinking are invoked under

different circumstances. For example, Hammond et al (1980) claimed that intuitive thinking is favoured when many cues are available. Dreyfus & Dreyfus (1986) argued that experience is crucial. An experienced clinician will resort to hypothetico-deductive thinking with an unfamiliar problem whereas novices must use it all the time until they acquire sufficient experience. Being on a cognitive continuum, these modes of thinking do not need to be mutually exclusive. The generation of a hypothesis may be intuitive and its subsequent testing can follow a more analytical path (Bradley 1993). Other authors (Higgs et al 2001) question the casual and pervasive use of the notion of intuition, regarding the use of advanced reasoning skills of experts to be a form of professional judgement and practice wisdom, grounded in deep experience-based knowledge, which is learned and is a highly refined form of reasoning ability. They see intuition as an important adjunct to reasoning.

MEDICAL DECISION THEORY

Another paradigm within clinical reasoning research dating back to the 1960s has been medical decision theory (e.g. Raiffa 1968, Sox et al 1988). This makes use of probability mathematics and logic as a theoretical lens and attempts to quantify the uncertainty of much clinical reasoning. Elstein et al (2002) maintained that such an approach encourages health professionals to adopt an evidence-based practice (EBP) approach. They asserted that even if a formal decision analysis is not possible this approach promotes a systematic appraisal of the trade-offs that need to be considered in a difficult decision. Medical decision theory has many attractions besides its associations with EBP. The possibility of making clinical decisions by calculation is seductive in an uncertain world where numbers appear to offer some degree of certainty. However, as Bradley (1993) pointed out, decision theory has drawbacks. Considerable skill and professional judgement are needed in formulating the decision trees that are a crucial part of the process. Croskerry (2005) showed that in medical specialties where decisions need to be routinely made in situations characterized by uncertainty, decision theory plays a negligible role. This was supported by Loftus (2006), who found that the health professionals in his study did not calculate medical decisions but articulated arguments in order to persuade patients, colleagues and themselves of a correct decision. It can be argued that a medical decision approach is useful for studying the optimal decisions for populations of patients, but has little place in the reality of clinical practice.

INTERPRETIVE RESEARCH APPROACHES

A recent alternative feature in the study of clinical reasoning has been the use of research approaches situated within the interpretive paradigm. Interpretive researchers have sought to study individuals within the context of their practice, thereby illuminating factors that individuals consider in their reasoning.

Our review of the history of clinical reasoning has thus far largely considered the history of clinical reasoning research as related to medicine. As health professions other than medicine have sought to understand the nature of their clinical practice and reasoning there has been an increasing use of interpretive research approaches. The use of these approaches has steadily increased since the early 1980s when Benner conducted seminal work into the nature of nursing expertise (Benner 1984) and later Gillette & Mattingly (1987) conducted a large scale ethnographic study of reasoning in occupational therapy. Jensen and associates (1992) added to the body of interpretive work by studying the nature of expertise in physiotherapy. These studies were followed by others that used interpretive approaches. However, much of this research has continued to focus on these same discipline areas (e.g. Titchen 2000 in nursing; Edwards et al 2004 and Resnik & Jensen 2003 in physiotherapy).

As suggested by the name, research within the interpretive paradigm seeks to interpret phenomena, in particular human phenomena (Higgs & Titchen 2000). Within the interpretive paradigm there is a major focus on preserving the context of the phenomenon and exploring its influence (Holman 1993). This is in contrast to the empirico-analytical paradigm where methods 'work best

when the context is defined, limited and perpetual' (Holman 1993, p. 30). Within the interpretive paradigm, clinical reasoning may be viewed as a human activity that is socially, historically and culturally constructed. Leonard (1989, p. 46) explained that 'to understand a person's behaviour or expressions, one has to study the person in context, for it is only there that what an individual values and finds significant is visible'.

Interpretive approaches use methods of data collection such as interview and observation to record practitioners' perspectives and descriptions of their clinical reasoning and associated actions. One advantage of these approaches over using paper-based cases is that it increases the likelihood that the research reveals practitioners' reasoning as used in practice as opposed to their espoused theory (Argyris & Schön 1974) such as might be revealed with questions based on a hypothetical situation (Eraut 2005).

An important contribution of interpretive approaches to the study of clinical reasoning has been in revealing clinical reasoning as a complex, multidimensional, integrated, task- and context-dependent process. Researchers in fields such as medicine have traditionally taken narrow perspectives to understanding decision making and clinical reasoning; seeking to identify *the* cognitive process used by expert decision makers. Norman (2005), in a review of clinical reasoning literature in medicine, challenged this assumption, suggesting that there may not be a single representation of clinical reasoning expertise or a single correct way to solve a problem. He commented (p. 426): 'the more one studies the clinical expert, the more one marvels at the complex and multidimensional components of knowledge and skill that she or he brings to bear on the problem, and the amazing adaptability she or he must possess to achieve the goal of effective care'. Interpretive approaches are grounded in a philosophical stance within which multiple interpretations of reality can exist. This philosophical stance results in the understanding of clinical reasoning pursued as a broad complex notion with multiple possible dimensions, and less in the realm of a single understanding to be discovered and tested.

The complexity of clinical reasoning revealed through interpretive approaches is evident in the findings of Smith (2006). Studying decision making by physiotherapists in acute care settings, she found that it was dependent upon the nature and complexity of the decision-making task, the attributes of the decision maker and the context in which the decisions were made. Further, Smith found that practitioners required complex cognitive, social, emotional and reflexive capabilities to integrate the multiple factors involved in clinical reasoning. Such a broad and dependent perspective would have been unobtainable with an approach that tested assumptions about the nature of factors affecting decision making, or viewed individuals apart from the contexts in which their decisions were made.

Further examples from interpretive approaches to the study of clinical reasoning reveal that in addition to diagnostic reasoning (which has been the predominant focus of medical research), practitioners engage in forms of reasoning such as narrative reasoning, reasoning about procedure, interactive reasoning, collaborative reasoning, reasoning about teaching, predictive reasoning, and ethical reasoning (Edwards et al 2004). In physiotherapy, broad dimensions of practice and reasoning have been identified, such as the individualized nature of care and expertise where the patient is the centre of decision making (e.g. Jensen et al 1992) and practice being characterized by reflexivity, contextual and task specificity and professional specificity of action (e.g. Beeston & Simons 1996, Jensen et al 2000, Resnik & Jensen 2003). Interpretive approaches have also revealed that clinical reasoning by individuals in acute care settings is socially and culturally determined and supported (Jette et al 2003).

The most important contribution of interpretive approaches to practice is in representing clinical reasoning as it occurs in real contexts. Therefore educational processes based on these approaches should result in novice practitioners who are better prepared for the reality of practice. This could avert the situation where novices acquire acontextual cognitive processes and conceptual frameworks which then have to be contextualized at the commencement of practice, with limited structured guidance and feedback as to how this is best achieved.

The contextualization of reasoning also has important implications for the current emphasis on EBP. The multidimensional understanding of clinical reasoning revealed by interpretive approaches suggests that the integration of evidence-based practice requires practitioners to balance EBP against other complex and at times competing influences on clinical reasoning. Much of the research produced and published under the rubric of EBP occurs with little reference to the context and broader factors that impact on its consumption by healthcare professionals (Rothstein 2004).

CONCLUSION

The history of clinical reasoning has resulted in a legacy of understanding that extends from discrete aspects of clinical reasoning, such as the use of hypothetico-deductive reasoning as a component in diagnostic decision making, through to representations of clinical reasoning as a multidimensional, complex phenomenon. Although we have argued for the advantages to be gained from interpretive approaches to the study of clinical reasoning it would be inappropriate to urge the exclusive use of these methods at the expense of approaches used in the empirico-analytical paradigm. The desired approach to the study of clinical reasoning is dependent upon the nature of the research question. When we seek to explore, describe and theorize about clinical reasoning as it occurs in the reality of practice, then interpretive approaches can be advocated as the approach of choice. When we seek to limit, control, test and compare aspects of reasoning this may be better achieved with experimental approaches. The combined use of different approaches to the study of clinical reasoning offers the challenge to bring the study of clinical reasoning out of paper-based cases which are acontextual into the realm of real practice.

As we saw with behaviourism, its limitations mean that it has largely been abandoned, but behaviourism has left us with a legacy of ideas that are still considered important and useful in medical education. A critical approach should be able to identify the difference between insights that are genuinely useful and those that are restricted to the philosophical assumptions of a particular field. For example, some of the insights of cognitivism, such as the use of the hypothetic-deductive method in clinical reasoning, seem to be robust findings, whereas the validity of the purported cognitive structures such as schemas and scripts is more questionable.

Our interpretation of this situation is that we are in a time of paradigm shift as described by Kuhn (1996). Some findings of cognitivism, such as the use of hypothetico-deductive reasoning with unfamiliar cases, may be subsumed by the newer interpretive approaches. However, there are fundamental conceptual differences between the older, more reductionist approaches and the newer interpretive approaches, and only time will reveal which paradigms prove to be more acceptable.

References

Argyis C, Schön D A 1974 Theory in practice: increasing professional effectiveness. Jossey-Bass, San Francisco

Barrows H S, Feltovich P J 1987 The clinical reasoning process. Medical Education 21:86–91

Beeston S, Simons H 1996 Physiotherapy practice: practitioners' perspectives. Physiotherapy Theory and Practice 12:231–242

Benner P 1984 From novice to expert: excellence and power in clinical nursing practice. Addison-Wesley, Menlo Park, CA

Bradley G W 1993 Disease, diagnosis and decisions. John Wiley & Sons, Chichester

Brooks L R, Norman G R, Allen S W 1991 Role of specific similarity in a medical diagnostic task. Journal of Experimental Psychology: General 120(3):278–287

Case R, Bereiter C 1984 From behaviourism to cognitive behaviourism to cognitive development: steps in the evolution of instructional design. Instructional Science 13(2):141–158

Croskerry P 2005 The theory and practice of clinical decision-making. Canadian Journal of Anesthetics 52(6):R1–R8

Custers E J F M, Boshiuzen H P A 2002 The psychology of learning. In: Norman G R, van der Vleuten C P M, Newble D I (eds) International handbook of research in medical education, vol 1. Kluwer Academic, Dordrecht, p 163–204

Dreyfus H L 1992 What computers still can't do: a critique of artificial reason, revised edn. MIT Press, Cambridge, MA

Dreyfus H L, Dreyfus S E 1986 Mind over machine: the power of human intuition and expertise in the era of the computer. Free Press, New York

Eddy D M, Clanton C H 1982 The art of diagnosis: solving the clinico-pathological exercise. New England Journal of Medicine 306:1263–1268

Edwards I, Jones M, Carr J et al 2004 Clinical reasoning strategies in physical therapy. Physical Therapy 84(4): 312–330

Elstein A S, Shulman L S, Sprafka S A 1978 Medical problem solving: an analysis of clinical reasoning. Harvard University Press, Cambridge, MA

Elstein A S, Schwartz A, Nendaz M R 2002 Medical decision making. In: Norman G R, Van der Vleuten C P M,

Newble D I (eds) International handbook of research in medical education. Kluwer Academic, Dordrecht, p 231–261

Engeström Y 1995 Objects, contradictions, and collaboration in medical cognition: an activity-theoretical perspective. Artificial Intelligence in Medicine 7:395–412

Eraut M 2005 Editorial: uncertainty in research. Learning in Health and Social Care 4(2):47–52

Ericsson K A, Simon H A 1993 Protocol analysis: verbal reports as data. revised edn. MIT Press, Cambridge, MA

Gillette N P, Mattingly C 1987 The foundation – clinical reasoning in occupational therapy. American Journal of Occupational Therapy 41:399–400

Greeno J G, Collins A M, Resnick L B 1996 Cognition and learning. In: Berliner D, Calfee R (eds) Handbook of educational psychology. Simon & Schuster-Macmillan, New York, p 15–46

Gruppen L D, Frohna A Z 2002 Clinical reasoning. In: Norman G R, Van der Vleuten C P M, Newble D I (eds) International handbook of research in medical education. Kluwer Academic, Dordrecht, p 205–230

Hamm R M 1988 Clinical intuition and clinical analysis: expertise and the cognitive continuum. In: Dowie J, Elstein A S (eds) Professional judgement: a reader in clinical decision making. Cambridge University Press, Cambridge, p 78–105

Hammond K R, McClelland G H, Mumpower J 1980 Human judgement and decision making. Hemisphere, New York

Higgs J, Titchen A 2000 Knowledge and reasoning. In: Higgs J, Jones M (eds) Clinical reasoning in the health professions, 2nd edn. Butterworth-Heinemann, Oxford, p 23–32

Higgs J, Burn A, Jones M 2001 Integrating clinical reasoning and evidence-based practice. AACN Clinical Issues: Advanced Practice in Acute and Critical Care 12(4): 482–490

Holman H R 1993 Qualitative inquiry in medical research. Journal of Clinical Epidemiology 46(1):29–36

Homa D, Sterling S, Treppel L 1981 Limitations of exemplar-based generalization and the abstraction of categorical information. Journal of Experimental Psychology: Human Learning and Memory 7:419–439

Jensen G M, Shepard K F, Hack L M 1992 Attribute dimensions that distinguish master and novice physical therapy clinicians in orthopedic settings. Physical Therapy 72:711–722

Jensen G M, Gwyer J, Shepard K F et al 2000 Expert practice in physical therapy. Physical Therapy 80(1):28–43

Jette D U, Grover L, Keck C P 2003 A qualitative study of clinical decision making in recommending discharge placement from the acute care setting. Physical Therapy 83(3):224–236

Kuhn T 1996 The structure of scientific revolutions, 3rd edn. University of Chicago Press, Chicago

Larkin J H, McDermott J, Simon H A et al 1980 Expert and novice performances in solving physics problems. Science 208:1335–1342

Laufer E A, Glick J 1996 Expert and novice differences in cognition and activity: a practical work activity. In: Engeström Y, Middleton D (eds) Cognition and communication at work. Cambridge University Press, Cambridge, p 177–198

Lemieux M, Bordage G 1992 Propositional versus structural semantic analyses of medical diagnostic thinking. Cognitive Science 16(2):185–204

Leonard V W 1989 A Heideggerian phenomenologic perspective on the concept of the person. Advances in Nursing Science 11:40–55

Loftus S 2006 Language in clinical reasoning: learning and using the language of collective clinical decision making. PhD thesis, University of Sydney, Australia. Online. Available: http://ses.library.usyd.edu.au/handle/2123/1165 3 July 2007

Norman D A 1980 Twelve issues for cognitive science. Cognitive Science 4:1–32

Norman G 2005 Research in clinical reasoning: past history and current trends. Medical Education 39:418–427

Norman G R, Schmidt H G 2000 Effectiveness of problem-based learning curricula: theory, practice and paper darts. Medical Education 34:721–728

Norman G R, Brooks L R, Colle C L et al 1999 The benefit of diagnostic hypotheses in clinical reasoning: experimental study of an instructional intervention for forward and backward reasoning. Cognition and Instruction 17(4):433–448

Patel V L, Arocha J F 2000 Methods in the study of clinical reasoning. In: Higgs J, Jones M (eds) Clinical reasoning in the health professions, 2nd edn. Butterworth-Heinemann, Oxford, p 78–91

Patel V L, Groen G J 1986 Knowledge-based solution strategies in medical reasoning. Cognitive Science 10:91–116

Patel V L, Groen G J, Arocha J F 1990 Medical expertise as a function of task difficulty. Memory and Cognition 18(4):394–406

Raiffa H 1968 Decision analysis: introductory lectures on choices under uncertainty. Addison-Wesley, Reading, MA

Resnik L, Jensen G M 2003 Using clinical outcomes to explore the theory of expert practice in physical therapy. Physical Therapy 83(12):1090–1106

Rimoldi H 1988 Diagnosing the diagnostic process. Medical Education 22:270–278

Rothstein J M 2004 The difference between knowing and applying. Physical Therapy 84(4):310–311

Smith M C L 2006 Clinical decision making in acute care cardiopulmonary physiotherapy. Unpublished doctoral thesis, University of Sydney, Australia

Smith C S, Irby D M 1997 The roles of experience and reflection in ambulatory care education. Academic Medicine 72:32–35

Sox H C Jr, Blatt M A, Higgins M C et al 1988 Medical decision making. Butterworth-Heinemann, Boston

Titchen A 2000 Professional craft knowledge in patient centred nursing and the facilitation of its development. Ashdale Press, Oxford

Vygotsky L S 1978 Mind in society: the development of higher psychological processes. Harvard University Press, Cambridge, MA

Vygotsky L S (trans A Kozulin) 1986 Thought and language. MIT Press, Cambridge, MA

Chapter 19

A place for new research directions

Joy Higgs and Stephen Loftus

> There are no facts, only interpretations
> (Nietzsche 1968, p. 267)

The previous chapter explored the history of clinical reasoning research, identifying trends in research that investigated and represented the nature of clinical reasoning and core issues such as novice/expert differences and the use of decision theory in clinical decision making. A broad transition and paradigm shift was identified from a focus on quantitative research to an increasing emphasis on qualitative research.

In this chapter we extend this discussion into four areas: reflections on the changing research questions that have been and are being addressed in this field; areas of clinical reasoning that require further research; factors influencing research directions; and an interpretation of the current direction that cutting edge clinical reasoning research is taking.

SETTING THE CONTEXT

Clinical reasoning is the core of clinical practice; it enables practitioners to make informed and responsible clinical decisions and address problems faced by their patients or clients. Around 20 years ago Schön (1987) pointed out that when a practitioner deals with new professional problems the first issue is 'problem setting'. This means choosing and naming the things that will be noticed and the things that will be ignored, which he described as 'naming and framing' (p. 4). The naming and framing process is essentially linguistic and discursive; it depends on factors such as 'disciplinary backgrounds, organizational roles, past histories, interests and political/economic perspectives' (p. 4). Schön indicated that this process of problem setting is also an ontological process. The professional is engaged in a localized and specialized form of world making and world interpretation. From this point of view, professional practice is much more than a straightforward epistemological or knowledge framing task, and practice involves much more than acquiring and mastering a body of propositional knowledge and learning how to apply it. From the interpretive viewpoint, mastering and applying a body of knowledge are still important, but being a professional such as a dentist or a physiotherapist is a much greater challenge. It is a way of being in the world.

This ontological idea of professionalism is echoed in the work of others, such as Thomas Kuhn (1996). Kuhn described how professionals (scientists, in his case) live in the world, and perceive it, in a way that is radically different from non-professionals, and that this comes about because they have internalized a particular way of perceiving the world. A layperson might see lines on paper whereas a cartographer instantly perceives a terrain (Kuhn 1996, p. 111). Kuhn also wrote that when scientists undergo a paradigm shift, that is, a radical change in the sets of ideas and assumptions they use to perceive and conceptualize the world, they talk of life after this experience as being like living in a new world.

Vygotsky (1978) noted that this internalization of particular ways of perceiving the world is true of all humans, starting at an early age. He used the example of a clock. When we see a clock, we learn to perceive it instantly as a clock, not something round and black-cased with hands, which is then consciously and deliberately interpreted as being a clock. If there is interpretation it is instantaneous and unconscious. Shotter (2000) realized that professional ways of seeing the world are extensions of this. Professional socialization shapes our attention and makes us see things in particular ways. For example, one medical student in a research project on learning clinical

reasoning (Loftus 2006, p. 199) spoke of being able to instantly recognize 'glaring cardiac signs' in a patient. Shotter (2000), following Vygotsky, maintained that it is through our language that this process occurs. These ways of responding to situations become embodied within us, and are therefore ontological rather than purely epistemological (i.e. words and knowledge). Professional ways of seeing the world are included among what Vygotsky (1978) described as higher mental functions. Such functions are the more complex and intellectually demanding skills that humans can develop, such as clinical reasoning, and they are qualitatively different from the lower mental functions or component cognitive skills (e.g. analysis) which they may incorporate.

KEY QUESTIONS

We identified four questions from this discussion:

1. What are the key questions about clinical reasoning that have been addressed in the past and are emerging in current research?
2. Which areas of clinical reasoning have been missing or under-researched in clinical reasoning research?
3. Which factors are influencing the direction of clinical reasoning research?
4. What is the shape of cutting edge clinical reasoning research?

THE CHANGING SHAPE OF RESEARCH QUESTIONS IN CLINICAL REASONING RESEARCH

Historically, in the majority of clinical reasoning research, researchers have stood outside the phenomenon of clinical reasoning, looking in, and addressed three key questions:

- What is clinical reasoning?
- How do experts reason?
- How can models of reasoning be used to teach students and novices to reason?

Not surprisingly, given the historical context of the scientification of health care and the dominance of medicine, these questions fit the expectations of the empirico-analytical research paradigm and the biomedical model. In both cases hypothetico-deductive reasoning or hypothesis generation and testing is the dominant mode of reasoning and decision making. The empirico-analytical research paradigm adopts a positivist philosophical stance where objectivity is the key issue and sense data determine reality; its goal is to measure, test hypotheses, discover, predict, explain, control, generalize and identify cause–effect relationships. Within the biomedical model the body is seen as a machine that can be adjusted or treated in seeking to cure (a person's condition) or restore the body to normal functioning. If this restitution narrative fails (which is common in chronic conditions) the patient may be labelled 'failed' or 'failing' or 'noncompliant' (Alder 2003). In the wellness model, in comparison, which fits with the interpretive and critical paradigms, the patient – the person – has greater initiative and support to write a different (e.g. ability) narrative.

When clinical reasoning research entered the interpretive paradigm the philosophical stance turned to idealism. In this philosophy the emphasis is on the actors' ideas or embodied knowing as the determinant of social reality, and multiple constructed or storied realities of the social world are recognized and acknowledged. Within this paradigm researchers seek to understand, interpret, seek meaning, describe, illuminate and theorize about lived experiences and actions. The context of human actions (including decision making) is seen as a vital influence on these actions and experiences. Hence, the way clinical reasoning came to be viewed changed towards a greater valuing of the narrative, contextual, conditional and interpersonal dimensions of practice. And the focus shifted onto the larger interactive phenomenon of making clinical decisions in the context of people with healthcare needs, their interests and concerns, their families, and the healthcare team.

Research in the interpretive paradigm has been conducted by Benner (1984) in nursing (with an emphasis on seeking understanding of behaviours and context), by Crepeau (1991) and Fleming (1991) in occupational therapy (with an emphasis on structuring meaning and interpreting the problem from the patient's perspective) and by Jensen et al (1992, 2007) in physiotherapy (with a focus

on elucidating the complex and unknown processes that occur during therapeutic interventions). The clinical reasoning processes which such approaches describe focus on seeking a deep understanding of patients' perspectives and the influence of contextual factors, in addition to the more traditional and clinical understanding of the patient's condition. The relevance of this broader perspective is evident in the growing body of research demonstrating that the meaning patients give to their problems (including their understanding of and feelings about their problems) can significantly influence their levels of pain tolerance, disability and eventual outcome (Borkan et al 1991, Feuerstein & Beattie 1995, Malt & Olafson 1995). As the volume and depth of research into clinical reasoning expands, it is becoming more and more apparent that traditional clinical reasoning models do not encompass the varying dimensions or reflect the diverse discipline-specific practice paradigms that exist across the health professions.

New questions being addressed in interpretive research include:

- What is involved in the professional socialization learning journey in which people learn to reason?
- What are the tools, particularly language and discourse tools, that need to be acquired and used when health professionals work in interactive decision-making situations?
- What are the contextual and personal factors that influence the way people learn to make decisions and the way they make decisions in healthcare settings?

Another emerging trend in seeking to enhance clinical reasoning is critical paradigm research. This paradigm is underpinned by the philosophical stance of historical realism in which it is recognized that social practices and culture shape practice over time. The goals of research in this paradigm are to improve, reform, empower, or change reality or a situation. Here we see the place of the individual as an agent of change, and action for self-enhancement as well as a change in the role of the health professional from provider to collaborator. Action research, collaborative inquiry and new paradigm research (Reason & Rowan 1981), with an emphasis on the researcher as the subject, means and object of his or her own research, are some of the strategies adopted here.

Limited research in this paradigm has been conducted specifically looking at clinical reasoning as a phenomenon. However, there is an emerging body of research, often blending interpretive and critical paradigm research (Charles et al 2005, McCormick 1998, Trede 2006), into the adoption of collaborative decision-making models and patient empowerment. In keeping with a growing interest in patient-centred care and in health practice models beyond the biomedical model, research questions in this category include:

- How can practitioners involve patients/clients in shared clinical decision making?
- What does clinical decision making mean and how can it be embodied in a person-centred framework?

AREAS OF CLINICAL REASONING NEEDING MORE RESEARCH

Returning to the notion of naming the things to be noticed about the problem to be solved and framing of the problem (e.g. within disciplinary backgrounds), we can identify a link between research paradigms and these actions (Table 19.1).

Naming and framing clinical problems depends to a large extent on the model of rationality underlying the particular health professions and the sciences they claim to be founded upon. The empirico-analytical paradigm uses a Cartesian approach to rationality. Descartes (trans. Clarke, 1999) claimed that the only rationality to be trusted was based upon mathematics and mathematical axioms. Despite the successes of the sciences built upon this form of rationality, it is increasingly recognized that Cartesianism demonstrates its limitations when applied to patient care. Wittgenstein (1958) argued that mathematical axioms are themselves conventions of language. From this viewpoint, language is more fundamental than mathematics. In fact, it can be argued that the way forward is, in a sense, a return to the past, provided we are willing to reconsider the ideas of such thinkers as Aristotle. Aristotle (trans.

Lawson-Tancred, 1991) maintained that there was more than one way to be rational, claiming that rhetoric and argumentation were important ways of being rational. He further stated that different problems needed different types of rationality if they were to be adequately dealt with. Some debates and differences of opinion are best settled with persuasive argument rather than by numbers and measurements. The interpretive and critical paradigms both embody important alternative ways of being rational.

FACTORS INFLUENCING RESEARCH DIRECTIONS IN CLINICAL REASONING

THE CONTEXT OF CLINICAL DECISION MAKING

A key aspect of planning future clinical reasoning research is understanding the context of healthcare practice and decision making. Challenges facing health care today include the need to:

- develop clinical decision-making strategies to recreate health care to encompass narratives suitable for ageing populations, increasing levels of co-morbidity and globalization of healthcare issues and systems
- address the demands for greater accountability and the explicit justification of clinical decisions
- make clinical decisions in workplace situations where cost-efficiency and evidence-based practice demand scientific rationales as a matter of priority
- recognize and honour the multitude of different cultural and situational contexts of clients and patients who seek healthcare services
- frame clinical decision making within models of practice that are compatible with practitioners' personal frames of reference, their professional codes of practice and the norms and regulations of their workplaces.

THE CONTEXT OF THE PROFESSION(S)

Another key factor influencing the directions of clinical reasoning research is the state of development of professions. Research into professional practice (e.g. Higgs & Titchen 2001) provides

Table 19.1 Research challenges across different research paradigms

Research paradigm	Language/discourse aspects of naming and framing the problem	Ontological aspects of problem setting	Aspects of clinical reasoning requiring further research
Empirico-analytical	Language and discourse focus on 'objectively real' clinico-pathological problems where the body is viewed as a machine and the mind as a computer and psychosocial aspects are discrete variables to be operationalized and statistically correlated with biomedical variables	The world/reality is as given to the senses within the biomedical/provided model with an assumption that generalizability and predictability will eventually be achievable and will then establish the best, externally referenced practice, independent of any bias or prejudice of the researcher or health professional	Questioning the underlying assumptions of traditional clinical reasoning strategies in different professions, e.g. narrow views of best practice and evidence-based practice. Language barriers in multidisciplinary teams. Patients' knowledge and opinions of their medical condition and its management. Pursuit of debate and research about generalization vs particularization of health care
Interpretive	Language and discourse focus on multiple interpretations of healthcare needs and strategies. Framing extends beyond disciplinary and biomedical limits to include sociocultural and personal interests	The world is interpreted and constructed within an experiential/lived model. This world, and best practice for individuals in this world, is contextualized and made meaningful through personal interpretation and particularization. Language (e.g. underlying metaphors) is used to rhetorically shape interpretive frameworks that then allow problems to be named and framed in ways that seem natural and obvious	Narratives for people with chronic conditions. Healthcare narratives for well people. Developing and interpreting common languages for health care beyond disciplinary boundaries. Collaborative decision making. Understanding in greater depth the nature of expertise and the capabilities of practitioners. Understanding more fully how decisions are made under conditions of uncertainty. Expansion of the place of changing community attitudes, interests and demographics and the impact these factors do and should have on clinical decision making. Expansion of teaching of these interpretations of clinical reasoning
Critical	Language and discourse here reflect critique of the status quo, emancipation and empowerment. The language of the client as well as the health professional is valued and included in collaborative decision making	The world is interpreted as a way of being that is socioculturally and historically constructed. Power relations between individuals are seen as crucial. In making sense of this world and in taking action, individuals need to be critical of taken-for-granted 'truths' and to seek liberation beyond received or accepted practices. Best practice includes both empowerment and particularization	Expansion in research in this area generally. Increase patient and client groups plus carers and advocacy groups in participative action research projects. Seek a deeper understanding of collaborative decision making and the factors that influence patient involvement in clinical decision making. Expansion of teaching of this way of being and critique in professional entry programmes

valuable insights into the nature of practice and factors influencing practice and reasoning. The professions are being shaped by external and internal forces such as demands for professional accountability and cost efficiency, driven by such factors as escalating healthcare costs, increasing public education and access to health-related information, technological advances and evidence-based practice. It is important to recognize that the outcomes of the clinical decisions practitioners make rest in their commitment to quality, relevant and accountable decision making. Such commitment is shaped by these contextual influences and also by the experiences of professionals and novices/students during their education and socialization. Research in education that is linked to clinical reasoning often examines the merits and challenges of problem-based learning. Medicine has the longest history of researching clinical reasoning, while nursing has a long history of workplace-based education. Further research into the context and education of professionals and their changing workplaces continues to be needed in support of quality health care and decision making.

THE NATURE OF THE PHENOMENON

Chapter 1 described clinical reasoning as both a simple and a complex phenomenon. Those researching clinical reasoning specifically and professional practice more generally must recognize the central role of clinical reasoning in practice. Clinical reasoning directs and informs the whole of clinical practice. Thus students of clinical reasoning must consider its nature and complexities. The following view of clinical reasoning demands research beyond the laboratory and involving multiple perspectives of the various participants in clinical decision making. Clinical reasoning is predominantly a human and social phenomenon that requires greater exploration through the human and social research paradigms.

Clinical reasoning (or practice decision making) is a context-dependent way of thinking and decision making in professional practice to guide practice actions. It involves the construction of narratives to make sense of the multiple factors and interests pertaining to the current reasoning task. It occurs within a set of problem spaces informed by practitioners' unique frames of reference, workplace contexts and practice models, as well as by patients' or clients' contexts. It utilizes core dimensions of practice knowledge, reasoning and metacognition and draws upon these capacities in others. Decision making within clinical reasoning occurs at micro-, macro- and meta-levels and may be individually or collaboratively conducted. It involves the metaskills of critical conversation, knowledge generation, practice model authenticity and reflexivity (Higgs 2006).

INTERPRETING DIRECTIONS OF CUTTING EDGE CLINICAL REASONING RESEARCH

A paradigm shift, as defined by Kuhn (1996), is a major and radical change in the conceptual basis underlying a discipline. Paradigm shifts are inevitable in response to changing circumstances which demand different ways of understanding and exploring these new realities. There have been a number of distinct paradigm shifts in clinical reasoning research, from early behaviourism which was superseded by cognitivism and the development of the separate paradigm of medical decision theory. These are discussed in more detail in Chapter 18. In this section we reflect on emerging changes of direction in research. These 'paradigm shifts' are also called 'turns' or 'moments', and we see three emerging turns in clinical reasoning research and practice.

The first of these turns we describe as the 'interdisciplinary turn'. In a previous edition of this book, Elstein & Schwarz (2000) recognized that the phenomenon we refer to as clinical reasoning is complex and multidimensional. They called for research into clinical reasoning that was informed by a range of academic disciplines. Social constructionism is one school of thought that synthesizes ideas from disciplines as diverse as philosophy, sociology and anthropology (Lupton 2003). Some research into clinical reasoning has been conducted from within the social constructionist worldview (e.g. Loftus 2006), with insights that would simply not have been possible with research from a strictly Cartesian point of view.

Interdisciplinary research also includes investigation of emerging and potential trends in clinical decision making that transcend professional groups (with their diverse backgrounds) and include patients as members of multidisciplinary teams (see Chapters 26, 27, 32, 34).

The second turn we see starting to emerge in clinical reasoning research relates to 'the linguistic turn'. The linguistic turn is the simple but profound recognition that our use of language is fundamental to what and who we are as human beings. Language is not merely a means of representing the world. Our use of language permits us, in a sense, to bring the world into being. As Gadamer (1989, p. 443) observed, 'Language is not just one of man's possessions in the world; rather, on it depends the fact that man has a *world* at all'. We are now beginning to appreciate the extent to which linguistic and discursive forms such as metaphor and narrative form a part of the phenomenon of clinical reasoning (Loftus 2006). An excellent and recent example of such an approach is Charon's (2006) study of narrative medicine, in which she argues that narratology can provide insights that enable practitioners to come to a deeper understanding of their patients' problems, and equip them with the cognitive tools to accompany those same patients on their journeys through illness and its treatment (see also Chapter 32).

Our third turn we call 'the meta turn'. It reflects cutting edge research which calls for clinical reasoning research and practice to be grounded in an understanding of reasoning as occurring within practice models and clinical reasoning models (see e.g. Trede 2006, Trede & Higgs 2003). This proposition calls for informed practice, that is, practice informed by these understandings. Practice, we contend, should seek to embody authentically the practitioner's chosen practice model, interests and clinical decision-making strategies. One such approach is the adoption of the critical social sciences as the basis for emancipatory practice (Trede et al 2003).

CONCLUSION

Clinical reasoning research is rapidly changing. While such research is still in the process of breaking away from and challenging the reductionist assumptions of much past research, the acceptance of new academic disciplines with different assumptions holds promise of providing exciting new insights into the ways in which clinical reasoning forms the basis of healthcare practice. As mentioned above, Elstein & Schwarz (2000) have called for research into clinical reasoning from different disciplines. We hope that they would be both pleased and surprised at the extent to which their call has been answered. We stand on the verge of a vital expansion in the scope of research in clinical reasoning that can go in many directions. There is much more to discover about clinical reasoning by pursuing promising new directions in research and by sharing across disciplines the findings of such research. This book is one means to that end.

References

Alder S 2003 Beyond the restitution narrative. Unpublished PhD thesis, University of Western Sydney, Sydney

Aristotle S (trans H C Lawson-Tancred) 1991 The art of rhetoric. Penguin Books, London

Benner P 1984 From novice to expert: excellence and power in clinical nursing practice. Addison Wesley, Menlo Park, CA

Borkan J M, Quirk M, Sullivan M 1991 Finding meaning after the fall: injury narratives from elderly hip fracture patients. Social Science and Medicine 33:947–957

Charles C, Gafni A, Whelan T et al 2005 Treatment decision aids: conceptual issues and future directions. Health Expectations 8(2):114–125

Charon R 2006 Narrative medicine: honoring the stories of illness. Oxford University Press, Oxford

Crepeau E B 1991 Achieving intersubjective understanding: examples from an occupational therapy treatment session. American Journal of Occupational Therapy 45:1016–1025

Descartes R (trans D M Clarke) 1999 Discourse on method and related writings. Penguin Books, London

Elstein A S, Schwartz A 2000 Clinical reasoning in medicine. In: Higgs J, Jones M (eds) Clinical reasoning in the health professions, 2nd edn. Butterworth-Heinemann, Oxford, p 95–106

Feuerstein M, Beattie P 1995 Biobehavioral factors affecting pain and disability in low back pain: mechanisms and assessment. Physical Therapy 75:267–280

Fleming M H 1991 Clinical reasoning in medicine compared with clinical reasoning in occupational therapy. American Journal of Occupational Therapy 45:988–996

Gadamer H-G 1989 Truth and method, 2nd revised edn. Continuum, New York

Higgs J 2006 The complexity of clinical reasoning: exploring the dimensions of clinical reasoning expertise as a situated, lived phenomenon. Seminar presentation at the Faculty of Health Sciences, University of Sydney, Australia, May 5

Higgs J, Titchen A 2001 Professional practice in health, education and the creative arts. Blackwell Science, Oxford

Jensen G M, Shepard K F, Hack L M 1992 Attribute dimensions that distinguish master and novice physical therapy clinicians in orthopedic settings. Physical Therapy 72:711–722

Jensen G M, Gwyer J, Hack L M et al 2007 Expertise in physical therapy practice: applications in practice, education and research, 2nd edn. Elsevier, Philadelphia

Kuhn T 1996 The structure of scientific revolutions, 3rd edn. University of Chicago Press, Chicago

Loftus S 2006 Language in clinical reasoning: learning and using the language of collective clinical decision making. PhD thesis, University of Sydney, Australia. Online. Available: http://ses.library.usyd.edu.au/handle/2123/1165 7 July 2007

Lupton D 2003 Medicine as culture: illness, disease and the body in Western societies, 2nd edn. Sage, London

McCormack B 1998 An exploration of the theoretical framework underpinning the autonomy of older people in hospital and its relationship to professional nursing practice. DPhil thesis, University of Oxford, England

Malt U F, Olafson O M 1995 Psychological appraisal and emotional response to physical injury: a clinical, phenomenological study of 109 adults. Psychiatric Medicine 10:117–134

Nietzsche F (trans W Kaufman, R J Hollingdale) 1968 The will to power. Vintage Books, New York [Opening chapter quotation based on Book 3, quotation no 481, p. 267]

Reason P, Rowan J (eds) 1981 Human inquiry: a sourcebook of new paradigm research. John Wiley, London

Schön D A 1987 Educating the reflective practitioner: toward a new design for teaching and learning in the professions. Jossey-Bass, San Francisco

Shotter J 2000 Seeing historically: Goethe and Vygotsky's 'enabling theory-method'. Culture and Psychology 6(2):233–252

Trede F 2006 A critical practice model for physiotherapy. Unpublished PhD thesis, University of Sydney, Australia

Trede F, Higgs J 2003 Re-framing the clinician's role in collaborative clinical decision making: re-thinking practice knowledge and the notion of clinician–patient relationships. Learning in Health and Social Care 2(2):66–73

Trede F, Higgs J, Jones M et al 2003 Emancipatory practice: a model for physiotherapy practice? Focus on Health Professional Education: A Multidisciplinary Journal 5(2):1–13

Vygotsky L S 1978 Mind in society: the development of the higher psychological processes. Harvard University Press, Cambridge, MA

Wittgenstein L (trans G E M Anscombe) 1958 Philosophical investigations, 3rd edn. Prentice Hall, Upper Saddle River, NJ

SECTION **4**

Clinical reasoning and clinical decision–making approaches

Chapter 20

Clinical reasoning in medicine

Alan Schwartz and Arthur S. Elstein

How do physicians solve diagnostic problems? What is known about the process of diagnostic clinical reasoning? In this chapter we sketch our current understanding of answers to these questions by reviewing the cognitive processes and mental structures employed in diagnostic reasoning in clinical medicine and offering a selected history of research in the area. We will not consider the parallel issues of selecting a treatment or developing a management plan. For theoretical background, we draw upon two approaches that have been particularly influential in research in this field. The first is problem solving, exemplified in the work of Newell & Simon (1972), Elstein et al (1978), Bordage and his colleagues (Bordage & Lemieux 1991, Bordage & Zacks 1984, Friedman et al 1998, Lemieux & Bordage 1992) and Norman (2005). The second is decision making, including both classical and two-system approaches, illustrated in the work of Kahneman et al (1982), Baron (2000), and the research reviewed by Mellers et al (1998), Shafir & LeBoeuf (2002) and Kahneman (2003).

Problem-solving research has usually focused on how an ill-structured problem situation is defined and structured (as by generating a set of diagnostic hypotheses). Psychological decision research has typically looked at factors affecting diagnosis or treatment choice in well defined, tightly controlled situations. A common theme in both approaches is that human rationality is limited. Nevertheless, researchers within the problem-solving paradigm have concentrated on identifying the strategies of experts in a field, with the aim of facilitating the acquisition of these strategies by learners. Behavioural decision research, on the other hand, contrasts human performance with a normative statistical model of reasoning under uncertainty. It illuminates cognitive processes by examining errors in reasoning to which even experts are not immune, and thus raises the case for decision support.

PROBLEM SOLVING: DIAGNOSIS AS HYPOTHESIS SELECTION

To solve a clinical diagnostic problem means first to recognize a malfunction and then to set about tracing or identifying its causes. The diagnosis is thus an explanation of disordered function, where possible a causal explanation.

In most cases, not all of the information needed to identify and explain the situation is available in the early stages of the clinical encounter. Physicians must decide what information to collect, what aspects of the situation need attention, and what can be safely set aside. Thus data collection is both sequential and selective. Experienced physicians often go about this task almost automatically, sometimes very rapidly; novices struggle to develop a plan.

THE HYPOTHETICO-DEDUCTIVE METHOD

Early hypothesis generation and selective data collection

Elstein et al (1978) found that diagnostic problems are solved by a process of generating a limited number of hypotheses or problem formulations early in the workup and using them to guide subsequent data collection and integration. Each hypothesis can be used to predict what additional findings ought to be present if it were true, and then the workup is a guided search for these findings; hence, the method is hypothetico-deductive. The process of problem structuring via hypothesis generation begins with a very limited data set and occurs rapidly and automatically, even if clinicians are explicitly instructed not to generate hypotheses. Given the complexity of the clinical situation, the enormous amount of data that could

potentially be obtained and the limited capacity of working memory, hypothesis generation is a psychological necessity. Novices and experienced physicians alike attempt to generate hypotheses to explain clusters of findings, although the content of the experienced group's productions is of higher quality.

Other clinical researchers have concurred with this view (Kassirer & Gorry 1978, Kuipers & Kassirer 1984, Nendaz et al 2005, Pople 1982). It has also been favoured by medical educators (e.g. Barrows & Pickell 1991, Kassirer & Kopelman 1991), while researchers in cognitive psychology have been more sceptical. We will examine these conflicting interpretations later.

Data collection and interpretation

Next, the data obtained must be interpreted in the light of the hypotheses being considered. To what extent do the data strengthen or weaken belief in the correctness of a particular diagnostic hypothesis?

A clinician could collect data quite thoroughly but could nevertheless ignore, misunderstand or misinterpret a significant fraction. In contrast, a clinician might be overly economical in data collection but could interpret whatever is available quite accurately. Elstein et al (1978) found no statistically significant association between thoroughness of data collection and accuracy of data interpretation. This was an important finding for two reasons:

1. *Increased emphasis upon interpretation of data.* Most early research allowed subjects to select items from a large array or menu of items. This approach, exemplified in patient management problems (Feightner 1985), facilitated investigation of the amount and sequence of data collection but offered less insight into data interpretation and problem formulation. The use of standardized patients (SPs) (Swanson et al 1995, van der Vleuten & Swanson 1990) offers researchers considerable latitude in how much to focus the investigation (or student assessment) on data collection or on hypothesis generation and testing. To deepen understanding of reasoning processes, investigators in the problem-solving tradition have asked subjects to think aloud while problem solving and have then analysed their verbalizations as well as their data

collection (Barrows et al 1982, Elstein et al 1978, Friedman et al 1998, Joseph & Patel 1990, Nendaz et al 2005, Neufeld et al 1981, Patel & Groen 1986). Considerable variability in acquiring and interpreting data has been found, increasing the complexity of the research task. Consequently, some researchers switched to controlling the data presented to subjects in order to concentrate on data interpretation and problem formulation (e.g. Feltovich et al 1984, Kuipers et al 1988). This shift led naturally to the second major change in research tactics.

2. *Study of clinical judgement separated from data collection.* Controlling the database facilitates analysis at the price of fidelity to clinical realities. This strategy is the most widely used in current research on clinical reasoning, the shift reflecting the influence of the paradigm of decision-making research. Sometimes clinical information is presented sequentially to a subject, so that the case unfolds in a simulation of real time, but the subject is given few or no options in data collection (Chapman et al 1996). The analysis can focus on memory organization, knowledge utilization, data interpretation or problem representation (e.g. Bordage & Lemieux 1991, Groves et al 2003, Joseph & Patel 1990, Moskowitz et al 1988). In other studies, clinicians are given all the data at once and asked to make a diagnostic or treatment decision (Elstein et al 1992, Patel & Groen 1986).

Case specificity

Problem-solving expertise varies greatly across cases and is highly dependent on the clinician's mastery of the particular domain. Differences between clinicians are to be found more in their understanding of the problem and their problem representations than in the reasoning strategies employed (Elstein et al 1978). Thus it makes more sense to talk about reasons for success and failure in a particular case than about generic traits or strategies of expert diagnosticians.

For evaluators in medical and other health professional education, this finding raises the practical problem of how many case simulations are needed to make a case-based examination a reliable and valid assessment of problem-solving skill. Test developers are now much more concerned about the number and content of clinical simulations in an examination than they were prior to this discovery (e.g. Page et al 1990, van der Vleuten & Swanson 1990).

DIAGNOSIS AS CATEGORIZATION OR PATTERN RECOGNITION

The finding of case specificity also challenged the hypothetico-deductive model as an adequate account of the process of clinical reasoning. Both successful and unsuccessful diagnosticians employed a hypothesis-testing strategy, and diagnostic accuracy depended more on mastery of the content in a domain than on the strategy employed. By the mid-1980s, the view of diagnostic reasoning as complex and systematic generation and testing of hypotheses was being criticized. Patel, Norman and their associates (e.g. Brooks et al 1991, Eva et al 1998, Groen & Patel 1985, Schmidt et al 1990) pointed out that the clinical reasoning of experts in familiar situations frequently does not display explicit hypothesis testing. It is rapid, automatic and often nonverbal. Not all cases seen by an experienced physician appear to require hypothetico-deductive reasoning (Davidoff 1996).

Expert reasoning in familiar situations looks more like pattern recognition or direct automatic retrieval from a well-structured network of stored knowledge (Groen & Patel 1985). Since experienced clinicians have a better sense of clinical realities and the likely diagnostic possibilities, they can also more efficiently generate an early set of plausible hypotheses to avoid fruitless and expensive pursuit of unlikely diagnoses. The research emphasis has shifted from the problem-solving process to the organization of knowledge in the long-term memory of experienced clinicians (Norman 1988).

Categorization of a new case can be based either on retrieval of and matching to specific instances or examplars, or to a more abstract prototype. In instance-based recognition, a new instance is classified by resemblance to memory of a past case (Brooks et al 1991, Medin & Schaffer 1978, Norman et al 1992, Schmidt et al 1990). This model is supported by the finding that clinical diagnosis is strongly affected by the context of events (for example the location of a skin rash on the body), even when this context is normatively irrelevant. Expert–novice differences are mainly explicable in terms of the size of the knowledge store of prior instances available for pattern recognition. This theory of clinical reasoning has been developed with particular reference to pathology, dermatology and radiology, where the clinical data are predominantly visual.

According to prototype models, clinical experience facilitates the construction of abstractions or prototypes (Bordage & Zacks 1984, Rosch & Mervis 1975). Better diagnosticians have constructed more diversified and abstract sets of semantic relations to represent the links between clinical features or aspects of the problem (Bordage & Lemieux 1991, Lemieux & Bordage 1992). Experts in a domain are more able to relate findings to each other and to potential diagnoses, and to identify what additional findings are needed to complete a picture (Elstein et al 1993). These capabilities suggest that experts are working with more abstract representations and are not simply trying to match a new case to a previous instance, although that matching process may occur with simple cases.

MULTIPLE REASONING STRATEGIES

Norman et al (1994) found that experienced physicians used a hypothetico-deductive strategy with difficult cases only, a view supported by Davidoff (1996). When a case is perceived to be less challenging, quicker and easier methods are used, such as pattern recognition or feature matching. Thus, controversy about the methods used in diagnostic reasoning can be resolved by positing that the method selected depends upon perceived characteristics of the problem. There is an interaction between the clinician's level of skill and the perceived difficulty of the task (Elstein 1994). Easy cases are solved by pattern recognition and going directly from data to diagnostic classification – what Groen & Patel (1985) called *forward reasoning*. Difficult cases need systematic hypothesis generation and testing. Whether a problem is easy or difficult depends in part on the knowledge and experience of the clinician who is trying to solve it (Figure 20.1).

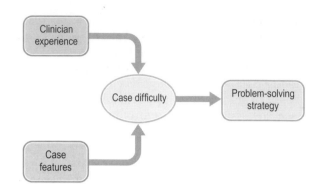

Figure 20.1 Impact on problem-solving strategy of case difficulty, clinician experience and case features

Both Norman and Eva have since championed the view that clinicians apply multiple reasoning strategies as necessary to approach diagnostic problems (Eva 2005, Norman 2005). Their research suggests that training physicians in multiple knowledge representations and reasoning modes may yield the best overall performance.

ERRORS IN HYPOTHESIS–GENERATION AND RESTRUCTURING

Neither pattern recognition nor hypothesis testing is an error-proof strategy, nor are they always consistent with statistical rules of inference with imperfect information. Errors that can occur in difficult cases in internal medicine were illustrated and discussed by Kassirer & Kopelman (1991) and classes of error were reviewed by Graber et al (2002). The frequency of errors in actual practice is unknown, but considering a number of studies as a whole, an error rate of 15% might be a good first approximation.

Looking at an instance of diagnostic reasoning retrospectively, it is easy to see that a clinician could err either by oversimplifying a complex problem or by taking a problem that could appropriately have been dealt with routinely and using a more effortful strategy of competing hypotheses. It has been far more difficult for researchers and teachers to prescribe an appropriate strategy in advance. Because so much depends on the interaction between case and clinician, prescriptive guidelines for the proper amount of hypothesis generation and testing are still unavailable for the student clinician. Perhaps the most useful advice is to emulate the hypothesis-testing strategy used by experienced clinicians when they are having difficulty, since novices will experience as problematic many situations that the former solve by routine pattern-recognition methods. In an era that emphasizes cost-effective clinical practice, gathering data unrelated to diagnostic hypotheses will be discouraged.

Many diagnostic problems are so complex that the correct solution is not contained within the initial set of hypotheses. Restructuring and reformulating must occur through time as data are obtained and the clinical picture evolves. However, as any problem solver works with a particular set of hypotheses, psychological commitment takes place and it becomes more difficult to restructure the problem (Janis & Mann 1977). Ideally, one might want to work purely inductively, reasoning only from the facts, but this strategy is never employed because it is inefficient and produces high levels of cognitive strain (Elstein et al 1978). It is much easier to solve a problem where some boundaries and hypotheses provide the needed framework. On the other hand, early problem formulation may also bias the clinician's thinking (Barrows et al 1982, Voytovich et al 1985). Errors in interpreting the diagnostic value of clinical information have been found by several research teams (Elstein et al 1978, Friedman et al 1998, Gruppen et al 1991, Wolf et al 1985).

DECISION MAKING: DIAGNOSIS AS OPINION REVISION

BAYES' THEOREM

In the literature on medical decision making, reaching a diagnosis is conceptualized as a process of reasoning about uncertainty, updating an opinion with imperfect information (the clinical evidence). As new information is obtained, the probability of each diagnostic possibility is continuously revised. Each post-test probability becomes the pre-test probability for the next stage of the inference process. Bayes' theorem, the formal mathematical rule for this operation (Hunink et al 2001, Sox et al 1988), states that the post-test probability is a function of two variables, pre-test probability and the strength of the new diagnostic evidence. The pre-test probability can be either the known prevalence of the disease or the clinician's belief about the probability of disease before new information is acquired. The strength of the evidence is measured by a *likelihood ratio*, the ratio of the probabilities of observing a particular finding in patients with and without the disease of interest. This framework directs attention to two major classes of errors in clinical reasoning: errors in a clinician's beliefs about pre-test probability or errors in assessing the strength of the evidence. Bayes' theorem is a normative rule for diagnostic reasoning; it tells us how we *should* reason, but it does not claim that we actually revise our opinions in this way. Indeed, from the Bayesian viewpoint, the psychological study of diagnostic reasoning centres on errors in both components, which are discussed below (Kempainen et al 2003 provide a similar review).

ERRORS IN PROBABILITY ESTIMATION

Many errors in probability revision result from simple heuristics that provide good estimates in most contexts, but may yield systematic biases in some contexts; Croskerry (2003) refers to such heuristics as *cognitive dispositions to respond*. For example, people are prone to overestimate the frequency of vivid or easily recalled events and to underestimate the frequency of events that are either very ordinary or difficult to recall (Tversky & Kahneman 1981). As a result of this 'availability heuristic', diseases or injuries which receive considerable media attention are often considered more probable than their true prevalence. This psychological principle is exemplified clinically in *overemphasizing rare conditions*. Unusual cases are more memorable than routine problems (Nisbett et al 1982).

People also overestimate the frequency of events that fit their ideas of a prototypical or representative case (Tversky & Kahneman 1974). When this 'representativeness heuristic' comes into play, the probability of a disease given a finding can be confused with the probability of a finding given the disease (Eddy 1982).

Small probabilities tend to be overestimated and large probabilities tend to be underestimated

(Tversky & Kahneman 1981). This results in strange discontinuities when probabilities are very close to 0 or 1. Cumulative prospect theory (Tversky & Kahneman 1992) and similar rank- and sign-dependent utility theories provide formal descriptions of how people distort probabilities in risky decision making. The distortions are exacerbated when the probabilities are vague and not precisely known (Einhorn & Hogarth 1986).

Many of the biases in probability estimation are captured by support theory (Redelmeier et al 1995, Rottenstreich & Tversky 1997, Tversky & Koehler 1994), which posits that subjective estimates of the frequency or probability of an event are influenced by how detailed the description is. More explicit descriptions yield higher probability estimates than do compact, condensed descriptions, even when the two would refer to exactly the same events (such as 'probability of death due to a car accident, train accident, plane accident, or other moving vehicle accident' vs 'probability of death due to a moving vehicle accident'). This theory can explain availability (when memories of an available event include more detailed descriptions than those of less available events) and representativeness (when a typical case description includes a cluster of details that 'fit', whereas a less typical case lacks some of these features).

ERRORS IN PROBABILITY REVISION

Conservatism

In clinical case discussions, data are commonly presented sequentially. In this circumstance, people often fail to revise their diagnostic probabilities as much as is implied by Bayes' theorem. This 'stickiness' has been called *conservatism* and was one of the earliest cognitive biases identified (Edwards 1968). A heuristic explanation of conservatism is that people revise their diagnostic opinion up or down from an initial anchor, which is either given in the problem or subjectively formed. Final opinions are sensitive to the anchor and the adjustment up or down from this anchor is typically insufficient, so the final judgement is closer to the initial anchor than would be implied by Bayes' theorem (Tversky & Kahneman 1974).

Confounding probability and value of an outcome

It is difficult for everyday judgement to keep separate accounts of the probability of a particular disease and the benefits that accrue from detecting it. Probability revision errors that are systematically linked to the perceived cost of mistakes demonstrate the difficulties experienced in separating assessments of probability from values (Poses et al 1985, Wallsten 1981).

Acquiring redundant evidence

In collecting data, there is a tendency to seek information that confirms a hypothesis rather than data that facilitate efficient testing of competing hypotheses. This tendency has been called 'pseudodiagnosticity' (Kern & Doherty 1982) or 'confirmation bias' (Wolf et al 1985).

Incorrect interpretation

The most common error in interpreting findings is over-interpretation: data which should not support a particular hypothesis, and which might even suggest that a new alternative be considered, are interpreted as consistent with hypotheses already under consideration (Elstein et al 1978, Friedman et al 1998). The data best remembered tend to be those that support the hypotheses generated. Where findings are distorted in recall, it is generally in the direction of making the facts more consistent with typical clinical pictures. Positive findings are overemphasized and negative findings tend to be discounted (Elstein et al 1978, Wason & Johnson-Laird 1972). From a Bayesian standpoint, these are all errors in assessing the diagnostic value of information, i.e. errors in subjective assessments of the likelihood ratio. These errors arise from an adaptive function, the need to keep problem representations simple enough to remain within the capacity of cognitive bounds (e.g. on working memory). Even when clinicians agree on the presence of certain clinical findings, wide variations have been found in the weights assigned to these findings in the course of interpreting their meaning (Bryant & Norman 1980, Wigton et al 1986).

Base-rate neglect

The basic principle of Bayesian inference is that a posterior probability is a function of two variables, the prior probability and the strength of the evidence. Research has shown that unless trained to use Bayes' theorem and to recognize when it is appropriate, physicians are just as prone as anyone else to misusing or neglecting base rates in diagnostic inference (Elstein 1988).

Order effects

Bayes' theorem implies that clinicians given identical information should reach the same diagnostic opinion, regardless of the order in which information is presented. Order effects mean that final opinions are also affected by the order of presentation of information. The information presented late in a case is given more weight than information presented earlier (Bergus et al 1995, Chapman et al 1996).

THE TWO-SYSTEM VIEW

Since the last edition of this book, the study of reasoning has been profoundly influenced by the 'two-system' or 'dual-process' theories of cognition (Hogarth 2005, Kahneman 2003, Stanovich & West 2000). Two distinct systems of judgement are posited. System 1 is a fast, automatic, and intuitive mode that shares similarities with perception. Judgements made using System 1 take advantage of the power of pattern recognition, prototypicality and the heuristics discussed earlier, and are susceptible to the associated biases and the impact of the emotional state of the judge and emotional content of the judgement. System 2 is a slow, effortful analytic mode that applies rules in an emotionally neutral manner (Figure 20.2). When appropriate data are available System 2 yields the most normatively rational reasoning, but it is easily disrupted by high cognitive load. Two-system accounts explain many puzzling findings about individual and contextual differences in reasoning, and can explain Norman's and Eva's findings of the value of multiple reasoning strategies, particular when different strategies (e.g. pattern recognition and hypothetico-deduction) may bring to bear the power of Systems 1 and 2, respectively.

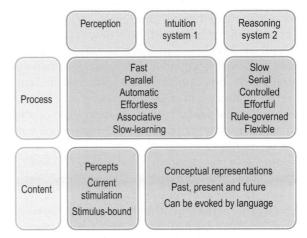

Figure 20.2 Characteristics of two cognitive systems for judgement (From 2003 (Fig. 1), The Nobel Foundation 2002, reprinted with permission)

EDUCATIONAL IMPLICATIONS

What can be done to help learners acquire expertise in clinical reasoning? Particularly in light of the two-system theory of cognition, we endorse the multiple reasoning strategies position espoused by both Norman and Eva, and seek to identify educational implications from both intuitive and analytical models in problem solving and decision making.

PROBLEM SOLVING: EDUCATIONAL IMPLICATIONS

Even if experts in non-problematic situations do not routinely generate and test hypotheses and instead retrieve a solution (diagnosis) directly from their structured knowledge, they clearly do generate and evaluate alternatives when confronted with problematic situations. For novices, most situations will initially be problematic, and generating a small set of hypotheses is a useful procedural guideline. Since much expert hypothesis generation and testing is implicit, a model that calls it to the novice's attention will aid learning. The hypothetico-deductive model directs learners toward forming a conception of the problem and using this plan to guide the workup. This plan will include a set of competing diagnoses and the semantic relationships that make it possible to order the diagnostic candidates as similar and different. This makes it possible to reduce unnecessary and expensive laboratory testing, a welcome emphasis in an era that stresses cost containment.

The instance-based model implies that clinical experience is needed in contexts closely related to future practice, because transfer from one context to another is limited. In one way, this model reinforces a very traditional doctrine in medical education: practical arts are learned by supervised practice and rehearsal combined with progressively increasing professional responsibility, supplemented by instruction in case conferences, clinical rounds, reading and the like. In another way, it conflicts with traditional training, since the model implies that trainees will not generalize as much from one context (say, hospitalized patients) to another (say, ambulatory patients) as has traditionally been thought.

The prototype position offers a more optimistic view, since it implies that clinical experience is necessary but needs to be reviewed and analysed so that the correct general models and principles are abstracted from the experience. Well-designed educational experiences can facilitate the development of the desired cognitive structures. Given the emerging consensus about characteristics distinguishing experts from novices, an effective route to the goal would be extensive focused practice and feedback with a variety of problems (Bordage 1987, Eshach & Bitterman 2003, Lemieux & Bordage 1992). Similarly, Rabinowitz & Glaser (1985) proposed that an adequate understanding of the expert's knowledge structure would lead to more effective instruction to assist novices in acquiring that structure.

DECISION MAKING: EDUCATIONAL IMPLICATIONS

If expert clinicians are not consistent in their approach across cases, what formal generalizable logic or operations can or should be taught to learners? In this section, we review some recent efforts to teach the logic of clinical decision making that have been strongly influenced by decision theoretic principles and research results.

Evidence-based medicine

Until recently, medical educators paid little attention to formal quantitative methods for dealing with these problems. It was implicitly assumed that the problems would become insignificant as clinical experience was acquired. Criticisms of clinical practice and efforts at controlling costs have both led to the rise of evidence-based medicine (EBM), an approach to clinical education and practice which reflects growing interest in applying formal quantitative methods to diagnosis and treatment choice (Evidence-based Medicine Working Group 1992, Sackett et al 1997). EBM emphasizes using the clinical literature to find answers to questions arising in clinical practice. The approach involves formulating a well-structured clinical question focused on such matters as the diagnostic value of a particular test or the expected outcomes of alternative treatments for well-defined conditions. Answers to these questions are sought in the medical literature. Individual studies are rigorously evaluated to determine how well the study responds to the clinical question that prompted the inquiry. This assessment considers soundness of research design, whether the findings apply to the patient of concern, trustworthiness of the conclusions, and limitations of the evidence. For integrating the results of diverse studies into a treatment recommendation or overall judgement of effectiveness of various treatments, there is a strong preference for meta-analysis (L'Abbe et al 1987, Oxman et al 1994, Rosenthal 1991), a more structured, quantitative form of literature review, rather than the traditional narrative review that embodies the subjective judgement of the experts who wrote the review. Meta-analyses have been particularly useful in integrating the results of clinical trials of new therapies because they use statistical measures, such as effect size, that can be combined across several studies to produce an overall estimate of effect. Whether meta-analyses will ultimately replace traditional reviews remains to be seen.

EBM is particularly relevant for the diagnostic inference process discussed in this chapter because it is, in our opinion, currently the most popular vehicle explicitly advocating a Bayesian approach to clinical evidence. Textbooks of EBM (Sackett et al 1991, 1997) show how to use prevalence rates and likelihood ratios to calculate posterior probabilities of diagnostic alternatives (predictive value of a positive or negative test), and at least one recent study suggests that prevalence data may be readily available in the medical literature for inpatient adult medicine problems (Richardson et al 2003). Formal statistical reasoning and decision analysis are likewise explained and advocated in an ever-growing number of works aimed at physicians (Kassirer & Kopelman 1991, Lee 2004, Mark 2006, Panzer et al 1991, Sox et al 1988, Weinstein et al 1980). Decision theory, decision analysis and evidence-based medicine seem to be on their way to becoming standard components of clinical education and training.

Decision support systems

Computer programs that run on microcomputers and can provide decision support have been developed (Applied Informatics 1990, de Bliek et al 1988). The role of these programs in medical education and in future clinical practice is still to be determined, but they hold out hope for addressing both cognitive and systemic sources of diagnostic error (Elstein et al 2004, Graber et al 2002).

A variety of paper, personal digital assistant (PDA), and online tools and spreadsheets have been developed to provide decision support or simplify EBM calculations. A typical example is the graphical Bayesian nomogram which permits quick calculation of posterior probabilities from prior probability and likelihood ratio information. Fagan (1975) published the best known nomogram, which is widely available on a pocket-sized card. Schwartz (1998) provides an on-line version.

Debiasing

A number of researchers have proposed methods for debiasing judgements without resorting to formal methods of probability estimation and

revision (Arkes 1991, Croskerry 2003, Keren 1990, Mumma & Wilson 1995). Debiasing methods include educating judges about common biases, encouraging judges to consider alternative hypotheses carefully and making judges more accountable for errors. Evidence for the effectiveness of these methods is mixed (Graber 2003).

CONCLUSION

Research on the clinical reasoning of physicians has a broad range, including but not limited to: differences between expert and novice clinicians; psychological processes in judgement and decision making; factors associated with non-normative biases in judgement; improving instruction and training to enhance acquisition of good reasoning; and the development, evaluation and implementation of decision support systems and guidelines. Many recent studies of physicians' decision making have sought to understand the process of clinical reasoning, improve instructional programmes designed for medical students and clinical training, assess competence at the level of medical licensure and certification, analyse the cognitive processes employed in specific clinical situations, and develop practice guidelines and standards.

Research on reasoning in medicine thus stands at the intersection of the interests of psychologists, medical sociologists, health policy planners, economists, patients and clinicians. Given this conjunction, both normative and descriptive studies of clinical reasoning in medicine, as well as studies to find practical methods of improving the level of reasoning, are still needed.

Acknowledgements

Preparation of this review was supported in part by grant RO1 LM5630 from the National Library of Medicine.

References

Applied Informatics 1990 ILIAD User manual. Author, Salt Lake City

Arkes H 1991 Costs and benefits of judgment errors: implications for debiasing. Psychological Bulletin 110(37):486–498

Baron J 2000 Thinking and deciding, 3rd edn. Cambridge University Press, New York

Barrows H S, Pickell G C 1991 Developing clinical problem-solving skills: a guide to more effective diagnosis and treatment. Norton, New York

Barrows H S, Norman G R, Neufeld V R et al 1982 The clinical reasoning process of randomly selected physicians in general practice. Clinical and Investigative Medicine 5(1):49–56

Bergus G R, Chapman G B, Gjerde C et al 1995 Clinical reasoning about new symptoms despite pre-existing disease: sources of error and order effects. Family Medicine 27(5):314–320

Bordage G 1987 The curriculum: overloaded and too general? Medical Education 21(3):183–188

Bordage G, Lemieux M 1991 Semantic structures and diagnostic thinking of experts and novices. Academic Medicine 66(9):S70–S72

Bordage G, Zacks R 1984 The structure of medical knowledge in the memories of medical students and general practitioners: categories and prototypes. Medical Education 18(6):406–416

Brooks L R, Norman G R, Allen S W 1991 Role of specific similarity in a medical diagnostic task. Journal of Experimental Psychology: General 120(3):278–287

Bryant G D, Norman G R 1980 Expressions of probability: words and numbers. New England Journal of Medicine 302(7):411

Chapman G B, Bergus G R, Elstein A S 1996 Order of information affects clinical judgment. Journal of Behavioral Decision Making 9(3):201–211

Croskerry P 2003 The importance of cognitive errors in diagnosis and strategies to minimize them. Academic Medicine 78(8):775–780

Davidoff F 1996 Is basic science necessary? In: Davidoff F (ed) Who has seen a blood sugar? Reflections on Medical Education. American College of Physicians, Philadelphia, p 18–23

De Bliek R, Miller R A, Masarie F E 1988 QMR user manual. University of Pittsburgh, Pittsburgh

Eddy D M 1982 Probabilistic reasoning in clinical medicine: problems and opportunities. In: Kahneman D, Slovic P, Tversky A (eds) Judgment under uncertainty: heuristics and biases. Cambridge University Press, New York, p 249–267

Edwards W 1968 Conservatism in human information processing. In: Kleinmuntz B (ed) Formal representation of human judgment. Wiley, New York, p 17–52

Einhorn H J, Hogarth R M 1986 Decision making under ambiguity. Journal of Business 59(4):S225–S250

Elstein A S 1988 Cognitive processes in clinical inference and decision making. In: Turk D C, Salovey P (eds) Reasoning, inference and judgment in clinical psychology. Free Press/Macmillan, New York, p 17–50

Elstein A S 1994 What goes around comes around: the return of the hypothetico-deductive strategy. Teaching and Learning in Medicine 6(2):121–123

Elstein A S, Shulman L S, Sprafka S A 1978 Medical problem solving: an analysis of clinical reasoning. Harvard University Press, Cambridge, MA

Elstein A S, Holzman G B, Belzer L J et al 1992 Hormonal replacement therapy: analysis of clinical strategies used by residents. Medical Decision Making 12(4):265–273

Elstein A S, Kleinmuntz B, Rabinowitz M et al 1993 Diagnostic reasoning of high- and low-domain knowledge clinicians: a re-analysis. Medical Decision Making 13(1):21–29

Elstein A S, Schwartz A, McNutt R 2004 Can metacognition minimize cognitive biases? Academic Medicine. Online (eLetters, now available from the authors)

Eschach H, Bitterman H 2003 From case-based reasoning to problem-based learning. Academic Medicine 78(5): 491–496

Eva K W 2005 What every teacher needs to know about clinical reasoning. Medical Education 39(1):98–106

Eva K W, Neville A J, Norman G R 1998 Exploring the etiology of content specificity: factors influencing analogic transfer and problem solving. Academic Medicine 73(10 Suppl):S1–S5

Evidence-based Medicine Working Group 1992 Evidence-based medicine: a new approach to teaching the practice of medicine. Journal of the American Medical Association 268(17):2420–2425

Fagan T J 1975 Nomogram for Bayes' theorem. New England Journal of Medicine 293(5):257

Feightner J W 1985 Patient management problems. In: Neufeld V R, Norman G R (eds) Assessing clinical competence. Springer, New York, p 183–200

Feltovich P J, Johnson P E, Moller J H et al 1984 The role and development of medical knowledge in diagnostic expertise. In: Clancey W J, Shortliffe E H (eds) Readings in medical artificial intelligence: the first decade. Addison-Wesley, Reading, MA, p 275–319

Friedman M H, Connell K J, Olthoff A J et al 1998 Medical student errors in making a diagnosis. Academic Medicine 73(10 Suppl):S19–S21

Graber M 2003 Metacognitive training to reduce diagnostic errors: ready for prime time? Academic Medicine 78 (8):781

Graber M, Gordon R, Franklin N 2002 Reducing diagnostic errors in medicine: what's the goal? Academic Medicine 77(10):981–992

Groen G J, Patel V L 1985 Medical problem-solving: some questionable assumptions. Medical Education 19(2): 95–100

Groves M, O'Rourke P, Alexander H 2003 The clinical reasoning characteristics of diagnostic experts. Medical Teacher 25(3):308–313

Gruppen L D, Wolf F M, Billi J E 1991 Information gathering and integration as sources of error in diagnostic decision making. Medical Decision Making 11(4):233–239

Hogarth R M 2005 Deciding analytically or trusting your intuition? The advantages and disadvantages of analytic and intuitive thought. In: Betsch T, Haberstroh S (eds) The routines of decision making. Lawrence Erlbaum Associates, Mahwah, NJ, p 67–82

Hunink M, Glasziou P, Siegel J et al 2001 Decision making in health and medicine: integrating evidence and values. Cambridge University Press, New York

Janis I L, Mann L 1977 Decision-making: a psychological analysis of conflict, choice, and commitment. Free Press, New York

Joseph G M, Patel V L 1990 Domain knowledge and hypothesis generation in diagnostic reasoning. Medical Decision Making 10(1):31–46

Kahneman D 2003 Maps of bounded rationality: a perspective on intuitive judgment and choice. In: Frangsmyr T (ed) Les Prix Nobel. The Nobel Prizes 2002. Almqvist & Wiksell International, Stockholm, p 416–499

Kahneman D, Slovic P, Tversky A (eds) 1982 Judgment under uncertainty: heuristics and biases. Cambridge University Press, New York

Kassirer J P, Gorry G A 1978 Clinical problem solving: a behavioral analysis. Annals of Internal Medicine 89:245–255

Kassirer J P, Kopelman R I 1991 Learning clinical reasoning. Williams and Wilkins, Baltimore

Kempainen R R, Migeon M B, Wolf F M 2003 Understanding our mistakes: a primer on errors in clinical reasoning. Medical Teacher 25(2):177–181

Keren G 1990 Cognitive aids and debiasing methods: can cognitive pills cure cognitive ills? In: Caverni J, Fabre J (eds) Advances in psychology, vol 68. Cognitive biases. North-Holland, Amsterdam, p 523–552

Kern L, Doherty M E 1982 'Pseudodiagnosticity' in an idealized medical problem-solving environment. Journal of Medical Education 57(2):100–104

Kuipers B J, Kassirer J P 1984 Causal reasoning in medicine: analysis of a protocol. Cognitive Science 8(4):363–385

Kuipers B, Moskowitz A J, Kassirer J P 1988 Critical decisions under uncertainty: representation and structure. Cognitive Science 12(2):177–210

L'Abbe K A, Detsky A S, O'Rourke K 1987 Meta-analysis in clinical research. Annals of Internal Medicine 107(2):224–233

Lee T H 2004 Interpretation of data for clinical decisions. In: Goldman L, Ausiello D (eds) Cecil textbook of medicine. 22nd edn. Saunders, Philadelphia, p 23–28

Lemieux M, Bordage G 1992 Propositional versus structural semantic analyses of medical diagnostic thinking. Cognitive Science 16(2):185–204

Mark D B 2006 Decision-making in clinical medicine. In: Kasper D L, Braunwald E, Fauci A S et al (eds) Harrison's principles of internal medicine, 16th edn. McGraw-Hill, New York

Medin D L, Schaffer M M 1978 A context theory of classification learning. Psychological Review 85(3):207–238

Mellers B A, Schwartz A, Cooke A D J 1998 Judgment and decision making. Annual Review of Psychology 49:447–477

Moskowitz A J, Kuipers B J, Kassirer J P 1988 Dealing with uncertainty, risks, and tradeoffs in clinical decisions: a cognitive science approach. Annals of Internal Medicine 108(3):435–449

Mumma G H, Wilson S B 1995 Procedural debiasing of primacy/anchoring effects in clinical-like judgments. Journal of Clinical Psychology 51(6):841–853

Nendaz M R, Gut A M, Perrier A et al 2005 Common strategies in clinical data collection displayed by experienced clinician-teachers in internal medicine. Medical Teacher 27(5):415–421

Neufeld V R, Norman G R, Feightner J W et al 1981 Clinical problem-solving by medical students: a cross-sectional and longitudinal analysis. Medical Education 15(5):315–322

Newell A, Simon H A 1972 Human problem solving. Prentice-Hall, Englewood Cliffs, NJ

Nisbett R E, Borgida E, Crandall R, Reed H 1982 Popular induction: information is not always informative. In: Kahneman D, Slovic P, Tversky A (eds) Judgment under uncertainty: heuristics and biases. Cambridge University Press, New York, p 101–116

Norman G R 1988 Problem-solving skills, solving problems and problem-based learning. Medical Education 22(4):279–286

Norman G 2005 Research in clinical reasoning: past history and current trends. Medical Education 39:418–427

Norman G R, Coblentz C L, Brooks L R et al 1992 Expertise in visual diagnosis: a review of the literature. Academic Medicine 67(10):S78–S83

Norman G R, Trott A L, Brooks L R et al 1994 Cognitive differences in clinical reasoning related to postgraduate training. Teaching and Learning in Medicine 6:114–120

Oxman A D, Cook D J, Guyatt G H 1994 Users' guides to the medical literature, no 6. How to use an overview. Journal of the American Medical Association 272(17):1367–1371

Page G, Bordage G, Harasym P et al 1990 A revision of the medical council of Canada's qualifying examination: pilot test results. In: Bender W, Hiemstra R, Scherpbier A et al (eds) Teaching and assessing clinical competence. BoekWerk Publication, Groningen, p 403–407

Panzer R J, Black E R, Griner P F 1991 Diagnostic strategies for common medical problems. American College of Physicians, Philadelphia

Patel V L, Groen G J 1986 Knowledge-based solution strategies in medical reasoning. Cognitive Science 10:91–116

Pople H E 1982 Heuristic methods for imposing structure on ill-structured problems: the structuring of medical diagnostics. In: Szolovitz P (ed) Artificial intelligence in medicine. Westview Press, Boulder, CO, p 119–190

Poses R M, Cebul R D, Collins M et al 1985 The accuracy of experienced physicians' probability estimates for patients with sore throats: implications for decision making. Journal of the American Medical Association 254(7):925–929

Rabinowitz M, Glaser R 1985 Cognitive structure and process in highly competent performance. In: Horowitz D F, O'Brien M (eds) The gifted and talented: developmental perspectives. American Psychological Association, Washington DC, p 75–98

Redelmeier D A, Koehler D J, Liberman V et al 1995 Probability judgment in medicine: discounting unspecified probabilities. Medical Decision Making 15(3):227–230

Richardson W S, Polashenski W A, Robbins B W 2003 Could our pretest probabilities become evidence based? A prospective survey of hospital practice. Journal of General Internal Medicine 18:203–208

Rosch E, Mervis C B 1975 Family resemblances: studies in the internal structure of categories. Cognitive Psychology 7(4):573–605

Rosenthal R 1991 Meta-analytic procedures for social research. 2nd edn. Sage, Newbury Park

Rottenstreich Y, Tversky A 1997 Unpacking, repacking, and anchoring: advances in support theory. Psychological Review 104(2):406–415

Sackett D L, Haynes R B, Guyatt G H et al 1991 Clinical epidemiology: a basic science for clinical medicine. 2nd edn. Little Brown, Boston

Sackett D L, Richardson W S, Rosenberg W et al 1997 Evidence-based medicine: how to practice and teach EBM. Churchill Livingstone, New York

Schmidt H G, Norman G R, Boshuizen H P A 1990 A cognitive perspective on medical expertise: theory and implications. Academic Medicine 65:611–621

Schwartz A 1998 Nomogram for Bayes' theorem. Online. Available: http://araw.mede.uic.edu/cgi-bin/testcalc.pl 7 July 2007

Shafir E, LeBoeuf R A 2002 Rationality. Annual Review of Psychology 53(1):491–517

Sox H C Jr, Blatt M A, Higgins M C et al 1988 Medical decision making. Butterworth-Heinemann, Boston

Stanovich K E, West R F 2000 Individual differences in reasoning: implications for the rationality debate? Behavioral and Brain Sciences 23(5):645–726

Swanson D B, Norman G R, Linn R L 1995 Performance-based assessment: lessons from the health professions. Educational Researcher 24(5):5–11

Tversky A, Kahneman D 1974 Judgment under uncertainty: heuristics and biases. Science 185(4157):1124–1131

Tversky A, Kahneman D 1981 The framing of decisions and the psychology of choice. Science 211(4481):453–458

Tversky A, Kahneman D 1992 Advances in prospect theory: cumulative representation of uncertainty. Journal of Risk and Uncertainty 5(4):297–323

Tversky A, Koehler D J 1994 Support theory: a nonextensional representation of subjective probability. Psychology Review 101(4):547–567

van der Vleuten C P M, Swanson D B 1990 Assessment of clinical skills with standardized patients: state of the art. Teaching and Learning in Medicine 2(2):58–76

Voytovich A E, Rippey R M, Suffredini A 1985 Premature conclusions in diagnostic reasoning. Journal of Medical Education 60(4):302–307

Wallsten T S 1981 Physician and medical student bias in evaluating information. Medical Decision Making 1(2):145–164

Wason P C, Johnson-Laird P N 1972 Psychology of reasoning: structure and content. Harvard University Press, Cambridge

Weinstein M C, Fineberg H V, Elstein A S et al 1980 Clinical decision analysis. W B Saunders, Philadelphia, PA

Wigton R S, Hoellerich V L, Patil K D 1986 How physicians use clinical information in diagnosing pulmonary embolism: an application of conjoint analysis. Medical Decision Making 6:2–11. In: Dowie J, Elstein A (eds) 1988 Professional judgment: a reader in clinical decision making. Cambridge University Press, New York, p 130–149

Wolf F M, Gruppen L D, Billi J E 1985 Differential diagnosis and the competing hypotheses heuristic: a practical approach to judgment under uncertainty and Bayesian probability. Journal of American Medical Association 253: 2858–2862. In: Dowie J, Elstein A (eds) 1988 Professional judgment: a reader in clinical decision making. Cambridge University Press, New York, p 349–359

Chapter **21**

Clinical reasoning in nursing

Marsha E. Fonteyn and Barbara J. Ritter

Clinical reasoning represents the essence of nursing practice. It is intrinsic to all aspects of care provision, and its importance pervades nursing education, research and practice. An understanding of nurses' clinical reasoning is important to nursing research because of the need for a scientific basis to evaluate nursing practice and education and a need to develop and test theories of nurses' cognitive processes and reasoning skills. Research is also needed to describe and explain the relationship between nurses' reasoning and patient outcomes, in order to demonstrate to society the essential role that nursing plays in the healthcare delivery system.

Knowledge about clinical reasoning is important to nursing education because education is expensive, and teaching that is based on inappropriate or irrelevant models of reasoning can not only lead to waste but also result in graduates who are ill-prepared to reason well in practice. Clinical reasoning is also important to nursing practice because patient care provision is becoming increasingly more complex and difficult, requiring sound reasoning skills to maintain patient stability, provide high quality care with positive outcomes, and avoid the costly, even deadly, mistakes that can occur from faulty reasoning and errors in decision making.

DEFINITION OF CLINICAL REASONING

The literature provides several definitions of nurses' clinical reasoning. Fonteyn (1991) defined nurses' clinical reasoning as the cognitive processes that nurses use when reviewing and analysing patient data to plan care and make decisions for positive patient outcomes. Gordon et al (1994) saw nurses' reasoning as a form of clinical judgement that occurs in a series of stages: encountering the patient; gathering clinical information; formulating possible diagnostic hypotheses; searching for more information to confirm or reject these hypotheses; reaching a diagnostic decision; and determining actions. Ritter (1998) viewed clinical reasoning as a process involving inclusion of evidence to facilitate optimum patient outcomes. Therefore, nurses' clinical reasoning can be defined as the cognitive processes and strategies that nurses use to understand the significance of patient data, to identify and diagnose actual or potential patient problems, to make clinical decisions to assist in problem resolution, and to achieve positive patient outcomes. According to O'Neill et al (2005), clinical decision making is a complex task geared towards the identification and management of patients' health needs that requires a knowledgeable practitioner along with reliable information and a supportive environment.

DISTINGUISHING BETWEEN NURSES' REASONING PROCESS AND THE NURSING PROCESS

Johnson (1959) used the term 'nursing process' to describe the series of steps that comprise the process of nursing. All the steps require reasoning skills. This concept of a five-step process, consisting of assessment, diagnosis, planning, implementation and evaluation, has become entrenched in both nursing practice and nursing education. In what has become a classic treatise, Henderson (1982) cautioned that the nursing process should not be confused with the process of clinical reasoning.

Although fundamental to providing care, nurses' reasoning and decision making has had limited explication in nursing research literature, but the descriptive work that has been done reveals a distinction between how nurses reason in practice and how they first learn to reason as an academic endeavour. In their classic study of nurses' clinical judgement, Benner & Tanner (1987) found

that with experience, nurses develop a method of reasoning that provides them with an 'intuitive grasp' of the whole clinical situation, without having to rely on the step-by-step analytic approach of the nursing process. They advocated the inclusion in nursing curricula of activities that would foster students' skills in intuitive judgement. Because the nursing process method teaches students to focus on individual patient problems and associated interventions separately, it may promote a less efficient way of reasoning and does not always reflect the realities encountered in actual practice, where one patient problem is often associated with another. In summary, when discussing the cognitive processes and strategies that nurses use to reason about patient care, it is important to clearly distinguish them from the nursing process, which represents one of the many approaches that nurses use in problem solving.

THEORETICAL PERSPECTIVES

Several different theoretical perspectives have helped provide an understanding of nurses' clinical reasoning, namely information processing, decision analysis and hermeneutics.

INFORMATION PROCESSING THEORY (IPT)

IPT was first described by Newell & Simon (1972) in their seminal work examining how individuals with a great deal of experience in a specific area (domain expertise) reasoned during a problem-solving task. A fundamental premise of IPT is that human reasoning consists of a relationship between an information processing system (the human problem solver) and a task environment (the context in which problem solving occurs). A postulate of this theory is that there are limits to the amount of information that one can process at any given time, and that effective problem solving is the result of being able to adapt to these limitations. Miller's (1956) earlier classic work had demonstrated that an individual's working, short-term memory (STM) can hold only $7 +/- 2$ symbols at a time. Newell & Simon showed that the capacity of STM could be greatly increased, however, by 'chunking' simple units into familiar patterns. Individuals with a great deal of knowledge and experience in a particular domain can more easily chunk information pertaining to that domain, and thus can make more efficient use of their STM during reasoning.

Another memory bank identified by Newell & Simon (1972) is long-term memory (LTM), which has infinite storage space for information. The theory proposes that information gained from knowledge and experience is stored throughout life in LTM, and that it takes longer to access LTM information than the small amount of information temporarily stored in STM. According to this theory, the information stored in LTM may need to be accessed by associating it with related information, which helps explain why experts reason so well within their domain. Indeed, cognitive research has demonstrated that experts possess an organized body of domain-specific conceptual and procedural knowledge that can be easily accessed using reasoning strategies (heuristics) and specific reasoning processes that are gradually learned through academic learning and through clinical experience (Glaser & Chi 1988, Joseph & Patel 1990).

DECISION ANALYSIS THEORY

Decision analysis theory (DAT) was introduced in medicine over 20 years ago as a method of solving difficult clinical problems. DAT methods include use of Bayes' theorem, use of decision trees, sensitivity analysis, and utility analysis. Bayes' theorem application involves the use of mathematical formulas, tabular techniques, nomograms, and computer programs to determine the likelihood of meaning of clinical data.

Several nursing studies have demonstrated the applicability of decision theory to nurses' decision making. In her classic study examining the relationship between the expected value (anticipated outcome) nurses assign to each of their outcomes and their ranking of nursing actions, Grier (1976) demonstrated that nurses select actions that are consistent with their expected values, which seems to support the use of decision trees in some instances of nurses' reasoning and decision making. Lipman & Deatrick (1997) found that nurse practitioner students who used a decision

tree made better decisions about diagnosis and treatment choices for both acute and chronic conditions. Lauri & Salantera (1995) studied decision-making models and the variables related to them. Findings were that the nature of nursing tasks and the context yielded the greatest difference in decision-making approach. Lewis (1997) found that conflict and ambiguity significantly increased task complexity. Therefore, recommendations are to consider task complexity during model design when developing decision models for use in nursing. Narayan et al (2003) examined decision analysis as a tool to support an analytical pattern of reasoning; they found that decision analysis is valuable in difficult and complex situations where there are mutually exclusive options and there is time for deliberation.

HERMENEUTICS

Hermeneutics is based on the phenomenological tradition that meaning is subjective and contextually constructed. The intent of studies of nurses' reasoning guided by this method is to understand the clinical world of nurses, including their reasoning as they make decisions about patient care. Benner et al (1992) used a hermeneutic approach to study the development of expertise in critical care nursing practice. Their findings indicated that nurses at different levels of expertise 'live in different clinical worlds, noticing and responding to different directives for action' (Benner et al 1992, p. 13). Findings from a later study by the same authors (1996) indicate that this clinical world is shaped by experience that teaches nurses to make qualitative distinctions in practice. They also found that beginner nurses were more task-oriented, while those with more experience focused on understanding their patients and their illness states.

RESEARCH FINDINGS OF STUDIES RELATED TO CLINICAL REASONING

Studies of nurses' clinical judgement, problem solving, decision making and intuition have contributed to the understanding of nurses' clinical reasoning.

CLINICAL JUDGEMENT STUDIES

Nurses' clinical judgement represents a composite of traits that assists them in reasoning (Tanner 1987). Benner et al (1992), in their hermeneutic study, described characteristics of clinical judgement exhibited by critical care nurses with varying levels of practice experience when they reasoned about patient care. Characteristics of clinical judgement identified in the most experienced subjects included: (a) the ability to recognize patterns in clinical situations that fit with patterns they had seen in other similar clinical cases; (b) a sense of urgency related to predicting what lies ahead; (c) the ability to concentrate simultaneously on multiple, complex patient cues and patient management therapies; and (d) an aptitude for realistically assessing patient priorities and nursing responsibilities.

The characteristics of clinical judgement identified by Benner & Tanner (1987) and Benner et al (1992) assist in our understanding of nurses' clinical reasoning by identifying and describing some of the cognitive traits or skills that nurses use during reasoning. Benner & Tanner's subsequent work with Chesla (Benner et al 1996) helps further the theoretical understanding of nurses' judgement that is needed to improve educators' ability to teach their students to reason better, and to provide nurses in practice with knowledge that will help them to problem-solve and to make better decisions about patient care.

PROBLEM-SOLVING AND DECISION-MAKING STUDIES

One of the primary objectives of clinical reasoning is to make decisions to resolve problems. Thus, research into nurses' problem solving and decision making provides understanding about the processes involved in their clinical reasoning. Fonteyn & Fisher (1995) examined nurses' decision making when monitoring unstable clients immediately after major surgery. The nurses used three types of reasoning in this situation: predictive reasoning (anticipating patient responses and outcomes based on the current status of a client and on previous experience with similar client cases); backward reasoning (searching the available data for support or substantiation of a clinical hunch when the working plan of care fails to provide an explanation for new data); and forward reasoning (incorporating new data into the working plan of care, while persisting with the plan that nurses commonly use to make clinical decisions). De la Cruz (1994) studied the problem-solving skills of home health nurses and identified three types of thinking style: 'skimming', 'surveying' and 'sleuthing'. De la Cruz defined skimming as a decision-making style that is used by experienced nurses who draw upon their previous knowledge and experience to quickly assess a clinical situation to expedite a predetermined and well-defined task. Surveying is a decision-making style that focuses on addressing distinct and specific patient problems which can be resolved using standardized nursing interventions. Sleuthing is used by experienced nurses when managing ambiguous, uncertain, complex problems, and involves the use of heuristics and inferencing (De la Cruz 1994).

A number of researchers have investigated the complexity of nurses' decision making tasks and situations and have identified a range of reasoning strategies, including hypothetico-deductive, intuitive and pattern recognition. These studies have emphasized the importance of consultation with experienced colleagues (Manias et al 2004) and the use of clinical supervision to facilitate review and feedback (Riley 2003).

INTUITION STUDIES

Several investigators have proposed that intuition is an important part of nurses' reasoning processes. A classic study that continues to guide nursing research on intuition was conducted by Pyles & Stern (1983) to explore the reasoning of a group of critical care nurses with varying levels of expertise. The investigators identified a 'gut feeling' experienced by the more seasoned nurse subjects, which they believed was as important to nurses' reasoning as their formal knowledge about patient cases. Subjects said they used these gut feelings to temper information from specific clinical cues; they also emphasized the importance of previous clinical experience in developing intuitive skills. Rew (1990) demonstrated the important role that intuition played in nurses' reasoning and decision making. Subjects described their intuitive experiences as strong feelings or perceptions about their patients, about themselves and responding to their patients, or about anticipated outcomes, that they sensed without going through an analytical reasoning process.

CLINICAL REASONING STUDIES

Fonteyn & Grobe (1993) showed that, unlike physicians' reasoning, most of nurses' reasoning tasks are not aimed at diagnosis and hypothesis generation. Rather, nurses reason to distinguish between relevant and irrelevant patient data, to determine the significance of patient data, and to make decisions that assist in accomplishing the overall treatment plan for each patient. Their study also provided a description of nurses' reasoning–thinking strategies (heuristics).

Heuristics are mental rules of thumb that assist in reasoning and are acquired over time through multiple experiences with similar patient cases (Fonteyn & Fisher 1995, Fonteyn & Grobe 1993). In a later study, Fonteyn (1998) provided a more complete description of the heuristics nurses use when reasoning about clinical dilemmas. They include recognizing a pattern, setting priorities, searching for information, generating hypotheses, making predictions, forming relationships, stating a proposition, asserting a practice rule, making choices, judging the value, drawing conclusions and providing explanations. Additional, less common thinking strategies were pondering, posing a question, making assumptions and qualifying and making generalizations. This evidence strengthens and expands previous clinical reasoning studies of nurses' use of heuristics. Cioffi & Markham (1997) found that advanced practice nurses relied on heuristics in clinical decision making when uncertainty was not resolved by information collected during an assessment, or to simplify task complexity which could lead to inaccurate diagnoses and treatment. Further research remains to be done on biases associated with nurses' heuristics use.

RESEARCH IN THE CLINICAL ARENA

Despite the research that has already been done, the nature of nurses' clinical reasoning requires further exploration. Beyond research conducted outside the clinical arena, using simulation, questionnaires or interviews, there is a need for more studies situated in the clinical arena to achieve the fullest and most accurate description of nurses' clinical reasoning. Fonteyn & Fisher (1995) demonstrated that it is both logistically possible and safe to study nurses' clinical reasoning in the clinical setting during the time that care is being given. Using a triangulated method consisting of guided interviews, participant observation and think-aloud technique, the investigators collected data from a group of expert critical care nurses while they were providing postoperative care to critically ill patients. Findings from this study suggest that a tremendous amount of rich, relevant data about nurses' reasoning can be obtained using this method. Moreover, studying nurses' reasoning in the clinical setting does not appear to compromise patient care or to disrupt either subject or unit functioning. Narayan & Corcoran-Perry (1997) demonstrated the feasibility of this methodological approach in a study examining how nurses with varying levels of expertise use knowledge to make a particular clinical decision.

Future studies of nurses' clinical reasoning undertaken in the clinical setting while care is being given to real (not simulated) patients will assist in completing the description of this phenomenon. Subsequently studies should be initiated that examine the relationship between nurses' clinical reasoning and other variables, such as level of expertise, domain knowledge, the climate in which the reasoning and decision making take place, patient stability and patient outcomes. Some of the important questions are:

- How is nurses' reasoning related to their sense of autonomy and job satisfaction?
- How is clinical reasoning related to expertise and level of knowledge within a domain?
- What factors are associated with optimal reasoning?
- What is the relationship between nurses' clinical reasoning and patient outcomes?

Later, as the state of the science evolves from research that provides answers to these questions, experimental studies can be undertaken to provide answers to additional questions, such as:

- Is nurses' reasoning improved with increased autonomy or job satisfaction?
- Can nurses be taught strategies that will improve their reasoning?
- Can methods be devised to improve nurses' reasoning outside their domain knowledge?
- Does improvement in nurses' reasoning result in improved patient outcomes?

EDUCATIONAL FOCUS ON CLINICAL REASONING

CRITICAL THINKING

Nurses increasingly need well developed reasoning skills to assist them in understanding and resolving the complex patient problems encountered in practice. In their text *Developing Clinical Problem-solving Skills*, Barrows & Pickell (1991, p. 3) remind us that 'ambiguities and conflicting or inadequate information are the rule in medicine'. This is equally true in nursing, where dealing with complex patient problems with uncertain and unpredictable outcomes requires continuous astute reasoning and accurate and efficient decision making. Thus, the ability to think critically is essential. Lee et al (2006) emphasize the importance of both cognitive and metacognitive skills in clinical reasoning and promote the use of self-regulated learning to facilitate the development of critical thinking and reflective practice abilities.

The roots of critical thinking (CT) can be traced back to the time of Aristotle and Socrates. Since then various authors have constructed definitions of critical thinking. The American Philosophical Association (APA) consensus panel (1990) recognized that divergent conceptualizations of CT have hindered research and education efforts. The expert panel worked toward development of a clear conceptualization of CT, as well as other critical factors, such as expertise, that have an influence on CT. A key result of the project was the conceptualization of CT in two dimensions, cognitive skills and affective dispositions. Firstly, the experts were virtually unanimous on including analysis, evaluation and inference as central to CT cognitive skills. Secondly, they found that one must have the affective dispositions to think critically about issues. Affective dispositions that characterize good critical thinkers include inquisitiveness, confidence in one's ability to reason, open-mindedness regarding divergent world views, flexibility, honesty, diligence and reasonableness.

Facione & Facione (1996) contended that the description of the ideal critical thinker resembles the descriptions of a nurse with expert clinical judgement. In the clinical context, the expert nurse adept in clinical reasoning draws judiciously on developed nursing knowledge in forming, evaluating or re-evaluating a purposeful clinical judgement. An expert nurse uses an organized and exhaustive approach to reflectively analyse, interpret, evaluate, infer and explain evidence and hypotheses. The Faciones pointed out that the APA consensus definition is consistent with descriptions of the nursing knowledge base which include carefully examining and delineating key concepts, constructing meaning, categorizing phenomena, identifying assumptions, testing relationships, hypotheses and theories, while formulating alternatives for justifying procedures and stating findings. All are manifestations of the CT skills needed for clinical decision making in situations that are often vital and time-limited. In addition, the Faciones indicated that the APA consensus definition of CT integrates consideration of contexts, criteria and evidence that are relevant to a given problem as well as organization of new information and reorganization of previously learned material into forms leading to new responses that can be applied to new situations. Thus, reasoned responses and actions are formulated for anticipated and unanticipated situations. This consensus definition aligns the conceptual definition of CT to nursing, as the definition incorporates descriptions of nursing practice wherein nurses need to make effective practice decisions, utilizing good judgement, in the context of uncertainty.

Gordon et al (1994) realized the complexities of operationalizing a broad concept such as CT and proposed a nursing model in which nursing judgement is the outcome of CT. Like the APA definition, the model focuses on CT as a process of purposeful judgement with emphasis on decision making, which can be placed in the context of the nursing process as an identified problem, goal and desired outcome. This conceptualization of CT as a cognitive skill and a disposition has implications for nursing curricula and instruction.

The cognitive skills that today's nursing students need to learn in order to reason accurately and make decisions effectively in practice have caused nurse educators to adjust their teaching methods. More creative teaching methods have been adopted that are designed to improve students' reasoning skills and furnish them with a repertoire of creative approaches to care (Norman & Schmidt 1993).

Much of nursing education literature has begun to focus on ways to teach CT. Fonteyn & Flaig (1994) proposed using case studies to improve nursing students' reasoning skills by teaching them to identify potential patient problems, suggest nursing actions and describe outcome variables that would allow them to evaluate the effectiveness of their actions. Case studies provide the advantage of allowing nurse educators to give continuous feedback in the safe environment of simulation and to provide reality-based learning (Manning et al 1995, Neill et al 1997, Ryan-Wenger & Lee 1997). Lipman & Deatrick (1997) found that beginning nurse practitioner students tended to formulate diagnoses too early in the data-gathering phase, thus precluding consideration of all diagnostic options. When they used a case study approach incorporating algorithms to guide the decision-making process, students developed a broader focus and diagnostic accuracy improved. To increase realism, case studies can be designed to provide information in chronological segments that more closely reflect real-life cases, in which clinical events and outcomes evolve over time (Fonteyn 1991).

Other methods that have been suggested by nurse educators to improve students' CT skills include clinical experience, conferences, computer simulations, clinical logs, collaboration, decision analysis, discussion, email dialogue, patient simulations, portfolios, reflection, role modelling, role playing and writing position papers (Baker 1996, Fonteyn & Cahill 1998, Kuiper & Pesut 2004, O'Neill et al 2005, Todd 1998, Weis & Guyton-Simmons 1998, Wong & Chung 2002).

Videbeck (1997b) indicated that as well as being effectively taught, CT must be assessed in an appropriate manner. She pointed out that standardized paper-and-pencil tests are often selected as an evaluation measure since normative data are available and reliability has been established. However, none of the available instruments is specific to nursing, and there is no consistent relationship between scores on this type of test and clinical judgement. The use of faculty-developed instruments to assess student outcomes is strongly recommended. Course-specific measures such as clinical performance criteria or written assignments have the advantage of being specific to nursing practice. Videbeck (1997a) suggested that a model which integrates CT in all aspects of the programme (definition, course objectives and evaluation) be used. Page et al (1995) advocated the use of key feature problem (case scenario) examinations to assess clinical decision-making skills.

In the future, educators must strive to devise additional methods to develop and improve nurses' clinical reasoning. Further changes will be required in the structure and function of nursing curricula. Students need to learn to improve the ways in which they identify significant clinical data and determine the meaning of data in regard to patient problems. They also need to learn how to reason about patient problems in ways that facilitate decisions about problem resolution.

O'Sullivan et al (1997) indicated that teaching strategies which promote clinical reasoning are ones in which the educator designs classroom activities to engage the students. Paul & Heaslip (1995) advocated that students need to reason their way critically through nursing principles, concepts and theories frequently, so that accurate application and transfer of knowledge occurs in an integrated and intuitive way. Computer-assisted instruction can provide high-quality instruction that is intellectually challenging (Junge & Assal 1993). Technological advances such as the internet, with access to online video conferencing, journals, websites, interactive programs and distance learning, hold rich promise for promoting creative and effective teaching environments (Fetterman 1996).

Problem-based learning (PBL) develops students' ability to reflect continuously on their reasoning and decision making during patient care, and leads to self-improvement through practice.

Evidence exists that PBL significantly increases CT, clinical reasoning, problem solving and transfer of knowledge gained (Schmidt 1993). Once students have developed their reasoning skills in this manner, they can then apply them while caring for real patients in the clinical setting. Fonteyn & Flaig (1994) suggested teaching students to reason and plan care in the same manner as practising nurses. In practice, nurses first identify (from data initially obtained in report form and confirmed by patient assessment) the most important patient problems on which to focus during their nursing shift. Information from the patient, the family and other members of the healthcare team should be included in a plan of care that will assist in resolving the problems identified. As the shift progresses, nurses continuously evaluate and refine their plan of care based on additional data obtained from further patient assessment, additional clinical data and information from all individuals involved in carrying out the plan of care.

PRACTICE

The ultimate goal of both research and educational endeavours related to clinical reasoning in nursing is to improve nurses' reasoning in practice and, ultimately, to achieve more positive patient outcomes. Nursing literature suggests that nurses' reasoning and interventions have a significant effect on patient outcome (Fowler 1994). The relationship between nurses' reasoning and patient outcomes requires identification of the specific patient outcome indicators associated with nurses' reasoning and explication of the measurements of these indicators. If nursing is to continue to play a proactive role in healthcare provision, it is essential to identify the role of nurses' reasoning and decision making in overall patient outcome.

A major difficulty in demonstrating the influence of nurses' reasoning on patient outcomes is the complex nature of the outcomes, which span a broad range of effects or presumed effects that are influenced not only by nursing and other healthcare providers but by many other variables, including time, environmental conditions, support systems and patient history. Decision support systems and expert systems are currently being developed to assist nurses in practice to reason more efficiently and to make better clinical decisions. Expert system development began in research laboratories in the mid-1970s and was first implemented in commercial and practical endeavours in the early 1980s (Frenzel 1987). Fonteyn & Grobe (1994) suggested that an expert system could be designed to represent the knowledge and reasoning processes of experienced nurses, and could then be used to assist less experienced nurses to improve their reasoning skills and strategies. 'Illiad' is one such expert system case-based teaching programme, which has been shown by Lange et al (1997) to be effective in improving nurse practitioner students' diagnostic abilities. Expert system shells, coupled with a focus on the concise nursing problems encountered within a specific area of nursing practice and a common taxonomy, provide a means to expedite and facilitate the growth and development of expert systems for use in nursing practice (Bowles 1997).

FUTURE DIRECTIONS IN PRACTICE RELATED TO NURSES' CLINICAL REASONING

The relationship between nurses' reasoning and patient outcomes should receive greater attention in future research, to demonstrate the important role that nurses play in healthcare delivery. There will be increasing need to develop meaningful data sets related to patient outcomes. These data sets should contain the actions that nurses commonly choose after reasoning about specific patient problems and intervention outcomes. Prior to the development of these data sets, the indicators of patient outcome that are related to nurses' reasoning and decision making need to be identified and described in a manner that facilitates their measurement. Computerized support systems will play a greater role in assisting nurses to reason, make decisions about appropriate nursing actions and evaluate their impact on patient outcome.

References

American Philosophical Association (APA) 1990 Critical thinking: a statement of expert consensus for purposes of educational assessment and instruction. Recommendations prepared for the Committee on Pre-College Philosophy. ERIC Doc. No. ED, 315–423

Baker C R 1996 Reflective learning: a teaching strategy for critical thinking. Journal of Nursing Education 35(1):19–22

Barrows H S, Pickell G C 1991 Developing clinical problem-solving skills: a guide to more effective diagnosis and treatment. W W Norton, New York

Benner P, Tanner C 1987 Clinical judgement: how expert nurses use intuition. American Journal of Nursing 87(1):23–31

Benner P, Tanner C, Chesla C 1992 From beginner to expert: gaining a differentiated clinical world in critical care nursing. Advances in Nursing Science 14:13–28

Benner P, Tanner C, Chesla C 1996 Expertise in nursing practice: caring, clinical judgment, and ethics. Springer, New York

Bowles K H 1997 The barriers and benefits of nursing information systems. Computers in Nursing 15:197–198

Cioffi J, Markham R 1997 Clinical decision-making by midwives: managing case complexity. Journal of Advanced Nursing 25:265–272

De la Cruz F 1994 Clinical decision making styles of home healthcare nurses. Image: The Journal of Nursing Scholarship 26(3):222–226

Facione N, Facione P 1996 Externalizing the critical thinking in knowledge development and clinical judgment. Nursing Outlook 44:129–136

Fetterman D 1996 Videoconferencing on-line: enhancing communication over the internet. Educational Researcher 24(4):23–27

Fonteyn M 1991 A descriptive analysis of expert critical care nurses' clinical reasoning. Unpublished doctoral dissertation, University of Texas, Austin

Fonteyn M 1998 Thinking strategies for nursing practice. Lippincott, Philadelphia

Fonteyn M E, Cahill M 1998 The use of clinical logs to improve nursing students' metacognition: a pilot study. Journal of Advanced Nursing 28(1):149–154

Fonteyn M, Fisher A 1995 An innovative methodological approach for examining nurses' heuristic use in clinical practice. Journal of Scholarly Inquiry, 9(3):263–276

Fonteyn M, Flaig L 1994 The written nursing process: is it still useful to nursing education? Journal of Advanced Nursing 19:315–319

Fonteyn M, Grobe S 1993 Expert critical care nurses' clinical reasoning under uncertainty: representation, structure and process. In: Frisse M (ed) Sixteenth annual symposium on computer applications in medical care. McGraw-Hill, New York, 405–409

Fonteyn M, Grobe S 1994 Expert system development in nursing: implications for critical care nursing practice. Heart and Lung 23:80–87

Fowler L 1994 Clinical reasoning of home health nurses: a verbal protocal analysis. Unpublished doctoral dissertation, University of Southern Carolina

Frenzel L 1987 Understanding expert systems. Howard W Sama, Indianapolis

Glaser R, Chi M T H 1988 Overview. In: Chi M T H, Glaser R, Farr M J (eds) The nature of expertise. Lawrence Erlbaum, Hillsdale, NJ, xv–xxviii

Gordon M, Murphy C P, Candee D et al 1994 Clinical judgement: an integrated model. Advances in Nursing Science 16:55–70

Grier M 1976 Decision making about patient care. Nursing Research 25(2):105–110

Henderson V 1982 The nursing process – is the title right? Journal of Advanced Nursing 7:103–109

Johnson D 1959 A philosophy for nursing diagnosis. Nursing Outlook 7:198–200

Joseph G M, Patel V L 1990 Domain knowledge and hypothesis generation in diagnostic reasoning. Medical Decision Making 10(1):31–46

Junge C, Assal J 1993 Designing computer assisted instruction programs for diabetic patients: how can we make them really useful? In: Frisse M (ed) Sixteenth annual symposium on computer applications in medical care. McGraw-Hill, New York, 215–219

Kuiper R A, Pesut D J 2004 Promoting cognitive and metacognitive reflective reasoning skills in nursing practice: self-regulated learning theory. Journal of Advanced Nursing 45(4):381–391

Lange L L, Haak S W, Lincoln M J et al 1997 Use of Illiad to improve diagnostic performance of nurse practitioner students. Journal of Nursing Education 36:35–45

Lauri S, Salantera S 1995 Decision-making models of Finnish nurses and public health nurses. Journal of Advanced Nursing 21:520–527

Lee J, Chan A C M, Phillips D R 2006 Diagnostic practice in nursing: a critical review of the literature. Nursing and Health Sciences 8(1):57–65

Lewis M L 1997 Decision-making task complexity: model development and initial testing. Journal of Nursing Education 36(3):114–120

Lipman L, Deatrick J 1997 Preparing advanced practice nurses for clinical decision making in specialty practice. Nurse Educator 22(2):47–50

Manias E, Aitken R, Dunning T 2004 Decision-making models used by 'graduate nurses' managing patients' medications. Journal of Advanced Nursing 47(3):270–278

Manning J, Broughton V, McConnel E 1995 Reality based scenarios facilitate knowledge network development. Contemporary Nurse 4:16–21

Miller G 1956 The magical number seven, plus or minus two: some limits on our capacity to process information. Psychological Review 63:81–97

Narayan S, Corcoran-Perry S 1997 Line of reasoning as a representation of nurses' clinical decision making. Research in Nursing and Health Care 20(4):353–364

Narayan S M, Corcoran-Perry S, Drew D et al 2003 Decision analysis as a tool to support an analytical pattern-of-reasoning. Nursing and Health Sciences 5(3):229–243

Neill K, Lachat M, Taylor-Panek S 1997 Enhancing critical thinking with case studies and nursing process. Nurse Educator 22(2):30–32

Newell A, Simon H A 1972 Human problem solving. Prentice-Hall, Englewood Cliffs, NJ

Norman G, Schmidt H 1993 The psychological basis of problem based learning: a review of the evidence. Academic Medicine 67:557–565

O'Neill E S, Dluhy N M, Chin E 2005 Modelling novice clinical reasoning for a computerized decision support system. Journal of Advanced Nursing, 49(1):68–77

O'Sullivan P, Blevins-Stephens W L, Smith F M et al 1997 Addressing the National League for Nursing critical thinking outcome. Nurse Educator 22(1):23–29

Page G, Bordage G, Allen T 1995 Developing key-feature problems and examinations to assess clinical decision-making skills. Academic Medicine 70:194–201

Paul R, Heaslip P 1995 Critical thinking and intuitive nursing practice. Journal of Advanced Nursing Practice 22:40–47

Pyles S, Stern P 1983 Discovery of nursing gestalt in critical care nursing: the importance of the grey gorilla syndrome. Image: The Journal of Nursing Scholarship 15(2):51–57

Rew L 1990 Intuition in critical care nursing practice. Dimensions of Critical Care Nursing 9:30–37

Riley M E 2003 Removing chest drains – a critical reflection of a complex clinical decision. Nursing in Critical Care 8(5):212–221

Ritter B 1998 Why evidence-based practice? CCNP Connection 11(5):1–8

Ryan-Wenger N, Lee J 1997 The clinical reasoning case study: a powerful teaching tool. Nurse Practitioner 22(5):66–70

Schmidt H 1993 Foundations of problem based learning: some explanatory notes. Medical Education 27:422–432

Tanner C 1987 Teaching clinical judgement. In: Fitzpatrick J, Tauton R (eds) Annual review of nursing research. Springer, New York, 153–174

Todd N 1998 Using e-mail in an undergraduate nursing course to increase critical thinking skills. Computers in Nursing 16(2):115–118

Videbeck S 1997a Critical thinking: prevailing practice in baccalaureate schools of nursing. Journal of Nursing Education 36:5–10

Videbeck S 1997b Critical thinking: a model. Journal of Nursing Education 36:23–28

Weis P, Guyton-Simmons J 1998 A computer simulation for teaching critical thinking skills. Nurse Educator 23(2):30–33

Wong T K S, Chung J W Y 2002 Diagnostic reasoning processes using patient simulation in different learning environments. Journal of Clinical Nursing 11(1):65–72

Chapter 22

Clinical reasoning in physiotherapy

Mark A. Jones, Gail Jensen and Ian Edwards

CHAPTER CONTENTS

INTRODUCTION

This chapter has undergone significant revision since the last edition of this book. We have retained the overview of clinical reasoning in physiotherapy being hypothesis-oriented and collaborative, along with discussion of key factors within the therapist influencing clinical reasoning. To this we have added discussion of the biopsychosocially oriented World Health Organization (WHO) framework of health and disability (WHO 2001) that depicts the scope of knowledge, skills and clinical reasoning focus physiotherapists must have. We present a biopsychosocial, collaborative hypothesis-oriented model of clinical reasoning in practice along with the notion of dialectical reasoning strategies, and a framework of different hypothesis categories that can operate within that model. We contend that these reasoning tools can assist therapists' application of biopsychosocial theory to practise in the spirit of the WHO framework and provide quality patient-centred physiotherapy services.

SITUATING PHYSIOTHERAPISTS' CLINICAL REASONING WITHIN A BROADER FRAMEWORK OF HEALTH AND DISABILITY

Whether working with patients having musculoskeletal/sports, neurological, oncological or cardiorespiratory problems from infants through to old age, or working in health promotion/injury prevention, physiotherapists must consider all factors potentially contributing to a person's health. Although physiotherapists are often perceived as having a focus on the 'physical', contemporary biopsychosocial understanding of health and disability (Borrell-Carrió et al 2004) requires that any attention to a patient's physical health include full consideration of environmental and psychosocial factors that may influence physical health, within the scope and limits of the therapists' education. This requires a holistic philosophy of health and disability, assessment and management knowledge (including referral pathways) and skills for all potential contributing factors. In addition, clinical reasoning proficiency is required to recognize whether these potential contributing factors are relevant to the individual patient, in order to make appropriate clinical judgements that will contribute to the patient's optimal health care.

The WHO has published a 'family' of international classifications to guide health services, such as the International Classification of Functioning,

Disability and Health (ICF) (WHO 2001). The ICF provides a standardized language and framework to facilitate communication about health and health care across professional disciplines and sciences. The ICF is based on a WHO framework of health and disability (Figure 22.1) that portrays a person's functioning and disability as outcomes of interactions between health conditions and contextual factors (both environmental and personal). 'Functioning' refers to all body functions, activities (a person's executions of tasks) and participation (a person's involvement in life situations such as work, family, leisure). 'Disability' is another umbrella term, referring to impairments in body function and structure, activity limitations and participation restrictions.

Thus patients' health conditions can be seen to both influence and be influenced by their body functions and structures (or physical status), their capacity and performance of functional activities of life, and their subsequent ability to participate in their family, work and leisure roles. People's physical

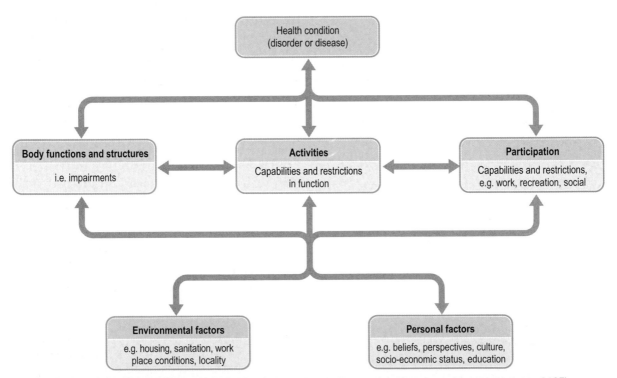

Figure 22.1   Framework of health and disability (adapted from 'Interactions between the components of ICF', World Health Organization 2001, p 18, with permission)

status, activities, participation and health condition can be positively or negatively influenced by a variety of factors, including environmental factors (e.g. social attitudes, architectural characteristics, legal and social structures, climate, terrain) and personal factors (e.g. gender, age, psychological features such as thoughts/beliefs, feelings and coping styles, health and illness behaviours, social circumstances, education, past and current experiences). This framework provides an excellent contextualization for physiotherapy practice.

THE CLINICAL REASONING PROCESS IN PHYSIOTHERAPY: HYPOTHESIS-ORIENTED AND COLLABORATIVE

Understanding the clinical reasoning underlying a physiotherapist's assessment and management of a patient requires consideration of the thinking process of the therapist, the patient and the shared decision making between the two. Figure 22.2 presents a biopsychosocial model of clinical reasoning as a collaborative process between physiotherapists and

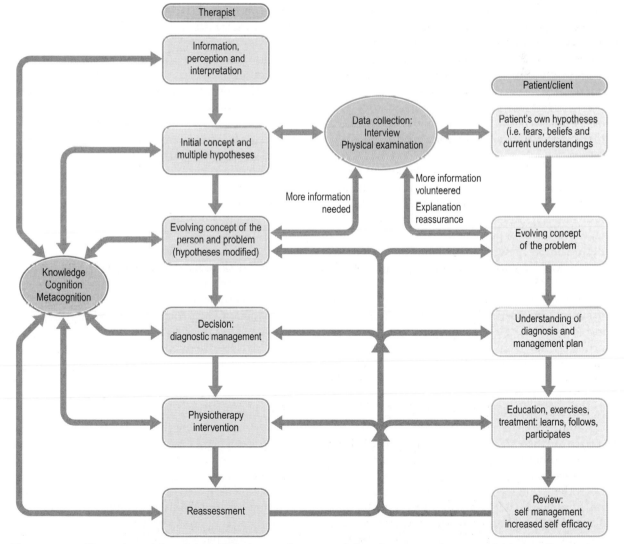

Figure 22.2 Biopsychosocial model of clinical reasoning as a collaborative process between physiotherapists and patients (adapted from Edwards & Jones 1995, with permission)

patients (Edwards & Jones 1995). In all physiotherapy settings, the physiotherapist's reasoning begins with the initial data/cues obtained (e.g. referral, observation of the patient). This preliminary information will evoke a range of impressions or working interpretations. While typically not thought of as such, they can be considered hypotheses in the sense that these initial interpretations are not fixed, final decisions. Instead, they are considered against subsequent information (data) obtained that may support or not support the initial impressions. Although this is similar to a process of hypothesis testing, depending on their education, not all therapists will be cognisant of this process, or indeed of their reasoning in general. Hypothesis generation involves a combination of specific data interpretations or inductions and the synthesis of multiple clues or deductions. In most settings the initial hypotheses are quite broad, for example in an outpatient setting: 'looks like a back or hip problem'. Initial hypotheses may be physical, psychological or socially related, with or without a 'diagnostic' implication.

All physiotherapists have an element of routine to their examination. Through professional education and clinical experience, they will have identified the categories of information which they have found to be particularly useful for problem identification and management decisions (e.g. environmental information along with subjective and physical features of the patient's physical impairments such as site, behaviour and history of symptoms, specific tests of function, structure and cognition). Beyond these routines, specific inquiries and tests are tailored to each patient's unique presentation. Initial hypotheses lead to certain inquiries and tests specific to each patient. This cognitive activity of 'hypothesis testing' ideally includes the search for both supporting and negating evidence. The resulting data are then interpreted for their fit with previously obtained data and hypotheses considered. Even routine inquiries, tests and spontaneous information offered by the patient will be interpreted in the context of initial hypotheses. In this way the physiotherapist acquires an evolving understanding of the patient and the patient's problem. Initial hypotheses will be modified and new hypotheses considered. This hypothesis generation and testing process continues until sufficient information is obtained to make a physiotherapy diagnosis regarding the physical and psychosocial presentation, appropriateness of physiotherapy and/or additional health professional referral, and the physiotherapy management that will be trialled.

The clinical reasoning process continues throughout ongoing patient management. Re-assessment either provides support for the hypotheses and chosen course of action or signals the need for hypothesis modification/generation or further data collection and problem clarification (e.g. additional physiotherapy examination or referral for other specialist consultation). Within a treatment session, therapists are constantly reading patient responses to guide their clinical decisions and reviewing treatment outcomes to test management hypotheses.

Equally important to the therapist's thinking are patients' thoughts about their problems, as reflected in the boxes on the right side of Figure 22.2. That is, patients begin their encounter with a physiotherapist with their own ideas of the nature of their problem, as shaped by personal experience and advice from medical practitioners, family and friends. Patients' understanding of their clinical problem has been shown to impact on their levels of pain tolerance, disability and eventual outcome (Flor & Turk 2006, Jones & Edwards 2006). Patients' beliefs and feelings which are counterproductive to their management and recovery can contribute to lack of involvement in the management process, poor self-efficacy and, ultimately, to a poor outcome. Conversely, patients who have been given an opportunity to share in the decision making have been shown to take greater responsibility for their own management and to have a greater likelihood of achieving better outcomes (Edwards et al 2004b). Patients' self-efficacy and the responsibility they take for their management can be maximized through a collaborative reasoning process with their therapists.

Through a process of evaluating patients' understanding of and feelings about their problems, through explanation, reassurance and shared decision making, patient and therapist jointly develop an evolving understanding of the problem and its management. Responsibility is shared between patient and therapist, with the patient taking an active role in the management.

Patient learning (i.e. altered understanding and improved health behaviour) is a primary outcome sought in the collaborative reasoning approach. When the patient is recognized as a source of knowledge for the therapist, reflective therapists will also learn from the collaborative experience. That is, when patients are given the opportunity to tell their story rather than simply answer questions, reflective therapists, who attend to individual patient presentations noting features that appear to be linked (such as increased stress affecting one patient's symptoms but not another's), will learn the variety of ways in which patients' health, cognition, behaviour, movement and pain can interact. And just as patients can be taught to problem-solve to recognize various physical and psychological stressors, therapists must continually reflect on their working hypotheses and the effects of their interventions to 'validate' their clinical patterns and procedural knowledge.

KEY FACTORS INFLUENCING CLINICAL REASONING

Clinical reasoning is influenced by factors relating to the specific task, the setting, the patient or client and the decision maker. For purposes of this discussion, we highlight certain critical aspects of those factors pertaining to the decision maker. The box to the left in Figure 22.2 highlights the strong relationship of the clinician's knowledge, cognition and metacognition within the process of clinical reasoning. Double-headed arrows are used to convey that these factors influence all aspects of the clinical reasoning process and in turn are strengthened by clinical reasoning experience, particularly when clinicians think or reflect about what they do during and after a clinical encounter.

KNOWLEDGE

Clinical reasoning requires rich organization of a wide range of knowledge including scientific and professional theory, procedural know-how and personal philosophy of practice, values and ethics.

The importance of knowledge to physiotherapists' clinical reasoning is highlighted in Jensen's expertise research, in which expert physiotherapists were seen to possess a broad, multidimensional knowledge base acquired through professional education and reflective practice where both patients and colleagues were valued as sources of learning (Jensen et al 2000). Physiotherapists utilize various forms of knowledge in their clinical reasoning including propositional ('knowing that') and non-propositional ('knowing how') knowledge (see Higgs & Titchen 2000, and Chapter 11). Identifying the use of these different types of knowledge in clinical practice reflects the tension between clinical reasoning that is focused on the clinical aspect of patient care and that kind of decision making that is identified in the current imperative for practitioners to serve as moral agents in assisting patients to negotiate the demands of increasingly complex healthcare systems (Nelson 2005).

COGNITIVE AND METACOGNITIVE SKILLS

Along with the different forms of knowledge associated with decision making, cognitive skills (e.g. data analysis and synthesis and inquiry strategies) and metacognitive skills (self-awareness and reflection) are key factors influencing physiotherapists' clinical reasoning. Physiotherapists must be able to identify and solve problems in ambiguous or uncertain situations.

Therapists' analysis of patients' presentations occurs at varying levels of complexity. Single bits of information that are perceived as potentially relevant (e.g. patients' description of symptoms, activity or participation restrictions, or understanding and expectations) must be understood in their own right, often requiring further clarification and 'validation' with the patient. Then, at a higher level of complexity, separate bits of information must be synthesized into a larger analysis of their meaning. In this way the addition of new information often alters a previous working interpretation. For example, on its own, tenderness to palpation and pain with physical testing may implicate specific somatic tissues. However, when these findings are considered alongside a long history of impairments and disability with what appear to be significant influences from psychosocial factors, the same physical signs may warrant an alternative interpretation such as central sensitization-induced mechanical hyperalgesia (Meyer et al 2006).

This synthesis of patient information is a form of pattern recognition. In both everyday life and in physiotherapy practice, knowledge is stored in our memory in chunks or patterns that facilitate more efficient communication and thinking (Anderson 1990, Rumelhart & Ortony 1977, Schön 1983). These patterns are prototypes in memory of frequently experienced situations that individuals use to recognize and interpret other situations. In physiotherapy, patterns exist not only in classic diagnostic syndromes and associated management strategies, but also in the pathobiological mechanisms associated with those syndromes and the multitude of environmental, physical, psychological, social and cultural factors that contribute to the development and maintenance of patients' problems. Physiotherapists must be able to recognize patterns of biomedical factors that contraindicate physiotherapy as clinical 'red flags' suggesting the presence of potentially serious organic pathology (Roberts 2000) and a range of psychosocial factors (conceptualized by the notion of yellow, blue and black flags (Kendall et al 1997, Main & Burton 2000, Main et al 2000)) that may predispose to chronic pain, prolonged loss of work and serve as potential obstacles to recovery.

Pattern recognition is required to generate hypotheses, and hypothesis testing provides the means by which those patterns are refined, proved reliable and new patterns are learned (Barrows & Feltovich 1987). Although expert therapists are able to function largely via pattern recognition, novices who lack sufficient knowledge and experience to recognize clinical patterns will rely on the slower hypothesis-testing approach to work through a problem. However, when confronted with a complex, unfamiliar problem, experts, like novices, will rely more on the hypothesis-oriented method of clinical reasoning (Barrows & Feltovich 1987, Patel & Groen 1991).

Physiotherapists are constantly faced with alternative choices of assessment, interpretation, and management action, the decisions about which may relate to their ability to synthesize the multitude of information obtained about a patient's presentation and the weighting they have given (consciously or unconsciously) to the various findings. Since therapists' cognition (perceptions, interpretations, synthesis and weighting of information) is directly related to their knowledge, faulty knowledge or personal biases and habits of practice can lead to errors in reasoning. Similarly, despite pattern recognition being a mode of thinking used by experts in all professions of life (Schön 1983), it also represents perhaps the greatest source of errors in our thinking (see Chapter 1).

METACOGNITION

Learning and being able to recognize common clinical patterns and their variations while minimizing the risks and limitations of pattern recognition requires metacognition. Metacognition, or reflective self-awareness, allows clinicians to monitor their data collection, clinical reasoning and clinical performance, also taking into account any knowledge limitations including their broader societal and cultural beliefs and values that, along with propositional and craft knowledge, underpin their practice.

Clinical reasoning models such as the one described here need further investigation to establish their validity in relation to actual practice, and to identify how clinical reasoning differs between expert (highly effective and efficient managers of patient problems) and non-expert clinicians. Although this biopsychosocial, collaborative, hypothesis-oriented model of clinical reasoning has not been formally evaluated, research in physiotherapy expertise does support key features of this model.

Key attributes of expert physiotherapists as identified by Jensen and colleagues (1992, 1999, 2000, 2006) and Resnik & Jensen (2003) that support explicit or implicit features of our model include the following:

- Expert physiotherapists have a patient-centred approach to care, in which patients are viewed as active participants in therapy and in which a primary goal of care is empowerment of patients achieved through collaboration between patient and therapist. This patient-centred process is grounded in a strong moral commitment to beneficence, or doing what is in the patient's best interest. Expert physiotherapists value the patient as the person in charge of his or her care and are willing to serve as a patient advocate or moral agent in helping them be successful. This is exemplified by therapists' non-judgemental attitude and strong emphasis on patient education.

- Expert physiotherapists use a collaborative problem-solving approach to help patients learn how to resolve their problems on their own, thereby fostering self-efficacy and empowering them to take responsibility.

- Expert physiotherapists' clinical reasoning is centred on the individual patient, enhanced by a broad, multidimensional knowledge base, skills in differential diagnosis, and self-reflection. Patients are seen as an important and valued source of knowledge. Recognition of their own limitations combined with reflection on practice enables therapists to refine and improve their approach to practice.

- Although not conceptualized as 'hypothesis testing', expert physiotherapists' individualized patient care, reflective practice and tendency to intertwine intervention and evaluation to fine-tune their patients' programmes are all consistent with our conception of hypothesis testing (with respect both to understanding patient presentations and individualizing patient care and to discovering, through reflection, improved ways to practise). This hypothesis testing is firmly grounded in a strong moral position that physiotherapists have the responsibility and authority for providing quality care.

FACILITATING THE APPLICATION OF BIOPSYCHOSOCIAL PRACTICE

Although many therapists will be familiar with our biopsychosocial model as illustrated in Figure 22.1, they may still struggle to apply this model in practice. Familiarity with the different clinical reasoning strategies and categories of decisions required may assist therapists in their application of the biopsychosocial model.

CLINICAL REASONING STRATEGIES IN PHYSIOTHERAPY

In a qualitative research study of clinical reasoning in physiotherapy, Edwards and colleagues (Edwards 2001, Edwards et al 2004a) identified patterns of clinical reasoning in expert physiotherapists in three different fields of physiotherapy (musculoskeletal, neurological and domiciliary care). They found that individual expert therapists in all three fields employed a similar range of clinical reasoning strategies, despite the differing emphases of their diagnostic and management strategies across the three settings. These clinical reasoning strategies were associated with a range of diverse clinical actions. They corresponded with various conceptions of clinical reasoning that have been identified by research, by theoretical proposition or by an exposition of the relevant skills in the literature of medicine, nursing, occupational therapy and physiotherapy.

These approaches are: diagnostic or procedural reasoning (Elstein et al 1978, Fleming 1991); interactive reasoning (Fleming 1991); conditional or predictive reasoning (Fleming 1991, Hagedorn 1996); narrative reasoning (Benner et al 1992, Mattingly 1991); ethical reasoning (Barnitt & Partridge 1997, Gordon et al 1994, Neuhaus 1988); teaching as reasoning (Sluijs 1991); and collaborative decision making (Beeston & Simons 1996, Jensen et al 1999, Mattingly & Hayes Fleming 1994).

DIAGNOSIS AND MANAGEMENT

Clinical reasoning strategies can be grouped broadly under 'diagnosis' and 'management'.

Diagnosis

- *Diagnostic reasoning* is the formation of a diagnosis related to physical impairments and functional limitation(s), with consideration of associated pain mechanisms, tissue pathology and the broad scope of potential contributing factors.

- *Narrative reasoning* seeks to map 'the landscape' between patients' actions and their intentions and/or motivations. This involves understanding patients' illness and/or disability experience, their 'story', context, beliefs and culture. In other words, what are patients' personal perspectives (or knowledge) regarding why they think and feel the way they do?

Management

- *Reasoning about procedure* is the decision making behind the determination and implementation of treatment procedures.
- *Interactive reasoning* is the purposeful establishment and ongoing management of therapist–patient rapport.
- *Collaborative reasoning* is the nurturing of a consensual approach towards the interpretation of examination findings, the setting of goals and priorities and the implementation and progression of treatment.
- *Reasoning about teaching* is the planning, carrying out and evaluating of individualized and context-sensitive teaching.
- *Predictive reasoning* is the envisioning of future scenarios with patients and exploring their choices and the implications of those choices.
- *Ethical reasoning* involves the apprehension and resolution of ethical dilemmas which impinge upon patients' ability to make decisions concerning their health and upon the conduct of treatment and its desired goals.

Edwards et al (2004a) found that expert physiotherapists used different processes of clinical reasoning, albeit in an often tacit manner, within each of the reasoning strategies. These processes express different forms of decision making and clinical action. Adopting the terminology of Mezirow's transformative learning theory (1991), Edwards et al (2004b) termed these different clinical reasoning and decision-making processes 'instrumental' and 'communicative' (see also Edwards et al 2004a, 2006). These terms also refer to the actions that result from two key forms of decision making: narrative and hypothetico-deductive reasoning.

These two forms of decision making and action are underpinned by different assumptions about knowledge and reality. Table 22.1 illustrates how these different assumptions are related in broad terms to quantitative and qualitative paradigms of research. The assumptions underlying quantitative research are also those underlying diagnostic (hypothetico-deductive) reasoning which are also those underlying the biomedical model of health care. Consider the diagnostic process in medicine where phenomena such as body temperature, blood pressure and blood counts are measured and the results analysed as deviations from an expected or normal value. As part of their physical examination, physiotherapists also quantify, measure and grade against normal values such aspects as muscle strength, ligament laxity or integrity and joint range of movement. Physiotherapists also compare the extent of any deviation between the affected and unaffected sides of the body.

The assumptions underlying diagnostic reasoning – namely that reality, truth and/or knowledge are best understood in an objective, measurable, generalizable and predictable framework – are very suited to the assessment and analysis of physical impairments. However,

Table 22.1 Assumptions underlying research paradigms, reasoning processes and decision making

Knowledge generation	Quantitative	Qualitative
Research paradigm	Scientific/experimental Positivist	Interpretive
Underlying assumptions about truth/reality	Objective Measurable Predictable Generalizable	Context-dependent Socially constructed Multiple realities
Reasoning processes	Hypothetico-deductive or diagnostic	Narrative
Forms of decision making and management	Instrumental	Communicative

involving the language of 'normality' and 'abnormality' as they do, these assumptions are less suited to reasoning focused on understanding the interpretation of illness or disability experience (Mattingly 1991) and the influence of those interpretations on such biological phenomena as movement (Edwards et al 2006). In the literature concerned with disability there is an emphasis on the social construction of disability (e.g. Imrie 2004, Johnson 1993, Werner 1998). That is, the 'construction' of disability has its genesis as much in the disabling effects of attitudes towards and beliefs about disabled persons, which exclude and marginalize them from participation in mainstream activities and roles in societies, as in the cumulative functional effects of their physical impairment(s). Hence, in Table 22.1, it can be seen that two of the important underlying assumptions of narrative reasoning (and the interpretive paradigm) are that reality is socially constructed and context-dependent (Higgs & Titchen 2000).

We contend that in every action of clinical practice physiotherapists can reason, make decisions and choose management strategies, using these two fundamentally different processes (with their contrasting underlying assumptions) in an intentional manner. With the increasing incidence of chronic conditions, it is becoming more imperative that physiotherapists are able to reason clinically in a manner that reflects understanding of both 'impairment' and 'disability' (WHO 2001) and the complexity of mind–body interaction (Edwards et al 2006). The two forms of reasoning and action are therefore intrinsically linked and should not be dichotomized or separated. The relationship between two fundamentally different forms of reasoning is also termed a dialectical model of reasoning and is further described in Edwards & Jones (2007).

HYPOTHESIS CATEGORIES

If clinical reasoning strategies can help in the organization of clinical reasoning for the various tasks in clinical practice, it is also important to consider how the clinical knowledge generated in and belonging to each of these settings is organized and thus made more explicit and accessible. There are implications for the teaching of students and inexperienced practitioners alike in each setting. Identification and organization of such knowledge would provide a framework through which experts in each field can share their clinical knowledge and insights, clinical patterns can be questioned and new patterns can be learned.

This question of the way in which specialty knowledge is organized has been addressed in the area of manual physiotherapy, where a set of hypothesis categories was introduced by Jones in 1987 (Jones 1987). Since that time the specific categories considered important and the terminology used to describe them have continued to evolve (Jones & Rivett 2004) to the most recent form (Box 22.1).

Some evidence is available to support these categories, demonstrating that therapists generate and test diagnostic and management hypotheses

---

Box 22.1 Hypothesis categories

Proposed categories of physiotherapists' judgments to assist their understanding and decision making regarding the patient as a person and their problem(s):

- *Activity capability/restriction* (abilities and difficulties an individual may have in executing activities) and *Participation capability/restriction* (abilities and limitations an individual may have with involvement in life situations)
- *Patients' perspectives on their experience*

- *Pathobiological mechanisms* (tissue healing mechanisms and pain mechanisms)
- *Physical impairments and associated structure/tissue sources*
- *Contributing factors* to the development and maintenance of the problem
- *Precautions and contraindications* to physical examination and treatment
- *Management and treatment*
- *Prognosis*

throughout their encounters with patients (Doody & McAteer 2002, Rivett & Higgs 1997). Also, anecdotal evidence from experienced physiotherapists and clinical educators has supported the relevance and use of these particular hypothesis categories across all areas of physiotherapy practice, with some variation in emphasis between therapists working in neurological, paediatric and domiciliary care settings compared to outpatient musculoskeletal and sports physiotherapy. We are not recommending these particular hypothesis categories for universal use, rather they are proposed as a useful means of assisting therapists to consider their clinical decisions. Whatever categories are used should be continually reviewed to ensure that they reflect contemporary practice.

Clinical reasoning and decision making across the different hypothesis categories occur simultaneously or with varying emphasis, depending on the context and nature of the clinical situation and problems encountered. That is, therapists recognize patient cues which in turn elicit hypotheses in one or more categories. Clinical patterns exist within all the hypothesis categories. As patient cues emerge and specific hypotheses are considered, the hypotheses should be tested for the remaining features of the pattern through further patient inquiry, physical tests and ultimately with the physiotherapy intervention.

We recommend that these categories be considered within broader conceptualizations of health and disability such as the WHO model (see Figure 22.1). In this way such hypothesis categories can assist therapists to relate the various components of the WHO model to the particular clinical decisions required in practice.

CONCLUSION

As experienced clinical educators of undergraduate and postgraduate physiotherapy students and practising clinicians, we have observed that understanding of clinical reasoning and conceptual models encourages therapists' conscious reflection about health, disability and the focus of reasoning and decision making that can be taken. In particular, we have found it beneficial

to use and teach clinical reasoning in the context of the WHO framework described above, our biopsychosocial, collaborative reasoning model, the notion of dialectical reasoning strategies, and the framework of different hypothesis categories. Collectively, these reflections and improved understandings should assist therapists' understanding of their patients and their patients' problems so that the most effective course of management can be pursued.

Regardless of any theoretical or working conceptual models which may be elaborated to explain or teach clinical reasoning, clinical reasoning without self-monitoring and reflection on the part of the therapist is sterile. That is, assessment and treatment 'rules' and procedures may be followed correctly but remain unfruitful. This impasse is especially likely to occur in complex or ambiguous patient presentations that comprise 'the swampy lowland ... (where) confusing problems defy technical solution' which Schön (1987, p. 3) described. These are precisely the indeterminate situations in which the experience and insights of experienced, senior and expert clinicians are often called upon.

To grow in expertise, professionals need self-monitoring skills in order to plan, control and evaluate problem-solving knowledge and methods (Hassebrock et al 1993), while reflection is critical if practitioners are to learn from experience. Whereas some clinicians learn little or nothing from their experience, instead relying on literature and continuing education to acquire new information, others continually revise and expand their clinical knowledge through their reflective approach to patient care.

In this chapter we have presented the WHO (2001) framework of health and disability as a means of highlighting the scope of knowledge, the skills and the clinical reasoning focus that physiotherapists must have in order to apply biopsychosocial theory to practice. This is particularly important in a profession such as physiotherapy, where clinicians are personally (physically, professionally, emotionally and socially) involved in the treatment of their patients. Therapists must attend to and search for cues, both diagnostic (suggesting source and cause of the patient's impairment and disability) and non-diagnostic (suggesting psychological, social and cultural aspects of the patient's problem), in order to arrive at management decisions that address holistically all relevant aspects of the individual's health and, as far as possible, the context in which that health or illness is experienced. Physiotherapists' clinical reasoning is portrayed as hypothesis-oriented and collaborative, requiring diverse and well-organized knowledge with good cognitive and metacognitive skills to facilitate the application and continual critique and revision of all forms of knowledge. Clinical reasoning strategies and hypothesis categories have been presented as valuable tools and approaches that can assist physiotherapists' application of biopsychosocial theory to practice. Although awareness and understanding of one's clinical reasoning is not essential to clinical practice, it is our view that by promoting awareness, reflection and critical appraisal, clinical reasoning can be enhanced.

References

Anderson J R 1990 Cognitive psychology and its implications, 3rd edn. Freeman, New York

Barnitt R, Partridge C 1997 Ethical reasoning in physical therapy and occupational therapy. Physiotherapy Research International 2:178–194

Barrows H S, Feltovich P J 1987 The clinical reasoning process. Medical Education 21:86–91

Beeston S, Simons H 1996 Physiotherapy practice: practitioners' perspectives. Physiotherapy Theory and Practice 12:231–242

Benner P, Tanner C, Chesla C 1992 From beginner to expert: gaining a differentiated clinical world in critical care nursing. Advances in Nursing Science 14:13–28

Borrell-Carrió F, Suchman A L, Epstein R M 2004 The biopsychosocial model 25 years later: principles, practice, and scientific inquiry. Annals of Family Medicine 2(6):576–582

Doody C, McAteer M 2002 Clinical reasoning of expert and novice physiotherapists in an outpatient orthopaedic setting. Physiotherapy 88(5):258–268

Edwards I 2001 Clinical reasoning in three different fields of physiotherapy: a qualitative study. Australian Digitized Theses Program Online. Available: www.library.unisa. edu.au/adt-root/18 Nov 2005

Edwards I C, Jones M A 1995 Collaborative reasoning. Unpublished paper submitted in partial fulfilment of the Graduate Diploma in Orthopaedics, University of South Australia, Adelaide

Edwards I, Jones M 2007 Clinical reasoning and expertise. In: Jensen G M, Gwyer J, Hack L M, Shepard K F (eds) Expertise in physical therapy practice, 2nd edn. Elsevier, Boston, p 192–213

Edwards I, Jones M, Carr J et al 2004a Clinical reasoning strategies in physical therapy. Physical Therapy 84(4):312–335

Edwards I, Jones M A, Higgs J et al 2004b What is collaborative reasoning? Advances in Physical Therapy 6:70–83

Edwards I, Jones M A, Hillier S 2006 The interpretation of experience and its relationship to body movement: a clinical reasoning perspective. Manual Therapy 11:2–10

Elstein A S, Shulman L S, Sprafka S A 1978 Medical problem solving: an analysis of clinical reasoning. Harvard University Press, Cambridge, MA

Fleming M H 1991 The therapist with the three track mind. American Journal of Occupational Therapy 45:1007–1014

Flor H, Turk D C 2006 Cognitive and learning aspects. In: McMahon S, Koltzenburg M (eds) Wall and Melzack's textbook of pain, 5th edn. Elsevier, Philadelphia, p 241–258

Gordon M, Murphy C P, Candee D et al 1994 Clinical judgement: an integrated model. Advances in Nursing Science 16:55–70

Hagedorn R 1996 Clinical decision making in familiar cases: a model of the process and implications for practice. British Journal of Occupational Therapy 59:217–222

Hassebrock F, Johnson P E, Bullemer P et al 1993 When less is more: representation and selective memory in expert problem solving. American Journal of Psychology 106:155–189

Higgs J, Titchen A 2000 Knowledge and reasoning. In: Higgs J, Jones M (eds) Clinical reasoning in the health professions, 2nd edn. Butterworth-Heinemann, Oxford, p 23–32

Imrie R 2004 Demystifying disability: a review of the International Classification of Functioning, Disability and Health. Sociology of Health and Illness 26(3): 287–305

Jensen G M, Shepard K F, Hack L M 1992 Attribute dimensions that distinguish master and novice physical therapy clinicians in orthopedic settings. Physical Therapy 72:711–722

Jensen G M, Gwyer J, Hack L M et al 1999 Expertise in physical therapy practice. Butterworth-Heinemann, Boston

Jensen G M, Gwyer J, Shepard K F et al 2000 Expert practice in physical therapy. Physical Therapy 80(1):28–43

Jensen G M, Gwyer J, Hack L M et al 2006 Expertise in physical therapy practice, 2nd edn. Saunders-Elsevier, St Louis

Johnson R 1993 'Attitudes just don't hang in the air...': disabled people's perceptions of physiotherapists. Physiotherapy 79:619–626

Jones M A 1987 The clinical reasoning process in manipulative therapy. In: Dalziel B A, Snowsill J C (eds) Proceedings of the Fifth Biennial Conference of the Manipulative Therapists Association of Australia. Manipulative Therapists Association of Australia, Melbourne, p 62–69

Jones M A, Edwards I 2006 Learning to facilitate change in cognition and behaviour. In: Gifford L (ed) Topical issues in pain 5. CNS Press, Falmouth, p 273–310

Jones M A, Rivett D A 2004 Introduction to clinical reasoning. In: Jones M A, Rivett D A (eds) Clinical reasoning for manual therapists. Butterworth Heinemann, Edinburgh, p 3–24

Kendall N A S, Linton S J, Main C J 1997 Guide to assessing psychosocial yellow flags in acute low back pain: risk factors for long term disability and work loss. Accident Rehabilitation and Compensation Insurance Corporation of New Zealand and the National Health Committee, Wellington, New Zealand

Main C J, Burton A K 2000 Economic and occupational influences on pain and disability. In: Main C J, Spanswick C C (eds) Pain management: an interdisciplinary approach. Churchill Livingstone, Edinburgh, p 63–87

Main C J, Spanswick C C, Watson P 2000 The nature of disability. In: Main C J, Spanswick C C (eds) Pain management: an interdisciplinary approach. Churchill Livingstone, Edinburgh, p 89–106

Mattingly C 1991 The narrative nature of clinical reasoning. American Journal of Occupational Therapy 45:998–1005

Mattingly C, Fleming M Hayes 1994 Clinical reasoning: forms of inquiry in a therapeutic practice. F A Davis, Philadelphia

Meyer R A, Ringkamp M, Campbell J N et al 2006 Peripheral mechanisms of cutaneous nociception. In: McMahon S, Koltzenburg M (eds) Wall and Melzack's textbook of pain, 5th edn. Elsevier, Philadelphia, p 3–34

Mezirow J 1991 Transformative dimensions of adult learning. Jossey-Bass, San Francisco

Nelson L 2005 Professional responsibility and advocacy for access: a case study in lymphedema services in Vermont. In: Purtilo R, Jensen G M, Brasic Royeen C (eds) Educating for moral action: a sourcebook in health and rehabilitation ethics. F A Davis, Philadelphia, p 107–120

Neuhaus B E 1988 Ethical considerations in clinical reasoning: the impact of technology and cost containment. American Journal of Occupational Therapy 42:288–294

Patel V L, Groen G J 1991 The general and specific nature of medical expertise: a critical look. In: Ericsson A, Smith J (eds) Toward a general theory of expertise: prospects and limits. Cambridge University Press, New York, p 93–125

Resnik L, Jensen G M 2003 Using clinical outcomes to explore the theory of expert practice in physical therapy. Physical Therapy 83(12):1090–1106

Rivett D, Higgs J 1997 Hypothesis generation in the clinical reasoning behavior of manual therapists. Journal of Physical Therapy Education 11(1):40–45

Roberts L 2000 Flagging the danger signs of low back pain. In: Gifford L (ed) Topical issues of pain 2. CNS Press, Falmouth, p 69–83

Rumelhart D, Ortony E 1977 The representation of knowledge in memory. In: Anderson R C, Spiro R J, Montague W E (eds) Schooling and the acquisition of knowledge. Lawrence Erlbaum, Hillsdale N J, p 99–135

Schön D A 1983 The reflective practitioner: how professionals think in action. Temple Smith, London

Schön D A 1987 Educating the reflective practitioner. Jossey-Bass, San Francisco

Sluijs E M 1991 Patient education in physiotherapy: towards a planned approach. Physiotherapy 77:503–508

Werner D 1998 Disabled persons as leaders in the problem solving process. In: Nothing about us without us: developing innovative technologies for, by and with disabled persons. Health Wrights, Palo Alto, CA

World Health Organization 2001 International classification of functioning, disability and health. World Health Organization, Geneva

Chapter 23

Clinical reasoning in dentistry

Shiva Khatami, Michael I. MacEntee and Stephen Loftus

Although clinical reasoning is a core competency for the healthcare professions, it is not always clear how the reasoning of one profession differs from that of another. This lack of clarity reflects our limited understanding of the clinical problems tackled by most professions and of the reasoning processes required to cope with such problems. Or perhaps, more precisely, it reflects lack of knowledge of the many factors used by clinicians as they unravel the myriad of clues and leads associated with most clinical problems.

Stemming from the historical relationship of dentistry with medicine, especially surgery, dental education and practice are based largely on a biomedical model of health care. In guiding clinicians, teachers and researchers through the process of diagnosing oral diseases, and in establishing clinical practice guidelines based on reliable evidence, dentistry has adopted in large part the analytical approaches of medicine, which are based on decision theory and information processing theory. However, the classical biomedical perceptions invoked by these theories are being challenged by more broadly based psychosocial models of health care (Evans et al 1994). Consequently, recent explorations of the psychosocial basis of diagnosis and treatment planning have been conducted through inductive or interpretive perspectives, unlike the deductive or hypothesis-based studies that dominate medical research in health care and clinical practice (Bryant et al 1995, Fleming 1991).

SYMBIOSIS OF DENTISTRY AND MEDICINE

During the 18th century in Europe, and about a century later in North America, dentistry embraced the responsibilities of a clinical profession somewhat differently than medicine, although it followed closely the educational and regulatory paths established by medicine (Adams 1999, Lafkin 1948). Dental educators in general adopted the classical medical model of professional education, with formal curricula based as much as possible on scientific enquiry and supplemented by a clinical apprenticeship under the guidance of experienced clinicians (Formicola 1991, Gies 1926). Indeed, this close affiliation with medicine was seen as the key to the survival and growth of dentistry as a 'respectable' clinical profession (Schön 1983).

The strength of the relationship between dentistry and medicine has served, and continues to serve, as the standard by which dental education, research and services are judged. However, it is not at all clear that this standard is a reasonable basis for exploring and explaining clinical reasoning in dentistry. The contact that most people have with surgeons is a 'one-off' relationship in which patient and surgeon may never see each other again. For example, patients may have their wisdom teeth removed by an oral surgeon whom they never see again. However, most dentists encourage patients to establish an ongoing relationship for routine dental care that will ideally last for many years. Healthy patients may see a general dentist more frequently and regularly than they see a physician, which is likely to influence the dynamics of the relationship and the clinical reasoning required. An ongoing relationship promotes an approach to care that is more problem-preventing than problem-solving, and is focused more on health than on disease.

INFLUENCE OF VARIOUS MODELS OF HEALTH

The emergence of science during the enlightenment period coincided with the development of hospitals and promoted a reductionist concept of disease and health (Foucault 1973). Disease was portrayed as a malfunction of biological systems, in which the mind had very little influence. Surgeons and physicians claimed the professional knowledge and authority to identify and diagnose malfunction and prescribe therapy. It followed, therefore, that health was simply the absence of disease (Davis & George 1988).

Parsons's theory of the 'sick role' challenged the medical model by introducing the social aspects of health and disease in relation to the patient's role in society. Accordingly, doctors were deemed by society as professionally responsible for recognizing disease and legitimizing patients' exemptions from their functional role in society due to sickness (Parsons 1951). Parsons' theory launched a move to explore the psychosocial aspects of medicine, from which emerged the biopsychosocial model of health care promoted by Engel (1977). Recent developments with interpretive methods have explored further the complexities of the interactions between clinicians, patients and society, and helped to redefine health and disease. Consequently, definitions of health have evolved from a simple perception of health as the absence of physical disease to the current view that health occurs when there is a general feeling of physical, psychological and social well-being. A good example of this is the research of Svenaeus (2000), who adopted an interpretive approach to studying the lived experience of health and disease based on hermeneutic phenomenology. He concluded that health is a sense of 'homelike being-in-the-world' (p. 173). He made the point, relevant to dentistry, that clinicians 'do not meet with agents [patients] who evaluate their pain and take a rational stand upon what they want to have done with their biological processes, but with worried, help-seeking persons, who need care and understanding in order to be brought back to a homelike being-in-the-world again' (p. 173–174).

How such care and understanding manifests itself depends on the interaction of all the biopsychosocial factors involved. At one extreme are casual patients, seeking immediate relief from toothache, who have little interest in ongoing dental care. These people appreciate an instrumental approach, with its emphasis on the technical expertise that will ease their suffering as quickly and painlessly as possible. At the other extreme are patients suffering from chronic orofacial pain, such as the so-called 'burning mouth syndrome'. These patients need a clinician who can listen to their stories of suffering and who can empathize with what they have been going through. Kleinman (1988) called this latter approach 'empathic witnessing'. Dentists need clinical judgement to recognize when a more instrumental approach is needed and when to be more empathic (Loftus 2006). This is not always easy for dentists because dental education has, in general, emphasized the more instrumental approach for the majority of oral problems.

Dental education has traditionally placed great emphasis on developing instrumental skills that are demanding and require a high level of manual dexterity and attention to detail. Such skills are developed only with time and under close supervision. However, this education tends to produce dentists who feel that they are truly practising dentistry only when they perform instrumental procedures such as surgery and fillings. Many dentists may feel that they are not doing real work if they are 'just' conversing with patients.

Dentists who work in an environment such as a multidisciplinary pain clinic have to make profound changes to their attitudes and approaches to care when their assessments and management must focus on a patient's history and psychosocial state rather than surgical or restorative needs (Loftus 2006). There may be none of the usual accoutrements of a dental clinic: no dental chair, light or instruments. Such management will normally entail an integrated approach, typically combining medication with psychological support.

Schön (1987) wrote that being a professional is ontological; it is a way of being in the world. For many dentists their sense of being a dentist is closely associated with the performance of instrumental tasks. This is reinforced in many countries by the remuneration systems for dentists, who are rewarded only for performing instrumental tasks. All this has the tendency to focus attention on the treatment of dental disease and away from the promotion of oral health.

The relationship between oral health and general health has been emphasized repeatedly in numerous reports (Field 1995, Gies 1926). The impact of change in theories of health surfaced in dental curricula during the latter part of the

20th century under the banner of the 'socially sensitive' movement (Formicola 1991). Consequently, dental curricula in most countries developed teaching of ethics and communication, to broaden the clinical competency of dentists beyond the more traditional instrumental psychomotor and technical skills that were the hallmark of previous curricula. Dentistry is now beginning to explore the psychosocial impact of oral health by adopting interpretive methods of research from sociology, psychology and other disciplines which have an explicit focus on human behaviour and belief. However, this shift in research methods has not yet had a major impact on studies of clinical reasoning in dentistry.

EXPLORING CLINICAL REASONING IN DENTISTRY

Psychometric measurement of how dentists diagnose clinical problems and decide on the appropriate treatment has shown how inconsistently dentists approach diagnosis and treatment (Kay et al 1992, Reit & Kvist 1998). Apparently, many diagnostic tests are both insensitive and non-specific, which might explain why dentists use specific tests inconsistently, and why there have been repeated calls for improved decision-support systems and practice guidelines. Since the 1970s there has been growing interest in how dentists could or should solve problems, and numerous conceptual explanations have been suggested, such as decision analysis, preference-based measurement, rating scales, standard gamble techniques, time trade-offs, quality-adjusted life (tooth) years, game theory, and Bayesian-based utility measures, all of which are known collectively as medical decision theory (Fyffe & Nuttall 1995, Matthews et al 1999).

Decision analysis considers diagnosis and treatment planning as a sequential process whereby dentists revise their decisions as they construct and proceed along the trunk and branches of decision trees. All decisions are weighted under the influence of Bayesian rules to: (1) identify expected outcomes; (2) estimate the probability of each outcome; (3) evaluate risks and benefits; and (4) assign a utility value for every possible outcome. Eventually, each branch offers a probability and utility value that together offer a value for the utility of each decision. This approach carries the authority of scientific and mathematical rationality for optimizing and justifying clinical decisions. It has been recommended as a means of evaluating clinical competency within a perceived range of normal or optimal decisions, as established by mathematical probability. However, a rational treatment decision based on the rules of decision analysis occasionally conflicts with a clinician's ethical principles or with a patient's preferences for treatment (Patel et al 2002). Moreover, the analyses based on Bayesian rules require comprehensive knowledge of all the available alternatives and their consequences, and these are not readily, if at all, accessible. Bradley (1993) noted that designing decision trees requires a certain degree of artistry and expertise. This is not a mechanical or automatic process. In other words, some interpretive creativity is required when constructing decision trees. It can be argued that decision theory implicitly relies upon such interpretive creativity, even though the conceptual framework and vocabulary of decision theory have no place for artistry. Consequently, there is little support for further development of decision support systems based on Bayesian rules.

Expert systems appeared in dentistry in the 1980s with a range of computer-based decision support systems for diagnosis and treatment planning in several dental specialties, such as orthodontics (Sims-Williams et al 1987), prosthodontics (Kawahata & MacEntee 2002) and oral medicine (Hubar et al 1990). Initially the systems were simplistic in scope and application, but recently there have been suggestions of applying more sophisticated systems based on the theory of fuzzy logic (Akcam & Takada 2002). There is now an awareness of the significance of language, symbols and semantics within the context of clinical situations where uncertainty is a dominant feature (Sadegh-Zadeh 2001). The relatively simple computation of numbers in Bayesian theory is being replaced by symbolic computations designed to address uncertainty, and by applications of heuristics or trial-and-error and the structure of knowledge and perception (Zadeh 2001). However, we are not aware of a practical application of these new ideas to analysing the clinical reasoning of dentists. Computerized decision-support systems are seen by some as overly reductionist, mechanistic, acontextual and value-free (Dreyfus 1992). Computerized systems cannot take account of the rich, complex and multi-layered meanings that patients can bring to any encounter with a doctor or a dentist. Humans, both clinicians and patients, live out complex narratives that can affect any clinical interaction (Charon 2006). However, it can be argued that clinical decision support systems may have a useful role in education (Gozum 1994). They can give students a degree of practice in solving simulated but realistic cases in a safe environment where patients will not be harmed.

The 1990s saw the beginning of exploration into the process by which dental clinical decisions are made, largely under the influence of the theory of information processing. The hypothetico-deductive (H-D) model (Elstein et al 1978) serves as the basis for problem-based learning in dentistry and in medicine. It identifies four stages in solving problems: cue acquisition, generation of hypothesis, cue interpretation and evaluation of hypothesis. A more elaborate model of H-D reasoning addresses the actual thinking process used when biomedical knowledge is applied to diagnose diseases (Gale & Marsden 1982). However, H-D models cannot adequately explain the diagnostic reasoning of dental students when confronted by a typically routine dental problem, such as managing a patient with caries. Apparently, students combine various strategies of H-D reasoning with aspects of pattern recognition to make diagnostic and therapeutic decisions (Maupome & Sheiham 2000).

Pattern recognition theory entails the assumption that the fast and efficient retrieval and processing of clinical information is related to the structure of knowledge in a person's memory. This is particularly evident among expert clinicians such as dermatologists and radiologists, who use visual cues from previous clinical experiences (Elstein & Schwartz 2000). Students, in contrast, store their knowledge in a more disorganized and disjointed pattern, and retrieve it in a process of trial and error to locate and connect isolated bits of information (Hendricson & Cohen 2001). From the perspective of cognitive psychology, it seems that experienced clinicians function unconsciously within the context of an 'illness script' that offers various cues or action 'triggers' based on previous experiences with similar patterns (Charlin et al 2000). From this viewpoint, caries, for example, is a visible disease that triggers the clinician to action based on a script describing the colour and size of the lesion and a hypothesis about whether or not the disease is present or absent (Bader & Shugars 1997).

EXPERTISE AND CLINICAL REASONING IN DENTISTRY

Most researchers who have compared the clinical reasoning of dentists with various degrees of expertise have focused on the outcome of the diagnostic and treatment decisions rather than on the process of reasoning used by the dentists (e.g. Balto & Al-Madi 2004, Knutsson et al 2001). Apparently, the outcomes and processes of reasoning by dentists are not very consistent. Comparing the reasoning processes of dentists with different levels of expertise showed that experts used 'forward reasoning' to identify relevant information, search for key information and organize the findings to form a diagnostic hypothesis. Students and less experienced dentists generated an initial hypothesis and then moved backward to confirm or reject it. However, at all levels of expertise, some clinicians moved back and forth between their original and revised hypotheses to come up with a final diagnosis. It seems that expert clinicians rely heavily on their clinical experience to explain the pathophysiological mechanisms underlying the disease, whereas students and inexperienced dentists rely more on textbooks and other information acquired from didactic courses. Crespo et al (2004) found the major difference between experts and novices to be the emphasis placed by experts on the impact of psychosocial issues such as the behaviours and beliefs of patients. Expert dentists seem to rely more on previous experience to construct an individualized treatment plan to address patients' special problems and needs, rather than working through a hypothetico-deductive process to an ideal treatment plan (Ettinger et al 1990).

One interpretation of these findings is that during the process of clinical reasoning, regardless of the level of expertise, clinicians use illness scripts, recognize patterns of conditions, and apply hypothetico-deductive reasoning in a forward or backward direction between hypotheses and data. Another interpretation is that clinicians use their narrative knowledge of previous situations (Charon 2006). Recent reviews of clinical reasoning in medicine endorse combining models of clinical reasoning to integrate the different strategies introduced earlier. In fact, combined use of different strategies seems 'superior' to the preferential application of one strategy over the others (Eva 2005, Norman 2005).

DEFINING PROBLEMS IN DENTISTRY: AN INTERDISCIPLINARY CALL

Medical models of clinical reasoning have focused mostly on the diagnostic process, which reflects an underlying assumption that treatment-planning automatically follows a 'correct' diagnosis (Elstein & Schwartz 2000). In acute settings with simple problems this may be true. However, dental problems range from acute to chronic conditions, such as acute toothache and chronic tooth loss, that usually have a significant impact on quality of life (MacEntee et al 1997). Management of chronic disease requires a sophisticated understanding of the experience of disease and of related psychosocial issues that complicate the problems. For example, the general health and psychosocial circumstances of elderly patients demand clinical decisions based on issues that extend beyond the confines of the biomedical model of disease (Ettinger et al 1990, MacEntee et al 1987). Dentists who provide care to frail elders have reported on ethical dilemmas such as obtaining consent for treatment when patients are cognitively impaired or when there is a conflict between a patient's autonomy and the dentists' ethical principles (Bryant et al 1995), and when care is rendered in the midst of conflicting priorities (MacEntee et al 1999). Cost of dental care is usually an important factor when selecting treatment options (Ettinger et al 1990). Financial issues can create a dilemma for dentists when there is a conflict of personal gain and social responsibility in relation to providing access to care for the disadvantaged (Dharamsi 2003).

Clinical problems can be complex and multidimensional. Clinicians interact with all such problems from within a context consisting of their own knowledge, values and experiences, the patient, and the healthcare system at large (Higgs & Jones 2000). With their recent hypothetical model of decision-making pertaining to diagnosis and management of caries and periodontal disease, White & Maupome (2003) made a good effort to integrate the various contexts within which clinical reasoning occurs, and to emphasize the dentist's previous experiences and feedback when making decisions. Included in the decision-making process are three pieces of evidence: (1) the patient's needs and preferences; (2) individual clinical expertise; and (3) external clinical evidence based on 'systematic reviews of the scientific literature'. All are incorporated to achieve the optimal oral health outcome within the biological, clinical, psychosocial and economic contexts.

To research such complex settings we need better models of rationality, other than the Cartesian reductionism typical of so much research in the literature. Montgomery (2006) has recommended the adoption of a new understanding of rationality based on Aristotle's notion of *phronesis*, or practical rationality, arguing that this provides a more realistic conceptual model for understanding clinical reasoning in medicine. It can be argued that the same applies to dentistry. Research based upon such ideas requires interpretive approaches. Recent adoption of interpretive inquiry in dental research offers a deeper understanding of dental practice and a more realistic appreciation of the complexities of clinical reasoning in dentistry. To understand the clinical reasoning of dentists we need to first explore the ways clinicians assess problems, in context, to construct a 'problem space'. Such understanding can eventually be used to guide curriculum development to simulate the contexts within which students can interact with a range of clinical problems and improve their reasoning skills by 'deliberate practice' of framing and solving problems and reflection on reasoning process (Eva 2005, Guest et al 2001, Norman 2005).

Research in clinical reasoning in dentistry has largely paralleled the equivalent research in medicine. This is understandable in view of the close historical relationship between the two professions. Medical decision theory has dominated much of the discourse, and has influenced such projects as computerized decision support systems. Other research traditions have included approaches that are strongly influenced by cognitive psychology, such as the hypothetico-deductive method and pattern recognition. Closely related to this is the research into differences characterizing experts and novices, such as those relating to forward and backward reasoning. More recently, there is a growing realization that interdisciplinary approaches that synthesize insights from the different research traditions offer exciting new ways of developing our understanding of clinical reasoning in dentistry. The more interpretive approaches of the social sciences, in particular, offer the means both to explore clinical reasoning in new ways and to integrate the findings from different research traditions into robust models that can improve the education of dentists and the care they provide to patients.

References

Adams T 1999 Dentistry and medical dominance. Social Science and Medicine 48:407–420

Akcam M O, Takada K 2002 Fuzzy modeling for selecting headgear types. European Journal of Orthodontics 24:99–106

Bader J D, Shugars D A 1997 What do we know about how dentists make caries-related treatment decisions? Community Dentistry and Oral Epidemiology 25:97–103

Balto H A, Al-Madi E M 2004 A comparison of retreatment decisions among dental practitioners and endodontists. Journal of Dental Education 68:872–879

Bradley G W 1993 Disease, diagnosis and decisions. John Wiley & Sons, Chichester

Bryant S R, MacEntee M I, Browne A 1995 Ethical issues encountered by dentists in the care of institutionalized elders. Special Care in Dentistry 15:79–82

Charlin B, Tardiff J, Boshuizen H P A 2000 Scripts and medical diagnostic knowledge: theory and applications for clinical reasoning instruction and research. Academic Medicine 75:182–190

Charon R 2006 Narrative medicine: honoring the stories of illness. Oxford Unversity Press, Oxford

Crespo K E, Torres J E, Recio M E 2004 Reasoning process characteristics in the diagnostic skills of beginner, competent, and expert dentists. Journal of Dental Education 68:1235–1244

Davis A G, George J 1988 States of health: health and illness in Australia. Harper & Row, Sydney

Dharamsi S 2003 Discursive constructions of social responsibility. Unpublished PhD thesis, University of British Columbia, Vancouver

Dreyfus H L 1992 What computers still can't do: a critique of artificial reason. rev edn. MIT Press, Cambridge, MA

Elstein A S, Schwartz A 2000 Clinical reasoning in medicine. In: Higgs J, Jones M (eds) Clinical reasoning in the health professions, 2nd edn. Butterworth-Heinemann, Oxford, p 95–106

Elstein A S, Shulman L S, Sprafka S A 1978 Medical problem solving: an analysis of clinical reasoning. Harvard University Press, Cambridge, MA

Engel G L 1977 The need for a new medical model: a challenge for biomedicine. Science 196:129–136

Ettinger R L, Beck J D, Martin W E 1990 Clinical decision-making in evaluating patients: a process study. Special Care in Dentistry 10:78–83

Eva K W 2005 What every teacher needs to know about clinical reasoning. Medical Education 39(1):98–106

Evans R G, Barer M L, Marmor T R 1994 Why are some people healthy and others not? The determinants of health of populations. Aldine de Gruyter, New York

Field M J (ed) 1995 Dental education at the crossroads: challenges and change. Institute of Medicine, National Academy Press, Washington, DC

Fleming M H 1991 The therapist with the three track mind. American Journal of Occupational Therapy 45:1007–1014

Formicola A J 1991 The dental curriculum: the interplay of pragmatic necessities, national needs, and educational philosophies in shaping its future. Journal of Dental Education 55:358–364

Foucault M (trans A M Sheridan Smith) 1973 The birth of the clinic: an archaeology of medical perception. Vintage Books, New York

Fyffe H E, Nuttall N M 1995 Decision processes in the management of dental disease. Part 1: QALYs, QATYs and dental health state utilities. Dental Update 22:67–71

Gale J, Marsden P 1982 Clinical problem solving: the beginning of the process. Medical Education 16:22–26

Gies W J 1926 Dental education in the United States and Canada: a report to the Carnegie Foundation for the advancement of teaching. Carnegie Foundation, New York

Gozum M E 1994 Emulating cognitive diagnostic skills without clinical experience: a report of medical students using quick medical reference and Iliad in the diagnosis of difficult clinical cases. In: Proceedings of the Annual Symposium on Computer Applications in Medical Care, p 991

Guest C B, Regehr G, Tiberius R G 2001 The life long challenge of expertise. Medical Education 35:78–81

Hendricson W D, Cohen P A 2001 Oral healthcare in the 21st century: implications for dental and medical education. Academic Medicine 76:1181–1206

Higgs J, Jones M 2000 Clinical reasoning in the health professions. In: Higgs J, Jones M (eds) Clinical reasoning in the health professions, 2nd edn. Butterworth-Heinemann, Oxford, p 3–14

Hubar J S, Manson-Hing L R, Heaven T 1990 COMRADD: computerized radiographic differential diagnosis. Oral Surgery Oral Medicine Oral Pathology Oral Radiology and Endodontics 69:263–265

Kawahata N, MacEntee M I 2002 A measure of agreement between clinicians and a computer-based decision support system for planning dental treatment. Journal of Dental Education 66:1031–1037

Kay E J, Nuttall N M, Knill-Jones R 1992 Restorative treatment thresholds and agreement in treatment decision-making. Community Dentistry and Oral Epidemiology 20:265–268

Kleinman A 1988 The illness narratives: suffering, healing and the human condition. Basic Books, New York

Knutsson K, Lysell L, Rohlin M 2001 Dentists' decisions on prophylactic removal of mandibular third molars: a 10-year follow-up study. Community Dentistry and Oral Epidemiology 29:308–314

Lafkin A W 1948 A history of dentistry. Lea & Febiger, Philadelphia

Loftus S 2006 Language in clinical reasoning: learning and using the language of collective clinical decision making. Unpublished PhD thesis, University of Sydney, Australia. Online. Available: http://ses.library.usyd.edu.au/handle/2123/1165 8 July 2007

MacEntee M I, Weiss R, Waxler-Morrison N E et al 1987 Factors influencing oral health in Vancouver's long-term care facilities. Community Dentistry and Oral Epidemiology 15:314–316

MacEntee M I, Hole R, Stolar E 1997 The significance of the mouth in old age. Social Science and Medicine 45:1449–1458

MacEntee M I, Thorne S, Kazanjian A 1999 Conflicting priorities: oral health in long-term care. Special Care in Dentistry 19:164–172

Matthews D C, Gafni A, Birch S 1999 Preference based measurements in dentistry: a review of the literature and recommendations for research. Community Dental Health 16:5–11

Maupomé G, Sheiham A 2000 Clinical decision-making in restorative dentistry: content-analysis of diagnostic thinking processes and concurrent concepts used in an educational environment. European Journal of Dental Education 4(4):143–152

Montgomery K 2006 How doctors think: clinical judgement and the practice of medicine. Oxford University Press, Oxford

Norman G 2005 Research in clinical reasoning: past history and current trends. Medical Education 39:418–427

Parsons T 1951 The social system. Free Press, New York

Patel V L, Kaufman D R, Arocha J F 2002 Emerging paradigms of cognition in medical decision-making. Journal of Biomedical Informatics 35:52–75

Reit C, Kvist T 1998 Endodontic retreatment behaviour: the influence of disease concepts and personal values. International Endodontic Journal 31:358–363

Sadegh-Zadeh K 2001 The fuzzy revolution: goodbye to the Aristotelian Weltanschauung. Artificial Intelligence in Medicine 21:1–25

Schön D A 1983 The reflective practitioner: how professionals think in action. Basic Books, New York

Schön D A 1987 Educating the reflective practitioner. Jossey-Bass, San Francisco

Sims-Williams J H, Brown I D, Matthewman A et al 1987 A computer-controlled expert system for orthodontic advice. British Dental Journal 163:161–166

Svenaeus F 2000 The hermeneutics of medicine and the phenomenology of health: steps towards a philosophy of medical practice. Kluwer Academic, Dordrecht

White B A, Maupome G 2003 Making clinical decisions for dental care: concepts to consider. Special Care in Dentistry 23:168–172

Zadeh L A 2001 From computing with numbers to computing with words: from manipulation of measurements to manipulation of perceptions. Annals of the New York Academy of Sciences 929:221–252

Chapter 24

Clinical reasoning in occupational therapy

Chris Chapparo and Judy Ranka

Occupational therapy (OT) in the 21st century is a complex and changing profession whose service provision has extended from medically based institutions to a variety of community, educational and social service agencies and private practice. Demands of consumer groups, expectation of documentation, the need for accountability of services and government intervention in service delivery have made an impact on every therapist. Within this context occupational therapists have a mandate to develop and implement therapy programmes aimed at promoting maximum levels of independence in life skills and optimal quality of life. The process of occupational therapy in this context consists of problem solving under conditions of uncertainty and change (Mattingly & Fleming 1994, Rogers & Masagatani 1982). Therapists collect, classify and analyse information about clients' ability and life situation and then use the data to define client problems, goals and treatment focus. The fundamental process involved is clinical reasoning.

The importance of reasoning in occupational therapy has been clearly established (Mattingly & Fleming 1994, Parham 1987, Rogers 1983, Unsworth, 2005). However, several questions remain unanswered in seeking to understand the nature of clinical reasoning. What personal and contextual elements are involved in the reasoning process? How do therapists combine science, practical knowledge and their personal commitments to make decisions about their actions? What is the range of elements involved in making judgements? Why do therapists make decisions the way they do?

In this chapter we examine clinical reasoning from three perspectives. First, a historical perspective of clinical reasoning in occupational therapy is outlined, and parallels with the development of the profession are drawn. Second, elements of therapist knowledge that have been found to influence the process of reasoning and ultimately determine occupational therapy action are examined. Third, alternative notions about the process of thinking that results in clinical decision making in occupational therapy are explored.

CLINICAL REASONING: A HISTORICAL PERSPECTIVE

Throughout the development of the occupational therapy profession, elements of what is termed clinical reasoning have been referred to as: treatment planning (Day 1973, Pelland 1987); the evaluative process (Hemphill 1982); clinical thinking (Line 1969); a subset of the occupational therapy process (Christiansen & Baum 1997); and problem solving (Hopkins & Tiffany 1988). The clinical reasoning process has been described as a largely tacit, highly imagistic and deeply phenomenological mode of thinking, 'aimed at determining "the good" for each particular client' (Mattingly & Fleming 1994, p. 13), 'thinking about thinking' (Schell 2003), and an example of behavioural intention that is based on salient beliefs, attitudes and expectancies held by the therapist (Chapparo 1999). Current descriptions and definitions of clinical reasoning have been influenced by the diverse nature and goals of occupational therapy practice, the philosophy of the profession itself, and the various epistemologies of individual researchers. A brief review of the development of the profession illustrates how its history has influenced various reasoning strategies in current practice as well as the methods that have been employed for studying them.

HUMANISM AND SOCIAL JUSTICE

Occupational therapy was founded on humanistic values (Meyer 1922, Slagle 1922, Yerxa 1991). The view of occupation that was accepted by the profession early in its development centred around the relationship between health and the ability to organize the temporal, physical and social elements of daily living (Breines 1990; Keilhofner & Burke 1977, 1983). This view of occupation and occupational therapy treatment was influenced by the theories and beliefs of the moral treatment movement of the 18th and 19th centuries (Harvey-Krefting 1985) which acknowledged people's basic right to humane treatment (Pinel 1948). A client-centred philosophy evolved which placed emphasis on the rights of all people to develop the skills and habits required for a balanced, wholesome life (Shannon 1977).

The profession subscribed to a belief in the unity of mind and body in action, and developed a philosophical approach to health through active occupation (Breines 1990). Influential in the creation of treatment principles was a thinking mode described by pragmatic theorist, John Dewey (1910), who claimed that actions of professionals depended on a unique mental analysis through which they sought to obtain an understanding of the significance and meaning in a person's everyday life. The criteria for judging this significance, meaning and worth were practical, largely arbitrary, qualitative rather than quantitative, nonspecialized and purposive (Stanage 1987). Clinical reasoning of the time took the form of commonsense inquiry and was structured around the goal of normalizing the activities and environments of people who had problems in daily living. This early pragmatic view of the subjective and individual reality of *knowing* is mirrored not only in contemporary occupational therapy practice (Yerxa 1991) but also in contemporary methods employed to study clinical reasoning which have focused on the examination of personal meaning of illness, disability and therapy action (Chapparo 1999, Crepeau 1991, Mattingly & Fleming 1994).

Remnants of past humanistic views of health are found in today's social theories of health and disability. Social disability theory lies at the heart of contemporary moves to redefine occupational therapy service delivery systems in community practice. It moves the focus of reasoning away from medical impairment by defining disability as a rights issue, locating the cause of disability and illness in exclusionary social, economic and cultural barriers to human occupation (Chapparo

& Ranka 2005, Peters 2000, Sherry 2002). The original humanistic values on which the professional thinking developed are seen in contemporary therapist thinking that is related to social and occupational justice (Wilcock 1998). *Health and ability for all* is conceptualized in this century as an issue that is not simply the concern of people with disabilities or those who are ill (Fawcett 2000). Therapists now think about social health and optimal occupational opportunities for all, thereby placing their reasoning within the realm of public health. Social justice is a vision of everyday life in which 'people can choose, organize and engage in meaningful occupations that enhance health, quality of life and equity in housing, employment and other valued aspects of life' (CAOT 1997, p. 182). Decision making focuses on issues such as maintaining well-being through occupation, enhancing people's unique capacities and potential, scaffolding occupational and social support for all people and communities, and advocating for politically supported and social valued occupational opportunities. Increasingly, therapists are required to think about structural social barriers in communities rather than behaviours in individuals. Public policy has become an everyday working arena for occupational therapists, who must use their reasoning skills to determine how occupational performance fits with social need.

SCIENCE AND EVIDENCE

During its early years, occupational therapy quickly expanded its services to a variety of medical facilities. Although everyday occupations remained the focus of therapy (Anderson & Bell 1988), there was an increased alliance to medical trends that focused on isolated cause-and-effect principles of illness. Growing pressure from medicine for a more scientific rationale for practice (Licht 1947) resulted in specialized interventions where scientific explanations and medical parallels existed (Keilhofner & Burke 1983). Occupational therapists turned to kinesiologic, neurophysiological and psychodynamic explanations of human function and dysfunction (Barris 1984, Keilhofner & Burke 1977). During this period, medical diagnosis permeated all aspects of occupational therapy

decision making. Clients' problems were viewed in terms of physical or psychiatric diagnosis rather than occupational need (Spackman 1968). Intervention focused on internal mechanisms (Jacob 1964). Clinical decision making became reductionistic, as evidenced by stated goals for intervention which were aimed at improving isolated units of function, such as particular physical or psychological attributes. The central concept of caring for self through a balanced sequence of activity found no place in the medical model and was discarded for many years. This type of reductionistic focus persists in a number of current clinical reasoning practices (Keilhofner & Nelson 1987, Neistadt & Crepeau 1998, Rogers & Masagatani 1982).

Elements of contemporary views of procedural reasoning emerged and reflected the scientific influence of the time. Reilly (1960), for example, proposed an early model of clinical reasoning for occupational therapy that was a type of procedural thinking process. She described its components using the formula: treatment plan equals the sum of the related raw data drawn from the data collecting instruments of observation, testing, interview and case history (Day 1973, Reilly 1960). During the 1970s this formula became formalized into the assessment and treatment planning part of the occupational therapy process.

From Reilly's work, and in keeping with the adoption of more scientific modes of thinking, systems approaches were applied to clinical reasoning (Line 1969, Llorens 1972). Day (1973), for example, created a model of decision making with the components of problem identification, cause identification, treatment principle or assumption selection, activity selection and goal identification. The circular model created depended on generating and testing a series of hypotheses about client problems and reactions to intervention, and contributed to our understanding of procedural reasoning today (Bridge & Twible 1997, Dutton 1996, Rogers & Holm 1991).

The last decade has seen a resurgence of scientific and reductionist thinking through the evidence-based practice movement (Taylor 2000). Contemporary authors lament the lack of appropriate evidence on which to base reasoning in occupational therapy (McCluskey 2003). Use of evidence in decision making is based in medicine. The original intention was that evidence-based medicine should base decisions on 'knowledge of individual client characteristics, and preferences in the formulation of clinical decisions' (Dubouloz et al 1999, p. 445), 'clinical experience' and 'clinical research' (Sackett et al 1996, p. 71). The reality, however, is that the current evidence-based practices demonstrate the dominance of reductionist science across health and disability services, including occupational therapy (Chapparo & Ranka 2005). Australia's National Health and Medical Research Council (1999), for example, outlined dimensions of evidence that call for and favour randomized controlled trials and statistical measurement (Dixon & Sibthorpe 2001). Assumptions that underpin this view of evidence include that health is a universal perfection and can be measured the same way for all people; that ill health and disability can be reduced to small units of measurement that accurately reflect a larger problem; and that what science chooses to and is able to measure is of primary relevance to people who experience complex problems of ill health and disability. The influence upon occupational therapy thinking is clear. Contemporary writers exhort a preferred thinking stratagem, with the systematic review of sanctioned information as its basis. This is reminiscent of the scientific dogma that 'derailed' the focus of the profession in the 1950s, 1960s and 1970s (Shannon 1977), leading therapists to think of client problems as single factors, and constraining therapy practice towards outcomes that can be precisely defined and statistically justified.

THEORY DEVELOPMENT AND CONFLICT

Occupational therapy practice since the 1970s has been characterized by theoretical conflict, as the profession universally re-examined its direction and focus. A number of theories, models and frames of reference emerged to explain the purpose of occupational therapy, with some emanating from other professions (Hagedorn 1992, Reed 1984). The result of this theoretical explosion is contemporary practice wherein various frames of reference are valued by different and substantial segments of the profession.

If theories, models and frames of reference are indeed the 'tools of thinking', as suggested by Parham (1987), the impact of this theoretical diversity on clinical reasoning is clear. By adhering to a specific frame of reference, therapists follow a particular line of thinking that translates knowledge into action. This specialized style of reasoning and action has been supported and fostered by current trends in health care and its specialties. Occupational therapists may refer to themselves variously as psychosocial therapists, physical disabilities therapists, hand therapists, or sensory integration therapists, to designate the area of specialty (Schkade & Schultz 1992). The existing pluralism appears to have defied attempts at synthesis (Katz 1985) and creates problems for those who seek an encompassing view of occupational therapy practice (Christiansen 1990, Van Deusen 1991). The present position is perhaps best described by Henderson (1988, p. 569) who urged the profession to 'be unified in ... [its] fundamental assumptions, but diverse in ... [its] technical knowledge'.

In summary, the nature of occupational therapy and the clinical reasoning processes that continue to form a basis for its identity are founded in the history and humanistic philosophy that shaped the profession's beginning. Continuation of the profession's original belief in health through occupation is reflected in preoccupation with the form, function and meaning of *doing* in contemporary clinical reasoning (Zemke & Clark 1996). The original belief in clients' rights to choice and autonomy is reflected in current phenomenological approaches to studying clinical reasoning (Chapparo 1999, Mattingly & Fleming 1994, Neistadt & Crepeau 1998).

The continuing impact of the reductionist and analytic orientation of medicine on current clinical reasoning in occupational therapy is illustrated by the prominent place of diagnosis and disease in the clinical reasoning process that is organized around notions of acceptable evidence (Bridge & Twible 1997, Rogers & Masagatani 1982, Taylor 2000). The influence of modes of scientific inquiry is reflected in a clinical reasoning style that involves systematic conceptualization and examination of clinical situations. Early scientific dogma has been tempered by the profession's emerging rejection of scientific dependency (Yerxa 1991, Zemke &

Clark 1996), resulting in modification of current concepts of clinical reasoning as being more than applied science (Mattingly & Fleming 1994).

Clinical reasoning is recognized as the core of occupational therapy practice. As a phenomenon for study, its contribution lies in describing the diversity, commonalities and complexities of therapists' thinking. Its importance in defining the professional identity of occupational therapy was summed up by Pedretti (1982, p. 12) who stated, 'perhaps our real identity and uniqueness lies not as much in what we do, but in how we think'.

THE CONTENT OF CLINICAL REASONING IN OCCUPATIONAL THERAPY

The therapy context, the client situation, theory, the identity of the therapist, attitudes about therapy and expectancies of OT outcomes impose powerful internal and external influences on the decisions therapists make about their actions. One way to describe these influences is to consider them as sources of knowledge and motivation for decision making (Chapparo 1997).

THE THERAPY CONTEXT

The organizational context contains powerful factors that establish conditions (e.g. organizational values) and constraints (e.g. human and financial resources, policies) on therapy. In many situations these elements determine therapy action (Schell & Cervero 1993). Within therapy contexts, therapists view themselves as autonomous individuals and reason according to their internalized values and theoretical perspectives, which may be consistent or at odds with the organizational influences. If practice beliefs and values of therapists fail to account for prevailing institutional contexts, therapy goals can come into direct conflict with organizational goals. The resulting dilemma for clinical reasoning is one of conflict between what therapists perceive should be done, what the client wants done, and what the system will allow.

Therapy experiences, including the organizational elements of therapy, contribute to the practical knowledge schemata that therapists develop. Therapy experiences are remembered by therapists as total contextual patterns of what is possible, involving people, actions, contexts and objects, rather than as decontextualized elements or rules (Gordon 1988, Schön 1983). Contextual patterns contribute to therapists' perceptions of the amount of control they have over their ability to carry out planned actions. These perceptions have a direct effect on their feelings of efficacy, self-confidence and autonomy (Ajzen & Madden 1986, Bandura 1997), all essential attributes for effective and creative reasoning. When therapists, because of organizational constraints, have a tenuous sense of efficacy and control, they have difficulty constructing images of how their actions can lead to a positive therapy outcome, and they will reason accordingly (Chapparo 1997, Fidler 1981).

CLIENTS AND THEIR LIFE CONTEXTS

Knowledge of clients and their life contexts is fundamental to the clinical reasoning process. A core ethical tenet of occupational therapy is that intervention should be in concert with clients' needs, goals, lifestyles and personal and cultural values (Chapparo & Ranka 1997, Christiansen & Baum 1997, Law 1998). To this end, Mattingly & Fleming (1994) described one of the primary goals of clinical reasoning as determining the meaning of disability from the client's perspective. At least five types of knowledge about the client are required to establish a picture of this meaning (Bridge & Twible 1997, Crepeau 1991, Dutton 1996, Robertson 1996). These are: (a) knowledge of the client's motivations, desires and tolerances; (b) knowledge of the environment and context within which client performance will occur; (c) knowledge of the client's abilities and deficits; (d) insight into the existing relationship with the client, its tacit rules and boundaries; and (e) a predictive knowledge of the client's potential in the long term. Knowledge from all these factors becomes a dynamic information flow during the process of assessment and intervention, demanding that therapists constantly update their understanding of how clients view themselves, how clients view therapy and the therapist, and what clients think should be done.

Elements of this knowledge are used by therapists in the reasoning process to build a conceptual model of the client (Mattingly & Fleming 1994, Rogers 1983). Commonly, therapists use themselves as referents during this model creation (Chapparo 1997), thereby ascribing meaning to the client's individual situation according to their own reality. Although this is viewed as a reasoning 'error' (Rogers 1983), it is debatable to what extent therapists are able to uncouple their own values and perspectives to reach a full understanding of the client's situation. Rather, what is probable is that therapists develop an internal model of what they believe is the client's perspective, and work from that belief system.

THEORY AND SCIENCE

Another source of motivation for clinical decision making is therapists' scientific knowledge about disease, human function and human occupation. Theory is purported to be useful because it gives direction for thinking, information about alternatives, and expectations of function and deficits (Mattingly & Fleming 1994, Parham 1987, Pelland 1987). Professional knowledge has been described as applied theory whereby a process of 'naming' and 'framing' the problem occurs (Schön, 1983). This process requires identifying and classifying abstract constructs according to some theory base (such as depression, motor control, occupational role, cognitive ability or social justice). The identified construct becomes a cognitive mechanism that can facilitate the selection of strategies for assessment and treatment (Christiansen & Baum 1997).

Theoretical knowledge alone, however, is an insufficient basis for effective clinical reasoning in occupational therapy. First, occupational therapy has a theory base that is incomplete and characterized by conflict. Second, therapists are required to make decisions in situations of uncertainty. Under these conditions, practical, intuitive knowledge is required. Such knowledge is tacit, founded in experience of clinical events (Gordon 1988, Mattingly & Fleming 1994, Rogers 1983). Practical knowledge is integrated with theoretical knowledge to form a reasoning strategy that has been termed 'deliberative rationality' (Dreyfus &

Dreyfus 1986). When listening to therapists talk through their treatments this strategy can be observed as a personal theory of why events occur in therapy (Chapparo 1999).

Therapists choose theories because of their potential to explain clients' problems. For instance, occupational therapists working with children are likely to choose developmentally based theories. However, therapists also choose one theory over another because of the congruence between the values implicit in the theory and the personal/professional values of the therapist, rather than because of any scientific merit. Many issues arising in conflicts between therapists and other professionals relate not to the logical soundness of the theoretical perspective but to the lines of thinking that arise from unspoken values embedded in the prescribed intervention approach (Parham 1987).

PERSONAL BELIEFS OF THE THERAPIST

The fourth source of motivation is personal beliefs and values of the therapist. These are the fundamental beliefs and assumptions we have about ourselves, others and occupational therapy. Related to personal values, they can be internalized at several levels, ranging from tentatively held beliefs to strong convictions. The strength with which a therapist adheres to a set of beliefs can differ from person to person as well as from situation to situation (Hundert 1987). The place of these beliefs in clinical reasoning is to define the limits of acceptable behaviour for an individual therapist in any given clinical situation. Chapparo (1997), for example, in studying therapist thinking over a 3-year period, was able to demonstrate that a set of 'personal norms' existed for each therapist studied. Moreover, there was a powerful causal relationship between these personal norms and clinical reasoning, as personal beliefs generated an expectation of personal behaviour during therapy and therefore expectations of personal satisfaction for the therapist.

Elements of each interpersonal interaction with a client are stored for use in future decision making. Knowledge that results from those personal experiences becomes personal knowledge and shapes what has been conceptualized as the architecture of self (Butt et al 1982, Fondiller et al 1990).

ATTITUDE, BEHAVIOURAL EXPECTANCY AND CLINICAL REASONING

After defining clinical reasoning as a purposive social interaction, Chapparo (1997) used elements of attitude-behaviour theory (Ajzen & Madden 1986) to demonstrate the effect of *attitude* on therapist thinking. In this model, actual therapy is found to be mediated through intention (what therapists choose to do) and expectancies (the perceived expectations of self and others). This refers to the extent to which therapists believe that their therapy will meet the expectations of other people whose opinions they value. These other people may be clients or family members, or other professionals. Attitude (what therapists expect as outcomes of therapy) develops from sets of beliefs derived from the personal, theoretical and contextual knowledge outlined above. This conceptual model of reasoning is an explanation, not of the effects of general beliefs and attitudes on clinical reasoning, but of the effects of attitude towards a specific behaviour; in this instance occupational therapy for a specific client. Attitudes of therapists about their actions are the primary driving force in decision making and are derived from salient beliefs triggered by specific and changing events in therapy. Although a new area of study in the area of clinical reasoning, these tenets find support in attitude-behaviour research (Ajzen & Madden 1986, Bandura 1997)

INTERNAL FRAME OF REFERENCE

The existence of a personal theoretical orientation (Hooper 1997), personal paradigm (Schell & Cervero 1993, Tornebohm 1991) or personal construct (Bruner 1990) is believed to underlie all decisions made in professional practice. Therapists hold certain pre-theoretical commitments about the world of therapy and disability that influence their service delivery. Clearly, clinical reasoning in occupational therapy is a phenomenon involving balancing a number of personal, client-related, theoretical and organizational sets of knowledge. How therapists orchestrate their knowledge to determine which element receives precedence in reasoning is not yet clear. One emerging hypothesis is that the knowledge used for clinical reasoning is housed within a highly individualized, complex internal framework structure, a personal internal frame of reference. Beliefs and attitudes are paramount sets of knowledge within this internal frame of reference, and represent the therapist's internal reality about any clinical event (Chapparo 1999). This knowledge is organized into facts about the therapist's everyday world of the clinic (external elements), perceptions of what is real within the everyday world of the clinic (internal elements), and judgements about the everyday world of the clinic that can be verified through action (attitude). Knowledge within this internal reality is viewed as a dynamic continuum of inquiry and is probably more correctly referred to as 'knowing' (Chapparo 1997, 1999; Mattingly & Fleming 1994). It is used during the clinical reasoning process to order, categorize and simplify complex data in order to develop a plan of action for intervention. In it resides the sum of the cultural and personal biases of the therapist which serve to colour and interpret clinical reality and, ultimately, clinical reasoning.

THE PROCESS OF CLINICAL REASONING

Considering the number of elements that impact on the decisions therapists make, it is not surprising to find researchers proposing that multiple reasoning processes are used by occupational therapists. In the third section of this chapter we explore the ways in which the various elements of knowledge involved in clinical reasoning, as described previously, are processed to form pictures of client problems, client potential, therapy action and outcome.

SCIENTIFIC REASONING

Occupational therapists are thought to use a logical process that parallels scientific inquiry when they try to understand the impact of illness and disease on the individual. Two forms of scientific reasoning identified by occupational therapy researchers are diagnostic reasoning (Rogers & Holm 1991) and procedural reasoning (Mattingly & Fleming 1994). These processes involve a progression from problem sensing to problem definition and problem resolution. Using information processing approaches put forward in medical models of clinical reasoning (Elstein & Bordage 1979), Rogers & Holm (1991) outlined a model of occupational therapy reasoning comprising cognitive operations identified as cue acquisition, hypothesis generation, cue interpretation and hypothesis evaluation.

As with earlier work (Rogers & Masagatani 1982), Rogers & Holm's (1991) notion of diagnostic reasoning begins even before the therapist approaches a client. A 'problem sensing' stage results in decisions being made concerning the information required to form an occupational diagnosis. It represents the therapist's interim, working and flexible identification of the general problem. It is probable that therapists have individual ideas about how well defined the problem should be before 'hypothesis generation' can begin.

Using procedural reasoning modes, therapists engage in a dual search for problem definition and treatment selection. Experienced therapists generate two to four hypotheses regarding the cause and nature of functional problems and several more concerning possible directions for treatment (Mattingly & Fleming 1994, Robertson 1999). Hypotheses generated are then subjected to a process of critical reflection. Newer therapists generate fewer hypotheses, the tendency being to jump to conclusions about the nature and direction of therapy without weighing the grounds upon which the conclusion rests (Unsworth 2005). The danger for experienced therapists is placing exclusive dependence on past experiences which have not been subjected to critical analysis through reflection. Without critical reflection, therapists forgo and cut short the act of inquiry that results in effective scientific reasoning (McCluskey 2003).

NARRATIVE REASONING

Implementing a therapy programme that will potentially change life roles and functions for the client, occupational therapists are faced with profound problems of understanding. Specifically, they involve understanding the meaning of illness, disability and therapy outcome from the client's perspective. Understanding the meaning of a situation involves making an interpretation of it. This interpretation leads to subsequent understanding, appreciation and therapy action. What therapists perceive and fail to perceive and what they think and fail to think in the interpretive process is powerfully influenced by sets of beliefs, attitudes and assumptions that structure the way they interpret clinical experiences (Crepeau 1991, Mezirow 1991).

Two dimensions of meaning making are involved in narrative reasoning. Meaning schemes are sets of related and habitual expectations governing if–then relationships. Mattingly (in Mattingly & Fleming 1994) cited Bruner (1990) in linking these meaning schemes to a paradigmatic mode of thinking. For example, an occupational therapist with experience in stroke rehabilitation expects to see signs of left hemiplegia when referred a client with diagnosis of right cerebrovascular accident. Meaning schemes are habitual, implicit rules for interpreting and are strongly linked to knowledge.

Meaning perspectives are made up of higher-order schemata, theories and beliefs. They refer to the structure of assumptions and beliefs within which new experiences are interpreted. For example, occupational therapists make interpretations about clients based on values espoused by the notion of a 'helping profession', and their judgements are focused on client performance and satisfaction with occupational roles and tasks. Both meaning schemes and meaning perspectives selectively order and delimit clinical reasoning. They define therapists' expectations and therefore their intentions, and affect the activity of perceiving, comprehending and remembering meaning within the context of communicating with clients (Chapparo 1997, Crepeau 1991).

Mattingly (in Mattingly & Fleming 1994) described how narrative thinking is central in providing therapists with a way to consider disability in phenomenological terms. She described two types of narrative thinking. One is a 'mode of talk' that therapists use to shift disability from a physiological event to a personally meaningful one. The second involves the creation of images of the future for the client. The result of this type of thinking is purposeful occupational therapy that creates therapeutic activities which are meaningful to the client's life.

ETHICAL REASONING

Evidence suggests that personal values impact substantially on clinical reasoning processes in occupational therapy (Chapparo 1997, Fondiller et al 1990, Haddad 1988, Mattingly & Fleming 1994, Neuhaus 1988, Rogers & Holm 1991). A clinical problem becomes an ethical *dilemma* when it seems that an occupational therapy treatment decision will violate the therapist's values (Tamm 1996). In the process of choosing a therapeutic action using the reasoning processes outlined above, occupational therapists are often forced to balance one value against another. While this process is typically unconscious, it appears to drive decision making at various points throughout the treatment programme (Jordens & Little 2004).

CONDITIONAL REASONING

Fleming (in Mattingly & Fleming 1994) described a third reasoning style, conditional reasoning, which involves projecting an imagined future for the client. Fleming used the term 'conditional' in three different ways. First, problems are interpreted and solutions are realized in relation to people within their particular context. Second, therapists imagine how the present condition could be changed. Third, success or failure is determined by the level of client participation. It is a circular process resulting in a flexible therapy programme, and is used by occupational therapists to assist clients to re-invent themselves through occupations. Chapparo (1999) extended the concept of conditional reasoning and described a thinking process whereby therapists reconcile the actual (therapy) and the possible (intention) in terms of therapy outcome. This involves *reflection*, whereby the therapist's action turns in on itself, *conflict*, whereby therapists seek to reconcile choices made, and *judgement*, whereby therapists weight the soundness of decisions.

PRAGMATIC REASONING

Pragmatic reasoning goes beyond the therapist–client relationship and addresses the contexts in which therapy occurs (Schell & Cervero 1993). Clinical reasoning focuses on practical action and therapists are compelled to think about what is achievable within their own or the client's world. As outlined above, these contexts include organizational constraints, values and resources, practice trends and reimbursement issues. Recent studies confirm that therapists' thinking is increasingly influenced by situations that occur in their practice world (Chapparo 1997, Strong et al 1995). Shepherd (2005), for example, demonstrated how therapists who worked in a brain injury rehabilitation setting thought about clients differently from those who worked with the same clients in a transitional residential situation. Using the terms 'house person' and 'hospital person' thinking, Shepherd showed that the context of thinking, rather than diagnosis, determined the type of decision that was made about the focus of intervention, and judgements about its worth.

Fleming (in Mattingly & Fleming 1994, p. 119) created an image of an occupational therapist with a 'three track mind'. The procedural track is used when therapists reason about the client's diagnosis. The interactive narrative track occurs when therapists focus on the client as a person. The conditional track creates an image of the client that is provisional, holistic and conditional on the client's participation. Alternatively, Chapparo (1999) used causal modelling to demonstrate that although therapists use multiple strategies (e.g. story-telling, testing, questioning, imagining, feeling and moving) to acquire the multidimensional knowledge needed for reasoning, one mode of thinking is used to draw together very disparate areas of consideration (e.g. personal–emotional, contextual rules of operation, client needs, and science) into a coherent, integrated judgement about the course of action in therapy. In this model, attitude-behaviour theory was used to demonstrate how reasoning was described as a thinking process that focused on reconciliation of the actual (*therapy*) and the possible (*intention*). Two aspects of this thinking process were apparent when studying reasoning of therapists during intervention for adults and children with chronic neurological impairments: 'thinking about' and 'thinking that'. Thinking about was descriptive, and held qualities of Mattingly's narrative reasoning. It was conscious thought that was continuous, streamed, and focused on contextualizing thinking for action. When therapists thought about, they related present to past, the particular client to all clients. Thinking about contained a time-gap quality whereby here-and-now thinking was connected to past realities of clients and therapy, and could be considered a precondition to therapists formulating propositions about action in a more focused way. Thinking that was propositional thought, and appeared to emerge from thinking about. It contained propositional episodes and scientific reasoning as outlined previously. As described by Chapparo, therapists' thinking flowed between thinking about (pre-conditional thought) and thinking that (propositional thought) as they funnelled their thoughts towards a conclusion culminating in action. The relationship between the two was conceptualized by Chapparo as a dynamic system which is sometimes, but not usually, linear, proposing instead that therapists may seem more rational in their decision making when interviewed after the fact because of the coherence that comes with reflection and the rules of narration.

It is unclear whether therapists use distinctly different types of reasoning that translate into mutually exclusive forms of thinking, or whether the different styles of reasoning that have been identified in each piece of research are images of thinking that have been constructed through the process of attempting to put words to a largely internal, tacit phenomenon. Descriptions of the different clinical reasoning processes that exist may actually be a reflection of the influence of the knowledge base of various researchers, such as anthropology (Mattingly & Fleming 1994), medicine (Dutton 1996, Rogers & Holm 1991), cognitive psychology (Bridge & Twible 1997), and social psychology (Chapparo 1999).

CONCLUSION

Clinical reasoning in occupational therapy, as in other health science professions, is a complex phe-

nomenon. It has been described as the use of multiple reasoning strategies throughout the various phases of client management. Procedural reasoning is used when therapists think about client problems in terms of the disease and within the context of occupational performance. Narrative reasoning (Mattingly & Fleming 1994), using interactive processes, involves developing an understanding of the meaning of existing problems from the client's perspective. Conditional reasoning (Mattingly & Fleming 1994) is a less definitive process by which occupational therapists imagine the client in the future and in so doing imagine the therapy outcome and the therapeutic action required to achieve that outcome. Additionally, there is evidence of processes of ethical and pragmatic reasoning that further frame decision making personally and contextually.

Many factors act as motivating forces for clinical decisions. Among them are organizational structures and expectations, client needs and expectations and theoretical and scientific knowledge about disease and human occupations. Within the therapist's internal frame of reference, perceptions of these external factors are integrated with personal beliefs about such things as perceived level of skill, personal knowledge, personal beliefs and perceived level of control. From this internal frame of reference, images of clients and their problems are created as well as plans for therapeutic action, all of which serve to direct clinical reasoning processes.

It is clear that current explanations and descriptions of clinical reasoning in occupational therapy are incomplete. Contemporary notions of clinical reasoning describe a highly individualistic mode of operation that is based in scientific knowledge and method, creative imagination, intuition, interpersonal skill and artistry, operating within the frame of reference of the occupational therapy profession.

References

Ajzen I, Madden T J 1986 Prediction of goal directed behaviour: attitudes, intentions and perceived behavioural control. Journal of Experimental Social Psychology 22:453–474

Anderson B, Bell J 1988 Occupational therapy: its place in Australia's history. NSW Association of Occupational Therapists, Melbourne, VIC

Bandura A 1997 Self efficacy: the exercise of control. W H Freeman, New York

Barris R 1984 Toward an image of one's own: sources of variation in the role of occupational therapists in psychosocial practice. Occupational Therapy Journal of Research 4:3–23

Breines E 1990 Genesis of occupation: a philosophical model for therapy and theory. Australian Occupational Therapy Journal 37:45–49

Bridge C E, Twible R L 1997 Clinical reasoning: informed decision making for practice. In: Christiansen C, Baum C (eds) Occupational therapy: enabling function and well being, 2nd edn. Slack, Thorofare, NJ, p 158–179

Bruner J 1990 Acts of meaning. Harvard University Press, Cambridge, MA

Butt R, Raymond D, Yamaguishi L 1982 Autobiographic praxis: studying the formation of teacher's knowledge. Journal of Curriculum Theorizing 7:87–164

CAOT 1997 Enabling occupation: an occupational therapy perspective. Canadian Association of Occupational Therapists, Ottawa

Chapparo C 1997 Influences on clinical reasoning in occupational therapy. Unpublished doctoral thesis, Macquarie University, Sydney

Chapparo C 1999 Working out: working with Angelica – interpreting practice. In: Ryan S E, McKay E A (eds) Thinking and reasoning in therapy: narratives from practice. Stanley Thornes, Cheltenham, p 31–50

Chapparo C, Ranka J (eds) 1997 Occupational performance model (Australia). Monograph 1. School of Occupational Therapy, University of Sydney

Chapparo C, Ranka J 2005 Theoretical contexts. In: Whiteford G, Wright-St. Clair V (eds) Occupation and practice in context. Elsevier, Sydney, p 51–71

Christiansen C 1990 The perils of plurality. Occupational Therapy Journal of Research 11:259–265

Christiansen C, Baum C (eds) 1997 Occupational therapy: enabling function and well-being. Slack, Thorofare, NJ

Crepeau E B 1991 Achieving intersubjective understanding: examples from an occupational therapy treatment session. American Journal of Occupational Therapy 45:1016–1025

Day D J 1973 A systems diagram for teaching treatment planning. American Journal of Occupational Therapy 27:239–243

Dewey J 1910 How we think. University of Chicago, Chicago

Dixon J, Sibthorpe B 2001 How can a government research and development initiative contribute to reducing health inequalities? NSW Public Health Bulletin July 12(7):189–191

Dreyfus H L, Dreyfus S E 1986 Mind over machine: the power of human intuition and expertise in the era of the computer. Free Press, New York

Dubouloz C J, Egan M, Vallerand J et al 1999 Occupational therapists' perceptions of evidence-based practice. American Journal of Occupational Therapy 65(3):136–143

Dutton R 1996 Clinical reasoning in physical disabilities. Williams and Wilkins, Baltimore

Elstein A S, Bordage G 1979 Psychology of clinical reasoning. In: Stone G, Cohen F, Adler N (eds) Health psychology: a handbook. Jossey Press, San Francisco, p 335–367

Fawcett B 2000 Feminist perspectives on disability. Pearson Education, New York

Fidler G 1981 From crafts to competence. American Journal of Occupational Therapy 35:567–573

Fondiller E D, Rosage L J, Neuhaus B E 1990 Values influencing clinical reasoning in occupational therapy: an exploratory study. Occupational Therapy Journal of Research 10:41–54

Gordon D 1988 Clinical science and clinical expertise: changing boundaries between art and science in medicine. In: Lock D, Gordon M (eds) Biomedicine examined. Kluwer Academic, Dordrecht, p 257–295

Haddad A M 1988 Teaching ethical analysis in occupational therapy. American Journal of Occupational Therapy 42:300–304

Hagedorn R 1992 Occupational therapy: foundations for practice. models, frames of reference and core skills. Churchill Livingstone, London

Harvey-Krefting L 1985 The concept of work in occupational therapy: a historical review. American Journal of Occupational Therapy 39:301–307

Hemphill B J 1982 The evaluative process. In: Hemphill B J (ed) The evaluative process in psychiatric occupational therapy. Charles Slack, Thorofare, NJ, p 17–26

Henderson A 1988 Eleanor Clarke Slagle lecture. Occupational therapy knowledge: from practice to theory. American Journal of Occupational Therapy 42:567–576

Hooper B 1997 The relationship between pretheoretical assumptions and clinical reasoning. American Journal of Occupational Therapy 51(5):328–338

Hopkins H L, Tiffany E G 1988 Occupational therapy – a problem-solving process. In: Hopkins H L, Smith H D (eds) Willard and Spackman's occupational therapy, 7th edn. Lippincott, Philadelphia, p 102–111

Hundert E M 1987 A model for ethical problem solving in medicine, with practical applications. American Journal of Psychiatry 144:839–846

Jacob F 1964 Occupational therapy in a psychiatric unit in a general hospital. Australian Journal of Occupational Therapy 11:10–16

Jordens C F C, Little M 2004 'In this scenario I do this, for these reasons': Narrative, genre and ethical reasoning in the clinic. Social Science and Medicine 58:1635–1645. Retrieved April 20, 2005 from Science Direct Elsevier Science Journals on-line database

Katz N 1985 Occupational therapy's domain of concern: reconsidered. American Journal of Occupational Therapy 39:518–524

Keilhofner G, Burke J 1977 Occupational therapy after 60 years: an account of changing identity and knowledge. American Journal of Occupational Therapy 31:675–689

Keilhofner G, Burke J 1983 The evolution of knowledge in occupational therapy: past, present and future. In: Keilhofner G (ed) Health through occupation. F A Davis, Philadelphia, p 149–162

Keilhofner G, Nelson C 1987 The nature and implications of shifting patterns of practice in physical disabilities occupational therapy. Occupational Therapy in Health Care 3(3/4):187–198

Law M (ed) 1998 Client-centered occupational therapy. Charles Slack, Thorofare, NJ

Licht S 1947 The objectives of occupational therapy. Occupational Therapy Rehabilitation 28:17–22

Line J 1969 Case method as a scientific form of clinical thinking. American Journal of Occupational Therapy 23:308–313

Llorens L 1972 Problem-solving the role of occupational therapy in a new environment. American Journal of Occupational Therapy 26:234–238

McCluskey A 2003 Occupational therapists report on low knowledge, skills and involvement in evidence-based practice. Australian Occupational Therapy Journal 50: 3–12

Mattingly C, Fleming M H 1994 Clinical reasoning: forms of inquiry in a therapeutic practice. F A Davis, Philadelphia

Meyer A 1922 The philosophy of occupational therapy. Archives of Occupational Therapy 1:1–10

Mezirow J 1991 How critical reflection triggers transformative learning. In: Mezirow J (ed) Fostering critical reflection in adulthood. Jossey-Bass, San Francisco, p 1–20

National Health and Medical Research Council 1999 How to review the evidence: systematic identification and review of the scientific literature. NHMRC Publications, Canberra, Australia

Neistadt M, Crepeau E B (eds) 1998 Willard and Spackman's occupational therapy, 9th edn. Lippincott, Philadelphia

Neuhaus B E 1988 Ethical considerations in clinical reasoning: the impact of technology and cost containment. The American Journal of Occupational Therapy 42:288–294

Parham D 1987 Toward professionalism: the reflective therapist. American Journal of Occupational Therapy 41:555–561

Pedretti L W 1982 The compatibility of current treatment methods in physical disabilities with the philosophical case of occupational therapy. Unpublished doctoral thesis, San Jose University

Pelland M J 1987 A conceptual model for the instruction and supervision of treatment planning. American Journal of Occupational Therapy 41:351–359

Peters S 2000 Is there a disability culture? A syncretisation of three possible work views. Disability and Society 15(4):583–601

Pinel P 1948 Medical philosophical treatise on mental alienation. In: Licht S (ed) Occupational therapy source book. Williams and Wilkins, Baltimore, p 19

Reed K L 1984 Models of practice in occupational therapy. Williams and Wilkins, Baltimore

Reilly M 1960 Research potentiality of occupational therapy. American Journal of Occupational Therapy 14:206–209

Robertson L J 1996 Clinical reasoning, part 1: the nature of problem solving, a literature review. British Journal of Occupational Therapy 59:178–182

Robertson L J 1999 Assessing Mabel at home: a complex problem-solving process. In: Ryan S E, McKay E A (eds) Thinking and reasoning in therapy: narratives from practice. Stanley Thornes, London, p 19–30

Rogers J C 1983 Clinical reasoning: the ethics, science, and art. Eleanor Clarke Slagle lecture. American Journal of Occupational Therapy 37:601–616

Rogers J C, Holm M 1991 Occupational therapy diagnostic reasoning: a component of clinical reasoning. American Journal of Occupational Therapy 45:1045–1053

Rogers J C, Masagatani G 1982 Clinical reasoning of occupational therapists during the initial assessment of physically disabled patients. Occupational Therapy Journal of Research 2:195–219

Sackett D L, Rosenberg W M, Gray J A et al 1996 Evidence based medicine: what it is and what it isn't (editorial). British Medical Journal 312(13 Jan):71–72

Schell B A B 2003 Clinical reasoning: the basis of practice. In: Crepeau E B, Cohn E S, Schell B A B (eds) Willard and Spackman's occupational therapy, 10th edn. Lippincott, Williams and Wilkins, Philadelphia, p 131–139

Schell B, Cervero R 1993 Clinical reasoning in occupational therapy: an integrative review. American Journal of Occupational Therapy 47(7):605–610

Schkade J K, Schultz S 1992 Occupational adaptations: toward a holistic approach for contemporary practice, part 1. American Journal of Occupational Therapy 46:829–837

Schön D A 1983 The reflective practitioner: how professionals think in action. Basic Books, New York

Shannon P 1977 The derailment of occupational therapy. American Journal of Occupational Therapy 31:229–234

Shepherd B 2005 Influences on residential care staff decision making. Unpublished PhD thesis, School of Occupation and Leisure Sciences, University of Sydney

Sherry M 2002 Welfare reform and disability policy in Australia. Just Policy 28:3–11

Slagle A C 1922 Training aids for mental patients. Occupational Therapy and Rehabilitation 1:11–14

Spackman C 1968 A history of the practice of occupational therapy for restoration of physical function: 1917–1967. American Journal of Occupational Therapy 22:67–76

Stanage S M 1987 Adult education and phenomenological research: new directions for theory, practice and research. Kreiger, Florida

Strong J, Gilbert J, Cassidy S, Bennett S 1995 Expert clinicians' and students' views on clinical reasoning in occupational therapy. British Journal of Occupational Therapy 58:119–123

Tamm M 1996 Ethical dilemmas encountered by community-based occupational therapists in the home care setting. Scandinavian Journal of Occupational Therapy 3:180–187

Taylor M C 2000 Evidence-based practice for occupational therapists. Blackwell Science, Oxford

Tornebohm H 1991 What is worth knowing in occupational therapy? American Journal of Occupational Therapy 45:451–454

Unsworth C A 2005 Using a head-mounted video camera to explore current conceptualizations of clinical reasoning in occupational therapy. American Journal of Occupational Therapy 59(1):31–40

Van Deusen J 1991 The issue is: can we delimit the discipline of occupational therapy? American Journal of Occupational Therapy 44:175–176

Wilcock A 1998 An occupational perspective of health. Slack, Thorofare, NJ

Yerxa E J 1991 Seeking a relevant, ethical and realistic way of knowing for occupational therapy. American Journal of Occupational Therapy 45:199–204

Zemke R, Clarke F (eds) 1996 Occupational science: the evolving discipline. F A Davis, Philadelphia

Chapter 25

Ethical reasoning

Ian Edwards and Clare Delany

CHAPTER CONTENTS

INTRODUCTION: WHAT IS ETHICAL REASONING AND WHY IS IT IMPORTANT?

Ethics has been defined as a systematic study of and reflection on morality. *Systematic*, because it is a discipline that uses special methods and approaches to examine moral situations, and a process of *reflection* because it consciously calls into question assumptions about existing components of our moralities, including our reasoning, that fall into the category of habits, customs or traditions (Purtilo 2005, p. 15). Ethics in professional practice has elements that go beyond just the reasoning and decision-making process and these are well summed up in a four component 'scaffold': moral sensitivity (the perception and recognition of ethical issues); moral judgement (making decisions about right and wrong); moral motivation (prioritizing ethical values in relation to other values); and moral courage (the taking of moral actions even in adversity) (Swisher 2005, p. 230). In this chapter we focus on the moral judgement component while recognizing that the ethical reasoning process cannot be separated from these other dimensions.

The component of ethical reasoning or making moral judgements can also be divided into four parts. They comprise first, a knowledge of ethical theory; second, a knowledge of the perspectives and values of those involved in the scenario; third, a knowledge of self as health practitioner;

and fourth, an ability to understand and articulate these different types of knowledge and associated values in the reasoning process.

In this chapter we present two research-derived perspectives from physiotherapy on ethical reasoning which we contend have relevance for debates on the practice of ethics within health professions other than physiotherapy. The first perspective (Delany 2005) is from a philosophical and normative ethical position, and proposes a re-consideration of the theory/ies underlying principles. Normative ethics expressed in the form of biomedical ethical principles continues to be the dominant form of bioethics and is characterized by a deductive logic or reasoning process (Fox 1994, Swisher 2002). The second perspective (Edwards et al 2005), is from a social science and descriptive ethical position, and describes the inductive reasoning processes of understanding patient/carer narratives as a counterpoint (but not as a substitute) for more traditional deductive processes of principles-oriented ethical reasoning. The ethical reasoning framework we propose seeks to recover, on the one hand, the rich ethical content underlying 'principles' within the principlist approach, and, on the other, the ethical values found in a richer understanding of patient perspective(s) in clinical practice (Edwards et al 2005). The two approaches together offer complementary sets of insights important for the development of skills in ethical reasoning, including accounting for moral judgements (Swisher 2005, Zussman 2000). We structure this chapter by first establishing links between the processes and underlying assumptions of clinical reasoning *and* the components and process of ethical reasoning. We contend that recognizing similarities between clinical and ethical reasoning processes enhances a deeper understanding, provides a more rigorous framework and facilitates an integrated implementation of ethical knowledge in everyday practice. We then examine two of the key components of ethical reasoning and their relationship in depth: the understanding and application of ethical theory/ knowledge and the understanding and application of knowledge of context, patient values and experience.

ETHICAL REASONING IN A CLINICAL REASONING FRAMEWORK

There has been a long expressed need for a better understanding of the relationship between ethical reasoning and clinical reasoning (Clawson 1994, Swisher 2002). One reason for this is so that clinicians can integrate and align their ethical reasoning with both a familiar and a rigorous method of clinical reasoning and problem solving in clinical practice. Another reason lies in the importance of understanding the assumptions or rationale underlying all types of decision making in clinical practice. Traditional understandings of clinical reasoning have emphasized the deductive process (commonly termed diagnostic and procedural reasoning) and described it as largely cognitive, occurring 'inside the head' of the health practitioner or clinician, generating and testing hypotheses in a unilateral manner. This understanding has now broadened and clinical reasoning is widely accepted as a collaborative and interactive process where two sets of understanding (the patient's and the practitioner's) are brought into a sense of coherence in the decision-making process in clinical practice. This inductive process of understanding particular patient beliefs and their interpretation of illness or disability experience in the clinical reasoning process has, therefore, assumed a more explicit and valued role in clinical reasoning.

There is a parallel situation in bioethics (Edwards et al 2005). The dominant form of bioethics, termed the *principlist approach* (Fox 1994, Swisher 2002), is a deductive approach which relies upon a theoretical framework of accepted biomedical ethical principles (Beauchamp & Childress 2001) to guide the development of ethical codes and ethical decision making. Codes of ethics in the caring professions in Australia (such as nursing, pharmacy, occupational therapy, physiotherapy, social work and medicine) are based on variations of the principlist approach (Hugman 2005). Although there continues to be a high degree of consensus regarding these principles as a foundation for ethics in the health professions (Hugman 2005), bioethics has shifted since the mid-1990s, in a similar way to contemporary understandings of clinical reasoning, towards hearing and interpreting a much richer and contextual variety of moral voices and approaches (Charlesworth 2005).

The importance of understanding ethical theory and ethical approaches and the different perspectives they offer for ethical decision making has been previously recognized in established models of ethical reasoning (Kerridge et al 2005, Purtilo 2005, Sim 2004, Swisher 2005). However, in the ethical reasoning literature, the way in which the different perspectives and ethical approaches might be incorporated into an ethical reasoning process has received less attention. For example, some authors have discussed making ethical decisions by following a particular step-by-step process in one or other direction (Sim 2004, Swisher 2005). A four-tiered process describes how therapists can defend or reason through an ethical decision in practice. Starting from the bottom tier, the practitioner's ability to trace the steps from a case-based decision through to ethical theory provides an 'objectivity' or rationale to ethical decision making (Sim 2004, p. 230). These steps begin with a specific contextually based ethical decision which can be defended by reference to different ascending, as it were, tiers of knowledge; professional rules or codes of practice, then ethical principles, and finally ethical theory/philosophy. This four-tiered model is portrayed by Sim (2004) as a bottom up, inductive process. Other authors have found that therapists make decisions from the top down. For example, in a study of how physiotherapists implemented the ethical obligation to obtain patients' informed consent to treatment, Delany (2006) found that therapists' reasoning processes moved from an interpretation of an ethical principle *downwards* to a particular clinical scenario. Specifically, their implementation of the ethical obligation to obtain their patients' informed consent to treatment was derived or deduced from their interpretation and analysis of their obligation to provide an overall benefit for the patient (the principle of beneficence). In an earlier study, Barnitt & Partridge (1997) also found that physiotherapists used a top down, deductive process (described as a diagnostic or procedural reasoning approach) when reasoning through ethical problems. This compared with a narrative (inductive) approach used by occupational therapists.

A key difference which has developed between the clinical reasoning literature and the ethical reasoning literature is the identification of underlying *epistemological* bases. Epistemology refers to the study of knowledge and how knowledge is constructed. In contemporary models of clinical reasoning (Edwards et al 2004, Jensen et al 1999, Mattingly 1994) epistemological bases underlying particular reasoning processes have been identified and the relevance of understanding these differences is made explicit. Existing models of ethical reasoning recognize reasoning approaches but do not explicitly require an epistemological basis for therapists' adoption of a particular approach. Moreover, they tend to leave the choice of an ethical approach in the process of ethical decision making as an ontological enterprise rather than an epistemological one. By this we mean that the choice and direction of application of which ethical approach to use as a primary tool to both gather and analyse data concerning the ethical problem is left, even implicitly, to the practitioner's views concerning the nature of truth or reality. That is, the models have not focused on practitioners providing an epistemological rationale of different bases of knowledge and values. For example, it has been implied that practitioners may see themselves as being intrinsically more orientated towards a benefit- or outcome-driven (utilitarianism) approach as opposed to a duty-driven (deontological) approach (e.g. Sim 2004). And yet, the manner in which practitioners' views of professional and practice realities (including ethics) are formed is a complex process and one that draws from many realms of knowledge. It may be learned socially, within practice communities, or personally derived from an individual ontological perspective (Abrandt Dalhgren et al 2004, Barnitt & Partridge 1997, Benner et al 1996, Edwards 2001). In addition, in many clinical situations there is scope for more than one ethical interpretation. Our contention is that in the same way that practitioners are required to account for clinical decisions on an epistemological basis, they should also be aware of and able to defend or account for the underlying epistemological framework informing (in both directions) their ethical reasoning process and decisions. To this end, and in agreement with Swisher (2005), we emphasize the importance of practitioners having a critical awareness of *both* inductive (bottom up) and deductive (top down) processes of clinical and ethical reasoning. We also advocate that practitioners have a thorough understanding of both the top end (ethical principles and their theoretical bases) and the bottom end (patient values and clinical contexts) in order to justify and recognize how the two ends might contribute and interact when they make ethical judgements.

CONSTRUCTING KNOWLEDGE IN TWO DIRECTIONS: INDUCTIVE AND DEDUCTIVE REASONING

To understand the nature and scope of knowledge which might influence ethical reasoning processes, and to appreciate the rationale for the place of both deductive and inductive reasoning, we suggest the inclusion of an epistemological approach in addition to an ontological understanding. In this book there is a recurrent theme concerning 'how we know what we know' for decision making in clinical practice. There is now consensus that this occurs, at least in part, through an appreciation of several different types of knowledge which, in turn, are constructed based on different assumptions of reality (see Chapter 45). We propose that in ethical reasoning (as for clinical reasoning) practitioners should have the capacity to engage in *applied epistemology* by understanding how the various types of knowledge (and values) in a situation which involves ethical issues are constructed.

The rationale for an applied epistemology has to do with the basis on which health practitioners make decisions in practice, and this is not always explicitly understood by the practitioners themselves. For example, practitioners may conduct the important processes of data gathering and analysis in practice from a particular paradigm of practice (as observed by Barnitt & Partridge (1997) in relation to ethical problem solving by physiotherapists and occupational therapists), without being aware of the implications of how a paradigm shapes the resultant decision-making processes. One of the mandates of clinical reasoning is that practitioners understand the assumptions upon which they gather data and

then make decisions from their chosen analysis of the data in clinical practice. Few clinical educators would accept the notion of clinical decision making on the basis of personal inclination rather than through critical reflection of assumptions underlying the reasoning process which is in use. For example, it would be hard to defend the choice of a narrative form of reasoning in order to determine the possible structures at fault in an impingement of the shoulder. Alternatively, choosing a hypothetico-deductive (biomedical) reasoning approach to understand the cultural influences on decisions made by patients regarding their health would be of limited value.

Deductive and inductive processes of reasoning, just as deductive and inductive forms of research, have quite different underlying assumptions regarding the nature of truth, reality and knowledge (Edwards 2001). Both contribute quite different forms of valuable knowledge in the clinical reasoning process, and this is equally true in ethical reasoning (Edwards et al 2005). The relationship of deductive and inductive forms of ethical reasoning can be described as the crossing and re-crossing of a bridge by the practitioner (Hudson Jones 1997). In the next two sections we discuss the two sides of the bridge (or two ends of the reasoning spectrum) in greater depth. We demonstrate how an awareness of the ethical theories underlying principles on one side, and ethical value found within patient perspectives on the other, can enhance and enrich the reasoning process.

ETHICAL THEORY AND ETHICAL PRINCIPLES

Beauchamp & Childress (2001) are the leading proponents of a principles approach to biomedical ethical thinking. Their account of the meaning and application of the four principles (autonomy, non-maleficence, beneficence and justice) has been a major influence in biomedical ethics literature. In the four tiered steps used to defend an ethical decision, the principles are the middle tier (see Figure 25.1). These middle tier ethical concepts and principles have been posited as the best course for teaching ethics in preparation for

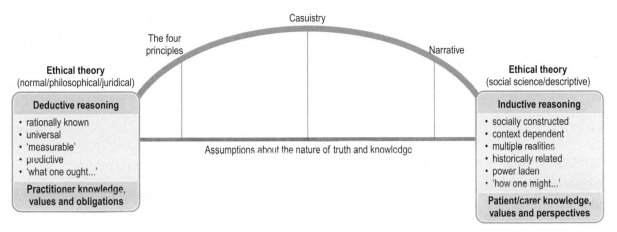

Figure 25.1   The ethical reasoning bridge – an epistemological framework

professional practice (Beauchamp & Childress 2001, Bebeau & Thoma 1999, Swisher 2005). In this section we highlight a potential danger in focusing on middle-range ethical concepts. We contend, as others have previously (Charlesworth 2005, Spriggs 2005), that there are limitations in ethical decision making which result from the unexamined application of normative principles without both an understanding of the depth of their philosophical meaning and an understanding of the complexity of different clinical situations. We believe that an understanding of the philosophical meaning underlying ethical principles provides a deeper and ultimately more flexible basis for ethical reasoning than the understanding and application of these principles alone. We discuss the principle of respect for autonomy as an example of how knowledge of underlying ethical theory can enrich the process of ethical reasoning by providing greater depth of knowledge about the meaning and application of middle tier ethical principles. We have chosen autonomy as the paradigm principle, because respect for a patient's autonomy, in some form, is central to clinical decision making in most healthcare contexts (Gillon 2003, Rothman 2001).

THE THEORY BEHIND THE PRINCIPLE: RESPECT FOR AUTONOMY

Beauchamp & Childress (2001) have suggested that the principle of respect for autonomy should be grounded in conditions of intention, understanding and lack of controlling influences. In defining autonomy, one of their main concerns is to reduce what they regard as an aspirational account of autonomy to an achievable account of autonomy, one which is within reach of normal choosers (Beauchamp & Childress 2001, p. 59). The focus of this definition or middle tier perspective is on what might be recognized as an autonomous choice rather than on the meaning of autonomy derived from its history and origins in ethical theory. Underlying this definition of autonomy, the notion of autonomy is honoured in different forms in all major moral theories in the Western analytic tradition (Hardin 1989). The theories and positions taken by the philosophers Immanuel Kant (1785/1998) and John Stuart Mill (1865/1991) provide the moral basis or foundational moral arguments for the principle of respect for autonomy. Kant's theory of respect for autonomy is grounded in metaphysical considerations of what it means to be a rational agent and to do what is right. Within that theory, Kant highlighted the importance of each person's inherent ability to reason and reflect as a basis of action. The consequences of this conception of autonomy in practice mean that respect for autonomy requires self-knowledge, self-reflection and reasoning which (grounded in metaphysical concepts) are able to withstand or rise above the influence of external forces.

Mill viewed autonomy differently. He was less concerned about the personal reasoning and reflective abilities of an individual. His conception of autonomy encompassed its value in maximizing happiness. He emphasized an individual's right to be free from interference in attaining happiness or pleasure. Respecting autonomy according to this consequentialist theory requires a focus on freedom of action to pursue individually based optimal outcomes. It is important to note that neither Kant nor Mill discussed ideas of autonomy as they might relate to clinical decision making or the process of ethical reasoning. They provided an ethical structure rather than specific guidelines for practical clinical action. The works of Gerald Dworkin (1988) and Robert Young (1986) are more useful in providing conceptual, interpretive and practical links from the underlying theories of Kant and Mill. Dworkin's theory of autonomy is grounded in the capacities and characters of individuals. He suggested that autonomous actions or choices should be made on the basis of critical reflection of a primary desire with a higher order desire. That is, such actions are characterized by a person who exercises capacities of thinking and reflection to define, and these actions 'give meaning and coherence to their lives' (Dworkin 1988, p. 20). In Young's view, the idea of autonomy should not be so individualistic that it neglects the reality of the often collaborative needs of people. He suggested that the idea of autonomy should bring coherence into the relationship between a person's general purposes and his or her particular actions (Young 1986, p. 12). An autonomous action, according to this view, equips a person to critically assess the advice tendered by others.

From these theories and conceptual explanations of autonomy it can be seen that respecting a patient's autonomy or even acting to benefit the patient is meaningless unless some attempt is made to examine the patient's capacities and desires to reason, to make decisions and to give preferences. By understanding that the philosophical meaning of autonomy requires both freedom of choice (Mill), reasons for choosing (Kant), evidence of reflection (Dworkin) and relevance to both short and long term goals (Young), healthcare practitioners have a number of ways of meeting their obligations to respect a patient's autonomy in a given situation. Spriggs (2005) proposed five criteria as a more useful way to understand and apply the philosophical ideal of respect for a patient's autonomy in clinical practice (Table 25.1). These criteria explicitly draw from underlying ethical theories of autonomy, and they promote a particular way of thinking for practitioners, rather than a list of duties with which practitioners must comply.

Table 25.1   A description of autonomous action based on ethical theories of autonomy (after Spriggs 2005)

Autonomous action	Explanation and application
1. Involves thinking	People are acting autonomously if they can be assessed as making a reasoned decision. That is, they must be able to demonstrate that they are able to understand and appreciate the circumstances of their decision
2. Involves critical reflection	People's decisions are autonomous if they can be justified and defended in terms of their own values or in terms of congruence with the kind of life they want to lead
3. Reflects a fundamental commitment about the way one's life is lived	This means that the specific content of an autonomous decision is not as important as the extent to which the decision demonstrates this feature of commitment
4. May not necessarily be a good choice	An autonomous choice should not be judged according to whether it is a wise choice or whether the consequences are disagreeable or unpalatable to another person. An autonomous choice is one that is based on criteria of reason, reflection and individual congruence
5. Is made deliberately and with an awareness of external influences	People who make autonomous choices should be aware of influences on their deliberation

INDUCTIVE APPROACHES TO ETHICS: NARRATIVE AND CASUISTRY

In a shift from thinking about and understanding how the top tier of ethical theory might influence and interact with the middle tier of ethical principles, we turn our attention to thinking ethically in terms of narrative. This shift involves health practitioners moving from a concern with philosophical and professionally based values to a concern with understanding patients' values and interpretations of experience. In this section we concentrate on the bottom tier of clinical experience, stories and cases. We highlight how narrative and casuistry as approaches to ethics are paradigmatic of the concerns of a number of social science derived approaches to ethics. Social science (with its many fields and disciplines of inquiry) has furthered an understanding of the importance of narratives as a form of socially constructed knowledge, a form of knowledge which encapsulates interpreted experience.

NARRATIVE AS SOCIAL SCIENCE ETHICS

In narrative ethics approaches, the emphasis is upon understanding the meaning of the situation for those involved (Brody 2003). Narratives (patient stories) are particularly rich forms of data in clinical practice (Greenhalgh 1998) and are understood by an inductive form of data gathering and analysis (Mattingly 1994). This form of inquiry and reasoning is concerned with understanding a patient's interpretation of experience, expressed through story, in contrast to a form of inquiry and reasoning that seeks to deductively confirm or disprove the conformity of data to a general norm, premise or principle. In narrative approaches to ethical dilemmas it is in the retelling of the story (often from the many perspective of the different protagonists) which finally brings a sense of who the participants really are and what the moral considerations are which ought to be brought to bear in the situation (Lindemann Nelson 2002, p. 45).

There is also the recognition in narrative approaches of the manner (often negative) in which dominant narratives (or accounts of social reality)

shape how both individuals and communities learn to interpret their experiences, express their stories and, in turn, form identities (e.g. feminist studies – 'ethics of care', Gilligan 1982; indigenous peoples – Bruner 1986, Dulwich Centre Newsletter 1995; disability – Mattingly 1998). The study of narratives is essentially about discovering how certain voices and groups in society may be marginalized while others are privileged. This has a particular relevance and significance in health systems, 'colonized' (Habermas 1984) and 'controlled' (Foucault 1980) as they are by medical and allied health professions, raising the question: what roles might we have as health practitioners in either evoking or extinguishing the voices of our patients and the perspectives they represent? There is a diversity of assumptions underlying the kinds of social science described above and the ethics they produce, and yet there is a reasonable agreement in how each emphasizes the importance of context and discourse, and the way in which truth is contested (Hugman 2005).

CASUISTRY

Casuistry is also a case-based form of ethics. It relies on paradigm cases or precedents (exemplar cases which are widely agreed on) in order to give substance and example to ethical principles (Toulmin 1994). This case-based ethical approach parallels the case-based nature of clinical practice. Casuistry in bioethics is similar to 'pattern recognition' in the clinical reasoning literature (Edwards 2001). Both are forms of reasoning which recognize features concerning a case and then attempt to confirm or verify those features. In clinical reasoning the process of pattern or case validation takes place by either a hypothetico-deductive process requiring hypothesis testing (tantamount to Beauchamp & Childress weighing the features of a case against known principles). Casuists maintain that comparisons of cases provide a means of apprehending unique or different features or issues and their possible solutions (Toulmin 1994). In casuistry, therefore, there is an appeal, in the manner of legal precedent, to the outcome of previous paradigm cases and the way in which a particular ethical issue has been previously identified, argued and resolved in these paradigm cases. The particular circumstances of the present particular case are then compared for their fit to the more universally agreed values expressed in identified paradigm cases. Casuistry, therefore, falls somewhere between deductive and inductive methods of analysis (Edwards 2001). That is, one case is likely to invoke the recall of others, thereby generating hypotheses inductively which may then be weighed against more universal principles of decision making (Jonsen 1986).

THE ETHICAL REASONING 'BRIDGE'

We observed earlier, when discussing the relationship between deductive and inductive reasoning, that normative- and principles-oriented ethics and social science, narratively-oriented ethics inform each other (Childress 1997, Hudson Jones 1997). The two ends of the four-tiered reasoning spectrum which we earlier labelled as the top end (beginning with principles and theories) and the bottom end (beginning with the specifics of a case) can also be visualized as two sides of a bridge (Figure 25.1).

The pylons on the one side are constructed from the richness of ethical theory, with assumptions based on the universal applicability of moral truths and values; understood by rationalist, abstract thought; and measurable in conformity with normative principles and legal or juridical processes. Using these assumptions, this perspective teaches and predicts what one 'ought' to do. The pylons on the other side, social science theory, are constructed from assumptions about reality which hold that it is socially constructed, context-dependent; that there are multiple realities; that knowledge has a historical construction and is produced from privileged positions of power to the advantage of some and the disadvantage of others. Using these assumptions, this perspective inductively teaches about the uniqueness and particularity of an individual and the context of the case, exploring 'how one might ...' instead of 'what one ought ...' in relation to interpretations of experience and the meaning(s) for that person.

On one side we find a reasoning process utilizing the ethical and professional values and knowledge of the practitioner encapsulated in but not confined to normative, professional and legal codes of conduct. On the other side is a reasoning process apprehending and utilizing the values and knowledge of the patient and the context in and by which the patient interprets his or her lived experience(s). In using deductive reasoning, the practitioner begins with ethical theory/ies and crosses the bridge seeking to determine the extent to which universal or normative moral (or ethical) values or theories apply to particular cases. In using inductive (or narrative) reasoning, the practitioner begins with a particular person or case, and crosses the bridge seeking to determine, from the particularities of that lived experience and interpreted meaning, how the details of this case qualify and provide deeper understandings of generalized ethical norms or principles. Casuistry may represent an initial response to a case, just as pattern recognition is often the initial reasoning process in a clinical presentation. However, casuistry, as an ethical reasoning approach, is only a point in the crossing described above, linking narrative and principles and inductive and deductive reasoning processes. The relationship between the inductive and deductive reasoning and their contribution to the development of ethical knowledge can be expressed in terms of the commentary and qualifications which a particular case (or narrative) can bring to bear on the application of normative principles, codes of conduct and even legislation:

> Legislation to improve compensation rights of asbestos victims passed through State Parliament in record time this week. ... Asbestos victims, unions and lawyers yesterday welcomed the passage of the Dust Diseases Bill, which was rushed through Parliament following a plea in *The Advertiser* by dying mother of nine-year-old triplets Melissa Haylock. An emotional Mrs Haylock, 42, of Lockleys, said yesterday she was relieved that she would be able to gain compensation for her children. 'It's peace of mind not only for my family, but for other families in the future,' she said. (The Advertiser 2005)

In this example the actual effects of current legislation relating to compensation for asbestos victims (and the way it is applied) are made accessible and more meaningful through the story of this young woman and the predicament of her three young children. The detailing of her story in the newspaper provided qualifying data for a reconsideration of existing principles of justice and eventually led to a change in legislation. This case then becomes a *paradigm* case of asbestos victim compensation. The underlying principle of justice combined with the individual circumstances of the family will be appealed to, in a casuistic manner, as precedent in the resolution of other asbestos victims' compensation cases.

FACILITATING REFLECTION ON ETHICAL KNOWLEDGE AND DECISION MAKING

A key component of ethical reasoning involves reflection on knowledge and decision making. Reflecting on knowledge requires an epistemological understanding of the diversity of knowledge, as exemplified in the typology outlined by Higgs & Titchen (1995): propositional, professional and personal knowledge. In the ethics context, philosophical ethical theory such as proposed by Kant

Casuistry (pattern recognition)

Does this situation or issue look or sound familiar?

- If it is familiar how has it generally been acceptably dealt with in the past? Does the resolution represent a particular ethical approach?
- If it isn't familiar what is different about it?
- Who appears to mostly benefit from the accepted method/outcome?
- Should I re-examine whether such a method/outcome is still appropriate here?

The four principles approach (deductive reasoning)

Which of the four ethical principles might be applicable in this situation?

- With respect to underlying ethical theory, what form would the most relevant principle take in this situation?
- What would the application of the most relevant principle 'mean' for this person(s) in this context?
- If more than one principle is relevant, does one principle have greater priority? If so, why?
- Do particular principles clash? How do I weight them?

Knowledge of personal and professional values

- Did my professional obligations and personal values 'meet' or clash in this scenario?
- If there was a clash, did I resolve it?
- Did the course of action I embarked on cause me to reflect on or change a previously held view, value or belief?
- What have I learned about myself (as a person, as a practitioner) through engagement in this ethical issue or situation?

Narrative ethics (inductive reasoning)

Whose voice (story or perspective) is coming through most clearly?

- Whose voice may not come through as well?
- What factors influence its expression or lack of expression?
- How can we better hear that voice?
- What factors influence its 'tone' (e.g. anger, fear, scepticism, frustration, passivity)?
- What qualifications/commentary does this perspective/story have on the application of any of the relevant principles?

Knowledge of others' values and relationships

- How would I characterize the main relationships in the situation (including my own role) – warm/cold, caring/indifferent, suspicious/trusting, hostile/conciliatory?
- Is the ethical dilemma made more complex by a lack of understanding of others' perspectives in one or more of the relationships in this situation?
- What communicative actions are required?

Figure 25.2   Examples of stimulus questions to facilitate deductive and inductive ethical reasoning

and Mill, or mid-range theories such as the four principles approach (Beauchamp & Childress 2001) would be examples of propositional knowledge. Professional craft knowledge might include a knowledge of professional codes of conduct and also clinical skills such as how to conduct an informed consent protocol for particular procedures. Communication skills such as conflict resolution might also be considered in this category. Personal knowledge would include an explicit understanding of the values and beliefs one holds, outside of codified professional values, and the ability to evaluate these in the light of new experiences and situations. Figure 25.2 outlines examples of stimulus questions designed to facilitate reflection on various areas of knowledge in ethical reasoning and also to assist practitioners to distinguish between inductive and deductive reasoning. The ethical reasoner is encouraged to move from one side to the other and back again, moving from the knowledge of one 'pylon' to the other, reflecting on answers to questions in the light of *both* ongoing data gathering *and* preliminary decisions and/or actions. It is important to consider the questions as representative of particular ways of thinking, more than as checklists to be instrumentally 'ticked off'.

CONCLUSION

In this chapter we have argued that ethical reasoning is best conducted by understanding the richness of ethical theory underlying middle tier concepts such as the four principles and, at the same time, understanding the ethical value of a rich understanding of patient perspectives. This involves two fundamentally different reasoning processes, both of which should be utilized by practitioners. It is our contention that in the ethical reasoning process what is important is not so much where we ontologically reside (that is, either on the side of positivist, universal norms or on the side of constructivist, socially constructed realities). What matters is that as practitioners we cross and re-cross the bridge in our ethical decision making in practice, reasoning on the basis of the widest set of data possible. Such diverse data encompass knowledge which is produced by different sets of assumptions and from different contexts and perspectives and so represents an epistemological approach.

References

Abrandt Dalhgren M, Richardson B, Kalman H 2004 Professions as communities of practice. In: Higgs J, Richardson B, Abrandt Dalhgren M (eds) Developing practice knowledge for health professionals Butterworth Heinemann, London, p 21–88

Barnitt R, Partridge C 1997 Ethical reasoning in physical therapy and occupational therapy. Physiotherapy Research International 2:178–194

Beauchamp T, Childress J 2001 Principles of biomedical ethics, 5th edn. Oxford University Press, Oxford

Bebeau M J, Thoma S J 1999 'Intermediate' concepts and the connection to moral education. Educational Psychology Review 11(4):343–360

Benner P, Tanner C, Chesla C 1996 Expertise in nursing practice: caring, clinical judgment, and ethics. Springer, New York

Brody H 2003 Stories of sickness, 2nd edn. Oxford University Press, Oxford

Bruner E M 1986 Ethnography as narrative. In: Turner V W, Bruner E M (eds) The anthropology of experience. University of Illinois Press, Urbana, p 139–155

Charlesworth M 2005 Don't blame the 'bio' – blame the 'ethics': varieties of (bio)ethics and the challenge of pluralism. Journal of Bioethical Inquiry 2(1):10–17

Childress J 1997 Narrative(s) versus norm(s): a misplaced debate in bioethics. In: Nelson H L (ed) Stories and their limits: narrative approaches to bioethics. Routledge, New York, p 252–272

Clawson A L 1994 The relationship between clinical decision making and ethical decision making. Physiotherapy 80:10–14

Delany C 2005 Respecting patient autonomy and obtaining their informed consent: Ethical theory – missing in action. Physiotherapy 91:197–203

Delany C 2006 Informed consent: ethical theory, legal obligations and the physiotherapy clinical encounter. Unpublished PhD thesis, University of Melbourne. Online. Available: http://eprints.unimelb.edu.au/archive/00001865/ 9 July 2007

Dulwich Centre 1995 Reclaiming our stories, reclaiming our lives. Part one. Dulwich Centre Newsletter, Adelaide, South Australia, 1:2–22

Dworkin G 1988 The theory and practice of autonomy. Cambridge University Press, Cambridge

Edwards I 2001 Clinical reasoning in three different fields of physiotherapy: a qualitative study. Australian Digitized Theses Program. Online. Available: www.library.unisa.edu.au/adt-root/18 Nov 2005

Edwards I, Jones M, Carr J et al 2004 Clinical reasoning strategies in physical therapy. Physical Therapy 84(4):312–335

Edwards I, Braunack-Mayer A, Jones M 2005 Ethical reasoning as a clinical-reasoning strategy in physiotherapy. Physiotherapy 91:226–236

Foucault M 1980, (trans C Gordon) Power/knowledge. Harvester Wheatsheaf, Brighton

Fox R C 1994 The entry of U.S. bioethics into the 1990s: a sociological analysis. In: Dubose E R, Hamel R, O'Connell L J (eds) A matter of principles: ferment in U.S. bioethics Trinity Press International, Valley Forge, PA, p 21–71

Gilligan C 1982 In a different voice. Harvard University Press, Cambridge, MA

Gillon R 2003 Ethics needs principles – four can encompass the rest – and respect for autonomy should be 'first among equals'. Journal of Medical Ethics 29:307–312

Greenhalgh T 1998 Narrative based medicine in an evidence based world. In: Greenhalgh T, Hurwitz B (eds) Narrative based medicine: dialogue and discourse in clinical practice. BMJ Books, London, p 247–265

Habermas J (trans T McCarthy) 1984 The theory of communicative action, vol 1. Reason and the rationalization of society. Polity Press, Oxford

Hardin R 1989 Autonomy, identity, and welfare. In: Christman J (ed) The inner citadel: essays on individual autonomy. Oxford University Press, New York, p 189–199

Higgs J, Titchen A 1995 The nature, generation and verification of knowledge. Physiotherapy 81:521–530

Hudson Jones A 1997 Literature and medicine: narrative ethics. Lancet 349:1243–1246

Hugman R 2005 New approaches in ethics for the caring professions. Palgrave Macmillan, Hampshire

Jensen G M, Gwyer J, Hack L M et al 1999 Expertise in physical therapy practice. Butterworth-Heinemann, Boston

Jonsen A R 1986 Casuistry and clinical ethics. Theoretical Medicine 7:65–74

Kant I 1998 Groundwork of the metaphysics of morals (1785). In: Gregor M (ed). Immanuel Kant: groundwork of the metaphysics of morals. Cambridge University Press, Cambridge

Kerridge I, Lowe M, McPhee J 2005 Ethics and law for the health professions, 2nd edn. Federation Press, Sydney

Lindemann Nelson H 2002 Context: backward, sideways and forward. In: Charon R, Montello M (eds) Stories matter: the role of narrative in medical ethics. Routledge, New York, p 39–47

Mattingly C 1994 Clinical revision: changing the therapeutic story in midstream. In: Mattingly C, Hayes Fleming M (eds) Clinical reasoning: forms of inquiry in a therapeutic practice. F A Davis, Philadelphia, p 270–291

Mattingly C 1998 Healing dramas and clinical plots: the narrative structure of experience. Cambridge University Press, Cambridge

Mill J S 1991 On liberty (1865). In: Gray J, Smith G (eds) On liberty in focus. Routledge, London, p 23–129

Purtilo R 2005 Ethical dimensions in the health professions, 4th edn. Elsevier Saunders, Boston

Rothman D 2001 The origins and consequences of patient autonomy: a 25 year retrospective. Health Care Analysis 9:255–264

Sim J 2004 Fundamentals of moral decision-making. In: French S, Sim J (eds) Physiotherapy: a psychosocial approach, 3rd edn. Elsevier, Edinburgh, p 221–236

Spriggs M 2005 Autonomy and patients' decisions. Lexington Books, Oxford

Swisher L 2002 A retrospective analysis of ethics knowledge in physical therapy. Physical Therapy 82:692–706

Swisher L 2005 Environment, professional identity, and the roles of the ethics educator: an agenda for development of the professional ethics curriculum. In: Purtilo R, Jensen G, Brasic Royeen C (eds) Educating for moral action: a sourcebook in health and rehabilitation ethics. F A Davis, Philadelphia, p 225–238

The Advertiser (December) 2005 Record time, asbestos victims' rights legislation passed, key bills put on ice until after March election. Adelaide, Australia

Toulmin S 1994 Casuistry and clinical ethics. In: Dubose E R, Hamel R, O'Connell L J (eds) A matter of principles: ferment in U.S. bioethics. Trinity Press International, Valley Forge, PA, p 310–318

Young R 1986 Personal autonomy beyond negative and positive liberty. Croom Helm, London

Zussman R 2000 The contributions of sociology to medical ethics. Hastings Center Report 30(1):7–11

Chapter 26

Multidisciplinary clinical decision making

Anne Croker, Stephen Loftus and Joy Higgs

Clinical decision making (CDM) often occurs in multidisciplinary modes, with collaboration among health professionals being required to make clinical decisions including diagnoses, treatment goals, management plans and evaluation of progress. A common context for multidisciplinary CDM is the healthcare team. The aim of this chapter is to consider: (a) the nature and place of multidisciplinary CDM in health care; (b) organizational parameters of decision making in multidisciplinary teams; and (c) interpersonal aspects required of health professionals participating in multidisciplinary CDM.

In this chapter we draw on the findings of two doctoral research projects (by the authors Anne Croker and Stephen Loftus) investigating multidisciplinary CDM using a phenomenological approach. The focus of the first project is collaboration in rehabilitation healthcare teams (Croker & Higgs 2005). Quotes below marked (AC) are derived from this research project. The second project (Loftus 2006; Loftus & Higgs 2004, 2005) involved a study of CDM in a multidisciplinary pain clinic.

MULTIDISCIPLINARY CDM, ITS NATURE AND PLACE IN HEALTH CARE

The growing complexity of health care, involving escalating healthcare costs, rapid technological advances and the proliferation of highly accessible internet medical information, as well as the increasing incidence of co-morbidities and chronic conditions in ageing populations, have together resulted in increased opportunities for and reliance on multidisciplinary CDM. Two areas in particular where collaborative decision making is prominent are multidisciplinary pain centres and rehabilitation teams. There has been a dramatic increase in the number of multidisciplinary pain centres around the world in recent decades (Loeser et al 2001); this has been attributed to a growing realization that management of problems experienced by patients with chronic pain, such as physical deconditioning complicated by psychosocial issues, are beyond the capability of a single health professional and need a coordinated team approach to be adequately addressed. Rehabilitation teams, although not a recent phenomenon, are much in evidence in 21st century health care, for today they face challenges such as coping with economic restrictions and accountability, and dealing with issues of specialization alongside difficulties in recruiting team members for remote and rural workplaces (Australian Health Workforce Advisory Committee 2006, Gans 2003).

MULTIDISCIPLINARY CDM

The term multidisciplinary CDM refers to the process in which individuals from different healthcare disciplines collaborate to diagnose problems and manage patients' care. In this chapter, collaboration is understood to be the cooperative act of working with one another. Multidisciplinary CDM is collaborative in nature; however, we use the term *multidisciplinary* here to distinguish this process from collaborative decision making (as discussed in Chapter 4), where the focus is on direct collaboration between one or more practitioners and a patient and where the goal is to engage in participative decision making with the patient. The context of collaborative decision making is emancipatory practice. In multidisciplinary CDM, the patient may or may not be seen as a team member and the practice model may vary from biomedical to biopsychosocial to emancipatory approaches; the focus of multidisciplinary CDM is on collaboration among practitioners to make decisions that build on their various disciplinary strengths and expertise.

Multidisciplinary CDM is a complex process in which many factors must be coordinated,

including the different skills and experience of a number of health professionals, in order to address the complexity of patients' problems and organizational contexts. For example, an established team of experienced health professionals, with a clear understanding of disciplinary roles, responsibilities and communication styles, can plan and coordinate the clinical management of an uncomplicated patient condition with ease and familiarity, perhaps initially via a team meeting followed up by informal discussions and emails. Such collaboration may appear deceptively straightforward. However, even apparently straightforward collaboration for multidisciplinary CDM relies extensively on the participating health professionals' prior experience of practice and collaboration, together with knowledge of self, other disciplines in the team, individuals in the team, team procedures and context. Collaborative processes may be more challenging when collaborating individuals are dealing with complex patient situations or are establishing their understanding of their discipline, self, others, team and context, or when the focus of the multidisciplinary CDM involves areas of conflict or territorial issues. In these situations, multidisciplinary CDM may require skilled communication and negotiation.

PROVISION OF HEALTH SERVICES BY TEAMS

With the increasing specialization of health professions, job transferability and demand for coordination of healthcare services, health professionals may be required during their career to collaborate in a range of different types of teams in different organizational contexts. Multidisciplinary CDM commonly occurs in the context of healthcare teams. Teams of health professionals from different disciplines work in various contexts to provide a range of health service functions. A team is considered here in its broadest sense to be a collective of health professionals regularly collaborating for patient care. Accordingly, teams can take on different structures, memberships and modes of operation, such as:

- a team comprising an informal network of health professionals working together intermittently and requiring special arrangements to meet in order (for example) to coordinate a range of ambulatory services for patients with chronic conditions (Suber 1996)

- a team with core members such as a physician and nurse working with the patient and family in an acute care setting, expanding to include other disciplines as the need arises (Baggs et al 2004)
- a formally managed team, such as a stroke rehabilitation team, identifying patients' goals and coordinating management of physical, vocational and social functions through regular team meetings (Bates et al 2005).

MULTIDISCIPLINARY CDM: ORGANIZATIONAL PARAMETERS

Organizations have systems and processes that support (or at times inhibit) sharing of information, team structures, and departmental boundaries, all of which impact on multidisciplinary CDM. An understanding of different organizational features assists health professionals to adapt to and negotiate different processes of multidisciplinary CDM.

ORGANIZATIONAL SYSTEMS AND PROCESSES THAT SUPPORT SHARING OF INFORMATION

Multidisciplinary CDM requires effective use of available communication processes and procedures. Sharing of information between collaborating health professionals is a basic requirement of multidisciplinary CDM. The means by which information is formally and informally shared within an organization may depend on available resources, employer and employee preferences, and ethical and legal obligations. For example, assessments, diagnostic reports, progress reports, discharge reports and referrals are different formal written systems that fulfil the dual purpose of information sharing and organization or discipline accountability (McAllister et al 2005). Case conferences and team meetings are formal processes for verbal information sharing, and facilitate face-to-face concurrent multidisciplinary CDM.

Informal communication systems are also used to share information and build relationships between disciplines; these include phone, email, shared work spaces and opportunities for socializing. For example, Cook et al (2001) reported that geographical proximity of a shared open-plan office enhanced timely sharing of information between members of a community health team, and Ellingson (2003) highlighted the importance of 'backstage communication' in building collegial relationships in a geriatric oncology team. Informal communication systems also provide a more flexible means of communication than formal case conferences and can facilitate micro-negotiations between team members (Ellingson 2003). There can also be a purposefully opportunistic element in informal communications systems, as evidenced by a rehabilitation team member's comment: 'I guess in terms of interaction with the other team members it would be more be bumping into each other and having a quick chat about things.' (AC)

TEAM STRUCTURES WITHIN ORGANIZATIONS

Underpinning multidisciplinary CDM is a range of factors supporting communication which need to be understood and mastered. One of these is the structure of the team itself. Structures are commonly either distributed (e.g. horizontal) or hierarchical. The decision-making power within a team is more evenly spread when the team's structure is horizontal and supportive of egalitarian, cooperative teamwork compared with a hierarchical structure with bureaucratic channels of decision making controlled by higher status professionals (Cook et al 2001, Cott 1998). A rehabilitation doctor described decision making at a team meeting as follows, providing an example of shared control for team decision making: 'We all have an understanding of what everyone else's thoughts and approach are to a patient, and what our individual goals are, so that we can all sit down and work out together what our overall goals are, to incorporate that together as a joint approach, and get the best outcome for a patient.' (AC)

Acute care hospital teams tend to work within a more task-oriented hierarchical structure in which the primary CDM control is commonly held by medical staff. Research into collaborative decision making in acute care situations has predominantly focused on intensive care situations. For example, Baggs & Schmitt (1997, p. 76) reported that medical residents in an acute medical intensive care unit saw themselves as the primary decision makers, one saying: 'The ultimate responsibility, legally and, you know, emotionally lies with the house officer'. Other researchers have reported low levels of collaboration between nurses and physicians, with collaboration tending to be the exception rather than the dominant practice, and with nurses providing input into physicians' decisions rather than collaborating in the decision-making process (Chaboyer & Patterson 2001, Higgins 1999, Kennard et al 1996, Thomas et al 2003).

Low levels of collaboration for decision making can also be found in rehabilitation teams. In Anne's study a rehabilitation specialist reported, 'I can remember distinctly, when I was an intern, the consultant telling the therapists exactly what was going to happen.' However, his experience in another team was different: 'the therapists ran the whole [meeting], the consultant gave advice when requested', and he subsequently preferred 'the unobtrusive approach, the consultant that sits there and is willing to listen more than talk'. (AC)

Power differences between professions within a hierarchical structure have been identified as contributing to low levels of collaboration between medical and nursing staff, and medical and social work staff in acute care settings (Abramson & Mizahi 2003, Baggs & Schmitt 1997). However, such power differences are not necessarily consistent across professions. Abramson & Mizahi found that, although not the dominant pattern, some physicians in metropolitan hospitals did share responsibility and decision making with other professional groups. An awareness of power differences within a team and the implications of these differences for decision making, enables team members to understand their 'allocated' role in multidisciplinary CDM, and may provide the basis for negotiation of decision-making roles within the team.

Team supervision or management can influence decision making in teams (Hyrkas & Appelqvist-Schidlechner 2003). There does not appear to be one ideal team management structure for enhancing decision making for all teams. For example, Cook et al (2001) noted that community primary health teams demonstrated an evenness of power distribution in decision making when the teams moved from a nurse manager model to a self-managed model. In contrast, Hyrkas & Appelqvist-Schidlechner found that some health professionals perceived an improvement of joint decision making following the introduction of team supervision. There is no guarantee that an egalitarian approach to teamwork will result in shared leadership and decision making; it could result in chaos, ineffectual decision making and disorder as people jockey for power or sit back and provide no leadership input. Improving collaboration in multidisciplinary CDM may require a review of team management in relation to the model of team management used, the context of the team and the power relationship between team members.

Some healthcare teams rely on clinical practice guidelines to standardize decision-making points and thus decrease the need for collaborative decision making. Grumbach & Bodenheimer (2004) claimed that a single specialty primary care practice with clear role delineation and clear divisions of labour can minimize the collaborative component of multidisciplinary CDM by ensuring that team members have defined tasks, task training, systems to support practice tasks, effective communication, on-the-job team training and time for team training. They reported that in this context, cohesive primary care teams could be formed where 'team members do not attend endless team meetings' (p. 1248). However, for many healthcare teams the diversity of clinical situations and patient needs precludes such a task-oriented structure, and regular team meetings provide a welcome and positive avenue for the dialogue required for collaborative multidisciplinary CDM.

ORGANIZATIONAL AND DEPARTMENTAL BOUNDARIES

Some teams are composed of members from separate organizations or departments. Straddling organizational and departmental boundaries adds another challenge to multidisciplinary CDM, as team members may be required to deal with different models of care and different organizational or departmental cultures and processes (Boaden & Leaviss 2000). For example, the work rehabilitation centre team described by Lingard et al (2004) faced inter-organizational challenges when collaborating with external stakeholders. Obstacles identified included lack of understanding of patients' programmes and decisions being made without consulting the team. Conversely, the community mental health teams studied by Carpenter et al (2003) placed more value on shared responsibilities between mental and health services when those services were integrated. An understanding of obstacles to inter-organizational or interdepartmental collaboration provides a basis for team members to develop strategies to straddle or minimize organizational boundaries. Thus we see that multidisciplinary CDM can also include multisectoral decision making on organizational matters and also on matters that directly relate to patient care.

INTERPERSONAL ASPECTS OF MULTIDISCIPLINARY CDM

The process of multidisciplinary CDM depends on the participating professionals' understanding of discipline differences, the dynamics of their team, and their skills in communication and interpersonal interactions.

DISCIPLINE DIFFERENCES

Achieving an understanding of the roles of different disciplines is an important precursor to decision making in teams. The socialization process involved in preparing to enter a particular profession means that each new member tends to adopt the views and identity of their professional culture. Members of each discipline have 'common experiences, values, approaches to problem solving and language for professional tools' (Hall 2005, p. 190), as well as 'distinct models of care, different skills sets ... and diverse political agendas' (Lingard et al 2004, p. 407). With different disciplines perceiving issues differently, teams can view issues from a wider perspective than is achieved by

one discipline alone (Cook et al 2001). However, health professional cultures can also act as barriers to collaboration; members of different professions use different jargon, have different priorities and meanings for tasks and events, and have different expectations of their roles in patient care. For example, Abramson & Mizahi (1996) found that social workers tended to seek a higher degree of shared responsibility and mutuality with interdisciplinary care than was sought by physicians.

The extent to which discipline differences inhibit collaboration can be minimized by clarifying and negotiating disciplines' and team members' roles. However, such negotiations may require confidence, assertiveness and an openness to the views of others, as evidenced by comments from rehabilitation team members in Anne's study:

> I think it's a positive thing that you can bring in different views and just work your way through treatment issues and I think it's only going to benefit the client in the long run but I guess you need to be confident enough to work in a team [in that way]. (AC)

> I'm happy to talk through rationales and theories and I'm always open to learning more if they've got a different approach, a different theory base. (AC)

An example of successful collaboration was demonstrated in Stephen's research by an experienced multidisciplinary pain team with a well-established routine for coordinating their assessment findings (Loftus 2006). In this team, separate assessments of new patients by the doctor, physiotherapist and psychologist were followed by a case conference. The format of the case conference required the findings of the hour long assessment to be reduced to a 1 or 2 minute summary. In addition, to avoid needless repetition of findings and to ensure key points were emphasized, the physiotherapist and psychologist were required to dynamically alter their summaries as they listened to their predecessors' summaries. At a deeper level the team members were also coordinating different perspectives of patient care into the CDM process. The doctors tended to adopt a pathophysiological paradigm of health care, looking for identifiable pathology that could be definitively treated. The other health professionals tended to adopt a more functional paradigm, identifying disability and ways of improving function. The team members recognized that the two paradigms were superficially opposed to each other. However, in practice the multidisciplinary approach allowed the two paradigms to be dialectically combined, bringing their strengths together.

WORKING IN TEAMS

Organization theory and management practice, when considered in the context of patient care, can provide frameworks for understanding and developing teams in health care (Shortell & Kalunzy 1994). The stages of 'forming, storming, norming and performing' (Tuckman 1965, Tuckman & Jensen 1977) are frequently used to describe team development. When groups of undergraduates used these stages as a basis for developing multidisciplinary teams to implement a health-related community action project, they reported improved skills in conflict resolution, collective decision making, action implementation and respect for individual team members, as well as improved understanding of the function of other disciplines (Hope et al 2005). However, in clinical practice not all healthcare teams have sufficiently stable membership to allow progression through the stages of team development. Rather, a team may be described as 'a complex and fluid entity composed of core and expanded groups' (Lingard et al 2004, p. 404). Teams may have to continually adapt to changes of membership. In some of the rehabilitation teams in Anne's project the staff continually rotated: 'We've had OTs come and go, physios come and go, they do their stint and then they move on' (AC). As well as impacting on team development, constant staff changes also disrupt the continuity of the collaborative relationships underpinning multidisciplinary CDM, as described by a physiotherapist in a rehabilitation team: 'I was negotiating to find out what they had on their mind, because I'm happy to work with [new] people but it gets a bit tiring when you've just got to do that over and over and over and over' (AC). It can be argued that the multidisciplinary pain team in Stephen's study could attribute a large part of its success to the stability of its core membership.

Lingard et al (2004) contended that for individuals to function as a collaborative team they each need to understand the 'rules of the game', which involves negotiating ownership of roles and 'trading' of equipment, resources, knowledge and goodwill. These authors contended that the aim of this negotiation should not necessarily be to overcome tensions, but rather to acknowledge and articulate these tensions in an effort to 'sustain the delicate balance between achieving a shared goal and competing for agency and status in the interprofessional setting' (Lingard et al 2004, p. 407). In Anne's project an awareness of role tension was expressed by an occupational therapist in reflecting on how a new team member was going to fit in with the team: 'Is she going to tread on our toes?' (AC). Having an awareness of the 'rules of the game' and being able to negotiate role ownership and boundaries are important precursors of multidisciplinary CDM.

An awareness of appropriate styles of interaction between team members provides a good basis for negotiation of team roles and resources. Team members' personal characteristics may influence team dynamics via preferred communication styles. McKinnon (1998) provided a classification system, proposing that team members can be: (a) *introverts*, preferring written communication to talking, and needing time to consider issues; (b) *extroverts*, making instant decisions and being energized by being with other people; (c) *'feeling' people*, valuing harmony and considering the implications on others in decision-making; and (d) *thinking–logical people*, using logic as a basis for decision making and being unaware of the emotional issues surrounding decisions. Although it is a simplistic representation of complex individual situations and interpersonal relationships, McKinnon's classification provides a basis for developing appropriate styles of interaction between individual team members during role negotiation and for the process of multidisciplinary CDM.

COMMUNICATION AND INTERRELATIONAL SKILLS

Communication in teams has a dual role of sharing of information and building working relationships

(Wicke et al 2004). To facilitate adequate sharing of information for multidisciplinary CDM, health professionals need to write clearly, succinctly, informatively and in a timely manner (McAllister et al 2005) and to be competent in the generic communication skills of listening, questioning, clarifying and explaining for verbal interactions. A rehabilitation team speech therapist highlighted the need for communication skills in collaborative relationships: 'You have to be able to listen effectively, and I guess with the consideration [that] your views might differ to other people's, but understanding where they're coming from, you need good communication skills to be able to express your views and your goals, and how you're feeling about certain issues.' (AC)

When performed sensitively, the dialogue between health professionals working in multidisciplinary CDM can produce a rich and multidimensional picture of a patient that is both a thorough assessment and paves the way to humane and comprehensive management (Loftus 2006).

CONCLUSION

Multidisciplinary CDM adds another layer of complexity to clinical reasoning and requires effective understanding of the implications of the organizational and team environment. It also requires communication skills that facilitate navigation through 'an environment charged with professional, temporal and financial tensions' (Lingard et al 2004, p. 404).

An understanding of organizational parameters and discipline differences provides an important basis for multidisciplinary CDM in teams. Multidisciplinary CDM also relies on team members' interpersonal and communication skills to share information and resolve conflicts.

References

Abramson J, Mizahi T 1996 When social workers and physicians collaborate: positive and negative experiences. Social Work 41(3):270–281

Abramson J, Mizahi T 2003 Understanding collaboration between social workers and physicians: application of a typology. Social Work in Health Care 37(2):71–100

Australian Health Workforce Advisory Committee 2006 The Australian allied health workforce: an overview workforce planning issues. AHWAC Report 2006.1, Sydney

Baggs J, Schmitt M 1997 Nurses' and resident physicians' perceptions of the process of collaboration in an MICU. Research in Nursing and Health 20(1):71–80

Baggs J, Norton S, Schmitt M et al 2004 The dying patient in the ICU: role of the interdisciplinary team. Critical Care Clinics 20:525–540

Bates B, Choi J, Duncan P et al 2005 Veterans Affairs/ Department of Defence clinical practice guideline for the management of adult rehabilitation care. Stroke 36 (Sep):2049–2056

Boaden N, Leaviss J 2000 Putting teamwork in context. Medical Education 34:921–927

Carpenter J, Schneider J, Brandon T et al 2003 Working in multidisciplinary community mental health teams: the impact on social workers and health professionals of integrated mental health care. British Journal of Social Work 33:1081–1103

Chaboyer W, Patterson E 2001 Australian hospital generalist and critical nurses' perceptions of doctor–nurse collaboration. Nursing and Health Sciences 3:73–79

Cook G, Gerrish K, Clarke C 2001 Decision-making in teams: issues arising from two UK evaluations. Journal of Interprofessional Care 15(2):141–151

Cott C 1998 Structure and meaning in multidisciplinary teamwork. Sociology of Health and Illness 20(6): 848–873

Croker A, Higgs J 2005 Collaboration in rehabilitation teams. In: Proceedings of the Association for Qualitative Research Conference, Melbourne, July 14–16, p 22

Ellingson L 2003 Interdisciplinary health care teamwork in the clinic backstage. Journal of Applied Communication Research 31(2):93–117

Gans B M 2003 Creating the future of PM&R: building on our past. Archives of Physical Medicine and Rehabilitation 84(7):946–949

Grumbach K, Bodenheimer T 2004 Can health care teams improve primary care practice? Journal of the American Medical Association 291:1246–1251

Hall P 2005 Interprofessional teamwork: professional cultures as barriers. Journal of Interprofessional Care 19 (Suppl 1):188–196

Higgins L 1999 Nurses' perceptions of collaborative nurse–physician transfer decision making as a predictor of patient outcomes in a medical intensive care unit. Journal of Advanced Nursing 29(6):1434–1443

Hope J, Lugassy D, Meyer R et al 2005 Bringing interdisciplinary and multicultural team building to health care education: the Downstate Team Building Initiative. Academic Medicine 80(1):74–83

Hyrkas K, Appelqvist-Schidlechner K 2003 Team supervision in multiprofessional teams: team members' descriptions of the effects as highlighted by group interviews. Journal of Clinical Nursing 12:188–197

Kennard M, Speroff T, Puopolo T et al 1996 Participation of nurses in decision making for seriously ill adults. Clinical Nursing Research 5(2):199–220

Lingard L, Espin S, Evans C et al 2004 The rules of the game: interprofessional collaboration on the intensive care team. Critical Care 8(6):403–408

Loeser J D, Butler S H, Chapman C R et al 2001 Bonica's management of pain. 3rd edn. Lippincott Williams and Wilkins, Philadelphia

Loftus S 2006, Language in clinical reasoning: learning and using the language of collective clinical decision making. Unpublished PhD thesis, University of Sydney, Australia. Online. Available: http://ses.library.usyd.edu.au/handle/2123/1165 9 July 2007

Loftus S, Higgs J 2004 In: Learning and using the language of collaborative clinical reasoning, From Cell to Society 4, 4th Research Conference, College of Health Sciences, University of Sydney, Leura, Nov, p 29/9

Loftus S, Higgs J 2005 Learning decision making in interprofessional settings. Proceedings of the EdHealth Conference, College of Health Sciences, University of Sydney, Terrigal, 16–17 Nov, p 23

McAllister L, Hay I, Street A 2005 Writing records, reports, and referrals in professional practice. In: Higgs J, Sefton A, Street A et al (eds) Communicating in the health and social sciences. Oxford University Press, Melbourne, p 105–119

McKinnon S 1998 Team play: strategies for successful people management. Lothian Books, Melbourne

Shortell S, Kalunzy A 1994 Organization theory and health services management. In: Shortell S, Kalunzy A (eds). Health care management: organisation design and behaviour. Delmar Publishers, Albany

Suber R 1996 Chronic care in ambulatory settings: components of an integrated system. American Journal of Behavioural Scientist 39(6):665–675

Thomas E, Sexton J, Helmreich R 2003 Discrepant attitudes about teamwork among critical care nurses. Critical Care Medicine 31(3):956–959

Tuckman B W 1965 Developmental sequences in small groups. Psychological Bulletin 63:384–399

Tuckman B W, Jensen M C 1977 Stages of small-group development revisited. Group and Organisational Studies 2(4):419–427

Wicke D, Coppin R, Payne S 2004 Teamworking in nursing homes. Journal of Advanced Nursing 45 (2):197–204

Chapter 27

Treatment decision making in the medical encounter: the case of shared decision making

Cathy Charles, Amiram Gafni and Tim Whelan

CHAPTER CONTENTS

INTRODUCTION

Over the last two decades, there has been increasing interest among health researchers, clinicians and ethicists in the general topic of treatment decision making between patients and physicians and, more recently, in shared treatment decision making in particular. In this chapter we describe some of the reasons for this interest, the meaning of shared decision making, physician attitudes towards shared decision making and the development and use of decision aids to promote shared decision making. In doing so, we draw heavily on our own conceptual and empirical research on the topic of shared treatment decision making conducted over a period of more than 10 years (Charles et al 1997, 1999a).

THE DEVELOPMENT OF THE SHARED DECISION MAKING APPROACH

Prior to the 1980s, the most prevalent approach to treatment decision making in North America was *paternalistic*, with the physician assuming the dominant role in the medical encounter (Levine et al 1992). Underlying this deference to professional authority were a number of assumptions (Charles et al 1999a). The first was that for most illnesses, a single best treatment existed and that clinical expertise and experience provided the basis for making the 'right' decision. Second, physicians were assumed to consistently and uniformly apply this clinical judgement when selecting treatments for their patients. Third, because of their expertise, physicians were assumed to be in the best position to evaluate treatment benefits and risks for the patient. Finally, professional ethics enjoined physicians to put the patient's welfare first – a kind of 'doctor knows best' mentality.

After 1980, these assumptions began to break down. It became apparent that for an increasing number of illnesses there was no one best treatment, and a more complex decisional context emerged wherein different treatments (including the 'do nothing' option) had different types of trade-off between benefits and risks. Because the patient had to live with the consequences, the assumption that physicians were in the best position to evaluate these trade-offs for the patient was increasingly challenged (Eddy 1990, Levine et al 1992, Lomas & Lavis 1996). Moreover, the burgeoning literature in North America on small area variations in medical practice was beginning to show consistent evidence that physician treatments for the same disease often varied considerably across small geographic areas, and that these variations were unrelated to differences in the health status of the respective populations (Chassin et al 1986, 1987; Roos et al 1988; Wennberg et al 1987). These findings called into question the precision of medical practice, including the assumption that physicians uniformly provided the best treatment to patients with a similar disease.

Two other system level trends also cast a negative light on the autonomy of physicians in clinical practice. The first was concern over rising healthcare costs which raised the issue of accountability of physicians to patients, governments and, in the case of the US, to third party payers for clinical decisions (Katz et al 1997). The second and even more direct influence was the rise of consumerism and consumer/patient sovereignty (Charles & DeMaio 1993; Haug & Lavin 1981, 1983) in particular, as manifested in new government legislation safeguarding the rights of patients to be informed about all available treatment options (Nayfield et al 1994) and in the growing interest among many individuals and groups (e.g. physicians, patients and ethicists) to develop and advocate new approaches to treatment decision making which would incorporate a greater role for patients in this process (Gafni et al 1998).

As a result of these and other trends, the appropriateness of the paternalistic model of treatment decision making began to be questioned, and other models, such as the *informed* and *shared* approaches, were identified and advocated as potentially preferred options for treatment decision making (Charles et al 1997, 1999a; Gafni et al 1998). One major problem with this emerging literature, however, was that these concepts themselves were not clearly defined; the same words (for example 'shared decision making') were used to mean different things, and different labels (such as 'informed', 'shared') were used without clear distinctions in their application. Thus, while more patient involvement in treatment decision making was being advocated, it was not clear exactly what this meant or how it could be implemented. To shed light on these issues we wrote two papers in the late 1990s (Charles et al 1997, 1999a) attempting to clarify the meaning of shared decision making, to define the key components of this approach and to compare them with those of the informed and paternalistic models of treatment decision making.

THE MEANING OF SHARED DECISION MAKING

Both the informed and the shared decision making models were developed to compensate for alleged flaws in the paternalistic approach. These three models are the most widely discussed in the literature on treatment decision making. The different stages of the treatment decision making process in general are identified in Table 27.1. These stages are: information exchange, deliberation about treatment options and deciding on the treatment to implement (Charles et al 1999a). We have identified these as distinct stages, although in reality they may occur together or in an iterative process. Table 27.1 identifies the 'ideal type' roles that both physicians and patients play at each decision-making stage and how these differ by decision-making approach.

INFORMATION EXCHANGE

Information exchange refers to the type and amount of information exchanged between

Table 27.1   Treatment decision making approaches (Charles et al 1999b)

Analytical stages		Paternalistic model	Intermediate approaches	Shared model	Intermediate approaches	Informed model
Information exchange	Flow Direction	One way (largely) Doctor→patient		Two way Doctor↔patient		One way (largely) Doctor→patient
	Type	Medical		Medical and personal		Medical
	Minimum amount	Legal requirement		Anything relevant to decision making		Anything relevant to decision making
Deliberation		Doctor alone or with other doctors		Doctor and patient (plus potential others)		Patient (plus potential others)
Who decides what treatment to implement?		Doctors		Doctor and patient		Patient

physician and patient and whether information flow is one way or two way. In the paternalistic model, the exchange is largely one way and the direction is from physician to patient. At a minimum, the physician must provide the patient with legally required information on treatment options and obtain informed consent to the treatment recommended. The patient is depicted in this model as a passive recipient of whatever amount and type of information the physician chooses to reveal. In general, this model assumes that the physician knows best and will make the best decision for the patient, without necessarily requiring any patient input.

In an informed model, information exchange is one way, from physician to patient. The physician is assumed to be the primary source of information for the patient on medical/scientific information about the disease and the treatment options. Beyond information transfer, the physician has no further role in the decision-making process. The tasks of deliberation and decision making are the patient's alone.

In a shared decision-making process, information sharing is a two way process. At a minimum, the physician must inform the patient of all the relevant information about available treatment options, the benefits and risks of each and the potential effects of these on the patient. However, for a meaningful deliberation and agreement on the treatment of choice, the physician should

describe his/her preferences, values and beliefs. The patient needs to provide the physician with information on her/his values, preferences, lifestyle and social context, beliefs and knowledge about the illness and its treatment. It is assumed in this model that both sets of information (technical/scientific) and subjective (values/preferences) are necessary to make the best treatment decision for any given patient.

DELIBERATION

The deliberation stage of decision making refers to the process of expressing and discussing treatment preferences. The minimum requirement as to which person/s are involved in the process varies across the three decision-making approaches. In the paternalistic approach, the physician weighs the benefits and risks of each option alone or in consultation with other physicians while the patient passively listens. In the extreme case of this model, the physician may verbally communicate to the patient only the ultimate treatment decision(s) selected, without soliciting patient input or describing the rationale for that decision.

In the informed model, the physician's role is limited to information transfer, that is, providing the patient with information about the relevant treatment information and the risks and benefits of each. The patient alone or with input from friends and family undertakes the deliberation process to arrive at an informed decision reflecting personal values and preferences. Underlying this approach are two key assumptions. The first is that information is both necessary and sufficient to enable the patient to make the best decision. The second is that the physician should not have an investment in the decision-making process or the decision made. In other words, patient sovereignty reigns in this approach, with the physician providing technical input only, in the form of relevant scientific information.

In a shared approach both patient and physician deliberate about treatment options in an interactive process where it is assumed that both parties have a legitimate investment in the treatment process and outcome. This emphasis on interaction ensures patient input, but also makes the process potentially more cumbersome and time-consuming than the other approaches. In a shared process both parties need to be willing to engage with each other, exchanging both information and treatment preferences. The physician can legitimately give a treatment recommendation to patients and try to persuade them to accept the recommendation. However, physicians using this approach would also have to listen to patients and try to understand why they might prefer a different option. If no agreement can be reached, several possibilities can occur. The physician would need to decide whether to endorse a particular patient's choice as part of a negotiated agreement in which patients' views count, or whether the strength of the physician's own views precluded agreement with any other treatment option. The patient would need to decide whether to stay with this physician or to seek advice elsewhere.

DECIDING ON THE TREATMENT TO IMPLEMENT

The final stage in the treatment decision-making process is choosing a treatment to implement. In the paternalistic and informed models, the decision maker is one person; in the first case it is the physician and in the second, the patient. However, neither party is totally autonomous because each faces constraints in implementing the decision. The physician must have the patient's informed consent prior to giving the treatment, and the patient needs authorization from a physician to receive the preferred treatment.

In the shared approach both parties, through the process of deliberation, work towards reaching an agreement that both can live with. As noted above, if agreement cannot be reached the process may terminate at this point unless one party can be persuaded to adopt the other's preferred option.

The different approaches described above are 'ideal types' in the sense that the role depictions for physician and patient in each model are defined as invariant, predictable and distinct from one another. In reality the boundaries around the role behaviour of physicians and patients in each model are rarely so clear-cut. There are various 'in-between' approaches to treatment decision making which do not conform precisely to one of the ideal types but rather lie somewhere in-between and may be characterized as shades of grey. For example, starting with the paternalistic model, the more that each stage moves from a physician-dominated encounter to one where the patient's input is recognized, nourished and valued, the more the model evolves into a shared approach. In fact the majority of physician–patient treatment decision-making processes are likely to reflect some form of in-between approach rather than a pure type.

Even in a single interaction, the decision-making approach used at the beginning of the discussion may evolve into one of the other approaches as the consultation progresses. It should be noted that we have described only the most simple type of interaction, that between one patient and one physician. We have done this to keep our analysis as clear as possible, but we recognize that many decision-making processes involve multiple participants and can take place over time, greatly complicating the process and allowing for the development of coalitions around treatment preferences. Nonetheless, the framework provides an analytic tool for articulating the different stages in treatment decision making, identifying the defining characteristics of the paternalistic, informed and shared approaches to undertaking this task and clarifying the differences between them.

PHYSICIANS' ATTITUDES TOWARDS SHARED TREATMENT DECISION MAKING

The conceptual model of shared decision making referred to here was developed over several years (Charles et al 1997, 1999a). Since then, a citation analysis undertaken by Makoul & Clayman in 2006 suggests widespread dissemination of and references to this model in the international treatment decision making literature. Our goal in developing this model was to focus on treatment decision making for serious (potentially life-threatening) illnesses, where several treatment options exist with different possible outcomes and substantial uncertainty, where there is often no right or wrong answer, and where treatments vary in their impact on the patient's physical and psychological well-being (Charles et al 1999b).

Early on, we also wanted to know how well this model resonated with practising physicians and in particular the extent to which the role expectations that we defined for patients and physicians in a shared approach coincided with those that

physicians themselves would define as generic to each approach. As a first empirical exploration we decided to undertake a cross-sectional survey of all Ontario-based medical and radiation oncologists and surgeons treating women with early stage breast cancer as an example of a decision-making context to which our model could be applied. Our goal was to assess the degree of congruence in the meaning of shared decision making as defined in our conceptual model and as perceived by these physicians (Charles et al 2004).

Of 322 eligible surgeons, 232 (72.0%) completed and returned our questionnaire. One hundred and two (78.5%) of the 130 eligible oncologists responded. In the questionnaire we included four clinical treatment decision-making examples or scenarios in which the roles of the patient and the physician were systematically varied. We then asked physicians to read each scenario (see Box 27.1) and identify which one(s) they thought reflected a shared approach to treatment decision making.

Example 1 was constructed as a paternalistic approach in which the physician dominated the

---

Box 27.1 Decision-making examples

Example 1
After looking at your medical records and examining you the doctor presents a treatment that he/she thinks is best for you. The doctor gives you information about the treatment including the risks and benefits. You accept the treatment that the doctor recommends.

Example 2
After looking at your medical records and examining you the doctor presents you with the treatment choices. Information about the risks and benefits of each choice is given and discussed with you. You ask questions and obtain all the information you want from the doctor. The doctor recommends a treatment that you accept.

Example 3
After looking at your medical records and examining you the doctor presents you with the treatment

choices. Information about the risks and benefits of each choice is given and discussed with you. The doctor asks you to decide on a treatment and states that you are the best person to make the decision. You decide and inform the doctor of the treatment you prefer.

Example 4
After looking at your medical records and examining you the doctor presents you with treatment choices. Information about the risks and benefits of each choice is given and discussed with you. You ask questions and obtain all the information you want from the doctor. The doctor asks you about your preferences for treatment given your lifestyle and the issues that are important to you. Together you decide on the treatment that is best suited to you.

process. In example 2, information was shared between patient and physician but the physician alone made the treatment decision (what we call some sharing). In example 3, the physician provided information to the patient but the latter was the sole decision maker (what we call an informed approach). In example 4, the patient and physician both participated in all phases of the decision-making process and together negotiated a treatment to implement (what we call a pure shared approach). None of the examples had any labels attached so physicians were unaware that we had deliberately constructed each scenario to represent a particular type of decision-making approach.

The study results indicated that over 95% of both oncologists and surgeons felt that a shared decision-making approach was illustrated in at least one of our clinical scenarios. Few physicians (less than 5%) described example 1, the paternalistic scenario, as shared. Example two, constructed to reflect a two way sharing of information but a single decision maker (physician) was identified as a shared approach by approximately 28% and 34% of surgeons and oncologists respectively. Example 3, constructed to reflect a two-way sharing of information but with a single patient decision maker, was considered shared by 27% of surgeons and 21% of oncologists. Example 4, illustrating a pure shared approach as defined in our model, was identified as shared by 94% of surgeons and 87% of oncologists.

From these results, we concluded that substantial congruence was found between the meaning of shared decision making as defined in our conceptual model and as perceived by study physicians. In recent years we have worked with physicians in other clinical areas such as general practice and diabetes to further refine our model and modify certain aspects of it to fit the respective decision-making contexts of different clinical areas (Montori et al 2006, Murray et al 2006).

The model can be used as a conceptual tool to guide research, compare different treatment decision-making approaches, clarify the meaning of shared decision making and enhance its translation into practice.

In the same study referred to above (Charles et al 2004), we also asked Ontario surgeons and oncologists the extent to which they practised shared decision making with their patients, their comfort level with this approach and perceived barriers and facilitators to implementation. More physicians from each specialty (89% of surgeons and 87% of oncologists) reported high comfort levels with example 4 (the pure shared approach) than with any other of the examples presented. Similarly, more surgeons and oncologists reported that their usual approach to treatment decision making was like example 4 than any other example presented (69% of surgeons and 56% of oncologists). Interestingly, reported comfort levels with example 4 were 20% higher for surgeons and 31% higher for oncologists than their reported use of this approach.

Physicians identified numerous barriers to implementing shared decision making, including lack of time, patient anxiety, patient lack of information or misinformation, and patient unwillingness or inability to participate. The latter barrier could be attributed to many factors, for example patient lack of interest and/or limitations in personal capacity, which in turn may be influenced by social circumstances, patient understanding, and the physician's skill/ability to inform patients of relevant treatment options and to create an environment conducive to shared decision making. Many of the above factors and others (including physician factors) have also been identified in other studies as barriers to implementing a shared approach (Gwyn & Elwyn 1999, Stevenson et al 2000).

Based on the above results, it seems that there is still much to do to create clinical practice environments that are conducive to shared decision making between physicians and patients. Moreover, despite attempts like ours and those of others (Deber 1994, Edwards & Elwyn 2001) to clarify the meaning of shared decision making, there are still different perspectives on what it means and entails at the practice level.

THE DEVELOPMENT AND USE OF TREATMENT DECISION AIDS

There has been increasing interest and activity in the development, use and evaluation of decision aids as instruments or tools to assist patients to participate in the treatment decision-making process with their physicians (Whelan et al 2002). Whereas some studies (Whelan et al 2002, 2003, 2004) have shown that such tools improve patients' knowledge and comfort with decision making, others have not (Goel et al 2001). The term *decision aid* is a general term applied to a broad array of different tools. Such tools are generally intended to help patients by providing them with evidence-based information about relevant treatment options and their risks and benefits, to structure the decision-making process in what the designers hope will be a useful and logical way, and to encourage patients to think about their treatment preferences and participate in the decision-making process. The number, types, formats, purposes and clinical contexts of their use have proliferated over the last 10 years (Charles et al 2005). Some of the more common formats include decision boards, interactive videos, pen and paper exercises, and coaching exercises to help patients interact with their physicians.

The development of decision aids, mostly by university academics or professional associations, has been so prolific that this growth has outpaced our ability to evaluate the rigor and success of such tools in achieving their stated goals. To help remedy this situation an international collaboration of scholars in different countries has been assembled to develop critical appraisal criteria (primarily methodological) for evaluating such aids, but this movement is still in its infancy (O'Connor et al 2005).

Methodological issues are not the only issues that need to be carefully thought through when developing and using various forms of decision aids. Other issues include, for example, the degree of fit of different aids with a variety of clinical and cultural contexts. Currently tool developers seem to commonly assume that a single type of aid will fit multiple contexts without the need for modification (a kind of 'one size fits all' mentality), but in reality this is unlikely to be the case. In addition, the theoretical underpinnings and assumptions underlying the development of such interventions often vary, may not be made explicit, or may be absent completely as a foundation on which applied decision-making tools are built. This is a little like putting the cart before the horse. No matter how rigorous the methodological steps are in developing a decision aid, the resultant tool will still be flawed if not guided initially by a clear statement about the goals of the instrument and a conceptual foundation of hypotheses and assumptions about the mechanisms to incorporate in the tool that are intended to produce the desired results. Unless these analytical processes are made clear, it is difficult for others to judge the thinking behind the development process or the extent to which such tools will resonate with physicians and patients. Finally, it is sometimes the case in this field of research that what we *can* measure drives what we *should* measure. However, more appropriately, desired goals of decision aids should drive measurement and not the other way round (Charles et al 2005).

One of the more recent developments in the design of decision aids is the attempt to structure into these tools exercises intended to help patients clarify their values (O'Connor et al 1999). Such exercises typically involve asking patients to evaluate the importance of various potential treatment risks and benefits and then to make, either implicitly or explicitly, trade-offs among them (for example, the importance of body image versus survival) to come up with a preferred decision. There are many variations on this exercise. The goal is to help patients assess whether the treatment decision they are leaning towards is consistent with the priorities they have identified in the exercise. This type of exercise assumes that undertaking a preference-based trade-off is the best method for determining individual treatment decisions.

There are several problems with such exercises that need to be addressed (Charles et al 2005). First, it is often not clear what the designers of such exercises mean by the concept of *values* and their various types and levels. Second, the alleged need for such exercises assumes that patients on their own do not know and cannot articulate their own values related to the desirability or undesirability of various treatments and need help to identify and weigh these. It is further assumed that all patients use a similar (universalistic) method to weigh the benefits and risks of various treatments, an assumption that may or may not be true. We wonder whether it is even possible to construct a valid test to assess the superiority of an explicit values clarification exercise over implicit methods. To do so would require that we first know what the patient's true values are so that we could use them as a 'gold standard' by which to judge which approach resulted in a treatment decision most congruent with these values. But if we knew what the patient's true values were in the first place, we would not need any explicit exercise to help the patient define them. Finally, the exercise of helping patients clarify their values may act inadvertently as an intervention, changing patients' values through the exercise itself. Thus, while laudable in intent, many current values clarification exercises are fraught with difficulties and assumptions that require further evaluation.

CONCLUSION

There are a number of outstanding issues, both conceptual and empirical, that require further investigation in the field of shared decision making between physicians and patients. These include: the definition, types and levels of patient values to be considered when attempting to help patients clarify their preferences for different treatment decisions; the definition and influence of culture on patients' preferences for decision-making processes and outcomes (Charles et al 2006); the fact that measurement activities often drive goal-setting activities for decision aids rather than the other way round; and the lack of precision in the stated rationale for and meaning of various goals suggested for decision aids, and for mechanisms through which they are intended to have an impact.

Further exploration of the above issues will enhance the development of practical tools to support shared decision making between clinicians and patients. We hope that this chapter has helped to inform readers of the many challenges facing researchers and clinicians working in this important field.

References

Charles C A, DeMaio S 1993 Lay participation in health care decision-making: a conceptual framework. Journal of Health Policy and Law 18(4):881–904

Charles C, Gafni A, Whelan T 1997 Shared decision-making in the medical encounter: what does it mean? (or, it takes at least two to tango). Social Science and Medicine 44:681–692

Charles C., Gafni A, Whelan T 1999a Decision-making in the physician-patient encounter: revisiting the shared treatment decision-making model. Social Science and Medicine 49:651–661

Charles C, Whelan T, Gafni A 1999b What do we mean by partnership in making decisions about treatment? British Medical Journal 319:780–782

Charles C, Gafni A, Whelan T 2004 Self-reported use of shared decision-making among breast cancer specialists and perceived barriers and facilitators to implementing this approach. Health Expectations 7 (4):338–348

Charles C, Gafni A, Whelan T et al 2005 Treatment decision aids: conceptual issues and future directions. Health Expectations 8(2):114–125

Charles C, Gafni A, Whelan T et al 2006 Cultural influences on the physician-patient encounter: the case of shared treatment decision-making. Patient Education and Counseling 63(3):262–267

Chassin M R, Brook R H, Park R E 1986 Variations in the use of medical and surgical services by the Medicare population. New England Journal of Medicine 314:285–290

Chassin M R, Kosecoff J, Park R E et al 1987 Does inappropriate use explain geographic variations in the use of health services?: a study of three procedures. Journal of the American Medical Association 258:2533–2537

Deber R 1994 The patient–physician partnership: changing roles and the desire for information. Canadian Medical Association 151:171–176

Eddy D M 1990 Anatomy of a decision. Journal of the American Medical Association 263(3):441–443

Edwards E, Elwyn G 2001 Evidence-based patient choice. Oxford University Press, Oxford

Gafni A, Charles C A, Whelan T 1998 The physician–patient encounter: the physician as a perfect agent for the patient versus the informed treatment decision-making model. Social Science and Medicine 47:347–354

Goel V, Sawka C A, Thiel E C et al 2001 Randomized trial of a patient decision aid for choice of surgical treatment for breast cancer. Medical Decision Making 21(1):1–6

Gwyn R, Elwyn G 1999 When is a shared decision not (quite) a shared decision? Negotiating preferences in a general practice encounter. Social Science and Medicine 49:437–447

Haug M R, Lavin B 1981 Practitioner or patient – who's in charge? Journal of Health and Social Behaviour 22:212–229

Haug M, Lavin B 1983 Consumerism in medicine. Sage, Beverly Hills, CA

Katz S J, Lomas J, Charles C et al 1997 Physician relations in Canada: shooting inward as the circle closes. Journal of Health Policy and Law 22(6):1413–1431

Levine M N, Gafni A, Markham B et al 1992 A bedside decision instrument to elicit a patient's preference concerning adjuvant chemotherapy for breast cancer. Annals of Internal Medicine 117:53–58

Lomas J, Lavis J 1996 Guidelines in the midst. CHEPA Working Paper #96-23, Centre for Health Economics and Policy Analysis, McMaster University, Hamilton, Ontario

Makoul G, Clayman M L 2006 An integrative model of shared decision making in medical encounters. Patient Education and Counseling 60(3):301–312

Montori V, Gafni A, Charles C 2006 A shared treatment decision-making approach between patients with chronic conditions and their clinicians: the case of diabetes. Health Expectations 9(1):25–36

Murray E, Charles C, Gafni A 2006. Clinical decision making in U.K. primary care. Patient Education and Counseling 62:205–211

Nayfield S G, Bongiovanni G C, Alciati M H et al 1994 Statutory requirements for disclosure of breast cancer treatment alternatives. Journal of the National Cancer Institute 86:1202–1208

O'Connor A, Wells G, Tugwell P et al 1999 The effects of an explicit values clarification exercise in a women's

decision aid regarding postmenopausal hormone therapy. Health Expectations 2:21–32

O'Connor A, Llewellyn-Thomas H, Stacey D 2005 International patient decision aid standards collaboration (IPDAS) collaboration background document. Online. Available:http://ipdas.ohri.ca/IPDAS_Background.pdf 27 Feb 2005

Roos N P, Wennberg J E, McPherson K 1988 Using diagnosis-related groups for studying variations in hospital admissions. Health Care Finance and Review 9:53–62

Stevenson F A, Barry C A, Britten N et al 2000 Doctor–patient communication about drugs: the evidence for share decision-making. Social Science and Medicine 50:829–840

Wennberg J E, Freeman J L, Culp W J 1987 Are hospital services rationed in New Haven or over-utilized in Boston? Lancet 329(8543):1185–1189

Whelan T, O'Brien M A, Villasis-Keever M et al 2002 Impact of cancer-related decision aids. Evidence Report/Technology Assessment (Summary) 46:1–4

Whelan T J, Sawka C, Levine M et al 2003 Helping patients make informed choices: a randomized trial of a decision aid for adjuvant chemotherapy in lymph node-negative breast cancer. Journal of the National Cancer Institute 95:581–587

Whelan T, Levine M, Willan A et al 2004 Effect of a decision aid on knowledge and treatment decision-making for breast cancer surgery: a randomized trial. JAMA 292 (4):435–441

Chapter **28**

Algorithms, clinical pathways and clinical guidelines

Karen Grimmer and Stephen Loftus

GUIDELINE HISTORY

In the medical profession, the development of clinical guidelines was first documented in the mid-1970s. Interest in guidelines which specifically address allied health practice took another 10–15 years to emerge. Guidelines were initially produced as statements of best practice regarding the structure and organization of healthcare facilities, and were usually associated with hospital accreditation programmes (Donabedian 1992). These guidelines dealt with issues such as staff registration and training, hygiene, safety and business management. They also highlighted adverse events, events that should not happen in a safe healthcare environment, such as avoidable deaths, unplanned readmission to hospital for the same condition within a specified time period, infections, falls and other avoidable injuries. In the Western world, public and private hospitals are expected to be accredited with a national body to demonstrate how they comply with specified standards of best practice relating to quality care. Compliance with accreditation guidelines is usually measured by performance indicators and benchmarking (within or between organizations), adjusted for size, staffing complement and location.

In the mid-1980s, the Australian Physiotherapy Association led the physiotherapy world, developing a private physiotherapy practice accreditation programme that specified quality frameworks for allied health service delivery (Grimmer et al 1998). This programme has gone from strength to strength in Australia and has formed the basis of accreditation programmes for private and public physiotherapy services in many other countries. Operating on the understanding that quality structural elements of care will produce good health outcomes, the accreditation programme applies consensus standards to each element involved in delivering high-quality physiotherapy service, including staff training, record keeping, length of appointments, regulating the performance of equipment, safety and cleanliness of premises, access, accounting systems and other business practices.

In recent years, academic and clinical interest has turned to developing recommendations to assist in the delivery of high-quality health care as a mechanism to improve health outcomes, reduce adverse events and variations in clinical practice and contain costs (Anderson & Mooney 1991, Antman et al 1992, Sackett et al 2000, Wilson & Harrison 1997). These recommendations have variably been called clinical guidelines, clinical (or care) pathways, care decision-making processes, algorithms or flowcharts. Whatever the nomenclature, these recommendations usually address aspects of clinical decision making such as what care should be provided, how it should be delivered, by whom it should be delivered, where it should be delivered, what equipment is required, and how much care should be provided (Hill 1998).

In this chapter we explore clinical guidelines within a clinical decision-making framework. The usefulness of clinical guidelines should be monitored by process indicators that answer questions such as, 'Was the guideline, or guideline elements, applied using appropriate clinical reasoning approaches?', or 'Did the application of the guideline achieve desired health and cost outcomes?' (Burgers et al 2003). Thus the application of any clinical guideline should include monitoring processes that allow reflection on both the processes and the outcomes of care (Wilson & Harrison 1997), the quality of care provision (Donabedian 1992) and stakeholder satisfaction with the care encounter (Cleary & McNeil 1988).

There has been a recent explosion of allied health clinical guidelines around the world, either as discipline-specific recommendations or as multidisciplinary approaches. Underpinning the development of quality allied health guidelines is the recently published 'Framework for clinical guideline development in physiotherapy' (Van der Wees & Mead 2004), which specifies the processes of guideline development relevant to any allied health discipline.

THE LINK WITH CLINICAL REASONING AND PATIENT OUTCOMES

Evidence-based medicine was famously discussed by Sackett et al (2000) as the judicious use of current best evidence in making decisions about individual patient care. Clinical guidelines are a synthesis of current best evidence, 'systematically developed statements to assist practitioner and patient decisions about appropriate health care for specific clinical circumstances' (Field & Lohr 1990, p. 38). Resistance to implementing clinical guidelines by clinicians is believed to reflect a fear that guideline use will undermine the autonomy of their clinical decision making (Grol & Grimshaw 1999). It seems that social factors have a strong influence on compliance. Thus guidelines are more likely to be accepted if produced locally, and if they reinforce local consensus rather than requiring a change in routine (Fairhurst & Huby 1998). Unfortunately, this is somewhat counterproductive. Guidelines are intended to promote better clinical reasoning and better care on a community-wide basis. Merely reinforcing local practice may not lead to practice according to the best available evidence.

Other barriers to implementing guidelines have been outlined by Entwistle & Shiffman (2005, p. 1), including:

> guideline-related obstacles, both extrinsic to the guideline (organizational and provider specific obstacles) and intrinsic to the guideline (such as failure to meet adequate standards in guideline development and format, identification and summary of evidence, and formulation of recommendations), electronic decision support issues which include such factors as: the extreme complexity of integrated decision support systems; poor alignment of the goals of different players; complex technical requirements; and complex content requirements.

Guideline-based care is meant to provide a framework for decision making by clinicians, not replace the clinician–patient interactions and decision-making processes.

The most useful clinical practice guidelines should be comprehensive, based on valid sources of high-quality research evidence, regularly updated and widely disseminated for comment prior to implementation (Feder et al 1999, Grol et al 1998). Clinical guidelines provide recommendations for the management of specific conditions, based on current best evidence. Best evidence could either reflect the highest available level of research evidence or, in the absence of such evidence for a specific clinical question, could draw on expert or consensus opinion. Best evidence may also change from day to day, based on findings from new research, or debate on interventions with equivocal evidence. The Australian National Health and Medical Research Council (NH&MRC) provides a comprehensive guide for guideline developers, identifying the levels and strength of evidence that should be considered for guidelines (NH&MRC 1998), how recommendations should be framed, and the process of obtaining stakeholder (clinicians, patients, referrers) feedback on the guidelines prior to implementation. Guidelines need to reflect best practice, applied appropriately within the local environment, which addresses patient choice and values.

Much continues to be written about the need for guideline development processes that are rigorous and transparent, as well as for ongoing research to test whether guidelines actually influence clinical practice decisions, improve patient outcomes or contain costs (Grol 2000, Haycox et al 1999, Margolis 1999). There is continuing debate about whether or not guidelines really do improve patient outcomes and decrease costs. These concerns are particularly relevant when guideline recommendations contradict current clinical practice, or when significant change in practice behaviours is required in order to implement guidelines in a sustainable manner (Feder et al 1999, Grimmer et al 2003, Shekelle et al 1999).

ACCESSING GUIDELINES

Finding clinical guidelines requires careful searching of published research in library databases and internet sites. The majority of clinical guidelines have not been published in peer-reviewed journals because they are too long (word count, reference lists, flowcharts and diagrams, etc). Health practitioners interested in clinical guidelines would be wise to bookmark websites with high-quality international guideline sites and regularly search these sites for new guidelines, as guideline development in therapy is an increasing area of activity. Using web search engines to find additional or updated guideline sites is highly recommended in order to keep abreast of changes in guideline development.

CONSTRUCTING GUIDELINES

Guideline users should be provided with sufficient information by guideline developers to demonstrate the validity and clinical utility of the recommendations (NH&MRC 1998), and to allow those users to access the recommended evidence sources to make up their own minds about the validity of recommendations. Guideline information should be presented simply and should fully document both the process of developing the guideline and the sources of supporting evidence. Guidelines should be based on current best practice and recognition of therapist and patient autonomy in decision making (Sackett et al 2000), thus presenting clinicians with fewer barriers to their implementation (Feder et al 1999, Haycox et al 1999, NH&MRC 1998).

GRADING THE EVIDENCE

Most guidelines deal with the effectiveness of specific approaches to treatment, and hence seek to provide users with information from secondary research (systematic reviews or meta-analyses of experimental studies) or from primary research of individual experimental studies, quasi-experimental studies or case studies. However, as guidelines become more sophisticated, they more frequently contain recommendations on diagnosis and risk assessment, drawn from epidemiological and diagnostic classification studies, as well as recommendations on cost-effectiveness of interventions drawn from studies that have investigated some manner of cost–benefit analysis.

A recommended process in developing guidelines is to evaluate the relevant literature using several evidence dimensions (NH&MRC 2000, Sackett et al 2000). This approach provides a framework for establishing the strength of a body of evidence. The NH&MRC guideline development recommendations suggest that the two primary evidence dimensions are first, the hierarchy (or level of evidence which ranks the study design based on potential for error in interpreting findings), and second, the methodological quality of the study. The method of evaluation may be chosen from one of the already published critical appraisal tools (Katrak et al 2004) or by establishing key quality criteria relevant to the topic (Higgins & Green 2005).

HIERARCHY OF EVIDENCE

The lack of international consensus about appropriate ranking of systematic reviews, experimental studies, epidemiological studies, case studies, and expert opinion could result in a situation where two guidelines derived from the same literature could produce two completely different sets of recommendations underpinned by the same evidence, albeit ranked differently with respect to hierarchy and importance. This raises a deeper philosophical point about the ways in which different kinds of evidence are privileged. Evidence-based medicine tends to privilege randomized control trials over case studies, in the belief that such trials bring us accurate knowledge. However, there is increasing support for the case that clinical reasoning is largely based on narrative knowing (Greenhalgh 1998). The proponents of narrative knowing argue that experts are experts and provide better care because they are familiar with a greater number of cases and the subtle differences between them, and that novices learn their practical clinical reasoning by building up their own case knowledge. Therefore, case studies should enjoy a higher status than they do at present within evidence-based medicine theory. Greenhalgh (1999) argued that clinical reasoning is a combination of narrative and the best evidence.

METHODOLOGICAL QUALITY OF EVIDENCE

A recent review of over 100 currently available critical appraisal instruments (Katrak et al 2004) demonstrated that, as with the many and varied ways of describing the hierarchy of evidence, there is no standard appraisal approach to evaluating the methodological quality of studies. Few critical appraisal instruments have been developed along rigorous scientific lines, and few have demonstrated psychometric properties of validity and reliability. The largest number of critical appraisal instruments have been developed for effectiveness studies (experimental/case studies). A small number of generic critical appraisal instruments have been developed in an attempt to provide a standard platform for evaluating methodological quality across the hierarchy of study designs. Using scoring systems to assess methodological quality also raises issues about the appropriateness of weighting all quality-based criteria similarly, and whether an overall methodological score is the most appropriate way to compare studies (Higgins & Green 2005).

DETERMINING THE BEST EVIDENCE

A source of frustration to many guideline developers is determining what is current 'best evidence'. The nature of research into questions about the effectiveness of health care often reflects the need to consider findings from a range of research designs of variable quality. As previously reported (Katrak et al 2004), many critical appraisal instruments do not assess the appropriateness of subject inclusion criteria for the clinical questions, details of interventions, or the importance placed by stakeholders on the measures of outcome. Consequently guideline developers could confront the situation where for a clinical question they may find a small number of trials of poor to moderate quality and inconsistent findings, and a larger number of case studies of a lower hierarchy but with higher methodological quality, with consistent findings. Which evidence should be denoted 'best evidence'?

WEIGHT/STRENGTH OF EVIDENCE

In the absence of standard classifications of study level and quality, guideline developers have taken novel approaches to determining the weight and strength of evidence for effectiveness with which to underpin guideline recommendations. A range of grading systems is found which variously use signs, numbers or alphabetical letters to denote good quality evidence. The disparity between grading systems makes it almost impossible accurately to compare the evidentiary bases of different guidelines.

APPRAISING GUIDELINE QUALITY

The importance of critically appraising guideline quality has been raised by many researchers and clinicians in order to ensure that the recommendations made by the guidelines are credible. In the first instance, guidelines should not be considered by clinicians unless they are available in full text, with a full reference list underpinning the recommendations, so that users can track the source of recommendations for themselves. It is also important to consider guideline development issues relating to:

- *Validity* – does the guideline tell you who was involved in the development? Can you determine the evidence sources? Could you reproduce the guideline development process?
- *Reliability* – would another guideline group, given the same evidence and methodology, produce the same recommendations? Will guideline users interpret them in the same way?
- *Representation* – did all key groups participate in developmental process?
- *Clarity* – is the language in guidelines clear and unambiguous?
- *Clinical flexibility* – is the patient group for whom the guideline was developed the same as the one on which research has been undertaken, which allows extrapolation of findings?
- *Scheduled review* – is there a stated review date so that the evidence can be updated?

Important elements of guideline quality were framed by Cluzeau et al (1997) to help clinicians

to identify areas which may diminish the trustworthiness of guidelines. These questions were:

- *Objectives of the guideline* – are these clearly defined?
- *Context* – is there an explicit description of the patient population and circumstances to which the guideline applies?
- *Responsibility for guideline development* – was there any potential for bias from funding sources?
- *Content of the guideline development group* – were all relevant groups, including consumers, involved in the guideline development process?
- *Identification and interpretation of the evidence* – is there a description of the sources of evidence and methods used to interpret and assess the strength of evidence?
- *Formulation of the recommendations* – are the methods used described?
- *Peer review and piloting of the guideline* – are the methods used described, and how were comments dealt with?
- *Likely costs and benefits* – are the health benefits, costs, potential harms and risks described?
- *Dissemination and implementation* – are methods for these described?

From this work emerged the AGREE instrument (AGREE Collaboration 2001, 2003), which has been used regularly by physiotherapy researchers and clinicians to assess guideline quality (Grimmer et al 2003, MacDermid et al 2005, Van Tulder et al 2004). The AGREE instrument requires at least two assessors and provides formulae to calculate standardized (percentage) scores for six guideline quality domains.

1. *Scope and purpose* reflects information on the overall aim of the guideline, the specific clinical questions and the target patient population.
2. *Stakeholder involvement* deals with the extent to which the guideline reflects the views of its intended users.
3. *Rigour of development* considers the process used to gather and synthesize the evidence, and the methods to formulate the recommendations and update them.
4. *Clarity and presentation* refer to the language and format of the guidelines.

5. *Applicability* relates to the likely behavioural, organizational and cost implications of implementing the guidelines.
6. *Editorial independence* reflects the independence of the guideline recommendations, and acknowledgement of any conflict of interest of guideline developers.

The AGREE instrument has one significant drawback, however, in that it does not take into account the level or strength of evidence used in guidelines. This limits the guideline users' capacity to evaluate the strength of guideline recommendations without undertaking a more in-depth analysis of the evidence that underpins the recommendations (MacDermid et al 2005, Vlayen et al 2005).

GUIDELINE ELEMENTS

Clinical guidelines generally provide two streams of recommendations. These are: (a) care management processes (usually presented as algorithms); and (b) care decision-making processes (usually presented as statements of current best evidence, or clinical recommendations).

CARE MANAGEMENT PROCESSES

Care management processes are generally the least evidence-based aspect of clinical guidelines for health practitioners because of the lack of research underpinning the construction of the episode of care. Clinicians, funders and patients frequently ask 'How much treatment is enough?' (Grimmer et al 2000). Algorithms assist clinicians in evidence-based decision-making processes within an episode of care, where patients' treatment plans may change throughout the episode as a result of their response to intervention. The questions 'How much treatment is enough?' and 'When does a specific intervention stop being effective?' require further research to underpin algorithms of best evidence management. Using the example of acute low back pain, a time-based algorithm was published in the New Zealand College of General Practitioners Clinical Guideline (2003) outlining evidence-based care management

approaches for GPs, using relevant time periods for decision making. One of the oldest guidelines for acute low back pain (Agency for Health Care Policy and Research 1994) provides three congruent algorithms (initial assessment of low back symptoms, further care of acute low back problems, and evaluation of the slow-to-recover patient – still requiring treatment after 4 weeks), which provide reasonable guidance on the progressive treatment of acute low back pain.

CARE DECISION-MAKING PROCESSES

Care decision-making processes reflect evidence-based treatment recommendations. As indicated earlier in this chapter, there is no standard manner in which recommendations are framed on the strength of evidence. Consequently, care decision-making recommendations in one guideline may well be framed differently from those in another guideline because of different language, and different descriptions of the strength of evidence underpinning the recommendation.

REGULARITY OF UPDATE

The regularity of guideline updates depends on the volume of research being published in the clinical area and its relevance (Feder et al 1999, Margolis 1999, NH&MRC 1998, Shekelle et al 1999). Thus guidelines for which there is a consistently large volume of primary research should be revised at least every 2 years in order to identify when recommendations should change as a result of recent research findings. Where primary research is less frequently conducted, guidelines could be revised in longer time frames, but in no case should this be longer than 5 years (Grol 2000).

ADOPTING A GUIDELINE

Adopting a guideline in clinical practice requires systematic decision making and planned implementation strategies. The decision making relates to the choice of guidance and its appropriateness for clinicians, referrers and patients. A commonly adopted theory for guideline implementation is that clinicians should adopt guidelines only for commonly treated conditions which can have variable outcomes, or conversely, for conditions which incur a high cost if treatment is ineffective (Field & Lohr 1990). This relates to the reasons for guideline development – to reduce variability in practice and to improve the likelihood of patients achieving good outcomes. If a clinical department has guidelines in place for common or high cost conditions, then it is believed that treatment for other conditions (not guideline-based) will also improve because of the underlying acceptance of the value of evidence-based practice (Sackett et al 2000, Shekelle et al 1999).

Choosing guidelines to adopt in clinical practice relates to the way that guidelines are framed and worded, in order to obtain maximum impact and minimum confusion regarding interpretation. Consequently, critical appraisal of guideline content and construction is vital. Clinicians should consider how much information they require in order to underpin treatment recommendations. (Do you want to make your own decisions based on the available literature? Do you trust the guideline developers to interpret the literature for you?) The layout of the guideline is also important in facilitating ease of use. (Should the algorithm and recommendations on care decisions be printed on one sheet such as a wall chart, or be provided in readily accessed booklet form, desktop charts or some other readily accessed medium?)

Organizations and health practitioners need to make decisions about whether it is the individual's responsibility to adopt a guideline, or whether the entire organization will adopt the guideline. In both cases, demonstrating group compliance with guidelines requires formal behaviour change mechanisms, such as regular education sessions about guideline construction and content; a clear understanding of current (pre-guideline) practice related to clinical decision making, patient outcomes and stakeholder satisfaction; and regular meetings to debrief about post-implementation interpretation, successful patient outcomes associated with guideline implementation or difficulties with applying

the guideline. Among the reported barriers to the ready acceptance of evidence-based practice are lack of access to readily absorbed information, difficulty in understanding the quality and clinical implications of research findings, lack of understanding of the relative merits of different research designs and uptake of evidence-based recommendations not supported by clinical leadership or formal change management processes (Metcalfe et al 2001).

QUALITY IMPROVEMENT PRACTICES

To measure change which could be attributed to implementing a guideline, implementation processes must include strategies that monitor pre- and post- implementation practices. This information demonstrates whether or not practice and patient outcomes improve with the use of guidelines, or whether guideline implementation needs to be enhanced by activities such as education sessions or introducing standard outcome measures to track change in patient outcomes. Accurate and comprehensive record keeping in clinical practice is essential for high-quality management and clinical review, regardless of whether guidelines are in place. As well as patient details, information such as diagnosis and clinical reasoning prompts, potential risk factors, the interventions that were applied and the outcome measures used should be recorded in full on patient notes at every contact with the patient. For example, there is now a plethora of standard outcome measures available to evaluate the effectiveness of management for most conditions that present to healthcare practitioners. Thus it is a matter for individual practitioners or clinicians in group practice to identify useful outcome measures and implement them on a regular basis throughout the episode of care. Outcome measures need to be applied at least twice to demonstrate change (such as on first and last contact with the patient at a minimum). Outcome measures need to reflect issues that are important to therapist, patient and referrer. In some circumstances they should also reflect issues that are important to the family (or carer) and to the employer.

SUMMARY

High-quality, full text, fully referenced, non-biased clinical guidelines offer health professionals a comprehensive vehicle with which to evaluate and improve their practice. These clinical guidelines provide clinicians with summaries of the current best evidence in the form of algorithms and care-decision-making recommendations, to assist clinicians, patients and referrers to determine best practice care for individual patients. In addition to the wealth of guidelines for medical practitioners there is an increasing number of clinical guidelines developed specifically for allied health practitioners by allied health practitioners, and this initiative is to be welcomed. High-quality guidelines contain the most recent best evidence and are constructed using transparent processes that evaluate the volume and quality of available evidence, framing the recommendations in the context of patient choices and clinical reasoning. Health professionals should consider using high-quality clinical guidelines to underpin their practice, as these guidelines can be applied to develop individual care plans for patients. In a world where 'evidence-based practice' is a common catch-phrase, high-quality clinical guidelines provide allied health practitioners with a persuasive, cost-efficient and effective mechanism with which to evaluate and improve practice.

References

Agency for Health Care Policy and Research (AHCPR) 1994 Acute lower back problems in adults. Clinical Practice Guideline 14, AHCPR Publication No 95–0642. Online. Available: http://www.ncbi.nlm.nih.gov/books/bv.fcgi?rid=hstat6.chapter.25870 10 July 2006

AGREE Collaboration (Appraisal of Guidelines for Research and Evaluation) 2001Online. Available: www.agreecollaboration.org 1 June 2006

AGREE Collaboration 2003 Development and validation of an international appraisal instrument for assessing the quality of clinical practice guidelines: the AGREE project. Quality and Safety in Health Care 12:18–23

Anderson T F, Mooney G 1991 Medical practice variations: where are we? In: Anderson T F, Mooney G (eds) The challenges of medical practice variations. McMillan Press, London, p 1–15

Antman E M, Lau J, Kupelnick G et al 1992 A comparison of meta-analysis of randomised control trials and recommendations of clinical experts. Journal of the American Medical Association 268:240–248

Burgers J S, Grol R P T M, Klazinga N S et al 2003 AGREE Collaboration. Towards evidence-based clinical practice: an international survey of 18 clinical guideline programs. International Journal of Quality in Health Care 15:31–45

Cleary P D, McNeil B J 1988 Patient satisfaction as an indicator of quality care. Inquiry 25:25–36

Cluzeau F, Littlejohns P, Grimshaw J et al 1997 Appraisal instrument for clinical guidelines. London, St George's Hospital Medical School, Online. Available: http://www.sgul.ac.uk/1 June 2006

Donabedian A 1992 The role of outcome in quality assessment and assurance. Quarterly Research Bulletin 18(2):356–360

Entwistle M, Shiffman R N 2005 Turning guidelines into practice: making it happen with standards. Health Care and Informatics Review Online [HCRO] March. Online. Available:http://hcro.enigma.co.nz/website/index.cfm?fuseaction=articledisplay&FeatureID=050305 and http://hcro.enigma.co.nz/website/index.cfm?fuseaction=articledisplay&FeatureID=060305 1 June 2006

Fairhurst K, Huby G 1998 From trial data to practical knowledge: qualitative study of how general practitioners have accessed and used evidence about statin drugs in their management of hypercholesterolaemia. British Medical Journal 317:1130–1134

Feder G, Eccles M, Grol R P T M et al 1999 Using clinical guidelines. British Medical Journal 318:728–730

Field M J, Lohr K N 1990 Clinical practice guidelines: directions for a new program. Institute of Medicine, National Academy Press, Washington DC

Greenhalgh T (ed) 1998 Narrative based medicine: dialogue and discourse in clinical practice. BMJ Books, London

Greenhalgh T 1999 Narrative based medicine: narrative based medicine in an evidence based world. British Medical Journal 318(7179):323–325

Grimmer K, Hughes K, Kerr J et al 1998 An overview of the Australian Physiotherapy Association accredited practice data collection 1995–1996. Australian Journal of Physiotherapy 44:61–63

Grimmer K, Bowman P, Roper J 2000 Episodes of allied health outpatient care: an investigation of service delivery in acute public hospital settings. Disability and Rehabilitation 22:80–87

Grimmer K, Milanese S, Bialocerkowski A 2003 Clinical guidelines for low back pain: physiotherapy perspective. Physiotherapy Canada 55:185–194

Grol R P T M 2000 Between evidence-based practice and total quality management: the implementation of cost-effective care. International Journal of Quality in Health Care 12:297–304

Grol R P T M, Grimshaw J 1999 Evidence-based implementation of evidence-based medicine. Joint Commission Journal on Quality Improvement 25:503–513

Grol R P T M, Mokkink H G A, Dalhuijsen J et al 1998 Dissemination of guidelines: which sources of physicians use in order to be informed? International Journal of Quality in Health Care 10:135–140

Haycox A, Bagust A, Walley T 1999 Clinical guidelines: the hidden costs. British Medical Journal 318:391–393

Higgins J P T, Green S (eds) 2005 Cochrane handbook for systematic reviews of interventions 4.2.5 [Updated May 2005]. In: The Cochrane Library issue 3. Online. Available: www.cochrane.org/resources/handbook/hbook.htm 1 June 2006

Hill M 1998 The development of care management systems to achieve clinical integration. Advanced Practice Nursing Quarterly 4:33–39

Katrak P, Bialocerkowski A, Massy-Westropp N et al 2004 The content of critical appraisal tools. Biomedcentral Research Methodology 4:22. Online. Available: http://www.biomedcentral.com/1471-2288/4/22 11 July 2006.

MacDermid J C, Brooks D, Solway S et al 2005 Reliability and validity of the AGREE instrument used by physical therapists in assessment of clinical practice guidelines. Biomedcentral Health Services Research 5:18. Online. Available: http://www.biomedcentral.com/1472-6963/5/18 11 July 2006.

Margolis C Z 1999 Clinical practice guidelines: methodological considerations. International Journal of Quality in Health Care 11:303–306

Metcalfe C, Lewin R, Wisher S et al 2001 Barriers to implementing the evidence base in four NHS therapies. Physiotherapy 87:433–440

National Health and Medical Research Council 1998 A guide to the development, implementation and evaluation of clinical practice guidelines. Canberra, NH&MRC. Online. Available: http://www.nhmrc.gov.au/publications/synopses/cp30syn.htm 1 June 2006.

National Health and Medical Research Council 2000 How to use the evidence: assessment and application of scientific evidence. Australian Government Publisher, Canberra. Online. Available: http://www.nhmrc.gov.au/publications/synopses/cp30syn.htm 1 June 2006.

New Zealand College of General Practitioners 2003 New Zealand acute low back pain guide, incorporating the guide to assessing psychosocial yellow flags in acute low back pain. Online. Available: http://www.emia.com.au/MedicalProviders/EvidenceBasedMedicine/nzgg/nzgg.html 1 June 2006.

Sackett D L, Richardson W, Rosenberg W et al 2000 Evidence-based medicine: how to practice and teach EBM. Churchill Livingstone, Edinburgh, p 3–15

Shekelle P G, Woolf S H, Eccles M et al 1999 Clinical guidelines: developing guidelines. British Medical Journal 318:593–596

van der Wees P, Mead J 2004 Framework for clinical guideline development in physiotherapy. European Region of the World Confederation for Physical Therapy, general meeting, May

Van Tulder M, Tuut M, Pennick V et al 2004 Quality of primary care guidelines for acute low back pain. Spine 29: E357–E362

Vlayen J, Aertgeerts B, Hannis K et al 2005 A systematic review of appraisal tools for clinical practice guidelines: multiple similarities and one common deficit. International Journal of Quality in Health Care 7: 235–242

Wilson R M, Harrison B T 1997 Are we committed to improving the safety of health care? Medical Journal of Australia 166:452–453

Chapter 29

Clinical reasoning to facilitate cognitive–experiential change

Mark A. Jones and Ian Edwards

CHAPTER CONTENTS

HEALTHCARE PRACTITIONERS ARE TEACHERS

Healthcare practitioners across all disciplines, areas of practice and practice settings assess and collaboratively manage (independently and in conjunction with other health professionals) patients' physical impairments, environment and psychosocial status. This holistic approach to understanding patients and their problems is consistent with the World Health Organization (WHO) model of health and disability (WHO 2001). Healthcare management regularly includes facilitating patients' learning, including under standing of their health condition and factors either predisposing or contributing to the maintenance of their health problems, understanding management options and understanding prognosis. An example of learning commonly required within physiotherapy is patients' awareness of habits in body posture and movement and alternative or more effective strategies, and their understanding and performance of general and specific exercises and self-management strategies. Ideally, clinicians' approach to promoting patient learning is tailored to the individual patient (in terms of expectations and goals, clinical presentation, cognitive and physical capabilities) and to the nature of the learning desired (e.g. technicalities of a specific exercise versus construction of a revised health and disability belief). However, the skill and effectiveness of clinicians in this important aspect of management varies enormously (Payton et al 1998). Ineffectiveness in facilitating patient learning can stem from a multitude of clinician, patient/family/carer, resource and policy factors. Here we focus on factors relating to the clinician, particularly clinicians' understanding and philosophy of health and disability and their approach to promoting patient learning, especially with respect to changing beliefs regarding health and disability.

PHILOSOPHY OF PRACTICE

Healthcare practitioners' philosophy of practice and their world view in general influences their perceptions and their approach to practice (Cusick 2001, Higgs et al 1999, Hooper 1997, Jensen et al 2000, Unsworth 2004). For example, based on research into expert physical therapy practice, Jensen and colleagues' model of expert practice in physical therapy has the therapist's philosophy of practice as the core ingredient of expert practice that both influences and is influenced by four additional integrated dimensions of expert practice: a dynamic, multidimensional knowledge base; a clinical reasoning process embedded in a collaborative, problem-solving approach; a central focus on movement assessment linked to patient function; and consistent virtues seen in caring and commitment to patients. The patient-centred expert practice evident in the findings of this research (see Chapter 11 for further details) is consistent with the intent and requirements of practising within a biopsychosocial as opposed to biomedical philosophy of health care (Borrell-Carrió et al 2004; Engel 1977, 1978; Waddell 1987).

BIOPSYCHOSOCIAL MODEL

The biopyschosocial model as it was originally proposed 'dispenses with the scientifically archaic principles of dualism and reductionism and replaces the simple cause-and-effect explanations of linear causality with reciprocal causal models' (Engel 1978, p. 175).

The WHO model of health and disability (WHO 2001; see also Chapter 22) reflects this biopsychosocial perspective whereby patients' clinical presentations (their body functions and structures or physical status; their capacity and performance of functional activities of life; and their subsequent ability to participate in their family, work and leisure roles) are portrayed as the result of influences (both positive and negative) of their health condition, environment and personal factors. Importantly, the contributions of the physical/biomedical, environmental and psychosocial influences to a particular patient are individual and complex. That is, the individual factors not only combine in determining a patient's disability experience, they also directly influence each other (Borrell-Carrió et al 2004).

However, some clinicians' personal and professional philosophies of practice are clearly more biomedically than biopsychosocially based, leading either to a lack of attention to these influences on patients' presentations (for example the view that 'psychological' aspects of patients' problems are separate from the physical and it is not the clinician's role to manage psychological issues) or to an overly superficial and hence less effective assessment, reasoning and management of psychosocial barriers. This may also be associated with a view that psychosocial factors only become relevant when working with patients in chronic pain and disability and are not relevant to the more acute patient presentations. Further, while health professionals may claim to be biopsychosocially oriented in their assessment, reasoning and management, espoused philosophies of practice do not always reflect actual practice attitudes and behaviours (Argyris & Schön 1978, Jorgensen 2000, Mattingly & Hayes Fleming 1994). In a critical review of cognitive-behavioural theory and practice, Sharp (2001) argued that the cognitive dimension of cognitive-behavioural therapy for chronic pain as reported in the literature is inadequate and that behavioural management inappropriately dominates the cognitive-behavioural interventions. The conception of *biopsychosocial* for some remains dualistic, in that either (a) the patient's presentation is viewed as a combination of biomedical and psychosocial problems, rather than construing biopsychosocial as a genuine integration of mind and body where each influences the other (Borrell-Carrió et al 2004, Duncan 2000, Engel 1978, Pincus 2004), or (b) appreciation and focus are given to psychological factors without appropriate recognition and attention to the social circumstances that have contributed to shaping those cognitions and that remain as barriers to change (Osborn & Smith 1998, Sim & Smith 2004).

Cognitive–behavioural approach

The cognitive-behavioural approach situated in the biopsychosocial model is increasingly put forward as the preferred approach for the management of chronic pain and disability and associated psychosocial influences (e.g. Main et al 2000, Morley et al 1999, Turk & Flor 2006). The evolution of this approach is described elsewhere (Gamsa 1994a, 1994b), but in general it is based on the theory that patients' thoughts, feelings and behaviours are interrelated in their pain or disability experience. Turk & Flor (2006, p. 340) explain that the cognitive-behavioural perspective is based on five central assumptions:

1. People are active processors of information and not passive reactors.
2. Thoughts (e.g. appraisals, expectancies and beliefs) can elicit and influence mood, affect physiological processes, have social consequences, and also serve as an impetus for behaviour; conversely, mood, physiology, environmental factors and behaviour can influence the nature and content of thought processes.
3. Behaviour is reciprocally determined by both the individual and environmental factors.
4. People can learn more adaptive ways of thinking, feeling and behaving.
5. People should be active collaborative agents in changing their maladaptive thoughts, feelings and behaviours.

Based on individual patient assessment, cognitive-behavioural management then draws on a combination of explanation and education directed at facilitating restructuring of unhelpful or maladaptive thoughts and associated feelings, and operant behavioural techniques to strengthen patients' constructive thoughts, self-efficacy and active coping behaviours while discouraging the reverse (Jones & Edwards 2006). The aim is to assist patients in gaining control over the effects of pain and disability while also modifying the actual affective, behavioural, cognitive and sensory aspects of the experience (Turk & Flor 2006).

PSYCHOSOCIAL FACTORS CONTRIBUTE TO THE DISABILITY EXPERIENCE

In the biopsychosocial and WHO models of health and disability, patients' thoughts, feelings, self-efficacy and coping strategies contribute (positively and negatively) to their disability experiences (Craig 2006, Flor & Turk 2006, Gottlieb et al 2001, Jones & Edwards 2006, King et al 2002).

Psychosocial factors, of course, involve more than just the patient's own thoughts and feelings; the expressed or perceived thoughts and feelings and the behaviour of others (healthcare practitioners, family, friends, acquaintances and service representatives such as insurers and resource providers) also influence an individual's disability experience. For example, in a qualitative study investigating the personal experience and psychological processes involved in maintaining pain, distress and disability in subjects presenting with benign chronic low back pain, Osborn & Smith (1998) used an interpretative phenomenological analysis to identify four themes common to the participants: (a) searching for an explanation; (b) comparing this self with other selves; (c) not being believed; and (d) withdrawing from others. The frustrations regarding inadequate explanation from the medical system reported by these participants is well recognized as an iatrogenic contributing factor to maintained disability (e.g. Main et al 2000, Main & Watson 2002). The effect of these subjects' self-image was evident in their continuing comparisons to others and to their memory of their past selves while also projecting who they were likely to be in the future (Osborn & Smith 1998, p. 72):

> Their contemporary self-regard contrasted with a nostalgic recall of their past and those around them, and their comparisons served almost inevitably as an index of their sense of threat and loss. Attempts to buttress self-esteem by comparison with those more unfortunate often proved counterproductive and served only to remind participants of their own gloomy prognosis.

Sim & Smith (2004) noted that this loss of a former self is a common finding in people suffering with chronic disability and pain, and described the circumstances that leave these people with a fundamental choice of trying to maintain their former self in spite of the pain, to suspend the former self in the hope that it can be regained once the pain is gone, or to come to terms with a new painful self.

The third theme identified by Osborn & Smith (1998) of not being believed created for the participants a continual need to justify their pain, and the incongruity of being mobile or appearing healthy created a sense that they should appear ill in order to conform to the expectations of others. The participants' tendency to withdraw from others was the final theme. The researchers related this to participants' fear of misunderstanding and rejection, highlighting the various and complex forms which fear-avoidance may take (Phillips 1987). In other words, fear-avoidance may have a social basis and not just a biomedical one.

With recognition that the thoughts, feelings and behaviours of patients and others influence disability, healthcare practitioners clearly need strategies and skills in assessing and managing these influences within the limits of their professional training. The level of education health practitioners receive in this area varies enormously, both across and within professions. Although it is not realistic to refer all patients to healthcare practitioners with more extensive education in psychosocial assessment and management (e.g. psychologists), superficial assessments leading to superficial judgements and inappropriate management are equally inappropriate. All healthcare professions have their own body of literature to assist their members' understanding and application in this important area. For example, there is now very helpful physiotherapy literature providing suggestions on assessment and management strategies specifically targeting patients' unhelpful thoughts, feelings and behaviours (e.g. Harding 1998, Johnson & Moores 2006, Keefe et al 2006, Kendall & Watson 2000, Main & Watson 2002, Muncey 2002, Strong & Unruh 2002). However, as discussed above, many clinicians either have not incorporated this approach into their philosophy and application of practice or have acknowledged its importance but take a superficial approach to psychosocial assessment and management.

It is not uncommon to find recommended management strategies that selectively ignore patients'

maladaptive coping behaviours while reinforcing their adaptive responses *without* providing practitioners with explanation as to how judgements of adaptive versus maladaptive should be made. It is as though there is an assumption that maladaptive thoughts, statements and behaviours can be defined out of context and some sort of universal truth exists that defines for everyone what is normal versus abnormal. For example, praying is classically given as an example of a passive coping behaviour that should be challenged and ideally replaced with something more active. However, judgements such as this simply cannot be made out of context. Whereas for one person praying may well be a passive coping behaviour linked to an excessively negative perspective, for another it may function as an active coping mechanism with links to positive thoughts, providing a source of strength and conviction to fight on. We certainly take issue with such a positivist position regarding judgements about normality and motivation. Any assessment of a patient's beliefs, emotions and behaviours cannot be made without a deeper understanding of the person (including personal perceptions and social influences) and the basis for their perspectives. Kleinman et al (1992, p. 6) highlight the challenge this creates to the epistemological premise that underpins traditional biomedical theory and research, 'namely that there is objective knowledge, knowledge apart from subjective experience'. Although it may not be the intent of those promoting cognitive-behavioural therapy, it is very common to see such superficial judgements being made in practice.

SCHEMATA UNDERLYING PATIENTS' COGNITIVE/AFFECTIVE STATUS

Because disability is influenced by patients' past and present psychosocial circumstances, even with the same medical condition (e.g. low back pain, cardiorespiratory or neurological disorder), no two patients will have the same disability experience. Understanding what patients think and feel about their disability is an important first step in determining how their cognitive/affective status may be positively or negatively affecting them and their recovery. However, when patients with the same or similar medical conditions are viewed by the clinician as homogeneous, or when patients' disability experiences are superficially explored (either through questionnaires alone or through shallow questioning) without attending to the basis of their expressed thoughts and feelings, the result is incomplete understanding and either failure to address important cognitive/affective factors or superficial attention to these factors with less than optimal results.

A construct we find promising for encouraging clinicians to seek a fuller understanding of patients' disability experiences, so that patients' thoughts are not oversimplified as simply internal behaviours that can be managed solely through operant behavioural strategies, is the notion of illness, pain and self schemata and how they are influenced by a person's disability experience. Pincus & Morley (2001) reviewed the literature on selective information processing bias in chronic pain patients and, based on conflicting research findings related to attention, interpretation and memory bias, proposed that patients' cognitive/affective status can be portrayed as schemata comprising personal perspectives (conscious and unconscious) linked with internal (e.g. sensory) and external (e.g. past and present life and disability-specific experiences) stimuli that contribute to determining patients' attention, interpretations, behaviours and coping.

Illness schemata

Research in medical anthropology, medical sociology and cognitive psychology has contributed to the understanding of illness representations or schemata. In what is recognized as a seminal article, Leventhal et al (1980) put forward the notion that patients' mental representations of health threats determine how they respond to those threats. Illness schemata are defined as individuals' 'implicit theories of illness' that they use in order to interpret and respond to health threats. These illness representations are like imprints, or patterns of interconnected features, learned through social and personal experiences. Skelton & Croyle (1991, p. 4) reported on illness cognition research supporting the thesis that lay illness schemata comprise the following elements:

1. concrete *symptoms* and a *label* (e.g. common cold versus pneumonia) that facilitate identification of the health problem, beliefs about
2. the immediate and long-term *consequences* of the problem and
3. its *temporal course*, and attributions concerning
4. the *cause* of the problem and
5. the means by which a *cure* may be affected.

Pincus & Morley (2001) added to these elements evaluative dimensions relating to the disability, autonomous functioning, quality of life and emotional expectations. For example, Bishop (1991) identified a number of dimensions that people use in evaluating a medical condition, including such things as seriousness, social desirability, personal responsibility, controllability and changeability. Thus it is not only people's existing beliefs and assumptions that make up their illness schema and contribute to determining their coping but also their appraisal of the threat posed by their medical condition.

Pain schema

Pincus & Morley (2001) portrayed the pain schema as comprising the immediate sensory–intensity, spatial and temporal features of pain, along with the initial affective responses and self-protective behaviours that ensue.

Self schema

The self schema is a complex multifaceted construct that relates to *who you are* with reference to *who you used to be* (prior to your perceived change in self) and *who you would like to be* in the future. It includes an evaluative dimension that contributes to an individual's sense of self-worth. Disability has the potential to disrupt aspects of the self such that repeated failures to function 'normally', and the negative emotions that result, can lead to changes in a person's self-image (Osborne & Smith 1998, Sim & Smith 2004).

SCHEMA ENMESHMENT

Schemata evolve over time, and the repeated simultaneous activation of aspects from different schemata is thought to be a mechanism of learning that results in a blurring of representations such that elements from one schema become incorporated in another. This enmeshment of schemata is believed to be one explanation for the observation that events leading to activation of one schema with relatively benign consequences can develop into a schema evoking more significant effects (Pincus & Morley 2001). For example, enmeshment of the pain schema and the self schema could result in a patient's aggravation of pain, not simply evoking specific pain behaviours (e.g. grimaces or cessation of activity), but also activating the patient's negative self schema such that the pain provocation evokes negative thoughts and self-statements.

Pincus & Morley (2001) put forward examples of possible interrelationships that can exist between a person's pain, illness and self schemata (Figure 29.1). Figure 29.1A portrays the relationship in a healthy person, where there is only partial overlap. The extent of overlap in acute pain is reported to depend on the context, and the authors provide the example of pain occurring with needle

puncture during blood donation having no significance to general physical well-being and little relevance to the sense of self other than perhaps strengthening the person's sense of altruism. In contrast, the same needle puncture pain occurring with a blood test for a potentially fatal disease would clearly activate both pain and illness schemata but also contemplation of the self and what the future may hold. Figure 29.1B is suggested as an enmeshment that might be found with a chronic pain patient who is adaptively coping with the condition and whose 'self' is largely unchanged and self-worth is retained. Figure 29.1C portrays a situation where the pain and self schemata are enmeshed without change to the illness schema. Here Pincus & Morley offered the example of the athlete whose pain following a traumatic injury has impacted on self-identity but without any significant activation of illness scenarios. Lastly, in Figure 29.1D all three schemata are enmeshed, as might occur in the chronic pain patient who is not coping and where the threats associated with the pain/illness experience have led to serious changes in the patient's concepts of self and self-worth.

We present this schema theory not to suggest that new discrete psychological categorizations are needed. Rather, we put this theory forward as we feel it highlights that patients are clearly not homogeneous in their psychosocial presentations while illustrating examples of factors (schemata) and combinations of factors (schema enmeshment) that may contribute to a patient's disability experience. It is hoped that this deeper view of patients' thoughts and feelings will discourage clinicians from limiting themselves to superficial assessments and superficial judgements regarding patients' cognitions, emotions and disability behaviours.

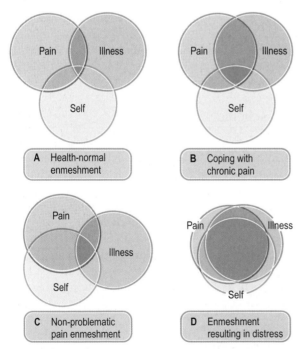

Figure 29.1 Variations in the overlap of pain, illness, and self schemata. (From Pincus & Morley 2001. Copyright © 2001 by the American Psychological Association. Reprinted with permission)

COGNITIVE–EXPERIENTIAL MANAGEMENT FOR FACILITATING PATIENT LEARNING

The interactions of patients' cognitions and emotions with their pain or disability experiences are well documented (e.g. Craig 2006, Flor & Turk 2006), and Turk & Flor (2006) have highlighted the growing body of evidence supporting the cognitive-behavioural approach in the management of a wide range of pain syndromes. However, we propose that a reconceptualization from cognitive-behavioural to *cognitive–experiential* may assist in discouraging superficial approaches to psychosocial assessment and cognitive-behavioural management. A cognitive–experiential approach requires a different focus of assessment than that traditionally used for determination of a physical diagnosis and requires management reasoning and action directed toward understanding and promoting change (i.e. learning) in patients' pain and disability experiences.

Clinical reasoning and the interpretation of experience

'Believing ... that man is an animal suspended in webs of significance he himself has spun, I take culture to be those webs, and the analysis of it to be therefore not an experimental science in search of law but an interpretive one in search of meaning' (Geertz 1973, p. 5).

In endeavouring to understand the decisions and actions that may arise from patients' interpretations of experience, models of reasoning which can embrace different paradigms of inquiry (as suggested by Geertz) are called for. We propose such a model of reasoning in this chapter (see also Chapter 22). Firstly, it is useful to reconceptualize one of the roles of clinical reasoning in clinical practice. Clinical reasoning is not only concerned with how clinicians interpret a broad range of data in the conduct of practice and then learn from their reasoning, through the 'outcomes' or consequences of their decision making; it is also concerned with fostering a process of adult learning in *and* together with patients regarding what can be learned to assist them to move from one place of understanding of their health to another place of understanding and therefore decision making. In the clinical practice context this will usually involve both an *instrumental* and a *communicative* form of learning. These two forms of learning are the products of different reasoning processes.

Instrumental learning arises from reasoning using assumptions that knowledge is objective, measurable, predictive and generalizable (Edwards et al 2006, Mezirow 1991). Some of the excellent behavioural strategies used in cognitive-behavioural therapy may fall within the process of instrumental learning, where patients are taught

particular ways of responding to and coping with pain; ways which might be useful for many other patients in a similar situation. The evaluation of such learning is amenable to an empirical evaluation in terms of performance or non-performance of particular tasks.

Unhelpful schema enmeshment is proposed to be a product of learning related to patients' pain and disability experiences (Pincus & Morley 2001). Understanding the interpretation of experience requires a communicative form of learning (Edwards et al 2006) arising from a narrative reasoning approach which utilizes assumptions about knowledge, including that knowledge is context-dependent, socially constructed, has multiple realities and is also irrevocably linked to historical, cultural and structural factors (Germov 2005). In other words, with respect to the latter factors, neither knowledge nor data can be understood apart from such contexts. For example, an understanding of the aetiology of the ongoing poor health of indigenous people in Australia cannot be separated from an understanding of their stories (narratives) and the history of Aboriginal people since European settlement began in 1788 (Gray & Saggers 2005).

Working with patients for better health, when framed in adult learning terms, involves another kind of skill building in addition to teaching behavioural strategies, relevant and constructive though they undoubtedly can be. It also involves patients learning how to reflect critically on their situations using both forms of learning – instrumental and communicative – and the understanding of knowledge associated with each. The term 'critical' in critical reflection does not mean necessarily reflecting more profoundly but reflecting with a critical examination of the assumptions underlying a presently held set of values and conclusions (or interpretations) from one's experiences (Brookfield 2000).

The adult learning process described here has been termed 'transformatory learning' (Mezirow 1991). In this chapter we also describe it as a *cognitive–experiential* approach to learning for better health. In using this term we wish to highlight what we consider an important element not necessarily captured in cognitive-behavioural approaches toward better health. The adult learning process of cognitive–experiential learning does not focus primarily on identifying, addressing and then modifying or changing identified activities and visible behaviours. Certainly, the aim or end result of such cognitive–experiential learning may well see the patient change unhelpful behaviours. Also, such identified data form an essential part of most health practitioners' assessment practices and help direct goal setting and collaborative processes. Notwithstanding, a cognitive–experiential learning process also focuses on how patients' interpretations of experience (pain, illness and/or disability) have created meanings which then inform their beliefs and, importantly, their decision making regarding their health. Using the quoted assertions of Geertz (1973), part of our inquiry, as a basis for further learning, is to understand 'the webs of significance' which patients have created for and about themselves. In certain circumstances such a web may be supportive, whereas in others it may enmesh patients, leaving them less able to function and participate in roles and activities than they would otherwise wish.

One of the most debilitating experiences of patients with chronic pain, as one increasingly common example of ill health, has been the so-called irrational and recalcitrant behaviour of such pain. In so-called 'central pain states', pain is no longer modulated by the same linear or cause-and-effect neurophysiological processes found in acute pain. Instead the pattern and behaviour of pain is less predictable, with secondary hyperalgesia creating false positive findings to traditional physical assessments that are often misinterpreted as indicative of local impairment and pathology (Fields et al 2006, Gifford et al 2006). Traditionally, such pain was difficult to validate on clinical examination, leading to a range of behavioural diagnoses based on an instrumental or biomedical form of reasoning (Gifford et al 2006, Main and Watson 2002, Waddell 2004). However, current pain research has provided patients with a plausible account of the 'irrationality' of chronic pain (Edwards et al 2006, Fields et al 2006, Gifford et al 2006). This research has been important because no longer are patients themselves held to be the primary source of irrationality in the situation (Steen & Haugli 2000). Instead of feeling compelled to act out particular social roles (such as the sick role) either successfully or unsuccessfully, as discussed earlier (Osborn & Smith 1998, Steen & Haugli 2000), patients are enabled to participate in more constructive learning processes. For example, patients are enabled to begin to identify the effects of the problem (e.g. pain) on their lives rather than viewing themselves and their pain as inextricable entities (Orchison 1997, White & Epston 1990). We see this as part of 'un-enmeshing' the enmeshed schemata discussed above.

CONCLUSION

The increasing body of evidence demonstrating significant influences of psychosocial factors on patients' pain and disability experiences has resulted in greater use of cognitive-behavioural approaches, particularly in therapies involved in the management of chronic pain and disability. However, the cognitive-behavioural approach has been criticized for its excessive focus on behavioural management, with a tendency for all patients with apparent psychosocial contributing factors to be treated as a single homogeneous group as though their cognitions, feelings and behaviours all had a similar basis that would be responsive to some generic application of cognitive-behavioural principles. Schemata and health representation theory provide some insight into how people structure their understanding of health, disability and pain which should discourage superficial approaches to the assessment and management of psychosocial factors. Cognitive–experiential learning represents a form of learning which utilizes reasoning processes from different paradigms of knowledge generation. To this extent we believe that it is a form of learning which expresses the underlying diverse scope of factors which influence and even 'construct' disability and which are, in turn, expressed in the WHO ICF model (2001) and the biopsychosocial model underpinning that (Imrie 2004). Cognitive–experiential learning has received more attention in terms of research in the field of adult learning than in health (Mezirow 2000). Our view expressed in this chapter is that cognitive–experiential learning holds significant promise in the area of persons learning to make constructive decisions regarding their health, particularly in situations of existing illness and the kinds of disability associated with chronic conditions. We have touched on chronic pain as one example of this. The measurement of outcomes from this type of learning related to patient decision making in health and disability remains a challenge for further research.

References

Argyris C, Schön D 1978 Organizational learning: a theory in action perspective. Addison-Wesley, Reading

Bishop G D 1991 Understanding the understanding of illness: lay disease representations. In: Skelton J A, Croyle R T (eds) Mental representation in health and illness. Springer-Verlag, New York, p 32–59

Borrell-Carrió F, Suchman A L, Epstein R M 2004 The biopsychosocial model 25 years later: principles, practice, and scientific inquiry. Annals of Family Medicine 2(6):576–582

Brookfield S 2000 Clinical reasoning and generic thinking skills. In: Higgs J, Jones M (eds) Clinical reasoning in the health professions, 2nd edn. Butterworth-Heinemann, Oxford, p 62–67

Craig K D 2006 Emotions and psychobiology. In: McMahon S, Koltzenburg M (eds) Wall and Melzack's textbook of pain, 5th edn. Elsevier, Philadelphia, p 231–239

Cusick A 2001 Personal frames of reference in professional practice. In: Higgs J, Titchen A (eds) Practice knowledge and expertise in the health professions. Butterworth-Heinemann, Oxford, p 91–95

Duncan G 2000 Mind–body dualism and the biopsychosocial model of pain: what did Descartes really say? Journal of Medicine and Philosophy 25:485–513

Edwards I, Jones M A, Hillier S 2006 The interpretation of experience and its relationship to body movement: a clinical reasoning perspective. Manual Therapy 11:2–10

Engel G L 1977 The need for a new medical model: a challenge for biomedicine. Science 196:129–136

Engel G 1978 The biopsychosocial model and the education of health professionals. Annals New York Academy of Sciences 310:535–544

Fields H L, Basbaum A I, Heinricher M M 2006 Central nervous system mechanisms of pain modulation. In: McMahon S, Koltzenburg M (eds) Wall and Melzack's textbook of pain, 5th edn. Elsevier, Philadelphia, p 125–142

Flor H, Turk D C 2006 Cognitive and learning aspects. In: McMahon S, Koltzenburg M (eds) Wall and Melzack's textbook of pain, 5th edn. Elsevier, Philadelphia, p 241–258

Gamsa A 1994a The role of psychological factors in chronic pain. I. A half century of study. Pain 57:5–15

Gamsa A 1994b The role of psychological factors in chronic pain. II. A critical appraisal. Pain 57:17–29

Geertz C 1973 The interpretation of cultures. Basic Books, New York

Germov J 2005 Imagining health problems as social issues. In: Germov J (ed) Second opinion – an introduction to health sociology, 3rd edn. Oxford University Press, Oxford p 3–27

Gifford L, Thacker M, Jones M A 2006 Physiotherapy and pain. In: McMahon S, Koltzenburg M (eds) Wall and Melzack's textbook of pain, 5th edn. Elsevier, Philadelphia, p 603–617

Gottlieb A, Golander H, Bar-Tal Y et al 2001 The influence of social support and perceived control on handicap and quality of life after stroke. Aging Clinical Experimental Research 13:11–15

Gray D, Saggers S 2005 Indigenous health: the perpetuation of inequality. In: Germov J (ed) Second opinion – an introduction to health sociology, 3rd edn. Oxford University Press, Oxford, p 111–128

Harding V 1998 Cognitive-behavioural approach to fear and avoidance. In: Gifford L (ed) Topical issues in pain 1 CNS Press, Falmouth, p 173–191

Higgs C, Neubauer D, Higgs J 1999 The changing health care context: globalization and social ecology. In: Higgs J, Edwards H (eds) Educating beginning practitioners: challenges for health professional education. Butterworth-Heinemann, Oxford, p 30–37

Hooper B 1997 The relationship between pretheoretical assumptions and clinical reasoning. American Journal of Occupational Therapy 51(5):328–338

Imrie R 2004 Demystifying disability: a review of the International Classification of Functioning, Disability and Health. Sociology of Health and Illness 26(3):287–305

Jensen G M, Gwyer J, Shepard K F et al 2000 Expert practice in physical therapy. Physical Therapy 80(1):28–43

Johnson R, Moores L 2006 Pain management: integrating physiotherapy and clinical psychology. In: Gifford L (ed) Topical issues in pain 5. CNS Press, Falmouth, p 311–319

Jones M A, Edwards I 2006 Learning to facilitate change in cognition and behaviour. In: Gifford L (ed) Topical issues in pain 5. CNS Press, Falmouth, p 273–310

Jorgensen P 2000 Concepts of body and health in physiotherapy: the meaning of the social/cultural aspects of life. Physiotherapy Theory and Practice 16(2):105–115

Keefe F, Scipio C, Perri L 2006 Psychosocial approaches to managing pain: current status and future directions. In: Gifford L (ed) Topical issues in pain 5. CNS Press, Falmouth, p 241–256

Kendall N, Watson P 2000 Identifying psychosocial yellow flags and modifying management. In: Gifford L (ed) Topical issues of pain 2. CNS Press, Falmouth, p 131–139

King G, Tucker M A, Baldwin P et al 2002 A life needs model of pediatric service delivery: services to support community participation and quality of life for children and youth with disabilities. Physical and Occupational Therapy in Pediatrics 22(2):53–77

Kleinman A, Brodwin P E, Good B J et al 1992 Pain as human experience: an introduction. In: Good M J D, Brodwin P E, Good B J, Kleinman A (eds) Pain as human experience: an anthropological perspective. University of California Press, Berkeley, p 1–28

Leventhal H, Meyer D, Nerenz D 1980 The common sense representation of illness danger. In: Rachman S (ed) Contributions to medical psychology, vol 2. Pergamon Press, New York, p 7–30

Main C, Watson P 2002 The distressed and angry low back pain patient. In: Gifford L (ed) Topical issues in pain 3. CNS Press, Falmouth, p 175–192

Main C J, Spanswick C C, Watson P 2000 The nature of disability. In: Main C J, Spanswick C C (eds) Pain management: an interdisciplinary approach. Churchill Livingstone, Edinburgh, p 89–106

Mattingly C, Fleming M H 1994 Clinical reasoning: forms of inquiry in a therapeutic practice. F A Davis, Philadelphia

Mezirow J 1991 Transformative dimensions of adult learning. Jossey-Bass, San Francisco

Mezirow J 2000 Learning to think like an adult: core concepts of transformation theory. In: Mezirow J (ed) Learning as transformation: critical perspectives on a theory in progress. Jossey-Bass, San Francisco, p 3–33

Morley S, Eccleston C, Williams A 1999 Systematic review and meta-analysis of randomized controlled trials of cognitive behaviour therapy and behaviour therapy for chronic pain in adults, excluding headache. Pain 80:1–13

Muncey H 2002 Explaining pain to patients. In: Gifford L S (ed) Topical issues in pain 4. CNS Press, Falmouth, p 157–166

Orchison R 1997 From pain-full narratives to pain-less lives. Dulwich Centre Newsletter. Adelaide. 4:31–35

Osborn M, Smith J A 1998 The personal experience of chronic benign lower back pain: an interpretative phenomenological analysis. British Journal of Health Psychology 3:65–83

Payton O D, Nelson C E, Hobbs M S C 1998 Physical therapy patients' perceptions of their relationships with health care professionals. Physiotherapy Theory and Practice 14:211–221

Phillips H C 1987 Avoidance behaviour and its role in sustaining chronic pain. Behaviour Research and Therapy 25:273–279

Pincus T 2004 The psychology of pain. In: French S, Sim J (eds) Physiotherapy: a psychosocial approach. Elsevier, Edinburgh, p 95–115

Pincus T, Morley S 2001 Cognitive-processing bias in chronic pain: a review and integration. Psychological Bulletin 127:599–617

Sharp T J 2001 Chronic pain: a reformulation of the cognitive-behavioural model. Behaviour Research and Therapy 39:787–800

Sim J, Smith M V 2004 The sociology of pain. In: French S, Sim J (eds) Physiotherapy: a psychosocial approach. Elsevier, Edinburgh, p 117–139

Skelton J A, Croyle R T 1991 Mental representation, health, and illness: an introduction. In: Skelton J A, Croyle R T (eds) Mental representation in health and illness. Springer-Verlag, New York, p 1–9

Steen E, Haugli L 2000 Generalised chronic musculoskeletal pain as a rational reaction to a life situation? Theoretical Medicine 21:581–599

Strong J, Unruh A M 2002 Psychologically based pain management strategies. In: Strong J, Unruh A M, Wright A, Baxter G D (eds) Pain: a textbook for therapists. Churchill Livingstone, Edinburgh, p 169–185

Turk D, Flor H 2006 The cognitive-behavioural approach to pain management. In: McMahon S, Koltzenburg M (eds) Wall and Melzack's textbook of pain, 5th edn. Elsevier, Philadelphia, p 339–348

Unsworth C A 2004 Clinical reasoning: how do pragmatic reasoning, worldview and client-centredness fit? British Journal of Occupational Therapy 67(1):10–19

Waddell G 1987 A new clinical model for the treatment of low back pain. Spine 12:632–644

Waddell G 2004 The back pain revolution, 2nd edn. Churchill Livingstone, Edinburgh

White M, Epston D 1990 Narrative means to therapeutic ends. W W Norton, New York

World Health Organization 2001 International classification of functioning, disability and health. World Health Organization, Geneva

SECTION 5

Communicating about clinical reasoning

SECTION CONTENTS

Chapter **30**

Learning to communicate clinical reasoning

Rola Ajjawi and Joy Higgs

CHAPTER CONTENTS

INTRODUCTION

In this chapter we present research (Ajjawi 2006; Ajjawi et al 2004, 2005a, b) investigating how practitioners develop the ability to understand and communicate their reasoning and the place of communities of practice in facilitating such learning journeys. There is no doubt that clear and effective communication of clinical reasoning is essential for all health professional practice, especially in the current healthcare climate. Increasing litigation leading to legal requirements for comprehensive information exchange between health professionals and patients (including their caregivers) and the drive for active consumer involvement are just two factors that emphasize the importance of clear communication and collaborative decision making. Health professionals are accountable for their decisions and service provision to various stakeholders, including clients, health sector managers, policy makers and colleagues. An important aspect of this accountability is the ability to clearly articulate and justify management decisions.

Because of its rapid, complex and often subconscious nature, clinical reasoning is not a skill that can be simply explained, understood and recalled. It is possible, however, to 'slow down' and systematically examine some of the processes involved in reasoning in order to reflect on them more clearly, thereby facilitating articulation of clinical reasoning. Effective communication of clinical reasoning involves a depth of knowledge and understanding of clinical reasoning and all the factors involved in and influencing the decision-making process. Practitioners must draw on formal, professional and personal knowledge to inform both the content and process of communicating reasoning (Siminoff & Step 2005). In addition, communication of clinical reasoning in practice is multifactorial, requiring cognitive and metacognitive processing of many factors about the co-communicator(s), the message to be communicated and the environmental context in which the communication takes place.

There has been little research in the health sciences into how health professionals learn to communicate clinical reasoning in practice. Learning of such a complex skill begins at university and continues following graduation in practitioners' chosen career paths. We propose that learning to communicate clinical reasoning is a journey of professional socialization that is supported and developed by communities of practice. A community of practice has been defined as a 'set of relations among persons, activity and world, over time and in relation with other tangential and overlapping communities of practice' (Lave & Wenger 1991, p. 98). Learning takes place through engagement in actions and interactions that are embedded in the culture and history forming the community of practice. Learning in communities of practice and the emphasis on the cultural learning process can be seen as essential parts of the broader concept and process of professional socialization (Abrandt Dahlgren et al 2004) that is based on learning the particular profession's socially constructed norms, values and beliefs through interaction within workplace and cultural situations (Richardson 1999). Thus, learning involves forming and developing professional identities with the embodied ability to behave and think as community members, along with the ability to communicate in the language of the community. Language, both spoken and written, is an important mediator of social interaction (Vygotsky 1978, Wells 1999).

RESEARCH DESIGN

In the first-named author's doctoral research (Ajjawi 2006) the goal was to investigate how experienced physiotherapists, having learned to reason, then learn to communicate their reasoning to patients and novice physiotherapists. A hermeneutic phenomenology approach was adopted. Participants were eight female and four male physiotherapists from major teaching hospitals in metropolitan Sydney, Australia. Their working experience ranged from 6 to 26 years, and their experience of supervising students or novice clinicians ranged from 2 to 24 years.

Data collection methods included observation, written reflective exercises and repeated semi-structured interviews. Data collection was spread over several months to enable participants to accommodate this additional task within busy work schedules and to promote reflection on the research phenomenon during daily work practices.

Data were collated, audiotapes were transcribed verbatim and a six-stage approach to analysing the transcripts was adopted, incorporating hermeneutic and phenomenological data analysis methods informed by the systematic data analysis methods developed by Titchen and colleagues (Edwards & Titchen 2003, Titchen & McIntyre 1993):

- immersion in the data and organization of data into texts
- identification of participants' interpretations and constructs (first order constructs)
- interpretation of these by the researcher (second order constructs)
- identification of sub-themes and themes
- elaboration of themes and clarification of relationships among themes
- integration of findings into a model.

The themes identified are listed in Box 30.1.

FINDINGS: LEARNING TO COMMUNICATE CLINICAL REASONING

For the participants in this study, learning to communicate clinical reasoning was part of a journey of professional socialization, situated and embedded in daily practices and supported by communities of practice. Working as practitioners provided them with opportunities to practise communication of clinical reasoning in their

Box 30.1 Themes identified: learning to communicate clinical reasoning (after Ajjawi 2006)

Learning to communicate clinical reasoning is:

1. Situated, embedded and enriched in practice
2. Driven by professional attributes and responsibilities
3. Supported, fostered and framed by communities of practice
4. Influenced by the workplace culture
5. Enhanced by experiential learning strategies
6. Promoted by self-evaluation and reflection on practice
7. Stimulated and deepened by reflexivity

everyday work with a wide variety of people, which aided in the development of their communication ability. These opportunities were often unplanned and revolved around 'authentic contribution' in work practices, communicating with patients about their conditions and management plans, educating students about reasoning, and communicating in team meetings and continuing education lectures. For example, participants spoke about learning to communicate reasoning:

> I think experience has had a lot to play with it, working with some senior therapists that have been involved in research and have a very good understanding of their area, . . . mentoring and modelling behaviour, I think that has really helped.

> I've had to think a lot about how I get the information across. We sometimes do group family education sessions about brain injury and [explaining] physiotherapy interventions involved . . . and I always have to think very carefully about how I say things because not only do I have to try and get really good clear, concise information across but I have to do it in lay terms . . . And at times answer challenging questions in lay terms as well.

Participants reported that learning to communicate their reasoning was often a subconscious and invisible process. They said they thought less often about communicating reasoning than about

reasoning itself, despite the fact that communication of clinical reasoning was a central feature of their practice with patients and with novice physiotherapists. Implicit learning has been identified as a feature of situated learning in the workplace (Billett 1996). Participants viewed learning to communicate reasoning as an inherent part of their professional development. In the research reported here, the structured reflective exercises and probing questions during interviews helped participants become aware of how they learned to reason and to communicate their reasoning, as demonstrated in the following quotations:

> You're probably changing [your communication] without thinking about why you're changing – you're changing because you're forced to change because your communication is not working. . . . with patients [and] with families, if something is not getting across to them then you've got to change the way you're getting it across and so you learn – and if that situation comes up again, [you remember that] 'it didn't work when I did it like that'.

> Through doing this research I've thought about some of the things that I ask myself [when reasoning] . . . where I've had to communicate, try and convey to someone else what things do I think about and probably don't even realize that I'm thinking about them . . . I realized that there is probably a lot of stuff that I think about . . . it was partly through doing this research and thinking a bit about what questions I ask myself that help me make decisions and how to communicate those to others, I realized that it's important that they [students] think those same questions.

Communities of practice were identified as supporting and fostering development of the skills required to communicate reasoning, including the ability to break down and 'unbundle' thinking processes, the ability to match co-communicators' frames of reference and to monitor and critique communication. Participants described periods or episodes in their careers when they were members of active learning communities. These experiences were consistently related to periods of accelerated development of communication of clinical reasoning. This social and socializing learning was recognized and valued by all the research participants, consistent with Wenger's (1998) observation that work team members gave priority to activities that addressed team goals or objectives and specific situation demands:

> I think we've got a good environment which is really important; I don't think I'd be able to communicate or educate people in the same way unless we've got the environment around us where we're really trying to get better at these things.

Learning from peers is a powerful way to learn to communicate through discussion, both formal and informal. Peer collaboration and support help to extend the abilities of team members to perform beyond what they could do on their own (see Vygotsky 1978). Participants learned to articulate, critique and defend their reasoning through conversations and reflections with peers about real patient cases. The process of articulating reasoning drew clinical reasoning, a skill that is often subconscious, to the participants' awareness, making it explicit, and thereby exposing it to critique by the participants as well as critique and feedback from others.

> Being in the environment where you talk to other experienced people and you listen to the way that they communicate ... working with clinical educators and listening to the way they work [with students] ... is a great time ... listening to other people going through their clinical reasoning ... I think you learn a lot about how to communicate reasoning by doing that.

The participants agreed that mentors and role models were invaluable in supporting and extending their learning. Participants learned to communicate reasoning by modelling their communication on that of others, usually seniors, mentors or role models with whom they were working.

> The acting senior ... was very good ... [at] justifying things and she was very good as a resource for [me] turning around and saying, 'I don't quite know what I'm doing, can you please help'. I guess because she was communicating to me it made it much easier for me to take on board what she was saying

and why she was saying [it], then impart that to others.

> Having mentors from within the university and also within your workplace ... really promotes lots of collegiate discussions ... about why you choose different things and why you don't and I think that really helps you to be able to communicate your reasoning processes.

Learning from patients and students was also a feature of learning within communities of practice.

> Sometimes some of the students give examples that help them, that you can take on board and that aids your communication [as a teacher] as well. Because they're giving you things that work for them, obviously it will work for others; you can take that on board and use that as well.

FACTORS AND STRATEGIES THAT FACILITATE LEARNING TO COMMUNICATE CLINICAL REASONING

Experiential strategies such as explicit guidance, observation, modelling, discussion and feedback are effective for the development of skills required to communicate reasoning. Participants found that learning to perform (and communicate) in the way the profession demanded of them involved active integration and participation rather than just passive internalization. Modelling was used in learning practical skills, communication skills and, importantly, reasoning skills, in a way similar to that of mentors and colleagues. This process is at the heart of professional socialization.

> [My mentor] helped guide me in terms of doing quality [research] projects ... which we were able to present at a couple of conferences. I think that started the whole process of really looking at what you do and analysing it and having a good look at the evidence behind what you do, and that's why I think I learned quite a bit in terms of reasoning and why we do different things.

> I'm working with other people that have students. I think that's probably the key, is watching other

people who teach and seeing how they do it, and picking up from the things that they do well and modifying your own practice.

Feedback from others about communication content and style was also a powerful strategy for learning, raising awareness and leading to critical thinking and change in behaviour or thinking.

Self-evaluation and reflection were strategies participants used to monitor and correct their reasoning and its communication. Professionals benefit from being aware of and observing how well they are interacting with others and how well their communication, content and style, are received by other people (Higgs et al 2005). Reflexivity was an embodied characteristic of some of the experienced participants and was evident in their heightened awareness and self-critique of practice, along with a genuine desire to continue to improve.

As a physio I don't want to be doing something that's not valid and I would hope that in the way that I do my own clinical work and the way that I talk about it that I would be questioning the validity of what I'm doing. So I hope that I would be teaching the students to question the validity of what they're doing as well.

Confidence, awareness and clarity about reasoning were considered useful in promoting learning to communicate reasoning for several reasons. When participants felt confident with their reasoning they were confident about communicating their thinking to others more easily and more frequently. By communicating their reasoning they became more aware of how they reasoned, which in turn improved their ability to reason and communicate their reasoning. Learning to communicate reasoning consistently lagged behind actual reasoning ability for all the participants, especially in the early stages of career development. Participants reported that they needed to be clear and confident about their own reasoning patterns before being able to communicate them, and also that there were limited opportunities for communicating reasoning early following graduation.

My knowledge base was increasing and I was getting more confident so I was able therefore to communicate it better.

I would say that as my clinical reasoning has ... gradually increased then my [communication of clinical reasoning] has increased in the sense that I then communicated that thinking and my patient management. As I became more aware or clearer on why I was doing things or what was really important for particular patients I think my ability to communicate that improved.

IMPLICATIONS FOR PRACTITIONERS

Findings from this research suggest that participants did not distinguish between learning to communicate reasoning and learning to be physiotherapists. Many of the participants lacked awareness of their communication of clinical reasoning; therefore, many of the learning opportunities were unplanned and opportunistic. Because communication of clinical reasoning is embedded in actions and interactions forming the community of practice, professional socialization is an appropriate framework for learning to communicate clinical reasoning. Understanding the powerful influence of the workplace culture on learning enables practitioners to adopt a critical and reflective stance with regard to the activities of their workplaces. This understanding also encourages them to be strategic in their learning and professional development, and to be active agents in choosing both what is learned and the process of learning within the community. Therefore, health professionals (novice and experienced alike) need to combine giving deliberate attention to their work activities with self-monitoring, rather than relying on routine and habit. Reflexivity goes beyond reflection, by bringing attention to learning and professional development as a result of reflection and critical self-assessment. Reflexivity is an essential characteristic of lifelong learning (Eraut 1994), requiring active awareness and engagement of learners in their communities of practice (Deakin Crick 2005); lifelong learning is widely recognized as an important goal for health professionals working in the current healthcare climate.

According to De Cossart & Fish (2005), three main processes that develop good reflective practice are: (a) following a rigorous process for reflection (particular to each individual); (b) engaging in dialogue with teachers and peers (including talking and writing as key means of developing reflection); and (c) recognizing proper ethical and moral obligations to patients and colleagues (for example, maintaining confidentiality). Strategies described in the literature to foster reflective practice are many; they include journal writing (Lincoln et al 1997, Williams et al 2002, Youngblood & Beitz 2001), portfolio development (Paschal et al 2002, Youngblood & Beitz 2001) and self-evaluation (Lincoln et al 1997). These strategies are likely to promote reasoning but are insufficient for learning to communicate reasoning. Individuals need to seek out opportunities to observe senior practitioners and educators and to seek feedback from various people, including their own patients. Discussions about learners' perceptions of their learning compared with observations of and by teachers at university or seniors in the workplace may aid the development of learners' critical self-assessment skills (Paschal et al 2002). Practitioners need to be responsible for their own learning through active participation in their communities and maintaining awareness of the influence of culture and the role of individual agency in the learning of clinical reasoning and communication.

IMPLICATIONS FOR THE UNIVERSITY

An important implication of this research is the need for explicit teaching of clinical reasoning and the role of communication of that reasoning in health sciences curricula, especially in the current healthcare climate. Recognition by faculty of the importance of learning and teaching of these two phenomena (reasoning and communicating reasoning) for future professionals, and their core place in the curriculum, is one key strategy to minimize the negative effect on student learning of the 'hidden curriculum' (for example prioritizing knowledge retention and technical skills). The hidden curriculum plays a role in the socialization of students, as they adopt values, beliefs and attitudes of educators and health professionals that may be inconsistent with the explicit curriculum objectives, and may be projected intentionally

or unintentionally (Shepard & Jensen 1990). It remains important to explicitly define the skills of clinical reasoning and its communication, raising them to learners' awareness and making them readily identifiable within the various units of study. The place of communication and clinical reasoning in university curricula needs to be clearly defined, with close integration between classroom activities and fieldwork placements/ clinical education. Universities should also aim to foster skills in collaboration and critical self-evaluation. Reflective learning should be built into the curriculum by making it an expectation and allowing time for it to occur, and should be modelled for students by academics and health professionals via articulation of thought processes, as recommended by Albanese (2006). A significant challenge for the design of learning and teaching activities in the classroom that promote reasoning and its communication (particularly with the increased use of information technology) is the preservation of context. Classroom teaching should aim to closely mimic the implicit, tacit cues and information learned from context and from being in the real situation observing experienced practitioners.

Sociocultural theory suggests that the goal of education should be to provide an environment in which learners can engage in purposeful activities and in the process learn to use the cultural tools and practices that have been developed to mediate the achievement of the goals of these activities (Wells 1999). The terminology used by health professionals in reasoning and communicating reasoning is an example of these culturally mediated tools. Brew (2003) argued for a reconceptualization of teaching and research in higher education to adopt a constructivist view of knowledge. She called for teaching to be student-focused and for knowledge to be viewed as constructed within a sociopolitical context. Adapting Lave & Wenger's (1991) model of learning in communities of practice, Brew claimed that research and teaching should both be viewed as activities where individuals and groups negotiate meanings, building knowledge within a social context. Academic communities of practice develop through engagement of academics and students in learning. Similarly, learning and teaching of clinical reasoning (and its communication) are optimized through participation in communities of practice, whether at university or in the workplace.

It is important to note that professionals learn from listening to others communicating their thoughts, and then critiquing and integrating what they consider of value to their own thinking. Therefore, communicating reasoning helps professionals to improve their thinking and its communication. Creating supportive opportunities for students to articulate their reasoning is essential, and may be achieved through the use of experiential learning methods in the classroom and during clinical education/fieldwork placements. Examples include role plays, vivas, conducting a history and physical examination with simulated or real patients, videotaping of the encounter and providing feedback. However, articulating reasoning does not necessarily reflect actual reasoning processes, because reasoning is rapid, situated and involves tacit knowledge; therefore, its communication represents a reconstruction of the main processes perceived as most relevant to the audience, framed and delivered to match the audience. Students need to learn to become aware of their thinking and to be given the necessary tools to construct their messages, including active listening, dealing with interpersonal difficulties and collaborating with others.

IMPLICATIONS FOR THE WORKPLACE

Workplace managers are responsible for promoting the development of clinical reasoning, including the ability to communicate reasoning, among staff. Communities of practice that adopt learning as their primary objective and that are supportive and offer guidance to extend the development of practitioners through all phases of their professional journeys are invaluable. Senior practitioners and managers should strive to build positive learning environments that support students and novice practitioners in their chosen career paths. Wenger & Snyder (2000) listed three important steps for managers to follow to cultivate communities of practice within their organizations. First, managers should identify potential communities that will enhance the organization's strategic capabilities. Second, managers should provide the infrastructure to support communities in effectively applying their expertise. Third, managers should aim to assess the value of the communities of practice using systematic, qualitative methods.

The knowledge base of a community of practice is largely tacit, created through participation and distributed through the community (Wenger 1998). Therefore, communities must recognize the value of informal learning and, in the health sciences context, must cultivate opportunities for open discussion of patient cases among staff (while maintaining patient confidentiality). This would help professionals learn the value of experiential and clinical knowledge as well as the research and propositional knowledge favoured in the current context of evidence-based practice. Personal and professional knowledge are essential for the building of collaborative relationships and the negotiation of meaning necessary for the communication of clinical reasoning.

Another finding from this research concerns the valuable role of mentors and role models in the development of communication abilities, particularly in the professional development of novice practitioners. This development may be spurred by generating regular opportunities for new graduates to discuss their reasoning about their patients and to ask questions of the senior practitioners. Seniors, educators and facilitators need to be aware of their professional responsibilities in guiding and mentoring novice practitioners, in creating a dynamic, responsible and supportive learning community of practice. These professional responsibilities extend beyond the possession of formal knowledge and technical skills to include attitudes, values and beliefs of senior colleagues or role models, which strongly influence the development of students' professional identities. This role transcends what is articulated explicitly; it encompasses the behaviour and values that embody a profession, which may be implicit or tacit, but which remain highly influential in learning and professional development.

CONCLUSION

Learning to communicate clinical reasoning in practice is a matter of professional socialization, of joining and participating in communities of practice, rather than the application of skills or principles that operate independently of social context. Learning to communicate reasoning is a contextualized and participation-focused activity. Fostering reflexivity and explicit learning of how to communicate clinical reasoning in the health professions is the responsibility of individuals, universities and the workplace. Strategies that promote this learning include practice, reflection, modelling, role play, self-appraisal and feedback from others, set in an overarching framework of adult learners and community members participating and learning in context.

References

Abrandt Dahlgren M, Richardson B, Sjostrom B 2004 Professions as communities of practice. In: Higgs J, Richardson B, Abrandt Dahlgren M (eds) Developing practice knowledge for health professionals. Butterworth-Heinemann, Edinburgh, p 71–88

Ajjawi R 2006 Learning to communicate clinical reasoning in physiotherapy practice. Unpublished PhD thesis, University of Sydney, Australia

Ajjawi R, Higgs J, Hunt A 2004 Learning to communicate clinical reasoning within communities of practice – the influence of Vygotsky and Wenger. In: ANZAME Conference Proceedings: Maintaining momentum: anticipating, innovating, facilitating, participating, evaluating. ANZAME: Association for Health Professional Education, Flinders Press, Bedford Park, SA, p 18

Ajjawi R, Higgs J, Hunt A 2005a Communicating clinical reasoning: a learning challenge. Proceedings of the Australasian New Zealand Association for Medical Education Conference, p 18

Ajjawi R, Higgs J, Hunt A 2005b Facilitating learning to reason within communities of practice. Proceedings of the EdHealth Conference, College of Health Sciences, University of Sydney, p 57

Albanese M A 2006 Crafting the reflective lifelong learner: why, what and how. Medical Education 40(4):288–290

Billett S 1996 Situated learning: bridging sociocultural and cognitive theorising. Learning and Instruction 6(3): 263–280

Brew A 2003 Teaching and research: new relationships and their implications for inquiry-based teaching and learning in higher education. Higher Education Research and Development 22(1):3–18

De Cossart L, Fish D 2005 Cultivating a thinking surgeon: new perspectives on clinical teaching, learning and assessment. tfm Publishing, Shrewsbury

Deakin Crick R 2005 Being a learner: a virtue for the 21st century. British Journal of Educational Studies 53(3): 359–374

Edwards C, Titchen A 2003 Research into patients' perspectives: relevance and usefulness of phenomenological sociology. Journal of Advanced Nursing 44(5):450–460

Eraut M 1994 Developing professional knowledge and competence, 2nd edn. Falmer Press, London

Higgs J, McAllister L, Sefton A 2005 Introduction: communicating in the health and social sciences. In: Higgs J, Sefton A, Street A et al (eds) Communicating in the health and social sciences. University Press, Oxford, p 3–12

Lave J, Wenger E 1991 Situated learning: legitimate peripheral participation. Cambridge University Press, Cambridge

Lincoln M, Stockhausen L, Maloney D 1997 Learning processes in clinical education. In: McAllister L, Lincoln M, McLeod S et al (eds), Facilitating learning in clinical settings. Stanley Thornes, Cheltenham, UK, p 99–129

Paschal K A, Jensen G M, Mostrom E 2002 Building portfolios: a means for developing habits of reflective practice in physical therapy education. Journal of Physical Therapy Education 16(3):38–51

Richardson B 1999 Professional development: professional knowledge and situated learning in the workplace. Physiotherapy 85(9):467–474

Shepard K F, Jensen G M 1990 Physical therapist curricula for the 1990s: educating the reflective practitioner. Physical Therapy 70(9):566–577

Siminoff L A, Step M M 2005 A communication model of shared decision making: accounting for cancer treatment decisions. Health Psychology 24(4Suppl):S99–S105

Titchen A, McIntyre D 1993 A phenomenological approach to qualitative data analysis in nursing research. In: Titchen A (ed) Changing nursing practice through action research report no 6. National Institute for Nursing, Centre for Practice Development and Research, Oxford, p 29–48

Vygotsky L S 1978 Mind in society: the development of higher psychological processes. Harvard University Press, Cambridge, MA

Wells G 1999 Dialogic inquiry: towards a sociocultural practice and theory of education. Cambridge University Press, Cambridge

Wenger E 1998 Communities of practice: learning, meaning, and identity. Cambridge University Press, Cambridge

Wenger E C, Snyder W M 2000 Communities of practice: the organisational frontier. Harvard Business Review 78(1): 139–145

Williams R M, Wessel J, Gemus M et al 2002 Journal writing to promote reflection by physiotherapy students during clinical placements. Physiotherapy Theory and Practice 18(1):5–15

Youngblood N, Beitz J M 2001 Developing critical thinking with active learning strategies. Nurse Education 26(1): 39–42

Chapter **31**

Learning the language of clinical reasoning

Stephen Loftus and Joy Higgs

CHAPTER CONTENTS

In this chapter we argue the case for a discursive view of clinical reasoning. We contend that becoming proficient at clinical reasoning is in large part a process of mastering, in particular, the language of a health profession and more broadly the language of healthcare systems. In learning to become competent in clinical reasoning, new practitioners must master a number of aspects of language; these include terminology, category systems, metaphors, heuristics, rituals, narrative, rhetoric and hermeneutics (Loftus 2006, Loftus & Higgs 2006). This interpretive view of clinical reasoning is in contrast to the current and more widespread view that clinical reasoning is, or should be, regarded as a phenomenon of computational logic and symbolic processing, combined with probability mathematics and statistics. The latter view is based within a more empirico-analytical paradigm and, we argue, is less useful as a conceptual model of clinical reasoning and how people come to learn this specialized skill. We draw both on the literature and on recent research (Loftus 2006) that utilized hermeneutic phenomenology to explore the nature of clinical decision making and how it is learned.

THE CENTRALITY OF LANGUAGE

Perhaps the most distinguishing feature of human beings is their use of language. A major problem with discussing language and its role in clinical reasoning is that for too many people language is mistakenly viewed as nothing more than a passive conduit by which meaning is transferred from the mind of one person to another. This is open to challenge. It can be argued that it is language that makes us human (Gadamer 1989). Language is central to human nature and to being human. Being immersed in a world of language allows us to construct meaning intersubjectively through the dialogue and interaction we have with others (Bakhtin 1986). The implication is that to understand reasoning of any kind, including clinical reasoning, we need to study the ways in which practitioners employ language and interaction to address clinical problems, rather than assuming that practitioners use objective mathematical methods to cope with tasks such as diagnosis.

In arguing for exclusively mathematical methods, Descartes (trans. Clarke 1999) made the error of rejecting Aristotle's notion that different fields of knowledge require different methods and different means of proof. Aristotle (trans. Lawson-Tancred 1991) asserted that mathematical proofs normally have no place in a speech meant to persuade others. It can be argued that clinical reasoning is largely a matter of persuading oneself and others that a particular diagnosis and management plan is correct. Clinical reasoning is therefore a discursive construction of meaning, negotiated with patients, their carers, other health professionals, but above all with oneself. To become proficient at clinical reasoning, health professionals must therefore become proficient in the language skills required to persuade people.

LANGUAGE SKILLS OF CLINICAL REASONING

In recent doctoral research Loftus (Loftus 2006, Loftus & Higgs 2006) sought to gain a deeper understanding of the place of language in clinical reasoning. He studied settings where health professionals and medical students engaged in clinical decision making in groups, including problem-based learning (PBL) tutorials and a multidisciplinary clinic.

The research showed that clinical reasoning can be visualized as a quest for meaning, using the language tools that are part of the interpretive repertoire provided by the community of practice

called a health profession. That is, communities of practice provide both the interpretive frames of reference and the language tools for meaning-making by their members. When working in these communities, health professionals need to learn a range of language skills to be used for clinical reasoning. These are represented in Figure 31.1. The skills include knowledge of, and ability to use, appropriate terminology, categories and category systems, metaphors, heuristics and mnemonics, ritual, narrative, rhetoric and hermeneutics. All these skills need to be coordinated, both in constructing a diagnosis and management plan and in communicating clinical decisions to other people, in a manner that can be judged intelligible, legitimate, persuasive, and as carrying the moral authority for subsequent action.

TERMINOLOGY/KEY WORDS

Mastering the terminology of a health profession is a basic skill in clinical reasoning, which forms the foundation for the other skills required. This is a matter not just of knowing particular words and phrases, but more importantly, of knowing how and when to use them appropriately. For example,

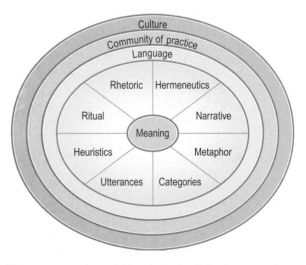

Figure. 31.1 A model for conceptualizing language in clinical decision making and communicating it. These are all embedded within a community of practice and the larger culture. This model emphasizes the construction of meaning through language. It applies to clinical decision making if we see clinical reports as a construction of meaning

one medical student spoke of acquiring basic skills in psychiatry:

> it [psychiatry] has its own little language for speaking to itself and you don't pick up on that unless you're using it every day in a group talking to someone ... we'd see patients together and we'd discuss the patients and run through it using our little list of jargon terms. ... So you got used to using the language and when it came time to sit your exam you felt quite comfortable. (Loftus 2006, p. 140)

Key words can also have profound effects on patients and the ways in which they interpret their illness experience. To a health professional, the expression 'degenerative changes' might be interpreted as a normal part of growing older and as something not to be taken too seriously. To patients, the phrase can sound disastrous and could encourage some patients to take on a 'sick role'. For example, in the multidisciplinary pain clinic studied in the current research, health professionals dealt with patients in chronic pain, and a large part of the clinical reasoning involved seeking out the beliefs that patients built up around such key terms, and the degree to which these beliefs then led into a spiral of deterioration. There was a need to be sensitive to this aspect of language in the world of patients, and the ways in which the narratives that patients lived out could be directed in self-destructive behaviours (or, with help, redirected into self-constructive lifestyles and health behaviours) based on the interpretation of key terms such as degenerative changes. To this extent it is clear that the meanings of these key words can be multilayered and contingent on context. Health professionals need awareness of these issues if they are to help and not hinder their patients' well-being.

CATEGORIES

Terminology, in turn, forms the basis for the various category systems that health professionals use to conceptualize clinical problems and their solutions. A large part of establishing a diagnosis is deciding upon a category for a patient's health complaint or need. The biomedical model provides a category system that is in widespread use. Within this model categories can provide a framework

that can be successfully refined. Basic frameworks that medical students learn to use might include:

- primary problems, risk factors, and co-morbidities
- critical problems and common problems
- active problems, complications and background problems.

Many student participants in Loftus's (2006) study found that a practice-based method of learning such as PBL gave them familiarity with a clinico-pathological category system that lent itself naturally to clinical practice. As one student observed, 'This year I've realized how helpful they [PBL tutorials] are because it gives you that approach to thinking about things in categories' (p. 143).

Many novice health professionals begin their clinical education already having learned the category systems of the basic medical sciences, and they find that these scientific categories can be quite different from the more practical categories of the real world of health professional practice. One student spoke of having to reorganize his knowledge in a case-based manner so that it was more fitting for the practice of medicine: 'I've gone through my old notes and progressively thrown them out as I've rewritten them into a different format ... now I approach learning the diseases in the same way that I would ... a patient' (Loftus 2006, p. 145). In other words, his biomedical knowledge was being reframed around patient narratives he had come across in clinical practice. The category systems used in clinical reasoning need to be appropriate for the practice situation. For example, typical diagnostic categories used by a doctor in chronic pain management were described thus: 'I think in three components. One is nociceptive ... and a neuropathic component ... [and thirdly] ... psychosocial contributors' (p. 146). A clinical psychologist, working in the same setting, spoke of three different categories: thought, feelings and behaviour. Categories provide a foundation for metaphors used in clinical reasoning.

METAPHOR

Lakoff & Johnson (1980) argued that thought and language are fundamentally metaphorical.

Metaphor is not simply an embellishment of language exploited by writers and poets. It can be argued that language and thought are intensely and inherently metaphorical and, because of this, metaphor use goes largely unnoticed as it is so completely natural to us (Ortony 1993). In recent years there has been a growing recognition of the extent to which metaphor underlies scientific and medical practice and shapes the ways in which both health professionals and their patients conceptualize their health problems and what can be done about them (e.g. Draaisma 2001, Reisfield & Wilson 2004).

A key metaphor underlying the biomedical model is 'The body is a machine'. This is also the underlying metaphor through which patients in Western societies tend to conceptualize their bodily problems (Hodgkin 1985). The implication of this metaphor is that we can always, in principle at least, repair a broken machine. In acute care this metaphor could be appropriate. However, the metaphor frequently falls down in the chronic situation where repeated attempts at repair fail, resulting in frustration and disappointment for both patients and health professionals. Often such patients are 'discarded' by the system as 'failed' patients (Alder 2003).

In the Loftus (2006) study the ways in which the staff of the multidisciplinary pain centre described their work indicated that the metaphors at work were more in keeping with caring for chronic patients. For example, one metaphor that suggested itself repeatedly was 'Life is a journey'. Rather than trying to cure patients, the staff provided interventions, from dorsal column stimulators to cognitive behavioural therapy, to help patients adjust their lives so that they could continue living a relatively normal life despite pain.

HEURISTICS/MNEMONICS

Heuristics and mnemonics are language tools that enable health professionals to manage an enormously complex and growing body of knowledge in ways that best suit the clinical reasoning required when dealing with patients in the real world. Student participants in the Loftus (2006) study who made maximum use of mnenonic and heuristic tools claimed that assessing complex

cases became relatively straightforward. Typical mnemonics include the well-known VITAMIN D memory aid used to assist novices in remembering the various disease categories. This particular mnemonic stands for **V**ascular, **I**nfectious, **T**raumatic, **A**utoimmune, **M**etabolic, **I**nflammatory/ **I**diopathic, **N**eoplastic and **D**rug-related. Another mnemonic is **D**ressed **I**n **A** **S**urgeon's **G**own, **M**ost **P**hysicians **I**nvent **D**iagnoses. This translates to: **d**efinition, **i**ncidence, **a**etiology, **s**ex, **g**eography, **m**acroscopic/**m**icroscopic changes, **p**resentation, **i**nvestigation, **d**rug treatment. For students, the PBL format itself can provide a heuristic for assessing patients. Medical students in the programme studied reported that by the third year they were entirely familiar with the PBL format. Most reported using the PBL format when assessing real patients, as they believed it was both a rigorous and a comprehensive approach to clinical reasoning. One student reflected: 'I think it's a really good idea. It's how you think clinically', and she was also persuaded of its normative nature: 'it's how you should think clinically' (p. 166).

Health professionals assessing complex chronic pain cases certainly found that they needed some format to guide assessment. As one physiotherapist said about teaching students: 'I encourage them [the students] to have a format to start with, because you can get lost with these patients because they can go off on many tangents' (Loftus 2006, p. 170). Heuristics and mnemonics also tend to be used in a ritualistic manner.

RITUAL

Ritual is closely related to heuristics and mnemonics and plays a part in at least two important aspects of clinical reasoning. The first is the ritual of assessment and the second is the performative aspect of presenting information to others. All health professionals are used to following protocols as frameworks for gathering information. Following a ritual allows the process of gathering relevant information, using the various heuristics and mnemonic devices, to become habitual and routine. Health professionals can then concentrate on diagnosing the patient's problem and planning treatment without having to be distracted with thoughts about what should be asked for next.

In a sense, the ritual guarantees that information gathering will happen appropriately and expeditiously; both are important factors in the busy world of practice accountability. Rituals are closely related to the category systems in use, together with the heuristics and mnemonics built on the categories. Medical students gradually come to realize that the ritualistic nature of PBL, for example, has real-world application in the clinical setting. As one student participant in the study observed:

> If someone was to come in with abdominal pain and they'll [senior doctors] ask you the causes of it . . . you can sometimes get a bit intimidated by it I suppose. There are so many structures in the abdomen. And you'll tell them the causes and they'll ask, 'What questions do you want to ask them [the patient] to eliminate those?' So you start asking questions, and then it's the PBL process. 'What investigations do you want to do?' And you realize you did know all the things you needed to know, but you forgot how to approach them. (Loftus 2006, p. 173)

In other words, the ritual of assessment is a means of coping with the complexity of practice. In presenting this observation, however, we emphasize two key matters. Firstly, routines should be tools and guides, not ends in themselves; they serve the needs of data collection, for example. Secondly, no matter how habitual a protocol becomes, it should not be implemented without critical attention to purpose, process and outcomes. Part of assessment, for example, is comparing anticipated to actual assessment findings and reflecting upon any discrepancies. Rituals should serve to decrease the chaotic or highly complex aspects of regular practices without reducing such input to 'white noise' within which errors or highly important information can go unnoticed.

Health professionals in multidisciplinary settings routinely have clinical meetings to compare assessment findings and negotiate management plans. These meetings tend to follow simple rituals of procedure that provide for smooth and rapid negotiation. For example, in the multidisciplinary pain clinic in the current study the doctor always presented a report first, followed by the physiotherapist and then a clinical psychologist, culminating in open discussion (Loftus & Higgs 2006). Atkinson (1995) and Hunter (1991) have also described the ritualistic nature, in medical practice, of delivering information to others. Mastering these discursive rituals is part of the process of socialization into a profession. The ritualistic delivery both helps the reporting health professionals to organize their information and, just as importantly, suggests to listeners (or readers of written reports) the systematic and thorough assessment that underlies the report. The ritualistic aspect thus reassures the recipients that the report is both legitimate and sound. As one medical student participant in the study remarked, mastering the rituals of clinical reporting began to make this complex experience seem easy: 'I gave a very templated response . . . I would go in and I would say "I spoke to Mr name, age and occupation" . . . and just have this template of rehearsed framework' (Loftus 2006, p. 176).

The same medical student echoed the words of Schön (1983, 1987) when he related that it was only the practical experience of following the rituals of assessment that eventually brought true understanding of what the students and clinicians were doing and why it was important to do it that way. Schön claimed that it was not possible for beginners in any profession to fully appreciate what the work involved until they had been completely immersed in the routines of that work for some time. Appreciating the power of routine and ritual in one's profession is an aspect of growing competence and expertise. Ritual establishes what the business at hand is to be about. As Perelman (1982, p. 10) wrote: 'Ritual . . . and rules of procedure fix, with more or less precision, the matters which are the objects of communication.' It can be argued that much more attention should be paid to the explicit teaching of thoughtful ritual to newcomers within health professions than occurs at present. Although ritual procedures are taught, the fact that they are rituals is often glossed over, and the value of clinical reasoning ritual as a tool to manage complex, disparate and changeable clinical data is underappreciated. If students were made aware of why rituals are so important they might appreciate their value more quickly.

NARRATIVE

A large part of clinical reasoning is the construction of a narrative about a patient within the conceptual framework of a health profession and the specific context of the patient and the workplace. There is a growing realization of the importance of narrative in therapeutic encounters (e.g. Charon & Montello 2002, Greenhalgh 1999). The construction of a clinical narrative is done in a manner that not only takes account of the past and present but also suggests the narrative trajectory that the patient's story might follow in the future, predisposing towards particular decisions about management. Such narratives can be diagnostic, prognostic and therapeutic. In multidisciplinary settings, patient narratives are best constructed jointly by the clinical team members. All the health professionals in the chronic pain clinic in the Loftus (2006) study needed to rapidly acquire the skill of reducing the findings of an hour's intensive assessment to a summary that could be delivered verbally in 2 minutes or less. This is a narrative skill requiring more than the ability to simply summarize findings. Health professionals in these settings realized that such a summary must be coherent with their colleagues' reports to create one comprehensive narrative, providing information that would permit the team to make complex decisions about patient management.

In addition, the physiotherapists and psychologists in that clinic had to acquire the skill of dynamically adjusting their summaries as they listened to their predecessors deliver reports about the same patient. They found that without such dynamic adjustment there would be three overlapping reports with much needless repetition and little cohesion. To prevent this from occurring, the health professionals would frequently dynamically adjust their own reports so that they delivered findings that constructively added to the collective narrative. If there was repetition then it would be deliberate, in order to emphasize an important point or to clarify any confusion. As one physiotherapist observed, 'your contribution is valid if you add 20 lines rather than repeat 40' (Loftus 2006, p. 184). Another physiotherapist reported that she had needed to learn 'what bit of information was it that they wanted from me . . . you don't

need to go into all the nitty gritty specific stuff that the doctor has already talked about. You're just basically covering ground that he hasn't covered' (p. 184).

Of particular interest is the extent to which this multidisciplinary pain clinic adopted a biopsychosocial approach in order to deal with patients in whom there was a complex interaction between medical, social and more existential issues. Most health professionals find such patients difficult to cope with, as they have such a bewildering array of problems, many of which are beyond the practitioner's expertise to solve because of their complexity or chronicity. The intense 3-hour multidisciplinary assessments in this particular clinic gave many patients the sense that they had been properly heard for the first time. There was time for Kleinman's (1988) 'empathic witnessing', which many patients found therapeutic in itself. It is encouraging that there is now a growing awareness of the importance of narrative in pain management (Carr et al 2005) and chronic conditions in general (Frank 1995). We hope that this will continue and lead to more attention being paid in practice and education to this aspect of health care, with the goal of a consequent improvement in practice.

RHETORIC

Rhetoric is the art of persuasive speaking or writing. A great deal of clinical reasoning is concerned with persuasion. Health professionals need to persuade other people, patients and their families, and other clinicians that a particular assessment and proposed course of action is both legitimate and sound. One medical student participant in the Loftus (2006) study realized the importance of this issue when reflecting on having to cope with an inadequate clinical report from a colleague: 'It's just being able to say what you find, and be able to say that . . . this person is in very dire straits. It's not making up stuff, but it's being able to present it in a convincing and competent manner that they [senior doctors] can say, "All right, this requires my attention"' (p. 190).

Two factors in the neglect of the role of language and the acts of persuasion and negotiation in clinical practice are the unchallenged rules of science and the equally unchallenged (although in a different frame of reference) rules of economics. In the biomedical sciences and the empirico-analytical paradigm there is a search for *the* truth, for justification of practice through the use of quantitative research evidence and for credible evidence in a science dominated field and a litigious society. Rather than persuasion, science talks of justification. In the healthcare marketplace 'the bottom line' drives much decision making; for example, how many treatments are allowed rather than optimal for the patient? Rather than persuasion, economics talks of financial or cost accountability. So where does the language of persuasion and negotiation fit into health care? Perhaps we need to listen to patients who want to be treated as individuals rather than cases. Perhaps we need to re-ground the acknowledged strengths of the biomedical sciences and technological advancement back into the intrinsic purpose of health services, to enhance the health of people.

Rhetoric, used appropriately, is something that senior practitioners expect from novices and learners. Part of demonstrating their learning, for instance, involves novices and students in persuading their teachers that they understand the clinical situation and the patient's needs sufficiently to have made a credible decision that goes beyond guesswork or practised answers. Senior doctors have to make decisions about patients based on clinical reports they receive from their juniors. In order to do this, the senior doctors must be persuaded that such reports are reliable and trustworthy. The reliability and trustworthiness come from a combination of the credibility of reported findings and the ritualistic, professional and persuasive manner of the reporting (Hunter 1991).

Atkinson (1995) claimed that rhetorical forms establish authority and attitudes to knowledge and uncertainty. After a 'long case' presentation in the Loftus (2006) study, one medical student was told by his examiners, 'you've got to get to the point now where you can lead us to where you want to go' (p. 192). It seemed that the student's clinical report needed to be more persuasive, even though the examiners were entirely satisfied that the diagnosis and treatment plan were correct. It is interesting to observe the varied attention that may be paid to students' decision making prior to graduation and prior to autonomous clinical practice, with all the responsibility for clinical decision making that the latter entails. Is it enough to have reached what the clinical educator sees as 'the right answer'? Does the student's management strategy for the patient or the intervention plan match the expectations of the educator, using familiar words and adopting compatible strategies? Beyond these matchings, does the student actually understand the rationale, the consequences and the justification of the chosen approach in comparison to others for this patient's or client's unique needs? We argue here that the skill of rhetoric, of presenting a sound argument, not just a solution, is required to examine each of these issues, along with the skill of critical appraisal by both learner and teacher.

In the multidisciplinary pain clinic reported in the Loftus (2006) study, one senior doctor spoke of the need for junior doctors to master the art of producing reports that were persuasive narratives that in turn permitted decisions to be made. 'The trainees [junior doctors] need to learn that [they have to] cut down the amount of information to a manageable summary for your colleagues ... and for yourself because ... at the end of the day ... you have to be able to isolate them [important findings] and make a decision on them' (p. 193). This ability is both a narrative and a rhetorical skill. In constructing a clinical report, a health professional is justifying a claim about a patient. The justification is supported by arguments that depend on the context of that patient, and that will stand up to reasonable criticism. As Perelman (1982, p. 162) argued: 'As soon as a communication tries to influence one or more persons, to orient thinking ... to guide their actions, it belongs to the realm of rhetoric.'

There is frequently uncertainty in clinical reasoning, uncertainty that is associated not with self-doubt or the inability to make sound decisions but rather with the 'greyness' or complexity of practice situations, the variability of patient's or client's needs and the presence in many situations of various acceptable solutions (e.g. management strategies). And, when there is uncertainty, judgements must be made in light of all the information available for that case. This is not done mathematically or statistically but persuasively and argumentatively. This is the essence of rhetoric and of pragmatism; not the abandonment of logic or professional judgement but the incorporation of these into the intensely practical and human world of health care.

HERMENEUTICS

Hermeneutics is the art and study of interpretation. Hunter (1991) argued a strong case that the practice of medicine is a hermeneutic art. Not only must health professionals master the art of constructing persuasive narratives for themselves and others, they must also master the ability of interpreting the reports of other people, whether these reports come from patients or other health professionals. A clinical encounter is a reinterpretation of the patient's narrative in professional terms. Svenaeus (2000) argued that the philosophical hermeneutics of Gadamer (1989) provides a powerful theoretical framework for conceptualizing clinical encounters. The assessment of a patient is not merely the gathering of objective data. Data have to be selected and *interpretively synthesized* into a coherent narrative. For example, a clinical psychologist in the Loftus (2006) study spoke of the need to interpret psychometric questionnaire data in the light of a clinical interview: 'You've just met with them, and spoken to them, and had an hour's discussion with them where they stayed on track, and yet, according to this questionnaire they should be lying in a vegetative state, catatonic. So it's expressions of need for help that come out of these things' (p. 203). Despite the claims of the validity and objective measurement of psychometric questionnaires, this health professional realized the need for the interpretation and integration of all findings into a narrative whole. This is a hermeneutic skill that builds upon all the language skills described and discussed so far.

Hermeneutics can also have an ontological aspect. The way we interpret the world can become an integral part of who and what we are. Schön (1983, 1987) recognized that being a professional is not simply knowing a body of knowledge and how to apply it, it is also a way of being in the world. Students have some sense of this when they realize that they can sometimes recognize clinical signs without having to ask certain questions. One student participant spoke of seeing 'glaring cardiac signs' (Loftus 2006, p. 199) in a patient. In other words, she did not need to ask herself if the patient had signs of heart disease. She could not stop herself from recognizing that the patient had heart disease. Seeing and recognizing these signs had now become a part of who and what she was. It was a part of her ontology. Mol (2002) discussed this issue at length in her examination of atherosclerosis. A patient's experience of atherosclerosis is different from that of the vascular surgeon who operates to remove atheromatous plaques. The surgeon's experience is different again from that of the pathologist who examines a pathological specimen in a laboratory. These people all coordinate their different perspectives and interpretations to produce the phenomenon we know as atherosclerosis.

IMPLICATIONS FOR LEARNING AND DEVELOPING CLINICAL REASONING ABILITIES

Acquiring the art of clinical reasoning is, to a large extent, acquiring mastery of the language of a health profession. Clinical reasoning is learned within the communities of practice (Lave & Wenger 1991) called health professions. A particularly powerful way of conceptualizing how clinical reasoning is learned is the 'zone of proximal development' (ZPD) first articulated by Vygotsky (1978). In the ZPD, with the aid of more competent members of the community of practice, students are helped to perform tasks at a level of competence above what they can achieve unassisted. Gradually, as students begin to acquire mastery, the assistance and scaffolding provided by the more competent people are withdrawn until the students are proficient on their own. A key aspect of the ZPD is that tasks are performed socially first. Mastery involves the gradual internalization of skills until students can perform alone. Intellectual tasks are performed inter-psychologically (with others) first and then increasingly intra-psychologically (self-directed). From this viewpoint, clinical reasoning is primarily a social skill.

Hutchins (1995) argued that there can be tasks that are so complex that no one individual is ever expected to master all the skills required and where a team approach is always necessary. Multidisciplinary clinics could be examples of such settings, where patients have such complex problems that a team of health professionals is needed to provide comprehensive assessment and management. Such settings could be said to form a permanent ZPD where team members are always scaffolding and supporting the work of others. This enables the team to perform at an expert level that none of its individual members could hope to emulate.

Many have argued, following Aristotle, that thinking is the internalization of talk we have with others, and that in learning to think we learn to have conversations with ourselves (Bakhtin 1984, 1986; Gergen 1999; Toulmin 1979; Vygotsky 1978, 1986). According to this argument we do not first have thoughts, which are then 'dressed up' in language. As Vygotsky (1986, p. 218) explained, 'Thought is not merely expressed in words: it comes into existence through them'. Wittgenstein (1921/1974, no. 5.6) was of the same opinion: 'The limits of my language mean the limits of my world.' Language serves as a means of controlling what we think and how we communicate. To speak a particular language is to inhabit a particular 'way of being' (Wittgenstein 1958). Language both shapes and limits how we construct our social realities (Higgs et al 2004).

From this viewpoint, language is of primary importance for understanding the nature of thought. According to Vygotsky, we learn at an early age to perceive the world as much through our language as through our eyes. Clinical reasoning is no exception. It is clear from Vygotsky's writing that language performs an integrative function. Other symbol systems and cognitive tools can have meaning because they are imbued with language and integrated within it. In the realm of clinical reasoning there are many symbol systems. These can include ECG traces, manual therapy symbols, dental notation, radiographs and MRI scans. Language, in Vygotsky's view, is the 'tool of tools' (Cole & Wertsch 1996) that allows us to bring other symbol systems together into a meaningful whole.

When health professionals assess patients they have a dialogue with the patient and an internal dialogue with themselves. Diagnoses and treatment plans are not statistically calculated, they are arrived at persuasively. This does not deny the importance of evidence-based practice. Rather, the information from the evidence base, like all relevant information about a patient, has to be integrated into the narratives we construct about our patients, and this is done persuasively with the linguistic skills outlined above. Clinical reasoning is a search for the meaning of a patient's complaint or healthcare need that can be expressed within a narrative form which integrates all the findings about the patient and persuasively suggests the future course. Similarly, for health professionals working with well populations or client groups, professional reasoning is a search for meaning, to produce with or for the client a health promotion strategy that persuasively addresses the client's needs.

In this view of clinical reasoning, its essence is the acquisition and integration of the various linguistic and discursive skills. If we wish to study how clinical reasoning works and how it is learned we need to look at the dynamics of language use as outlined above. Although all reasoning requires active thinking, we argue that analytic priority should go to the functioning of language, rather than being focused on cognitive mechanisms. Clinical reasoning is a social and linguistic phenomenon that may occur collectively, in conversation and negotiation, but may also be performed in silence by health professionals when working alone.

References

Alder S 2003 Beyond the restitution narrative. Unpublished PhD thesis, University of Western Sydney, Sydney

Aristotle (trans H C Lawson-Tancred) 1991 The art of rhetoric. Penguin Books, London

Atkinson P 1995 Medical talk and medical work: the liturgy of the clinic. Sage Publications, London

Bakhtin M 1984 Problems of Dostoevsky's poetics. University of Minnesota Press, Minneapolis

Bakhtin M (trans V W McGee) 1986 Speech genres and other late essays. University of Texas Press, Austin, TX

Carr D B, Loeser J, Morris D B (eds) 2005 Narrative, pain, and suffering. IASP Press, Seattle

Charon R, Montello M (eds) 2002 Stories matter: the role of narrative in medical ethics. Routledge, London

Cole M, Wertsch J V 1996 Beyond the social-individual antimony in discussions of Piaget and Vygotsky. Human Development 39(5):250–256

Descartes R (trans D M Clarke) 1641/1999 Discourse on method and related writings. Penguin Books, London

Draaisma D 2001 The tracks of thought. Nature 414(6860):153

Frank A W 1995 The wounded storyteller: body, illness, and ethics. University of Chicago Press, London

Gadamer H-G 1989 Truth and method, 2nd edn. Continuum, New York

Gergen K J 1999 An invitation to social construction. Sage Publications, London

Greenhalgh T 1999 Narrative based medicine: narrative based medicine in an evidence based world. British Medical Journal 318(7179):323–325

Higgs J, Andresen L, Fish D 2004 Practice knowledge – its nature, sources and contexts. In: Higgs J, Richardson B, Abrandt Dahlgren M (eds) Developing practice knowledge for health professionals. Butterworth-Heinemann, Edinburgh, p 51–69

Hodgkin P 1985 Medicine is war: and other medical metaphors. British Medical Journal 291(6511):1820–1821

Hunter K M 1991 Doctors' stories: the narrative structure of medical knowledge. Princeton University Press, Princeton, NJ

Hutchins E 1995 Cognition in the wild. MIT Press, Cambridge, MA

Kleinman A 1988 The illness narratives: suffering, healing and the human condition. Basic Books, New York

Lakoff G, Johnson M 1980 Metaphors we live by. University of Chicago Press, Chicago

Lave J, Wenger E 1991 Situated learning: legitimate peripheral participation. Cambridge University Press, Cambridge

Loftus S 2006 Language in clinical reasoning: learning and using the language of collective clinical decision making. Unpublished PhD thesis, University of Sydney, Australia. Online. Available: http://ses.library.usyd.edu.au/handle/2123/1165 9 July 2007

Loftus S, Higgs J 2006 Clinical decision making in multidisciplinary clinics. In: Flor H, Kalso E, Dostrovsky J O (eds) Proceedings of the 11th World Congress on Pain. International Association for the Study of Pain, IASP Press, Seattle, p 755–760

Mol A 2002 The body multiple: ontology in medical practice. Duke University Press, Durham, NC

Ortony A (ed) 1993 Metaphor and thought, 2nd edn. Cambridge University Press, Cambridge

Perelman C (trans W Kluback) 1982 The realm of rhetoric. Notre Dame University Press, Notre Dame, IN

Reisfield G M, Wilson G R 2004 Use of metaphor in the discourse on cancer. Journal of Clinical Oncology 22(19):4024–4027

Schön D A 1983 The reflective practitioner: how professionals think in action. Basic Books, New York

Schön D A 1987 Educating the reflective practitioner. Jossey-Bass, San Francisco

Svenaeus F 2000 The hermeneutics of medicine and the phenomenology of health: steps towards a philosophy of medical practice. Kluwer Academic, Dordrecht

Toulmin S 1979 The inwardness of mental life. Critical Inquiry 6:1–16

Vygotsky L S 1978 Mind in society: the development of higher psychological processes. Harvard University Press, Cambridge, MA

Vygotsky L S (trans A Kozulin) 1986 Thought and language. MIT Press, Cambridge, MA

Wittgenstein L (trans G E M Anscombe) 1958 Philosophical investigations, 3rd edn. Prentice Hall, Upper Saddle River, NJ

Wittgenstein L (trans D F Pears, B F McGuinness) 1921/1974 Tractatus logico-philosophicus. Routledge & Kegan-Paul, London

Chapter 32

Beyond the restitution narrative: lived bodies and expert patients

Suzanne Alder and Debbie Horsfall

Organic life is vulnerable; it inevitably ends in disintegration. This is part of its beauty.
(Tollifson 1997, p. 6)

In this book on clinical reasoning this chapter speaks of reasoning that goes beyond the practitioner's frame of reference and beyond the dominant medical paradigm. Our aim in this chapter is to explore what it means to be living beyond the restitution narrative (Frank 1995) in which the restoration of health, cure and medical science construct practitioners' behaviour and restrict the role of patients. In doing so we focus on practitioner–patient interactions. Our underlying belief is that even while people are chronically ill they can live a life worth living, and this is made easier when they are allowed to rise above 'patient' status, are seen as their own best experts about their bodies, and are treated with dignity and respect regardless of their 'failure' to get better. Essentially, what we want for patients living beyond the restitution narrative is the right to create a new 'normal' for themselves, even while medically speaking they can never be normal again. This is important because society looks to medicine to define 'normal' and 'abnormal', and therefore reinforces the right of a person to participate in life as a normal person or not. In keeping with the group whose experiences speak in this chapter, we refer to patients as female.

Our exploration is grounded in the research discussions of the Phoenix Rising group from the Blue Mountains Women's Health Centre, Katoomba, New South Wales, Australia. This group comprises 15 women living with chronic conditions and disabilities who have been meeting weekly for 2 years. They live with a wide range of chronic conditions, among them Parkinson's disease, cancer, stroke, multiple sclerosis, Huntington's disease, chronic fatigue syndrome, depression and chronic pain. None are curable, but all are determined to live as normal a life as possible. The meetings are facilitated by Suzanne. All vignettes in this chapter are either individual stories the women have told or composite stories that illustrate a theme. They have agreed to their stories being told in this chapter in this way. Paradoxically, what they are asking for from people working in the health professions seems surprisingly simple to give. What follows is what these women want us to tell you.

BEYOND THE RESTITUTION NARRATIVE

> Living with chronic illness is a long, arduous journey. The constant compromise and coping with developing disability is an ever-increasing challenge. The frustration of dealing with reducing activity, loss of previously held freedoms and the changing/shrinking world around me means dealing with an unknown situation, on a regular basis. The effort that has to go into finding information is an exhausting process and occurs at a time of low energy. The emotional impact of receiving a sympathetic and supportive response could play a strong part in the process of healing. Helplessness, the overwhelming loss and feelings of lack of control can be overcome somewhat when practitioners recognize that the way they respond to the panic, stress and trauma associated with life-challenging diagnoses have such a tremendous impact on survival. (Phoenix Rising participant)

Some people who are diagnosed with a chronic illness or disability do not get better, are not cured and never return to 'normal'. People working across the whole spectrum of the health professions both know and avoid acknowledging and dealing with this reality. The dominant narrative, or belief, is that once diagnosed you will be treated, and then you will be cured. All energies, all treatments and all interventions are geared to the goal that it is possible to get better. This is the promise

of science and medicine. Yet science and medicine do not completely understand how to prevent or cure a wide range of conditions that become chronic. There may be much that medicine can do to relieve symptoms and improve the prognosis, but the brute fact of chronicity and permanent illness identity remains. For these people, the restitution narrative has failed. They will not necessarily be 'restored' to heath.

THE PROBLEM OF CHRONICITY

When someone develops a chronic illness they need to work out an identity, a self narrative, that will enable them to continue living while under the constant physical, mental and emotional assaults of life-changing challenges that make it difficult to feel like themselves anymore. We include disability with chronic illness under the term 'chronic condition', by which we refer to any disease or impairment of body or mind that is not yet curable by any branch of medicine. This includes congenital forms of disability. We are aware that many people who see themselves as disabled resist being thought of as ill, even chronically ill. Our working definition of a chronic condition is that it is defined by medicine as an abnormal condition, and even if it cannot be cured medicine holds authority over it. Whether the patient resists the classification of disability as an illness, medicine still regards it as deviation from normal, and social attitudes to abnormal conditions follow the lead of medicine. This leads to the challenging issue of where patient narratives fit in the clinical decision-making process. On the one hand we challenge practitioners to listen well to the narratives and expert knowledge of people with chronic illnesses. On the other hand, perhaps we should replace the terms *clinical* (pertaining to biomedical pathology) and *decision making* (commonly implying a dominant role for, and expertise of, the practitioner) with *lifestyle negotiation*, where partners with different areas of expertise and potential contributions negotiate on ways of supporting the client's optimal lifestyle. In this way practitioners are recognizing and honouring the fact that, although stranded in illness as far as their medical status is concerned, people who live with a chronic condition try to create a way of life that makes them feel normal, autonomous and efficacious. The first step in this process is gaining an understanding of what it means to live, indeed flourish, beyond the restitution narrative. So how do people with chronic conditions try to create a new 'normal' for themselves? What are the supports and barriers in this re-narrativization process?

NEGOTIATING MULTILAYERED MEANINGS

A stroke patient is pleased at first that she has survived and appears to be getting better. As the medical efforts subside, however, she begins to see how stuck on her path she really is. She cannot imagine ever feeling normal again. There does not appear to be anything or anybody capable of restoring her to 'normality' if she cannot achieve complete cure. There are no maps except medical ones. The attitudes around her reflect her lost value to the community, her helplessness and the paucity of options available. Being cared for seems to be the best she can hope for.

A person living with an incurable illness is firmly located as abnormal, ill and disabled. As this person turned patient begins to negotiate the spatial layers of discourse, attitudes and assumptions concerning being ill and disabled, she encounters a sticky web of professional, social and cultural attitudes and practices that have been constructed based on the dualisms of health/illness, and the value that health is better than illness. Everything that now happens in the life of the patient is coloured by that dualism and those values. These values are deeply seated and reflect Western society's fears about decay and death (Garland-Thomson 1997).

Gender theorists suggest that we act out what it is to be male or female according to pre-written cultural scripts that tell us what to do, how to be, and that allow other people to read us and be able to tell who we are (Butler 1993, Connell 2002, Kimmel 2000). There are well-trodden paths that tell patients and doctors and the rest of the community how to think about being ill, what to do, and how to

behave towards illness. The mapping of those cultural ways is laid down in layers of meanings. There are many culturally approved layers that tell us what is 'really' happening to bodies and to the people who live in and around them. There are discursive layers where the rhetoric about health and illness is spun. There are political and economic layers which lay down the rules for how people may participate in community when they are ill. There are social layers that tell us how to behave with illness and around illness. These layers are the taken-for-granted assumptions we hold about health and illness in our society. Because they are taken for granted, seen as normal, they are mostly invisible. This invisibility makes it seemingly impossible to negotiate ways around and through them.

THE LIVED BODY

It is my body,
my life
I have to live with it
not you.
Expertise is supposed to rest with the professional entirely and not at all with the patient. The sheer weight of history that professionals have had with other patients works against an individually referenced perception being made. The system is unwieldy and inflexible. There is an appalling lack of imagination among health scientists and professionals that sometimes makes it hard for them to see outside the label box.

Medicine examines and treats bodies and minds (Fosket 2000; Foucault 1982; Illich 1977; Porter 1993, 1999). The status of these bodies and minds is determined by a series of tests which subject the body–mind to minute and objective surveillance (Foucault 1973). Classification by way of diagnosis follows. Ideally, diagnosis leads to treatment options and some idea of prognosis. This whole performance is theoretically independent of the subjective world of the patient. The patient is expected to render herself a passive recipient of professional care, acting only when asked to carry out medical instructions. Refusing to inhabit this passive role has its consequences:

> Having preferred to use alternative therapies all her life, a woman living with Huntington's disease alienates her medical carers when she refuses some medications on the basis that they will interfere with her preferred values. Consequently, she feels disapproved of and unable to return to their care.

Each instance of disease occurs in the lived body of a unique individual. Medicine often proceeds on the principle that all instances of disease are essentially the same. The *lived body* encompasses the idea that the body–mind under the medical gaze is not free of values, is not interchangeable with any other body–mind, and cannot be properly read without the original inhabitant and her life world. Whatever is going on in the body is influenced and affected by the subjectivity of the person who lives in it, and has to be incorporated into a particular life. It follows that any health care will be more or less successful depending on whether it takes the subjectivity of a lived body into account. The lived body is the sum of all the physical and mental signs and symptoms normally regarded as the proper focus for health care, plus the experiences of living those signs and symptoms in the day-to-day world. The lived body then encompasses the whole spectrum of bodily and mental experience and the subjective values that guide the life lived with/in that body. The lived body brings all its experiences into the surgery and refuses to be treated without these being part of the decision-making equation.

> After her stroke she was told by her doctors that there was little point in hoping for improvement beyond the 6 month mark. She was left to her own devices. She wanted to die because there was no hope. She never thought that her doctors might be wrong. When she found out that it was not true, that she could still work for improvement, she got her old sense of life back. 'It seems that it does not matter to my doctors that I have a life, just that I stay alive.'

Here is the difference between feeling like a body and feeling like a lived body. If all a professional is interested in is the drama of the fight to keep someone alive, regardless of how that saved life is lived out, the patient may be stranded in the black hole of recovery without direction or hope.

For practitioners, then, a serious shock and awakening is necessary. Have you caused or contributed to this black hole? Is your motivation the existence of life or the support of living?

THE EXPERT PATIENT

> If you do not know how to cure the disease
> I have to go on living with forever
> then maybe
> what I know about it is as valid and valuable
> as what you know about it
> perhaps my expertise
> in my life narrative
> is greater than yours

The lived body produces an expert patient. The expert patient accumulates an impressive research history as she works through the issues of her illness and begins to know what works for her and what does not. Along this journey to expertise there are many stages and many levels of self-empowerment and self-awareness. For those coming to terms with their new living reality, understanding and demands for acknowledgement are emergent rather than readily and ever-present. By comparison, the expert patient brings her lived body into every medical encounter and insists on its recognition in that environment. This insistence often meets resistance from professionals:

> Living with an atypical form of Parkinson's disease, a woman who lives alone needs medical reassurance when her breathing is threatened. She encounters different staff all the time at Accident and Emergency, all of whom insist on reading her body by the usual methods and not listening to her. She carries a letter from her GP to reinforce what she is trying to tell them about what works and what doesn't, but she is labelled hysterical and neurotic and the letter is often not referred to at all. The knowledge of the body possessed by the staff is supposed to be all that is required. She has refused certain medications because they have been poorly tolerated in the past. She is sidelined as a difficult patient.

The expert patient is not a bully. She lives in this ill or disabled body and she is trying to make a life with it. She knows that her disease is incurable. She wants the help of medicine insofar as it is able to help at all, and she wants to benefit from future developments. But for the time being, she is trying to live out a life that feels as normal and satisfying as possible. She is trying to bridge the narrative gap between the old life that she could live before illness or disability disrupted narrative flow and a new life that reflects as much of what is important to her as possible. So she brings her lived body into every decision-making arena because she needs her treatments to be consonant with her own needs and values. She knows things about living a particular life with this illness or disability that the professional cannot know. Both bring expertise to the encounter. The professional brings knowledge about the disease or impairment she is living with. However, professional expertise is culturally privileged over personal or subjective feelings and preference. This means that the expertise of a patient is rarely heard.

It can be difficult, perhaps impossible, for a patient who wants to share her expertise to do so when the power differential is very much tipped to the advantage of the professional (Bogoch 1994), when there is not much time for consultations, and when practitioners have been taught that the only important things to know about illness come from their own discipline and body of knowledge, and not from a patient (Atkinson 1997, Beckett & Wrighton 2000). A patient may feel fearful about being labelled a troublemaker or a difficult patient, so she may not insist on being heard. Assertiveness goes out the window in favour of maintaining the approval and cooperation of the practitioner. However, if her expertise can never be a part of decision making, then she may find her life hampered as much by health professionals as by the burden of disease alone.

NEGOTIATING THE PRACTITIONER SPACE

Prescribing treatments
that work against remaining quality of life
probably means
non-compliance with your instructions.

With/in the medical narrative, authority on the lived body of the chronically ill person is positioned with the practitioner, not with the patient. This authority enables the practitioner to tell the 'truth' about the patient's body. The authority is exercised through the use of a highly technical and specialized language that is valued over the subjective discourse of patients. Practitioners tell the truth, and patients tell 'stories'. The practitioner's truths are seen as the only useful knowledge about a person's condition and body.

She was an avid campaigner for valued causes but is no longer able to participate physically as she would like to. When she tries to explain her purposes to her specialist so that they can be made a part of decision making, he seems to feel uncomfortable and ignores the subjective side of her illness entirely. It is as if her story does not count. This means she feels invisible, and as if the only identity she can have is through her dysfunctional body.

However, practitioner truth about what is wrong with the patient is just a clinical story; perhaps no more true than any story the patient may be trying to tell. The clinical story bisects the life of the patient, and she needs time and a willing audience to help imagine a way to pick up the pieces and go on to make a new life. The clinical adventure, which so thrills many practitioners, can leave the patient abandoned in the black hole of narrative ruin.

Can we truly afford to listen to the patient's version of what is going on? Taylor & Brown (1988, 1989) made a case for the positive effects on the lived experience of illness of patients being able to develop and live out their illusions and representations, even if these are not medically 'factual', and Wiginton (1999) reported similar findings in a study of lupus patients. Illness representations appear to be important to outcome, and yet they are either entirely unacknowledged in the medical encounter or rejected as nonsense because they conflict with the medical story.

Foucault (1982) considered that where there is oppressive power there is always resistance. The power of the clinical expert's knowledge stories is resisted by expert patients who have a different story. But resisting the authority of the so-called truth tellers, because it does not accord with what the expert patient knows about her preferred lifestyle or choices, is fraught with difficulty.

> One woman was subjected to guardianship proceedings, and could have been scheduled, because she resisted the advice of specialists. Although she prevailed that time, she knows that she no longer has the sympathy of those practitioners. This worries her because she will probably need them as the disease progresses. All she wanted was to be able to choose treatments that reflected her own values for as long as possible.

Time and energy become fiercely guarded commodities when a person is chronically ill, yet medicine plunders both for its own ends. Many of the women in this chapter spend so much time waiting in waiting rooms, going for testing, and struggling to meet the endless expectations of government agencies to prove that they are ill, in need of some support, that they feel their illness is a full-time job. There is no time or energy for anything more meaningful when they eventually get home. They collapse, and feel even more hopeless about their ability ever to be able to live a participatory and contributing life. The time of a health practitioner always seems to be considered more important than the time of the patient. If a patient gets *impatient*, and leaves the surgery, she can be punished by disapproval and difficulty in making another appointment. If she is sent for more blood tests, or to see a specialist, on a day that clashes with her patchwork class, the decision to go to the class instead of the medical appointment is seldom sympathized with. When you are living with a permanent illness, the things that mark out your life that are not medical are vital to well-being. Patients need to be able to choose other or different commitments over medical ones and not risk losing medical support. Sometimes choices are about different sorts of treatment:

> A woman with metastatic cancer refused a second bout of chemotherapy in favour of Chinese herbal treatments. She does not know if these will 'work' for cure or not. But the practitioner who prescribes them makes her feel as though anything is possible. 'He chooses to reject my cancer as a clinical entity and instead sees it as a pilgrimage that is tied up intimately with my own

soul journey'. The way he explains health and illness captures the ecology of her whole life. That offers her more hope and sense of purpose. She knows that she can work for good things to happen in her life that have nothing to do with cure. Her oncologist speaks to her only about cells and cellular processes.

Medicine deals with the observable processes and dynamics of the clockwork body–mind (Broomfield 1997; Porter 1993, 1999; Wertheim 1997). Treatment aims to change the condition of the body–mind, much as a clockmaker fixes a clock by understanding exactly how every cog fits and works together. When that cannot happen because of insufficient knowledge or skill, many patients feel hopeless and bereft of direction for further action. If they can find a way to think about the illness that transcends the brute facts of the disease they often feel more positive and empowered. This is healing, not cure. Some would call this attitude being 'in denial', because the brute facts of the disease appear to be sidelined. The women in this chapter feel it is the opposite of denial.

Broyard (1992, p. 41) spoke of the need for practitioners to be able to see past their love affair with technology: 'The technicians bring in the raw material. The doctor puts them into a poem of diagnosis'. Refusing to be reduced to a mechanical body is an act of resistance and hope. It is not easy. Every time a diagnosis is made patients tend to take on that diagnosis as an identity. This can prevent practitioners and others from seeing the patient as a full human being, let alone an expert. It can prevent participation in community and work situations because the incompetence and dysfunction that goes with a disease or disability can generalize outwards to encompass the whole space the patient occupies.

> The label 'Parkinson's disease' had reached someone on an interviewing panel when a woman applied for a job which she knew she would be able to do for some time. She was not given the job. This was read by some as a good thing, because she clearly had to be protected from doing too much. There was an implicit judgment of incompetence to know what was best for her that went along with the potential dysfunctions that would come with her disease.

Labels can follow patients around for the rest of their lives in the form of case notes. Even after recovery is achieved, it is hard to see past the 'truths' written into the medical case notes.

> Misdiagnosed schizophrenic several years ago, this woman is now considered to have been suffering from a severe depression. After years of treatment she has recovered her confidence and ability enough to think about re-entering the world of work. Although her mental health workers individually agree with her, she cannot get her old identity back officially because of the label 'schizophrenic' recorded in her case notes. The official attitude is that the notes must be right, and her good performance now is just a temporary thing, she will probably relapse. The default setting is suspicion, not affirmation and celebration at recovery.

There seems to be little room for recognition of who the patient was before becoming ill, as well as who she is becoming now. Most of the women in our group enjoyed active and contributing lives and gained a large part of their sense of self from their work, paid and unpaid. Their practitioners rarely want to know who they used to be. The medical gaze is focused on the body–mind and its 'truths'.

CONCLUSION

> Dear practitioner,
> Chronically ill patients have to live their disease for the rest of their lives. The medical system often fails people like me by constantly re-engaging with the stubborn face of my disease and failing to engage with the lived body behind it. In your well-meaning campaign to re-seek success in terms of cure you shuffle me in and out of tests and treatments, expect me to comply and reject me if I don't pursue the goals of the clinicians, even when the probability of success is very low. Everyone is afraid when the restitution narrative fails.

> When you find you have strayed off the medical map and are floundering in the wasteland beyond the restitution narrative, remember that you have a guide with you. You have an expert patient who will show you what she needs and how you can best support her.
> Encourage me to reclaim my experience with vulnerability as normal. It is normal to be vulnerable, after all, and not the other way around. In our love affair with medicine we may have forgotten that.
> Sit with me. Listen to me as I tell you what's important for me to be able to re-engage with life. Reassure me of your support whenever I need it, whatever my decisions. Be honest with me about your distress and sense of helplessness, and let me know you will continue to be available as a resource to me. Be comforted by what can happen beyond the restitution narrative when I am allowed to rise above patient status and make decisions about my quality of life and the way it is storied. 'What do I want in a doctor? I would say that I want one who is a close reader of illness and a good critic of medicine' (Broyard 1992, p. 39).

In this chapter we have tried to make visible and clear the spaces that people living with chronic conditions both inhabit and learn to negotiate as they struggle to live a life beyond cure. Making negotiations and decision practices that are guided by expert patients and the needs of lived bodies can enable people to resist being captured by the inherent confusion and contradictions of lived illness and disability, particularly when chronic. The oppressive forces that keep patients with chronic conditions firmly pinned in their role as permanent passive patient stimulate resistance in patient groups like Phoenix Rising. That resistance must be nurtured to flow out into all the spaces inhabited by patients and within which they struggle to find a new 'normal' for themselves.

References

Atkinson P 1997 The clinical experience: the construction and reconstruction of clinical experience 2nd edn. Ashgate, Aldershot

Beckett C, Wrighton E 2000 What matters to me is not what you're talking about: maintaining the social model of disability in 'public and private' negotiations. Disability and Society 15(7):991–999

Bogoch B 1994 Power, distance and solidarity-models of professional–client interaction in an Israeli legal aid setting. Discourse and Society 5(1):65–88

Broomfield J 1997 Other ways of knowing: recharting our future with ageless wisdom. Inner Traditions International, Rochester, VT

Broyard A 1992 Intoxicated by my illness. Ballantine Books, New York

Butler J 1993 Bodies that matter: feminism and the subversion of identity. Routledge, London

Connell R W 2002 Gender: short introductions. Polity Press, Cambridge

Fosket J 2000 Problematizing biomedicine: women's constructions of breast cancer knowledge. In: Potts L K (ed) Ideologies of breast cancer: feminist perspectives. Macmillan Press, London, p 15–36

Foucault M 1973 The birth of the clinic. Vintage Books, New York

Foucault M 1982 The subject and power. Critical Inquiry 8:777–795

Frank A W 1995 The wounded story teller. body, illness and ethics. University of Chicago Press, Chicago

Garland-Thomson R 1997 Extraordinary bodies: figuring physical disability in American culture and literature. Columbia University Press, New York

Illich I 1977 Disabling professions. In: Illich I, Zola I K, McKnight J et al (eds) Disabling professions. Marion Boyars, London, p 11–40

Kimmel M 2000 The gendered society. Oxford University Press, New York

Porter R 1993 The body and the mind, the doctor and the patient: negotiating hysteria. In: Gilman S, King H, Porter R et al (eds) Hysteria beyond Freud. University of California Press, Berkeley, p 92–225

Porter R 1999 The greatest benefit to mankind: a medical history of humanity from antiquity to the present. Fontana Press, London

Taylor S E, Brown J D 1988 Illusions and well-being: a social psychological perspective on mental health. Psychological Bulletin 103:193–210

Taylor S E, Brown J D 1989 Maintaining positive illusions in the face of negative information: getting the facts without letting them get to you. Journal of Social and Clinical Psychology 8(2):114–129

Tollifson J 1997 Imperfection is a beautiful thing. In: Fries K (ed) Staring back: the disability experience from the inside out. Plume, New York

Wertheim M 1997 Pythagoras' trousers: God, physics and the gender wars. Fourth Estate, London

Wiginton K L 1999 Illness representations: mapping the experience of lupus. Health Education and Behavior 26 (4):443–453

Chapter 33

Facilitating clinical decision making in students in intercultural fieldwork placements

Lindy McAllister and Gail Whiteford

INTRODUCTION

Health professional education is increasingly being undertaken in intercultural settings, in both domestic and international contexts. Such intercultural contexts are both more complex and more demanding than the familiar environments in which students in the health professions typically find themselves. Clinical reasoning within such complex practice settings presents significant challenges for all healthcare practitioners, not only for students. Despite the challenges inherent in intercultural settings, there is a relative paucity of information on best practice in facilitation of clinical reasoning and decision making in such contexts. This chapter draws upon data gathered over several years spent developing, implementing and evaluating an interdisciplinary student fieldwork programme in Vietnam. Using extracts from research interviews undertaken with students about their learning experiences in Vietnam, the chapter illuminates the demands and tensions experienced by students. It also outlines processes and strategies employed by fieldwork educators to facilitate students' clinical reasoning in intercultural settings. We present recommendations for academics and fieldwork educators for facilitating the clinical reasoning of students in intercultural fieldwork placements, and conclude with reflections on the future of intercultural fieldwork, clinical reasoning and research.

THE CONTEXT OF THE DATA REFERRED TO IN THIS CHAPTER

Since 2001, the School of Community Health at Charles Sturt University's (CSU) Albury campus has been conducting an international multidisciplinary allied health fieldwork programme involving children with physical disabilities at Phu My orphanage in Saigon, Vietnam. Each March and April, up to 12 final-year occupational therapy, physiotherapy and speech pathology students, with rotating fieldwork educators from these disciplines, spend 6 weeks at the orphanage. One goal of the programme is to educate and train Vietnamese staff in the orphanage (Vietnamese-trained physiotherapists, paediatricians, teachers and carers) about optimizing feeding, communication, play, mobility and other activities of daily living with children with physical and intellectual impairments. The aim is not to 'treat' or provide direct therapy to individual children, except when modelling skills and supporting capacity development for Phu My staff. The second goal pertains to student learning issues. Students are expected to develop intercultural competence and a range of other basic competencies including Vietnamese language skills and knowledge of Vietnamese history and culture; skills in training and working with interpreters; working with children with physical and intellectual impairments; training and educating others (Vietnamese staff, other volunteers at the orphanage, CSU students from other disciplines); managing team dynamics and group processes; working in resource-poor environments. The term 'intercultural competence' refers to cultural self-awareness, knowledge of 'the other', and skill in mediating communication (Sodowski et al 1994).

An ongoing research programme has been in place since the inception of the Vietnam project, one aspect of which uses a critical incident approach (Fitzgerald 2000). We interviewed students in the country and/or upon return to Australia about their experiences in Vietnam. The critical incident approach, a specific narrative device through which meaning is ascribed to a significant event via guided reflection, was chosen because it provided a contextually sensitive means through which the students could make sense of both their clinical decision-making processes and their multilayered interactions with Vietnamese staff. Preliminary findings of this research have been reported elsewhere (McAllister et al 2006; Whiteford & McAllister in press).

CLINICAL REASONING IN THE INTERCULTURAL CONTEXT

Within the distinct milieu of Phu My orphanage, effective clinical reasoning and decision making are requisite to the success of the programme. As a fieldwork site it is complex and demanding because of the sociopolitical environment, the attendant intercultural interactions, the interdisciplinary nature of the placement and the complex needs of the children and staff of the orphanage. Students and fieldwork educators interact daily with large numbers of children and staff, responding to different and at times competing requests for help and advice. Higgs & Jones (2000) have described several approaches to conceptualizing clinical reasoning. Because they are neither fluent in the language (needed to elicit case histories) nor able to perform detailed diagnostic assessment, students appear not to use hypothetico-deductive and pattern recognition approaches to reasoning, which are perhaps more appropriate to the delivery of treatment in like cultures and treatment within medical contexts. Students and health professionals in intercultural contexts, such as that of the orphanage, need to use complex approaches to clinical reasoning and appear to use interpretive approaches, particularly the interactive, narrative, collaborative and ethical/pragmatic approaches to reasoning outlined by Higgs & Jones (2000), derived from research in occupational therapy (Fleming 1991) and physical therapy (Edwards et al 2004).

The client-centred model of clinical reasoning described by Higgs & Jones (2000) best describes the approach to clinical reasoning sought in the Vietnam placements. The client-centred approach involves the application and integration of cognition (thinking about the clinical problem), professional knowledge, considerations of the environment, clients' input (in this case preferences expressed by children and requests from staff), and metacognition (monitoring one's thinking and the interaction of all the factors mentioned earlier – especially important in the intercultural setting). In our case, the clinical problem might be a child's needs for mobilizing, play or self-care, carers' needs for training, or determining how to enrich the children's environment. Within the context of this client-centred reasoning model, students have relied most significantly upon processes of narrative reasoning (Mattingly 1991) to articulate and refine their clinical decision making. Narrative reasoning often entails practitioners creating or sharing stories about their work. The self-talk or talk with others involved can mediate metacognitive processing and promote deep learning through creating opportunities for critical reflection (Brookfield 1990). For students in the complex intercultural environment, narrative reasoning is particularly relevant and offers an appropriate medium through which to plan, articulate and evaluate both their professional goals and the overarching goals of the programme. Group reflection (discussed later in the chapter) is therefore an important aspect of the programme.

The propensity for students to employ narrative reasoning processes naturalistically, in response to the specific demands of the setting, reinforced the appropriateness of the adoption of a critical incident approach to programme evaluation. It allowed us to capture rich narratives and thick descriptions of intercultural interactions and the nature and demands of clinical reasoning and decision making in situ. An excerpt from one such critical incident interview is presented here as an exemplar of the experience of being in a complex intercultural environment and doing continuous reasoning.

ILLUSTRATING CLINICAL REASONING AND DECISION MAKING IN THE INTERCULTURAL CONTEXT

We present an excerpt from an interview with John, a physiotherapy student. This interview was conducted early in John's placement in Vietnam. The child John refers to has severe physical limitations due to cerebral palsy.

STOP, THINK AND SAY NO: JOHN'S STORY

... after doing a little bit of an assessment and playing with one of the children we began to feed the child and I was actually feeding the child and taking a lot of time because the child was feeding very slowly and then the carer came in and took over and said 'let me show you how to do it'. She then sort of grabbed the child's head, pushed his head back, shoved the spoon straight down his mouth and continued shovelling in and this was very disturbing for me and in fact I even had to leave the room. ... I found it upsetting, I felt helpless because I'd lost control. I also felt that I'd failed in my job of feeding the child in that the carer had to come in and take over. And I felt that I had sort of lost face through that. I've since repaired that, but it was difficult on that level, the relationship with the carer, but I also felt very much for the child. You could see the child protesting ... showing some obvious signs of distress. Hands

pushing away, head turning away, mouth clenched closed, all those things, but the food was going in there regardless. ... I wanted to step in but I had to recognize my professional boundaries. That was the sort of relationship that the child had with the carer and that's how he's probably fed a lot of the time, so I had to step back and that was very difficult to do because I would usually jump in there before I'd think about it. So I actually had to think and stop and say no, the right thing to do would be let him be fed by the carer as the carer wants to at this stage and slowly work at [changes] rather than try and change things all at once. It was difficult, it was difficult for me because I like to jump in there and do things. ... She's the chief carer in that room and someone we have now developed a really good relationship with and she's very receptive to the work that we're doing. I'm now regularly feeding a different child and she's allowing me much more

(Continued)

STOP, THINK AND SAY NO: JOHN'S STORY

time to feed with that child. There's food going everywhere, we're making a terrible mess but she's okay with it, she's fine because I'm cleaning it up. So I can see the benefits of what I did at that stage. If I had got upset in front of her or tried to change forcefully what she was doing that would have had a negative consequence. I can see now that she's much more receptive and she's come around to what we're doing. ... [On reflection] apart from the obvious language barrier there were the cultural issues, I think it was really the 'save face' kind of thing. I was aware of [it] in Asian cultures in terms of being seen to do something or recognizing your own limitations; I guess [there] is a point to it as well and being able to 'save face' rather than, you don't want to be humiliated. So the honourable thing I could do in that situation was to withdraw. If I hadn't I would have offended her, as I would have probably someone in any culture but particularly I think here, they are very sensitive to it. And probably then there would be the male... female dynamics as well, that would have definitely, definitely been an issue. Had I said anything at that stage she would have definitely resented it as to 'who are you? who do you think you are? you guys know nothing about what we're doing here'.

THE DEMANDS AND TENSIONS OF INTERCULTURAL PRACTICE AND COMMUNICATION

John's story is an honest and moving account of one person's cognitive and affective responses to the challenges inherent in working with children with severe impairments as well as working in a demanding intercultural environment. The experiences recounted here are commonly experienced by students and university fieldwork educators in their early weeks at the orphanage. As John's story illustrates, clinical reasoning in such intercultural contexts has added dimensions compared to that in one's home country. Intercultural clinical reasoning involves tracking interactions and communications at multiple levels. John spoke little Vietnamese; however, he was alert to the nuances of non-verbal communication and body language and relied on them to interpret what the carer might have been intending and doing. The nuances of verbal and non-verbal communication vary widely across cultures (McAllister & Street 2005) and the potential for miscommunication and misinterpretation is considerable. These misinterpretations can lead to conflict. Further, there is an aspect of immediacy in the intercultural context. It appeared that the carer misinterpreted John's request for assistance. It was early in the placement where a relationship had not yet been established with the carer, and John had no clear quick way to repair the miscommunication. John needed to make an immediate decision on how to avoid conflict and preserve the relationship he was developing with the carer. He acquiesced to the carer's taking over the task at hand, despite his distress at witnessing the carer's handling of the child. John sensed that he needed to give way, to avoid amplifying any consequences such as a breakdown in the relationship, loss of face for himself and the carer, and perhaps being unwelcome in future in the child's care room. The interaction was further complicated by the status of the carer who, as 'head carer' in the room, demanded respect and could not afford to lose face.

Ethical tensions add further complexity to intercultural practice. In John's story, he was torn between ensuring beneficence and non-maleficence for the child, while showing respect for the carer. In the interests of long-term good for both child and carer, he made an ethical decision to preserve the relationship with the carer. When such ethical reasoning has cultural overtones, it becomes even more challenging.

John's story highlights the importance of the affective dimension of clinical reasoning. Students and fieldwork educators working in intercultural contexts such as Phu My are emotionally vulnerable because of the unfamiliarity of contexts, communication and status issues, and the adjustment required to adapt to the culture of the country and the host organization. Fatigue and illness can exacerbate such vulnerability. John freely expressed his emotional response to the severity of the children's disabilities, their plight, and to the averted conflict with the carer. He effectively managed his emotions in ways that were not typical for him, but enabled him to use his clinical reasoning and make appropriate decisions.

STRATEGIES USED TO FACILITATE THE DEVELOPMENT OF CLINICAL REASONING AND DECISION MAKING IN INTERCULTURAL CONTEXTS

In the excerpt from John's story it is clear that he used a range of strategies we believe are powerful in assisting students to develop clinical reasoning and decision making in the intercultural context. Over the 5 years during which the Vietnam project at Phu My orphanage has been operating, the fieldwork educators have developed and refined a number of strategies which we believe support students' development of clinical reasoning and decision making in the intercultural context. The strategies are both direct, as described below, and indirect, arising from the very nature of living in another culture as well as living and working within a team setting.

PRE-DEPARTURE BRIEFING PROGRAMME

The structure of the Vietnam placement programme of itself facilitates clinical reasoning. A programme of pre-departure readings, meetings and team building activities forms the foundation for later, in-country clinical reasoning. Students begin their preparation 6 months before departure. After application and selection at the end of the third year of their courses, they meet two or three times with fieldwork educators to discuss bookings, costings and health requirements for the placement. They are assigned readings on Vietnam and on disability, and review videotapes of the orphanage and its children. Students plan activities (e.g. talks to service clubs, trivia nights) to raise funds for purchase of equipment for the orphanage; this starts the process of team bonding. In the 6 weeks between the start of their fourth year and departure for Vietnam

students attend seminars on a range of topics (e.g. working with children with cerebral palsy, the culture and history of Vietnam, working with interpreters). Fieldwork educators spend time clearly establishing expectations for students' learning and behaviour, both as individuals and as a team. Students analyse reports prepared by the previous group of students, and can talk to a new graduate who has participated in the programme. As a team, students also collate information or purchase materials as recommended by former groups at the orphanage or as requested by orphanage staff.

BUILDING IN OPPORTUNITIES FOR REFLECTION ON PRACTICE

The structure of the programme in Vietnam has been designed to maximize opportunities for reflection, a key process in the development of intercultural competence (McAllister et al 2006). Reflective thinking leading to reflective judgement appears to be an important aspect of cultural competence; in fact, it may be more critical than possessing specific knowledge or having a particular kind of attitude towards specific groups of people. Brookfield (1990) noted that the critical reflective thinker can identify assumptions that underlie their thoughts and actions, evaluate the accuracy and validity of these assumptions and, as necessary, reconstitute these assumptions.

Kitchener & King (1990) suggested that reflective judgement is developmental in nature, with discrete stages. Although their work is based on Western, reasonably well-educated populations, Kitchener & King's reflective judgement model has some utility for understanding cultural competence. There appear to be important similarities in the developmental processes associated with both reflective judgement and intercultural competence; in fact, the two appear to be intimately related. At each level are epistemological assumptions about the nature of knowledge and the ability and willingness to engage in information evaluation, enquiry and analytical processes, including the evaluation and analysis of profession-specific knowledge. In terms of intercultural competence, Kitchener & King's stages equate with ethnocentrism at the lowest level, progressing to cultural awareness, then to cultural particularism, and ultimately to increasing degrees of intercultural competence (Fitzgerald 2000). We considered this developmental sequence in developing the Phu My programme.

A STRUCTURED FIELDWORK PROGRAMME

In the first of the 6 weeks in Vietnam, students attend Vietnamese language classes in the mornings and visit the orphanage in the afternoons. These visits are designed to familiarize students with the culture and routines of the orphanage, with the children and their carers and environment, and to establish teamwork processes. This scaffolded introduction to the placement, with time for cultural adaptation and reflection, has been found to be crucial to reduction of culture shock and achievement of learning outcomes for the students. Having a designated room for use by fieldwork educators and students during the placement is very helpful. The university has equipped the room with a computer and printer, and there is also a large table for group meetings. At the end of each day, at least 1 hour is allotted for discussion and reflection on what has been seen and learned. This is important given the culture shock experienced by students, and indeed fieldwork educators, as they settle into Vietnam (Arthur 2001, McAllister et al 2006) and into the orphanage. Students read the files on what work has been done previously with target children and with staff training. They familiarize themselves with working with their interpreters. From week 2 onwards, the days at the orphanage are structured to maximize group learning and reflection.

INTERDISCIPLINARY TEAMWORK

A key aspect of the placement is its interdisciplinary nature. Student-run group meetings (with facilitation from fieldwork educators if needed) are vital to attainment of goals of the placement. Because programming goals must be developed and delivered in an interdisciplinary manner, students need to discuss children's intervention goals and carers' training needs from a holistic perspective. The students and fieldwork educators do not function only as 'OTs', 'physios' or 'speech paths', but must also work in a transdisciplinary manner. We believe this

significantly challenges and enhances clinical reasoning and decision making in the students as they articulate their discipline's perspectives and seek clarification of the perspectives of others. The group meetings also require reasoning and management of group processes, invaluable skills for professional practice. Students must also collaborate in the preparation of programmes, reports and resources. When requested by students, fieldwork educators deliver tutorials to assist the development of knowledge, practical skills and clinical reasoning on various topics; for example, handling children with cerebral palsy, positioning for feeding, engaging children with severe impairments in play. Where possible, students conduct the tutorials, sharing their discipline-specific knowledge with the other disciplines, so that multidisciplinary programme goals can be developed.

SUPERVISION, TEACHING AND SUPPORT FROM FIELDWORK EDUCATORS

Input from the fieldwork educators is critical to the development of students' clinical reasoning and decision making. Fieldwork educators provide both direct teaching and indirect support as commonly used in any clinical settings (McAllister et al 1997). They conduct tutorials on a range of topics and model techniques for working with children and interacting with staff. They provide online feedback to students, watching them work with children or carers, and stepping in to assist or comment as needed. They also provide formative feedback and summative assessment as required by the clinical subjects in which the students are enrolled. Perhaps most importantly, because of the complexities, tensions and demands involved in the intercultural setting, they ask critical questions which help students reason their way through professional and intercultural issues, and request clear articulation of clinical decision-making processes. When students struggle with clinical reasoning, fieldwork educators promote, probe and scaffold the process to assist students with their reasoning.

This critical questioning is also an important part of the peer learning dynamic in the interdisciplinary team context of the placement. A student from one discipline cannot assume shared knowledge, assumptions or perspectives from students in the other disciplines. Students must articulate their clinical reasoning in the group sessions and be prepared to defend, clarify or modify it, as the team develops multidisciplinary goals and programmes.

There are periods during the placement where more than one fieldwork supervisor is working alongside the students. The supervisors take these opportunities to openly discuss their questions, concerns and approaches with each other and their students. In doing so, they are actively sharing their clinical reasoning, and modelling for the students how to promote their own clinical reasoning. The students report finding this instructive and entertaining, to see staff openly challenging each other. We present here some extracts of students' reflections on the value of the multidisciplinary team in communicating, reasoning and decision making:

> Talking to everyone else in the team, that was good, just throwing ideas around and talking. 'OK, this is what I did, what would you have done, what choices would you have made?' . . . yeah things like that were good . . . I mean it was a steep learning curve, it was good and I'm glad that I was put in that situation and was able to do that. Yeah, I think a lot of it was a team effort with other students . . . we were always aware about how people were feeling. Molly (speech pathology student)

> I have actually learned a lot about myself and the way that I work with other people . . . the experience has given me way more confidence in that I know that If I have a team meeting and there are 10 physios sitting around me I know that I'm going to be able to speak up and have the confidence to say what I feel and believe because we did that on a daily basis. So I learned a lot about the way I work on a team. Louise (occupational therapy student)

One week without on-site supervision (typically week 4) is built into the programme. Although fieldwork educators are on call in Australia via distance supervision methods (email, text messaging, telephone), students tend to rely more on each other as resources to support their reasoning and clinical management skills. Fieldwork educators involved in the programme have consistently been impressed with the growth in clinical reasoning,

increased autonomy and accountability, and professional and self-management that occurs in this week before the final rotating university fieldwork educator arrives for the last week when the final assessments of learning outcomes occur.

CRITICAL INCIDENT INTERVIEWS

One final strategy used to promote clinical reasoning and decision making is the use of critical incident interviews. More specifically, critical incidents are 'distinct occurrences or events which involve two or more people; they are neither inherently negative nor positive, they are merely distinct occurrences or events which require some attention, action or explanation; they are situations for which there is a need to attach meaning' (Fitzgerald 2000, p. 190).

Shorter interviews occur in Vietnam during the placement and a more in-depth version is conducted upon return to Australia. The format is a semi-structured interview in which students are asked to discuss an event that was in some way significant for them during the placement. Sometimes this is personal in nature, sometimes professional, and sometimes the incidents chosen have both personal and professional connotations. The extracts from John's, Molly's and Louise's stories are from such critical incident interviews (for more information on the critical incident methodology used in this study of intercultural competence development see McAllister et al 2006). The in-country interviews assist students' reasoning and decision making about the incidents retrospectively. The interviews conducted when students return to Australia tap into deep learning from the intercultural experience, after a longer period of reflection. These interviews also illuminate how learning from the Vietnam placement can be integrated into professional practice in Australia, assisting with the sense-making of the experience and the generalization of learning to a new context.

RECOMMENDATIONS AND CONCLUSIONS

> Just having to deal with all the different structures and things in that [Vietnamese] culture

and trying to adjust your practice to fit in with those is a real challenge and I think it stretches you as a person and as a professional. A fantastic experience. I'd do it again if I had the option. Michelle (occupational therapy student)

Negotiating, securing and developing international intercultural placements is hard work. Time pressures, fiscal constraints and professional accreditation demands also add to the layers of complexity that fieldwork educators must actively manage in making real this opportunity for students. The value to both students and the stakeholders of the placement site, especially in resource-poor settings, however, is not insignificant, and is the primary motivator for the continuation of such programmes. Over time we have learned specific strategies that enhance the overall quality of the experience for students and facilitate the attainment of clinical reasoning and decision-making skills in the international and intercultural context. In addition to the strategies outlined above, two further strategies are key to the success of intercultural fieldwork programmes: curriculum content which supports the intercultural fieldwork and ongoing evaluation of the experience and learning outcomes.

Intercultural fieldwork needs to be strongly grounded in a curriculum that provides students with knowledge and skills for the placements and supports their experiences during placements. At a general level, the curriculum must address conceptual representations of 'the other', culture, ethnocentrism, understanding difference and cultural safety. Specifically, the curriculum must support clinical reasoning processes and skills development, and articulation of theory to practice in intercultural contexts. The fieldwork placement should not be an 'add-on' but should flow from the curriculum as a whole.

Intercultural placements need to be supported and refined through strong evaluative processes. Learning outcomes for students must be evaluated. In addition, we suggest that the processes of intercultural learning must be made transparent for students so they can appreciate the scope of their achievements and apply these processes to other contexts. Reflective journals, the critical incident interviews described above, and having students prepare assignments or deliver conference presentations derived from their experiences have proved helpful in this regard. Furthermore, the experiences and perspectives of stakeholders at the fieldwork site must be considered, and triangulated against students' reports, to ensure that the placements are beneficial for all concerned. Evaluation over the 5 years of the programme to date has assisted us to refine and develop the strategies we use to facilitate students' clinical reasoning in intercultural contexts.

Clinical reasoning in intercultural contexts is a complex and demanding professional skill. The facilitation of clinical reasoning in students in such contexts is challenging for fieldwork educators. In this chapter we have described several strategies that we have used successfully over time to support students' reasoning processes. The students' narrative excerpts illustrate the valuable learning through clinical reasoning that can be stimulated in intercultural practice settings.

Acknowledgements

The study from which narrative extracts in this chapter are drawn was supported by a multidisciplinary research grant from the Charles Sturt University Centre for Research and Graduate Training.

References

Arthur N 2001 Using critical incidents to investigate cross-cultural transitions. International Journal of Intercultural Relations 25:41–53

Brookfield S 1990 Using critical incidents to explore learners' assumptions. In: Mezirow J (ed) Fostering critical reflection in adulthood: a guide to transformative and emancipatory learning. Jossey-Bass, San Francisco, p 177–193

Edwards I, Jones M, Carr J et al 2004 Clinical reasoning strategies in physical therapy. Physical Therapy 84 (4):312–335

Fitzgerald M 2000 Establishing cultural competency for health professionals. In: Skultans V, Cox J (eds) Anthropological approaches to psychological medicine. Jessica Kingsley, London, p 149–200

Fleming M H 1991 The therapist with the three track mind. American Journal of Occupational Therapy 45:1007–1014

Higgs J, Jones M 2000 Clinical reasoning in the health professions. In: Higgs J, Jones M (eds) Clinical reasoning in the health professions. 2nd edn. Butterworth-Heinemann, Oxford, p 3–14

Kitchener K, King P 1990 The reflective judgement model: transforming assumptions about knowing. In: Mezirow J (ed) Fostering critical reflection in adulthood: a guide to transformative and emancipatory learning. Jossey-Bass, San Francisco, p 159–176

McAllister L, Street A 2005 Intercultural communication. In: Higgs J, Sefton A, Street A et al (eds) Communicating in the health and social sciences. Oxford University Press, South Melbourne, p 239–246

McAllister L, Lincoln M, McLeod S et al (eds) 1997 Facilitating learning in clinical settings. Stanley Thornes, Cheltenham

McAllister L, Whiteford G, Hill R et al 2006 Reflection in intercultural learning: examining the international experience through a critical incident approach. Reflective Practice 7(3):367–381

Mattingly C 1991 The narrative nature of clinical reasoning. American Journal of Occupational Therapy 45: 998–1005

Sodowski G, Taffe R, Gutkin T et al (1994) Development of the multicultural counselling inventory. Journal of Counselling Psychology 41(2):137–148

Whiteford G, McAllister L (in press) Politics and complexity in intercultural fieldwork: the Vietnam experience. Australian Occupational Therapy Journal Online. Available: http://www.blackwell-synergy.com/doi/abs/10.1111/j.1440-1630.2006.00607.x10 July 2007

Chapter 34

Using decision aids to involve clients in clinical decision making

Lyndal Trevena, Alex Barratt and Kirsten McCaffery

WHAT IS A DECISION AID?

As the term implies, *decision aids* are tools that are designed to facilitate health decision making between patient and practitioner. Probably the most widely used definition of decision aids is the following, from the Cochrane Library's systematic review:

> Decision aids are interventions designed to help people make specific and deliberative choices among options by providing information about the options and outcomes that is relevant to a person's health status. The specific aims of decision aids and the type of decision support they provide may vary slightly, but in general they are designed to enable people to:
>
> a) understand the probable outcomes of options by providing information relevant to the decision;
> b) consider the personal value they place on benefits versus harms by helping clarify preferences;
> c) feel supported in decision making;
> d) move through the steps in making a decision; and
> e) participate in deciding about their health care. (O'Connor et al 2006)

Although there is some variation in viewpoints, there is general consensus among international groups (IPDAS 2006) developing decision aids that, in the context of making decisions about health, such tools should be:

- explicitly evidence based in content
- evidence based in format and design
- balanced in presentation of options and information
- evaluated by experts for methodology
- evaluated with consumers for efficacy.

We propose that decision aids should also be accessible to people from a range of literacy levels, but the best mechanism for achieving this is still being determined. A more detailed list of quality criteria for decision aids is discussed later in this chapter.

Interest in clinical decision making has been increasing for some time. David Eddy wrote a significant series of essays over a decade ago in which he proposed that health decisions not only include analyses of scientific and clinical evidence but also patient preferences. He maintained that most decisions involved weighing up benefit against harm and that some judgement is involved (Eddy 1996). In the past, such a weighing up process might have been completed by the clinician on behalf of the patient. However, as this chapter will demonstrate, societal attitudes have changed substantially, and patients increasingly want to be involved in these decision-making processes. Clinicians may assume wrongly that their preferences are the same as those of their patients. There is now empiric evidence that consumers and clinicians value at least some treatment outcomes differently. For example, the value patients place on stroke prevention with anticoagulants is different from that of their physicians (Protheroe et al 2000), and families are content to discontinue antiepileptic drugs at different levels of risk than are their physicians (Gordon et al 1996). The concepts proposed by Eddy have been further developed by members of the Evidence-Based Medicine Working Group and others to suggest that research evidence should be combined with clinical expertise, the patient's clinical state and circumstances and the patient's preferences and actions (Haynes et al 2002, Trevena & Barratt 2003). Decision aids may be one mechanism by which this can be achieved.

A systematic review of effective strategies for communicating with patients about evidence showed that patients' understanding of evidence was improved by most structured tools but particularly if they were tailored, personalized and/or interactive. Decision aids have the capacity to achieve tailoring and also to facilitate the elicitation of patient preferences through personalized worksheets and value clarification exercises (Trevena et al 2005).

WHAT IS THE EFFECT OF DECISION AIDS ON PATIENT INVOLVEMENT?

A Cochrane systematic review of 32 decision aids concluded that decision aids increased patient knowledge of the options compared to usual care, with gains in such knowledge ranging from 9 to 30 percentage points (weighted mean difference (WMD) 19 points, 95% CI: 13 to 24). Studies also suggested that decision aids increased realistic expectations about the benefits and harms of different healthcare options as measured by patients' perception of the probability of outcomes. The review indicated improved patient satisfaction with the decision-making process and greater agreement between patient values and actual choice.

There is some evidence that decision aids increase the proportion of patients who are actively involved in decision making. The Cochrane systematic review included seven randomized controlled trials comparing decision aids against usual care. These trials covered a range of decisions such as prostate cancer screening, treatment of early prostate cancer, treatment of ischaemic heart disease, anticoagulation in atrial fibrillation, colorectal cancer screening and the use of hormone therapy during the menopause. The meta-analysis showed that people receiving a decision aid were 30% less likely to report having a passive (practitioner-controlled) role in their decision (RR 0.7; 95% CI: 0.5 to 0.9). The corollary of this is that decision aids were more likely to be associated with an active role in decision-making (RR 1.4, 95% CI: 1.0 to 2.3). The quality of the decision process was also significantly improved. In particular, uncertainty about decision making (decisional conflict) was significantly reduced (WMD −9.1 of 100, 95% CI: −12 to −6).

HOW CAN WE ASSESS PATIENT INVOLVEMENT?

The measurement of patient involvement in decision making has mainly used the Control Preferences Scale (Degner et al 1997). Patients usually assess their actual or preferred role from the five options shown in Box 34.1.

Although this scale continues to be widely used in many studies to measure patient involvement, some researchers have questioned its validity (Davey et al 2004; Entwistle et al 2001, 2004). A systematic review of instruments to measure patient involvement came to a similar conclusion, suggesting that *patient involvement* is a complex construct that requires more qualitative assessment (Elwyn et al 2001). As a result of this, other instruments have now been used and validated in analysing recorded consultations (Elwyn et al 2005, Shields et al 2005). Both of these instruments expand the Control Preferences Scale to assess whether patients were provided with a range of options, their pros and cons, whether the patient's preferred level of involvement was assessed, whether questions were invited and clarification

---

Box 34.1 Control Preferences Scale

Active role
A. I prefer to make the decision about which treatment I will receive.
B. I prefer to make the final decision about my treatment after seriously considering my doctor's opinion.

Collaborative role
C. I prefer that my doctor and I share responsibility for deciding which treatment is best for me.

Passive role
D. I prefer that my doctor makes the final decision about which treatment will be used, but seriously considers my opinion.
E. I prefer to leave all decisions regarding treatment to my doctor.

---

offered. The effect of decision aids on patient involvement as measured by these new instruments has not yet been published.

TO WHAT EXTENT DO PATIENTS WANT TO BE INVOLVED IN HEALTH DECISIONS?

There is increasing evidence that a high proportion of people want to be actively involved in a range of health decisions. A telephone survey of 8119 randomly selected adults from eight European countries showed some inter-country variability in the proportion of people wanting to be actively involved in healthcare decisions but overall, the majority preferring such a role. This was particularly so in people under the age of 35 years, of whom 74% indicated a preference for active involvement in treatment decisions (Coulter & Jenkinson 2005). Desire for greater participation in decision making was increased in people with higher socioeconomic status but there was still a substantial proportion of people wanting participation even in the lowest socioeconomic groups (McKinstry 2000). Similarly an Australian survey of 652 women showed that 94.6% preferred to share decisions about diagnostic tests and 91.2% to share treatment decisions (Davey et al 2002). The Australian study, however, showed no difference across age groups.

A closer look shows that what 'preference for involvement' actually means to patients can vary not only with culture and age, but also with the decision itself. Cancer patients in one study indicated that involvement for them meant having information but not necessarily making the decision about treatment. They perceived more opportunity for participation in decisions about adjuvant therapy than about definitive surgical management. They also considered that decisions about physical therapies such as stoma care and psychological therapies such as counselling were more amenable to active roles in decision making (Beaver et al 2005). Cancer patients also appear to have different levels of preferred involvement with respect to information needs about prognosis (Leydon et al 2000).

Despite a preference for active involvement, it seems that many patients continue to value the doctor's opinion in some circumstances. A study of 202 patients attending a general medicine clinic reported that 62.5% preferred shared, 22.5% physician-based and 15.5% patient-based decision making. More than half of respondents rated the doctor's opinion as the most important information for decision making. These patients were considering decisions about invasive medical procedures such as endoscopy, biopsy, interventional radiology and cardiac catheterization (Mazur et al 2005).

Studies of screening decisions appear to show a higher level of patient preference for involvement. A study of women aged 40–49 considering screening mammography showed that 46% preferred shared and a further 46% preferred patient-based decision making compared with 9% preferring physician-based decision making (Nekhlyudov et al 2005).

DOES PATIENT INVOLVEMENT IMPROVE HEALTH OUTCOMES?

This question has been the source of considerable debate (Coulter 2005). Given the evidence provided about societal attitudes towards involvement in health decisions, one could argue on ethical grounds that a relationship with improved health outcomes is not important. Some have suggested that 'effective decisions' are those which are consistent with the patient's values (Kennedy 2003). Yet others maintain that health care is primarily concerned with improving health and well-being, not just with the processes of decision making (Entwistle et al 1998). A direct link between patient involvement in decision making and improved health and well-being is not well documented.

McNutt (2004) succinctly argued that patient involvement in decision making is concerned with two things: (a) informing them of the consequences of the available options, including the probabilities of these where available; and (b) the opportunity to trade off the benefits and risks for them. This may not result in the patient actually making the final decision but does describe a process of involvement.

Involving patients in health decision making implies some level of choice and autonomy. In some circumstances, patient decisions may not be consistent with population level or policy recommendations. Concerns about this potential source of tension and conflict have been raised, particularly in relation to informed decisions by individuals not to immunize their children or not to participate in population screening (Entwistle 2001, Hargreaves et al 2005). Nevertheless, declining MMR (measles, mumps and rubella) vaccination rates in the UK may also be attributed to uninformed or ill-informed decisions in many cases (Coulter 2005, Parker 2001). As decision aids continue to be evaluated in these decision areas, it appears that involving patients through the use of evidence-based decision aids may facilitate informed decisions that are consistent with the evidence. For example, an online decision aid about the pros and cons of MMR vaccination improved parental attitudes towards vaccination (Wallace et al 2006) and a decision aid about prostate cancer screening reduced the proportion of men who had testing (Gattellari & Ward 2003). Similarly, a decision aid for women considering adjuvant breast cancer therapy showed a reduction in the proportion of women choosing adjuvant therapy in those with low tumour severity who would gain little or no benefit (Peele et al 2005).

WHAT MAKES A GOOD DECISION AID?

Given that decision aids can increase patient knowledge, satisfaction with decision making and involvement in healthcare decisions, and this appears to be consistent with societal attitudes and ethically desirable, we should consider criteria by which the quality of such tools can be appraised.

Internationally there has been a two-stage process to establish such criteria. Firstly, the Cochrane Review group developed the CREDIBLE criteria for evaluating decision aids included in their systematic review and inventory (Box 34.2).

Secondly, a recent international collaboration has been establishing a more comprehensive set of criteria for judging the quality of patient decision aids. The International Patient Decision Aid Standards (IPDAS) collaboration will make available a detailed list of criteria under the following broad headings (IPDAS 2006; Box 34.3). It is anticipated that the IPDAS criteria will supersede the earlier CREDIBLE checklist.

Box 34.2 Cochrane Review CREDIBLE criteria

C – Competently developed
  i. Credentials of developers were included; and
  ii. Development process was published or easily accessible.
R – Recently updated
  i. Decision aid was published or updated within the past 5 years; and
  ii. Update policy or statement was included or known.
E – Evidence-based
  i. Linked to an evidence review group or described the process that was used to identify and appraise evidence;
  ii. Used references to scientific studies or systematic overviews to support statements describing benefits/harms of treatment/ screening; and
  iii. Provided a description of the level of uncertainty regarding evidence.
DI – Devoid of conflicts of Interest
  i. Sponsorship was free from perceived conflict of interest.

BL – BaLanced presentation of options, benefits, and harms
  i. Presented all options (including, if appropriate, watchful waiting);
  ii. Presented potential harms as well as potential benefits; and
  iii. Data regarding user responses indicates at least 2/3 of users find it balanced.
E – Decision aid is Efficacious at improving decision making
  i. Evaluations show that decision aid improves knowledge of options;
  ii. Evaluations show that decision aid is acceptable to users;
  iii. Evaluations show other benefits;
  iv. Evaluations show that it was free from adverse effects; and
  v. Evaluations included a randomized controlled trial design.

Box 34.3 IPDAS standards: quality criteria subheadings

1. Using a systematic development process
2. Providing information about options
3. Basing information on up-to-date scientific evidence
4. Presenting probabilities
5. Clarifying and expressing values
6. Using patient stories
7. Guiding/coaching in deliberation and communication
8. Disclosing conflicts of interest
9. Delivering patient decision aids on the internet
10. Balancing the presentation of options
11. Using plain language
12. Establishing effectiveness

IPDAS SUBHEADINGS

Although the final and more detailed list of quality criteria is not yet available, it is worth considering briefly some of the issues that each of the 12 subheadings are concerned with, particularly to judge how these features might facilitate patient involvement in clinical decision making.

1. Using a systematic development process

Users of a decision aid should be able to view the credentials of the developers and authenticate them in some way. Since clinical decision making will involve both patients and practitioners (and sometimes family members as well), these user groups should be consulted about their information needs during development and should pilot test decision aids for acceptability. The development process should also be reviewed by expert peers.

2. Providing information about options

Unlike many traditional forms of patient information, decision aids involve patients by providing balanced information about a range of options (including what happens if you do nothing). In addition to providing background information about the disease and tests or treatments under consideration, they also explain the potential risks as well as the potential benefits of each.

3. Basing information on up-to-date scientific evidence

Decision aids should be based on high-quality evidence. The quality of the evidence and the method used to obtain it should be documented. If relevant, this should be applied to a specific population. It should report when the decision aid was last updated and references should be provided.

4. Presenting probabilities

Outcomes should be quantified (where available) using visual diagrams and presented using natural frequency formats over the same timeframe. Words should also explain the numbers. An example from a published decision aid about hormone therapy during the menopause is shown in Figure 34.1 (Sydney Health Decision Group (SHDG) 2005).

5. Clarifying and expressing values

The decision aid usually contains a personal worksheet or interactive section of a website which provides patients with the opportunity to think about the positive and negative aspects of each option and how important it is for them. This component of the decision aid is important for patient involvement, as it requires them to indicate their preferences. An example of this is given in Figure 34.2.

6. Using patient stories

Some decision aids include videos or written descriptions of patient experiences. If these are included they should represent a range of patient experiences.

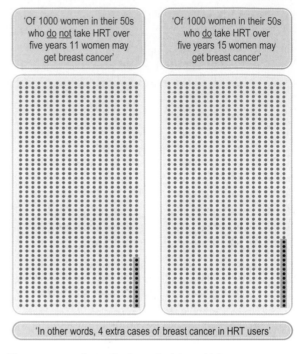

'Of 1000 women in their 50s who do not take HRT over five years 11 women may get breast cancer'

'Of 1000 women in their 50s who do take HRT over five years 15 women may get breast cancer'

'In other words, 4 extra cases of breast cancer in HRT users'

Figure 34.1   Example from decision aid for women considering hormone therapy for menopausal symptoms (SHDG 2005; copyright Commonwealth of Australia, reproduced by permission)

7. Guiding/coaching in deliberation and communication

Many decision aids facilitate decision making through a step-by-step approach to the personal worksheet.

8. Disclosing conflicts of interest

Funding sources should be stated, as should any relationship between decision outcomes and the authors. In other words, it should be stated if the authors might gain or lose by the choices patients make using the decision aid.

9. Delivering patient decision aids on the internet

This is an emerging area but a popular one, given the ability to make decision aids more interactive and tailored online. Security of information and clear design are important.

Benefits of taking HRT	Risks of taking HRT
Relief from menopause symptoms (hot flushes, night sweats, sleep disturbance, irregular periods)	Increasing my risk of breast cancer and/or an abnormal mammogram
Not at all important ☐ ☐ ☐ ☐ ☐ Extremely important	Not at all important ☐ ☐ ☐ ☐ ☐ Extremely important
Other reasons for taking HRT important to you	Increasing my risk of stroke
....	Not at all important ☐ ☐ ☐ ☐ ☐ Extremely important
....	Increasing my risk of blood clots
Not at all important ☐ ☐ ☐ ☐ ☐ Extremely important	Not at all important ☐ ☐ ☐ ☐ ☐ Extremely important
	Increasing my risk of nuisance symptoms (breast tenderness, spotting/periods returning)
	Not at all important ☐ ☐ ☐ ☐ ☐ Extremely important
	Other reasons for NOT taking HRT important to you
	....
	....
	Not at all important ☐ ☐ ☐ ☐ ☐ Extremely important

Which way are you leaning in your decision?

Fill in one of the squares below to indicate which way you are leaning in your decision.

☐	☐	☐	☐	☐	☐	☐	☐	☐	☐
HRT				Not sure					No HRT

Figure 34.2 An example of personal worksheet and values clarification

10. Balancing the presentation of options

Presentation of benefits and harms for each option should be consistent. Field testing with patients should assess whether they felt the decision aid was balanced.

11. Using plain language

Readability scores should be no higher than grade 8 and the decision aid should be written at a level that can be understood by at least half the target audience.

12. Establishing effectiveness

Evaluation of the decision aid is important. This should establish that patients understand the available options, are aware of their values associated with the possible outcomes, and appreciate that the decision aid helps them to become more involved in decision-making.

WHERE CAN DECISION AIDS BE FOUND?

The Cochrane systematic review group has established an inventory of decision aids within the Cochrane Library. Some of these can be accessed freely online. The poor accessibility of many decision aids is an issue that needs to be addressed. A number of research groups have links to their decision aids on their website and some of these are listed in Table 34.1.

Table 34.1   Decision aid sources

Group sources	URL
Cochrane Inventory	www.cochrane.org
Ottawa Health Research Institute	http://204.187.39.28/decaids.html
Sydney Health Decision Group	www.health.usyd.edu.au/shdg/
Specific examples	
MMR decision aid	http://www.ncirs.usyd.edu.au/decisionaid/index.html
HRT decision aid	http://www.nhmrc.gov.au/publications/_files/wh37.pdf
PSA for prostate cancer screen	http://www.prosdex.com/index_content.htm

DECISION AIDS: WHAT LIES AHEAD?

One of the main issues for future research into decision aids is how they can best be implemented within clinical practice to promote patient involvement in healthcare decisions. As this chapter has shown, there is evidence that decision aids increase patient involvement in clinical decision making by presenting options and helping patients to weigh up what is important for them. We have also highlighted that access to decision aids is not easy, although a highly motivated patient or practitioner could find some using standard search engines on the internet.

It is quite likely that decision aid use will vary depending on the patient and also the clinical decision. Decision aids about surgical treatment options for early breast cancer have included interactive desktop aids that breast surgeon and patient can discuss during the consultation (Whelan et al 2004). Other decisions may be considered by the patient at home before or after visiting a healthcare provider (SHDG 2005). There is probably also a need for information that independent consumers can access in response to concerns they may have, such as regarding the safety of childhood vaccinations (Wallace et al 2006).

Further research is also needed on the effect of decision aids on clinical consultation processes and duration. It is unclear whether patient involvement in this way is a cost-effective use of healthcare resources, albeit ethically desirable.

Nevertheless, the future of clinical decision making in health care is likely to be increasingly concerned with patient involvement. Decision aids appear to be one tool that can facilitate this process. Quality criteria will be important in maintaining the best possible outcomes, but strategies for facilitating access to decision aids and assessing their implementation in clinical practice remain an area of research activity.

The potential role for decision aids in clinical decision making of the 21st century is well described by Muir Gray & Rutter (2003):

> The fundamental contract between patient and clinician in the 21st century should start with the assumption that the patient is competent and responsible, providing they are given the resources to exercise that responsibility. There is a need to recognize that some patients would want to ask the clinician to take responsibility for, among other things, managing their records, arranging all aspects of their care, and taking the lead in decision-making. However, many patients would like to be more involved and to take more responsibility themselves. For those patients who wish to use the resources there will, however, be expectations: they will be expected to prepare for the consultation and, if necessary, do homework after it. (Muir Gray & Rutter 2003)

References

Beaver K, Jones D, Mazur M D et al 2005 Exploring the decision-making preferences of people with colorectal cancer. Health Expectations 8(2):103–113

Coulter A 2005 Shared decision-making: the debate continues. Health Expectations 8:95–96

Coulter A, Jenkinson C 2005 European patients' views on the responsiveness of health systems and healthcare providers. European Journal of Public Health 15(4):355–360

Davey H, Barratt A, Davey E et al 2002 Medical tests: women's reported and preferred decision-making roles and preferences for information on benefits, side-effects and false results. Health Expectations 5(4):330–340

Davey H, Lim J, Barratt A et al 2004 Women's preferences for and views on decision-making for diagnostic tests. Social Science and Medicine 58:1699–1707

Degner L F, Sloan J A, Venkatesh P 1997 The Control Preferences Scale. Canadian Journal of Nursing Research 29(3):21–43

Eddy D 1996 Clinical decision making: from theory to practice. A collection of essays from the Journal of the American Medical Association. Jones and Bartlett, Boston

Elwyn G, Edwards A, Mowle S et al 2001 Measuring the involvement of patients in shared decision-making: a systematic review of instruments. Patient Education and Counseling 43(1):5–22

Elwyn G, Hutchings H, Edwards A et al 2005 The OPTION scale: measuring the extent that clinicians involve patients in decision-making tasks. Health Expectations 8:34–42

Entwistle V 2001 Participation in screening programmes. Health Expectations 4:79–80

Entwistle V A, Sowden A J, Watt I S 1998 Evaluating interventions to promote patient involvement in decision making: by what criteria should effectiveness be judged? Journal of Health Service Research and Policy 3(2): 100–107

Entwistle V, Skea Z, O'Donnell M 2001 Decisions about treatment: Interpretations of two measures of control by women having a hysterectomy. Social Science and Medicine 53:721–732

Entwistle V A, Watt I S, Gilhooly K et al 2004 Assessing patients' participation and quality of decision-making: insights from a study of routine practice in diverse settings. Patient Education and Counseling 55(1): 105–113

Gattellari M, Ward J 2003 Does evidence-based information about screening for prostate cancer enhance consumer decision-making? A randomised controlled trial. Journal of Medical Screening 10(1):27–39

Gordon K, MacSween J, Dooley J et al 1996 Families are content to discontinue antiepileptic drugs at different risks than their physicians. Epilepsia 37(6):557–562

Hargreaves K M, Stewart R J, Oliver S R 2005 Informed choice and public health screening for children: the case of blood spot screening. Health Expectations 8:161–171

Haynes R B, Devereaux P J, Guyatt G H 2002 Physicians' and patients' choices in evidence based practice. British Medical Journal 324(7350):1350

IPDAS 2006 International patient decision aid standards. Online. Available: http://ipdas.ohri.ca/20 Sep 2006

Kennedy A 2003 On what basis should the effectiveness of decision aids be judged? Health Expectations 6:255–268

Leydon G M, Boulton M, Moynihan C et al 2000 Cancer patients' information needs and information seeking

behaviour: in depth interview study. British Medical Journal 320(7239):909–913

McKinstry B 2000 Do patients wish to be involved in decision making in the consultation? A cross sectional survey with video vignettes. British Medical Journal 321:867–871

McNutt R 2004 Shared medical decision making: problems, process, progress. JAMA 292(20):2516–2518

Mazur D J, Hickam D H, Mazur M D et al 2005 The role of doctor's opinion in shared decision making: what does shared decision making really mean when considering invasive medical procedures? Health Expectations 8:97–102

Muir Gray J, Rutter H 2003 The resourceful patient: 21st century healthcare. Online. Available: http://www.resourcefulpatient.org/ 13 Jul 2005

Nekhlyudov L, Li R, Fletcher S W 2005 Information and involvement preferences of women in their 40s before their first screening mammogram. Archives of Internal Medicine 165(12):1370–1374

O'Connor A M, Stacey D, Entwistle V et al 2006 Decision aids for people facing health treatment or screening decisions. Cochrane Database of Systematic Reviews 2006 (3):Online. Available: http://www.cochrane.org/reviews/en/ab001431.html 16 Oct 2006

Parker M 2001 The ethics of evidence-based patient choice. Health Expectations 4:87–91

Peele P B, Siminoff L A, Xu Y et al 2005 Decreased use of adjuvant breast cancer therapy in a randomised controlled trial of a decision aid with individualised risk information. Medical Decision Making 25(3):301–307

Protheroe J, Fahey T, Montgomery A A et al 2000 The impact of patients' preferences on the treatment of atrial fibrillation: observational study of patient based decision analysis. British Medical Journal 320(7246):1380–1384

Shields C G, Franks P, Fiscella K et al 2005 Rochester Participatory Decision-Making Scale (RPAD): reliability and validity. Annals of Family Medicine 3:436–442

Sydney Health Decision Group (SHDG) 2005 Making decisions: should I use hormone replacement therapy? Online. Available: http://www.nhmrc.gov.au/publications/synopses/wh35syn.htm 19 Sep 2006

Trevena L, Barratt A 2003 Integrated decision making: definitions for a new discipline. Patient Education and Counseling 50(3):265–268

Trevena L, Davey H, Barratt A et al 2005 A systematic review on communicating with patients about evidence. Journal of Evaluation in Clinical Practice 12(1):13–23

Wallace C, Leask J, Trevena L J 2006 A web-based decision aid pilot improves parental attitudes to MMR vaccination. British Medical Journal 332(7534):146–149

Whelan T, Levine M, Willan A et al 2004 Effect of a decision aid on knowledge and treatment decision making for breast cancer surgery: a randomized trial. JAMA 292(4):435–441

SECTION 6

Teaching and learning clinical reasoning

SECTION CONTENTS

Chapter 35

Teaching and learning clinical reasoning

Susan Ryan and Joy Higgs

CHAPTER CONTENTS

'Clinical reasoning is widely acknowledged by different healthcare professions as a vital part of health professional education and effective practice. In fact, we would argue that clinical reasoning should be central to a health professional's thinking development. It is now conventional wisdom that the term *clinical reasoning* and some of its associated vocabulary are included in major curriculum documents, in educational conversations and in practice descriptions. It has been incorporated into practice competency documents as a section in its own right (Bossers et al 2002). This chapter raises several key issues associated with teaching and learning clinical reasoning as a prelude to the more specific educational chapters to follow. They are:

- addressing new interpretations of clinical reasoning in curricula
- teaching reflexive learning and reasoning practices
- utilizing relevant educational philosophies
- explicit and integrated teaching of clinical reasoning in curricula
- facilitating clinical reasoning.

ADDRESSING NEW INTERPRETATIONS AND PARAMETERS OF CLINICAL REASONING

Often the first task that faces educators is to understand the nature and context of the phenomenon they wish to teach. This is very much the case with clinical reasoning education. Of particular interest are the emergence of new models of interpreting and explaining clinical reasoning and the importance of practice context in understanding, facilitating and teaching clinical reasoning.

CHANGING INTERPRETATIONS AND PRACTICE OF CLINICAL REASONING

As with any new corpus of work, authors and researchers in this new era are now critiquing previous studies (Harries & Harries 2001, Paterson & Summerfield-Mann 2006), adding on to or refining existing frameworks (Chapparo 1999, De Cossart & Fish 2005, Paterson et al 2005), producing new perspectives and models (Hooper 1997), and becoming more sophisticated in ways of researching clinical reasoning and constructing early theories (Unsworth 2004). But, most critically, authors are also integrating into this original work associated bodies of knowledge such as creativity (Andresen & Fredericks 2001), adult learning theories and reflection (Refshauge & Higgs 2000, Ryan 2003), reflexivity (Finlay 2002), and world view and client-centred practice (Precin 2002, Unsworth 2004). With these integrations new perceptions are being merged into the original topic area, resulting in other dimensions of viewing clinical reasoning development.

For educators in the academy and in practice, the ways of guiding learning and reasoning development and the choice of clinical reasoning models to use will become more sophisticated as our understanding of this complex capability grows from continuing research studies and theoretical development. As discussed in Chapter 1, there is a growing emphasis on narrative, collaborative and interactive models of clinical reasoning in keeping with changing attitudes of society toward the input of patients and carers in clinical decision making. This has implications for the ways clinical reasoning will be construed and taught in the future and the ways it will be presented in a multitude of learning opportunities.

THE IMPORTANCE OF CONTEXT IN CLINICAL REASONING

Major changes in the context of health professional practice are occurring worldwide (see Chapter 2).

Increasingly, practitioners and students need to be able to deal with uncertainty in practice and to change their thinking and reasoning between different contexts. A new conceptual and interpersonal frame of reference for clinical reasoning and decision making is being drawn. And, as health practitioners are becoming increasingly more globally mobile, it is becoming more important that they become critical of themselves and their thinking and reasoning in practice or education within a dual frame of reference: they need *to be locally informed and globally aware*. The importance of firmly embedding thinking and reasoning in context is strongly emphasized in recent publications (Whiteford & Wright-St Clair 2005) and greater interest is being given to understanding the contextual factors that impinge upon and that need to be considered during clinical reasoning (Smith 2006) (see Chapter 8).

In Figure 35.1 we provide a framework for contextual reasoning that draws together these multiple contextual factors. This framework is a useful way to help students learn to think about reasoning in context. The use of this framework when situating case stories and case studies in the curriculum helps teachers to stimulate learners' thinking about the wider implications of their practice decision making. The different levels of this framework range from broad to narrower contexts, from global to local. No levels are mutually exclusive. The complexities of the national and local picture surround the personal and professional frames of reference of individual students and practitioners.

Reasoning through these complex contexts and dealing with macro- and micro-dimensions of clinical reasoning calls for a more sophisticated mode of (and model for) reasoning than required by earlier interpretations of reasoning, such as problem solving and diagnostic reasoning. The psychologist Gelb (1996) has introduced the term *synvergent thinking*. This term describes this more sophisticated way of thinking, where there is a synergy between different levels of thinking and there is a synthesis of these in the reasoner's mind. Local considerations such as guidelines and local rules are not removable from the larger context. To hold one idea and set of thinking simultaneously with thinking in a wider framework is a sophisticated and complex reasoning approach that suits the

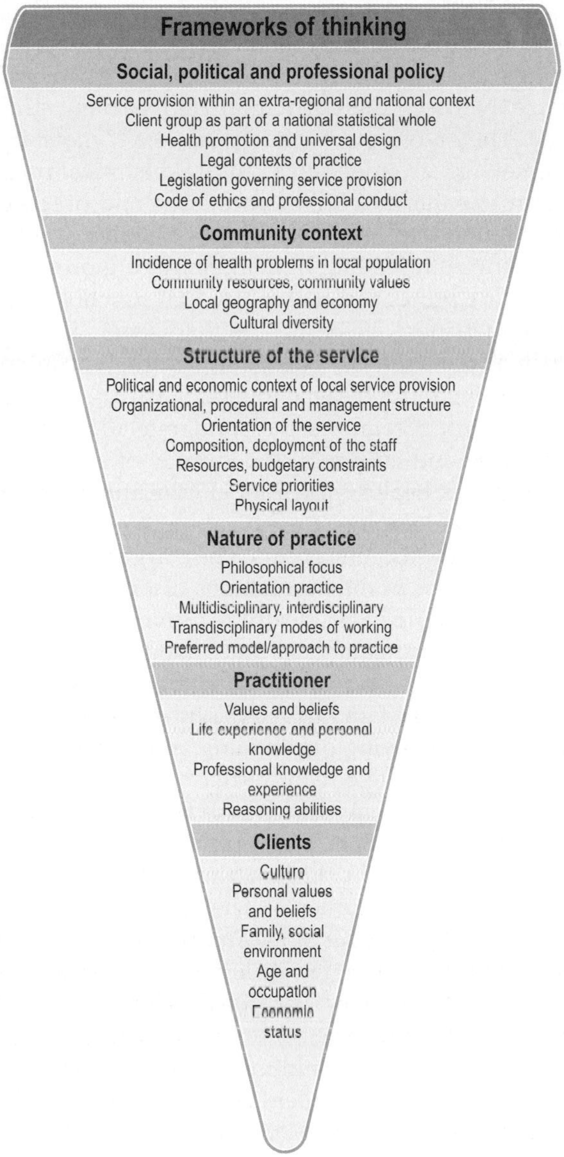

Frameworks of thinking

Social, political and professional policy

Service provision within an extra-regional and national context
Client group as part of a national statistical whole
Health promotion and universal design
Legal contexts of practice
Legislation governing service provision
Code of ethics and professional conduct

Community context

Incidence of health problems in local population
Community resources, community values
Local geography and economy
Cultural diversity

Structure of the service

Political and economic context of local service provision
Organizational, procedural and management structure
Orientation of the service
Composition, deployment of the staff
Resources, budgetary constraints
Service priorities
Physical layout

Nature of practice

Philosophical focus
Orientation practice
Multidisciplinary, interdisciplinary
Transdisciplinary modes of working
Preferred model/approach to practice

Practitioner

Values and beliefs
Life experience and personal
knowledge
Professional knowledge and
experience
Reasoning abilities

Clients

Culture
Personal values
and beliefs
Family, social
environment
Age and
occupation
Economic
status

Figure 35.1 A contextual framework for thinking in clinical reasoning

TEACHING REFLEXIVE LEARNING AND REASONING PRACTICES

Higgs (2006) has described parallels between reasoning, research and learning. One of the most

powerful opportunities for learning about clinical reasoning and continuing to develop practice capability is to recognize these synergies and to help students learn to transfer understandings and skills learned in one area of responsibility and practice to another. The ideas of learning from one area of research, learning and practice and of transferring this learning to another area, situation or practice challenge have been discussed by Higgs (2006) as an overall strategy of informed meaning-making, similar to the strategies inherent in the hermeneutic circle. Such practice requires heightened awareness, critical self-appraisal and development of ideas and practices.

These ideas are linked to the *prelude or prospective thinking approach* based on the *'WHOLE – PART – WHOLE'* way of thinking and learning from adult learning theory (Knowles et al 1998). The prelude, the first WHOLE, is what the practitioner brings to the clinical encounter. This is the *prospective section*. Often, this can be understood hypothetically in university before actual practice experience. The subsequent PARTS occur in actual practice and the final WHOLE is a new set of understandings. This 'final' (that is actually the next prelude) may happen at the end of a practice experience, either while still in practice or when the learner is back at university. Such reasoning is holistic; it helps the practitioner to form a new lens for future practice. It can also be called meta-reasoning since it looks beyond and across particular practice and learning episodes to broaden the horizons of a health practitioner's mind and help make subsequent practice episodes and experiences more realistic instead of idealistic.

UTILIZING RELEVANT EDUCATIONAL PHILOSOPHIES

There is considerable and ongoing debate in the literature and in educational practice about educational philosophies that can be used by teachers in the planning and implementation of health professional education to enhance the learner's ability to engage in clinical reasoning. For example, for many years problem-based learning (PBL) has been heralded as the learning philosophy and strategy of choice for developing clinical

complexities and challenges of the current clinical practice context.

reasoning. Learners have to search inductively for knowledge and then decide deductively and critically which material is relevant to use. In 2004, the European Network of Occupational Therapy in Higher Education (ENOTHE) espoused PBL as the learning method of choice. However, in Europe today, some of the first schools to adopt this PBL method, that have been using it for more than 20 years, are beginning to question its effectiveness. The practice competencies of these health practitioners are actually being questioned, as the learners struggle in practice settings to combine their largely academic reasoning with their actions.

This interesting debate needs closer and further examination. Savin-Baden (2000) determined that it was the way PBL questions were designed that lessened its effectiveness. Ryan (2003) found that while PBL helped to integrate knowledge better than subject-based learning, it was the way PBL was applied by educators that made the crucial difference between its being an effective learning philosophy or a waste of precious time.

One approach to addressing this dilemma is reshaping the teaching and learning strategy. Inquiry-based learning in Canada (Amort-Larson et al 1997) and task-based learning in Ireland (Ryan et al 2004) both integrate the PBL inductive methods of inquiry with new components added to the learning strategy; specifically, theoretical input from experts and required readings are incorporated, as well as an experiential element that is subsequently discussed and reflected upon in a feedback loop. These inquiries and tasks are set into guided learning experiences at regular intervals throughout the curriculum so that transferable knowledge, abilities and skills are developed alongside other transferable competencies. Learners appear to need these skills. As one student wrote: 'I realized that analysing clinical reasoning was something I had the capacity and potential to do once I understood it more and realized that there was skill involved in this process' (Student's reflective diary – University College Cork (UCC) Clinical Reasoning postgraduate module).

We suggest that many learning philosophies can achieve this awareness of clinical reasoning skills as long as the educators design ways of learning that embrace the body of clinical reasoning knowledge and facilitate its development in the learner. Loftus & Higgs (2005) assert that there is a need to revise the theoretical basis of PBL to optimize the use of this curriculum and learning strategy. They advocate the adoption of a Vygotskian framework grounded in a cultural historical paradigm to enhance PBL interpretation and practice, explaining that Vygotsky's ideas 'revolve around the central thesis that human beings are products of their culture, and that individual psychological characteristics, especially higher level abilities such as the ability to engage in clinical reasoning, are derived from social interaction' (p. 5). This framework recognizes the fundamental place of language and culture in the journey of acculturation that is health professional education, within which the learning of clinical problem solving and clinical reasoning occurs. These arguments support a review of the foundations of PBL to ensure that such curricula and learning activities are based on a solid foundation, an integrated approach to curriculum design and implementation.

Figure 35.2 (from Higgs 2004) provides a framework for reviewing or planning strategies to promote the learning of clinical reasoning by relating key educational questions to educational theory and principles that can provide answers and guidelines for curricula. Inherent in the framework are two main arguments. The first is that there needs to be coherence between the intention, guiding principles, design, implementation and evaluation of curricula. Secondly, such curricular dimensions need to be made explicit to ensure this coherence and to communicate, realize and critique the curriculum intent and achievements.

EXPLICIT AND INTEGRATED TEACHING OF CLINICAL REASONING IN CURRICULA

Although much credence is given to the value of clinical reasoning and in many courses the goal of developing clinical reasoning skills is made explicit, there is often a lack of explicit communication of how this goal is to be achieved in curricula in any coherent and integrated manner. Even in PBL courses that are built around the development of clinical problem solving ability there is a

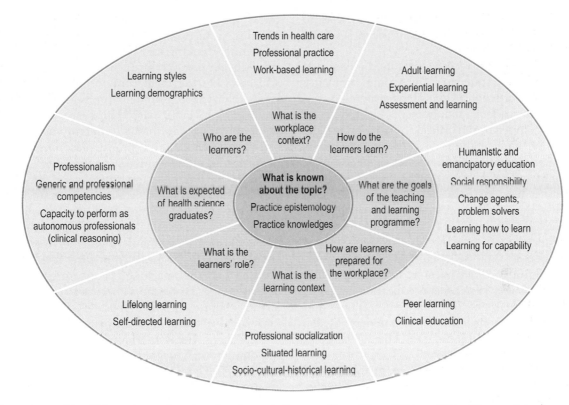

Figure 35.2 Identifying relevant learning theories and discourse (from Higgs 2004, p. 380, with permission)

need, as discussed above, for a greater explication and realization of educational principles and theory in curricula.

Clinical reasoning is at the *heart of practice thinking*. The ability to reason clinically demonstrates how practitioners or learners have assimilated, integrated and included all the various sets of knowledge they have developed cognitively and experientially. This ability should not be left to develop haphazardly or by chance, as occurred frequently in traditional curricula. We advocate the creation of curricula that infuse clinical reasoning principles throughout the entire programme. This process has been described as mainstreaming of the desired content, skills and learning process (in this case clinical reasoning) across the curriculum (Higgs & Boud 1991).

To effectively create such a curriculum the team of educators must be committed to this approach, rather than simply including clinical reasoning as a listed goal or isolated learning activity in their programme. To do so they need

to be knowledgeable about clinical reasoning literature and practices and be able to transfer conceptually the different reasoning ideas across the curriculum.

Activities and opportunities for delivering these principles of clinical reasoning as a transferable skill can be planned systematically. Whether the programme is modularized or not, this planning can be mapped out across the years (horizontal themes) as well as throughout one particular year (vertical themes). Within each year, generalized learning activities in the form of specific frameworks or guidelines can be used. These activities can be designed to be progressively more complex throughout the curriculum over the years. Such activities should include teaching about models of clinical reasoning, teaching different reasoning strategies, reflecting upon reasoning strategies experienced or modelled in clinical practicums, and classroom hypothetical or problem/case-based learning activities. Educators may consider implanting the reasoning processes first and defining the actual models later, to illustrate to learners how they have actually been working through these elements.

There is a need to facilitate a more sophisticated way of reasoning suited to today's complex practice world. It is worth noting that such reasoning is congruent with academic requirements for students to develop competence in critical thinking and in the integration and synthesis of cognitive awareness as they progress through the levels of an academic programme. We propose that an important meta-strategy in teaching reasoning is the promotion of reflective and interactional learning through such activities as using explicit discussion of the nature and challenges of reasoning in classroom learning. One example could be discussion of the implications of Figure 35.1 for clinical reasoning in practice. The goal of using these ideas as educational triggers is to enable learners to become interactional and transformational healthcare practitioners of the future, as espoused by Higgs & Hunt (1999) and Higgs & Edwards (1999).

Another valuable strategy we propose is to *make explicit the links between learning activities and clinical reasoning*. Opportunities for conceptualizing specifics of practice can be provided in the form of designing decision trees or spidergrams (Gelb 1996) where links and hierarchies are illustrated. Further, stories, always powerful, allow the exploration of clients' lived experiences, of treatment rationales and provisional outcome paths. Students who are exposed to these narratives instead of the more typical case studies begin to see the *complexities of practice being interwoven into their understandings* (Ryan & McKay 1999). In our experience, narratives have ignited passionate responses that have captivated learners' imaginations and developed their fascination with a particular practice area. In these cases their reasoning became sophisticated and profound. They *lifted something ordinary into the extraordinary*; such passion for the field in which one is practising has tremendous career motivation.

Specific 'linking learning' sessions (UCC Accreditation Document 2004) can be orchestrated in many creative ways at strategic points within the academic year, between years and before and after practice experiences. In this way novice healthcare practitioners can incorporate their personal and professional ideas and learning from experience into their repertoire of reasoning, thinking and reflecting practices. Practice education experiences, whether simulated or real, provide the ideal context and opportunity for verbalizing reasoning. This reasoning cross-linking or overlap also helps to reduce the theory–practice gap that is frequently observed.

Teaching models of clinical reasoning to students can be strategically interposed into the curriculum. By linking these models and theory to experiential learning of clinical reasoning in the classroom and the workplace, educators can give a shape and language to students' reasoning. One of the choices to be made is whether the theory should precede the practice or vice versa. It has been argued that teaching theory retrospectively acknowledges to learners that their reasoning is already happening and validates their existing knowledge as 'thinking therapists' (Butler 2002).

Achieving successful mainstreaming of clinical reasoning teaching requires documentation in module booklets and handouts using clear clinical reasoning terminology. Educators also need to articulate these ideas and use this vocabulary in the classroom regularly so that learners become familiar with the terms and transfer them to practice when they are describing patients'/clients' management needs and programmes and talking about their own clinical reasoning.

FACILITATING CLINICAL REASONING: APPROACHES

Learning opportunities and methods for facilitating clinical reasoning development can be used in many creative ways. In broad terms these can be thought of as activities that occur before, during and after workplace reasoning experiences. These help students to:

- learn the language and theory of clinical reasoning
- understand the process of reasoning as a prelude to workplace experience
- experience and gain understanding of clinical reasoning in action through workplace practice and feedback

- reflect upon their reasoning during and after practice to further understand, critique and develop their reasoning abilities.

Table 35.1 gives examples of these facilitation methods and their advantages and disadvantages. By examining and using this table critically, educators and researchers may choose appropriate methods

of capturing reasoning for particular contexts. At the very least, the advantages and disadvantages in all these methods need to be made explicit to the learners. The table illustrates how difficult it is to really capture reasoning that first has to be brought to awareness before it can be spoken or written. Thus, an important dimension of learning to reason is learning to articulate reasoning (see Chapter 30).

Table 35.1 Methods of learning about reasoning

Methods to promote	Advantages	Disadvantages
Prospective reasoning		
- Guided observation (viewing videos/actors/patients/documents) - Uses students' experiences/stories - Uses provocative readings	Learner focuses their thinking on a topic (*priming the mind*) Learner becomes aware of their *personal body of knowledge* – what they know and what they need to know in a *general sense* so they can act on this knowledge Learner becomes more aware of own *biases, values, attitudes* to be discussed Learners' reasoning can be challenged in a safe environment	The immediacy of the situation is not apparent The learner might still be really unaware of the recipient's feelings and actual conditions so their reasoning is not contextual but hypothetical As this experience is one-sided plans are not developed together as in client centred practice
Reasoning in-action		
- Guided observation/demonstration - Participant observation	Learner sees immediate reality but may need prompting/guiding Learner is aware of the *real context* with all the players involved in the scene Learner becomes aware of immediacy of critical incidents as they happen Learner is aware of the respondent's reactions, repertoires and emotions Learner may question on the spot	Learner needs to become a 'part of the scene' by a period of prolonged exposure to acclimatize everyone to his/her presence Learner may not know what to look for if this is not made explicit by others Learner might be unprepared for the reality of the situation Learner may need more time to assimilate thoughts before asking questions
- Reasoning with head mounted video-camera - Reasoning into a lapel microphone	Learner can capture their interactions and their spoken words from the immediate situation. *This may help recall retrospectively*	Learner is aware of the equipment and may have to manage it too Learner is not able to voice thoughts in the presence of the patient / client Learner may have to leave the room in order to say what they are really thinking
- Being videotaped / tape-recorded by someone else	Learner is not having to manage or manipulate equipment as above and can ignore it to a certain extent	Learner is aware of being videotaped which might inhibit performance Learner needs to be used to being videotaped

(Continued)

Table 35.1   Methods of learning about reasoning—cont'd

Methods to promote	Advantages	Disadvantages
Retrospective reasoning		
– Tape-recording thoughts, memories and accounts of situations alone or in an interview situation	Less effort for the learner than some other methods Captures immediate thinking – free thinking There is a record for further examination Gaps in learning and ability are identified when the script is transcribed Voice and story-telling acts as a trigger for other thoughts and memories The learner's tone of voice and mood is apparent	Learner feels foolish as most people are very unused to this Learner feels disorganized unless they can have prompt notes There are no visual prompts The process can appear to be too long The tape is open to legal interpretation You need privacy
– Talking with another person	Challenging questions need to be done in a particular way The other person can bring in related ideas you had not thought of You do not need any equipment Sometimes it is comforting that others think the same way	Others may interrupt the learner's thought patterns with questions Thoughts are not captured anywhere so there is no record to go back to Others may interrupt with different thought patterns or their own stories The learner can feel inhibited
– Writing retrospectively and reflectively	Logical and ordered process – you see an order and an image Free flow writing can capture ideas People are used to writing things down Learner may feel less inhibited than in other methods – may depend on audience Learners have time to review their ideas Learners can identify links between ideas	Many thoughts are lost in writing as each person edits their thinking Learner may feel lazy and not put in the necessary details Writing takes too much time Writing must be legible Writing is open to legal interpretation The learner may be very selective about what they write

Assessment of clinical reasoning can be accomplished in various ways and should involve reflection on reasoning, articulation of reasoning and feedback. Such processes can shape learners' ideas and enhance their confidence.

CONCLUSION

Clinical reasoning is becoming a primary educational goal; more attention, however, needs to be given to making clinical reasoning teaching and learning activities a mainstream part of health professional education. We have found that clinical reasoning learning can be facilitated by creating reflective and reflexive learning opportunities throughout health sciences curricula. We believe that it is essential, within curricula that incorporate clinical reasoning, that students develop their reasoning abilities, gain the capacity to articulate their reasoning convincingly, and develop a deeper understanding of the phenomenon of clinical reasoning and their own reasoning processes and abilities. Significantly, the benefits are not only for individual learners; developing the ability to talk succinctly about their practice allows both learners and their professions to gain credence in the eyes of listeners.

References

Amort-Larson G, Esmail S, Chan C 1997 Student simulated patients – an innovative approach to learning activity analysis. Paper presented at the Hong Kong International Occupational Therapy Congress: Key to Practice, 22–25 March

Andresen L, Fredericks I 2001 Finding the fifth player: artistry in professional practice. In: Higgs J, Titchen A (eds) Professional practice in health, education and the creative arts. Blackwell Science, Oxford, p 72–89

Bossers A, Miller L, Polatajko H J et al 2002 Competency based fieldwork evaluation for occupational therapists. DELMAR Thomson Learning, Australia

Butler J 2002 The *thinking* profession. British Journal of Occupational Therapy 65(7):305

Chapparo C 1999 Working out: working with Angelica – interpreting practice. In: Ryan S E, McKay E A (eds) Thinking and reasoning in therapy: narratives from practice. Stanley Thornes, Cheltenham, p 31–50

De Cossart L, Fish D 2005 Cultivating a thinking surgeon: new perspectives on clinical teaching, learning and assessment. tfm Publishing, Shrewsbury

Finlay L 2002 The practice of psychosocial occupational therapy, 3rd edn. Nelson Thornes, Cheltenham

Gelb M 1996 Thinking for a change. Aurum Press, London

Harries P, Harries C 2001 Studying clinical reasoning, part 1: have we been taking the wrong tack? British Journal of Occupational Therapy 64(4):164–168

Higgs J 2004 Educational theory and principles related to learning clinical reasoning. In: Jones M A, Rivett D A (eds) Clinical reasoning for manual therapists. Butterworth-Heinemann, Edinburgh, p 379–402

Higgs J, Boud D 1991 Self-directed learning as part of the mainstream of physiotherapy education. Australian Journal of Physiotherapy 37:245–251

Higgs J, Edwards H (eds) 1999 Educating beginning practitioners: challenges for health professional education. Butterworth-Heinemann, Oxford

Higgs J, Hunt A 1999 Rethinking the beginning practitioner: introducing the 'interactional professional'. In: Higgs J, Edwards H (eds) Educating beginning practitioners: challenges for health professional education. Butterworth-Heinemann, Oxford, p 10–18

Hooper B 1997 The relationship between pretheoretical assumptions and clinical reasoning. American Journal of Occupational Therapy 51(5):328–338

Knowles M, Holton E, Swanson R 1998 The adult learner, 5th edn. Gulf Publishing, Houston, TX

Loftus S, Higgs J 2005 Reconceptualising problem-based learning in a Vygotskian framework. Focus on Health Professional Education: A Multidisciplinary Journal 7(1):1–14

Paterson M, Higgs J, Wilcox S 2005 The artistry of judgement: a model for occupational therapy practice. British Journal of Occupational Therapy 68(9):409–417

Paterson M, Summerfield-Mann L 2006 Clinical reasoning. In: Duncan E (ed) Foundations for practice in occupational therapy, 4th edn. Elsevier, Edinburgh, p 315–335

Precin P 2002 Client-centred reasoning: narratives of people with mental illness. Butterworth-Heinemann, Oxford

Refshauge K, Higgs J 2000 Teaching clinical reasoning. In: Higgs J, Jones M (eds) Clinical reasoning in the health professions, 2nd edn. Butterworth-Heinemann, Oxford, p 141–147

Ryan S 2003 Voices of newly qualified occupational therapists: their practice and educational stories. Unpublished PhD thesis, School of Innovation Studies, University of East London

Ryan S, McKay E (eds) 1999 Thinking and reasoning in therapy: narratives from practice. Nelson Thornes, Cheltenham

Ryan S, Hunt E, Horgan L 2004 University College Cork as a learning environment. In: Hyland A (ed) Innovations in teaching learning and assessment: task based learning for occupational therapy. Cork University Press, Cork, p 59–65

Savin-Baden M 2000 Problem-based learning in higher education: untold stories. Society for Research into Higher Education and Open University Press, Buckingham

Smith M C J 2006 Clinical decision making in acute care cardiopulmonary physiotherapy. Unpublished doctoral thesis, University of Sydney, Sydney

UCC 2004 UCC accreditation document: Department of Occupational Therapy. University College Cork, Cork

Unsworth C A 2004 Clinical reasoning: how do pragmatic reasoning, worldview and client-centredness fit? British Journal of Occupational Therapy 67(1):10–19

Whiteford G, Wright-St Clair V (eds) 2005 Occupation and practice in context. Elsevier, Sydney

Chapter **36**

Helping physiotherapy students develop clinical reasoning capability

Nicole Christensen, Mark A. Jones, Ian Edwards and Joy Higgs

CHAPTER CONTENTS

A primary goal of professional entry programmes is to prepare graduates to practise effectively in today's complex healthcare system. The clinical reasoning and decision making of new graduates can be viewed as a practical demonstration, or outcome, of the professional entry education process. Therefore, we propose that the development of capability in clinical reasoning should be a priority for educators responsible for preparing new members of the profession for practice.

In Chapter 9 we introduced some of the findings of recent research (Christensen 2007) into clinical reasoning capability. Clinical reasoning capability involves integration and effective application of thinking and learning skills to make sense of, learn collaboratively from, and generate knowledge within familiar and unfamiliar clinical experiences. We also described four dimensions of clinical reasoning capability: reflective thinking, critical thinking, dialectical thinking and complexity thinking. We described capable clinical reasoners as having developed a justified confidence in their practice abilities and a strong motivation to learn from experience through intentional reflective processing of their reasoning in practice.

The doctoral research conducted by Nicole Christensen and supervised by the other authors of this chapter (Christensen 2007) used a hermeneutic approach (described in Chapter 9) to explore how the development of capability in clinical reasoning can be facilitated in the context of professional entry physical therapist education. In this chapter we again draw upon the findings of this research, and suggest some ways in which students can be guided towards the development of clinical reasoning capability during their professional entry educational journeys.

FACILITATING THE DEVELOPMENT OF CLINICAL REASONING CAPABILITY DURING PROFESSIONAL ENTRY EDUCATION

Current models of expert physiotherapists' practice and clinical reasoning (Edwards & Jones 2007, Jensen et al 1999) interpret this phenomenon as inherently complex, demonstrating characteristics of a complex adaptive system. A number of authors have advocated the adoption of a complexity perspective to facilitate understanding and coping with escalating complexity in all subsystems (social, political, professional, human) involved in health care today (e.g. Plsek & Greenhalgh 2001, Zimmerman et al 2001). Professional entry education systems therefore face great challenges in the endeavour adequately to prepare new practitioners who are capable of practising within their professional role and interacting effectively in the larger healthcare environment.

Long before they enter the practice environment, student physiotherapists must learn to successfully negotiate their professional entry education programmes. Graduate and professional education systems have been characterized as complex, inherently challenging and ultimately transformative for learners (Weidman et al 2001). For the student physiotherapist, then, the process of becoming a capable professional (and thus a capable clinical reasoner) depends upon becoming a capable learner within the professional entry education system. Physiotherapy students engage in learning experiences within academic classroom and clinical education settings in which individual students' learning experiences are quite variable, despite the efforts of individual programmes, national accreditation systems and international standards to provide some degree of consistency in curriculum content and expected outcomes. Both within and between academic programmes, there is considerable variability in the extent of integration of curriculum content (theoretical and technical) and the learning of processes,

including clinical reasoning, thinking and learning skills.

Christensen's (2007) research illustrated this variability in learning experiences, in both academic and clinical education settings, through the different contexts and ways the student participants described learning about clinical reasoning. For example, they described varying levels of explicit exposure to clinical reasoning theory (e.g. learning about what it is, what it involves), and variation in the number of opportunities and the quality and value of their learning experiences in relation to developing clinical reasoning skills. Most notably, these students experienced great variability in clinical education experiences. This is not surprising, since individuals in the programmes in the study (as with many such educational programmes) were commonly placed in different practice situations, under the supervision of a variety of clinical educators, all with different levels of skill in and understanding of clinical reasoning. The clinical educators also varied in their level of skill in facilitating students' clinical reasoning skills development through experiential learning opportunities and in enhancing their learning from clinical reasoning practice experiences.

Overall, Christensen (2007) found that the learning and practice of clinical reasoning was often a self-directed journey for the participants, some ultimately and inevitably more capable in their learning than others. Since the learning programmes studied largely devolved (mainly incidentally rather than intentionally) the responsibility for learning clinical reasoning to the students, the question of the responsibility of educators to teach clinical reasoning explicitly was highlighted. Another key finding was that the role of chance or 'luck of the draw' in providing students with opportunities to develop their clinical reasoning capability was even more influential than the students' own capabilities as learners in the professional education process. The role of chance was most evident in the context of clinical education, where some students benefited from the mentoring of self-reflective clinical educators who modelled clinical reasoning and made reasoning an explicit part of their teaching and feedback. In arguing that clinical reasoning is such an integral and complex component of effective, capable practice, we contend that the availability and quality of opportunities for facilitation of clinical reasoning capability need to be guaranteed for all students. Such learning should be a core rather than chance component of the professional education journeys of all health professional students.

In this chapter we identify several ways in which capability in clinical reasoning can be facilitated during the professional education process. We consider opportunities for such learning within the professional socialization process, academic classroom and clinical education learning contexts. Such strategies could also be employed in other curricula.

FACILITATING THE DEVELOPMENT OF CLINICAL REASONING CAPABILITY THROUGH PROFESSIONAL SOCIALIZATION

Professional socialization is a complex learning process that occurs throughout professional entry education (Cant & Higgs 1999, Clouder 2003, Weidman et al 2001). Upon graduation, students have learned how to *do* physiotherapy, but more importantly they have *become* physiotherapists – they have constructed their professional identity. As part of their professional identity formation, physiotherapy graduates have developed an understanding of their new professional role and a vision of how they should act and interact within the healthcare system, within the profession, and with their clients.

We contend that students' learning during their professional socialization, reflected in their construction of a professional identity, has direct implications for their clinical reasoning approach and capabilities as they enter the professional practice community. Graduates' interpretations of who they are and who they should be in their professional roles directly relate to how they frame situations or identify problems to be solved, and how they think through and act upon decisions they make (Schön 1987, Wenger 1998). Within clinical reasoning all elements of practice are integrated and put into action, including identity, philosophy of practice, profession-specific technical skills, communication, collaboration, and ethics. Successful completion of the professional entry educational process culminates in the transformation of

students to fully participating members of the professional community of practice (Lave & Wenger 1991, Wenger 1998). As Wenger (1998) stated, 'such participation shapes not only what we do, but also who we are and how we interpret what we do' (p. 4).

Key elements of capability are recognizable in the clinical reasoning of skilled physiotherapists, and best demonstrated in the clinical practice of skilled clinicians (Christensen 2007). Expert participants have been found to employ a collaborative approach in their clinical reasoning and to embody a patient-centred philosophy in their practice (Edwards et al 2004, Jensen et al 1999). In the USA, where Christensen's (2007) research participants were located, the adoption of patient-centred approaches to practice is an explicit requirement within the published professional entry curricula guidelines. This is consistent with the philosophy adopted by the American Physical Therapy Association (2003) and the World Confederation for Physical Therapy (2004) and is an expected element of the professional socialization of new physiotherapists in America. However, in her research Christensen (2007) found that although the participants recognized the value of being collaborative and patient-centred in practice, this was not universally reflected in their practice. In particular, some participants' ideas of their role as a physical therapist and the role of the patient were inconsistent with a patient-centred orientation to clinical reasoning. For example: 'I think my role is . . . to just kind of use your knowledge and apply it to them. And their role is, I guess, to trust you and then to follow your directions' (John).

In their clinical reasoning these students demonstrated beliefs and actions more consistent with therapist-centred approaches to practice, evidencing a belief that they were supposed to possess sufficient specialized physical therapist knowledge to independently reason through the problem, diagnose and prescribe to/for patients the proper plan of care (in contrast to collaborating with their patients in reasoning and decision making). On the other hand, some participants demonstrated views more consistent with a collaborative, patient-centred approach to reasoning in practice. One participant described his view as follows:

> That's why it's so important for you to define their goals from the outset, so then you can adjust your way of dealing with this patient or include things or exclude things from the programme. ... So it's kind of like an interplay between they're the ultimate decision maker, you teach them what to do, how to do it, help them do it, ... and I think everyone is happy, hopefully, at the end. (Frank)

These findings have direct implications for ways in which to increase the likelihood of facilitating development of capability in clinical reasoning within the professional socialization process, including the way this capability is influenced by the practitioner's practice model (e.g. patient-centred care). Educators can help students understand that the *whole* of the learning experience that is becoming a professional – a physiotherapist – is the bigger context within which the learning of how to be a physiotherapist (*part*) and of how to do physiotherapy (*part*) are interrelated and inseparable from each other. This is consistent with the suggestions by Bowden & Marton (1998) in the educational literature that the type of learning linked to being and becoming capable involves developing ways of experiencing and understanding phenomena (creating meaning) through a process of discernment of the 'parts and the whole, aspects and relations' (p. 33).

By making overt the hermeneutic nature of the learning involved in their professional development, educators can also facilitate development of some of the thinking and learning skills that we have proposed are key dimensions of capability in clinical reasoning (Christensen 2007). According to Davis & Sumara (2006, p. 167), critical reflection about one's pre-existing perceptions of reality and development of new perspectives through incorporation of new understandings (which is characteristic of hermeneutic inquiry) are 'deeply compatible' with complexity thinking.

We propose that capability in clinical reasoning can be facilitated by education which pays overt attention to the relationships between key elements of *who we are* as physiotherapists and how this can and should be reflected in our clinical reasoning and associated actions – congruent with *how we think* and *what we do* in practice. One key to guiding students' learning toward capability is the development of critical thinking skills and promoting students' pursuit of critical self-reflection on their reasoning and decision making. In particular, students should be encouraged to reflect on any inconsistencies between their professional identities, their reasoning and their clinical actions.

FACILITATING THE DEVELOPMENT OF CLINICAL REASONING CAPABILITY BY STRENGTHENING CONNECTIONS BETWEEN ACADEMIC AND CLINICAL EDUCATION CONTEXTS

Professional entry education of physiotherapists consists of two distinct components: that conducted in the academic classroom setting and that conducted in the clinical education setting. The clinical education context provides students with the opportunity to experience and practise putting into action what they have learned in the academic component of their education. It also provides unique and invaluable experiential learning opportunities where students' classroom knowledge is transformed and enhanced through experience, and their construction of practice knowledge begins (Higgs et al 2004). Both these learning contexts provide opportunities to reinforce, integrate and expand what is learned in the other, preparing students for real-world practice.

Christensen's research (2007), in contrast, showed that many student physical therapists in the programmes studied experienced a lack of coherence between the academic and clinical educational settings in relation to the teaching and learning of clinical reasoning. She found that the development of clinical reasoning capability can be facilitated by the creation of more overt integration of the teaching and learning occurring in these two learning settings.

When considering how to facilitate this integration we find particular relevance in Wenger's (1998) discussion of the ways in which communities of practice develop and socialize new members to negotiate meaning from experiences in practice. According to Wenger, practice involves the negotiation of meaning through the interaction of two constituent processes, *reification* and *participation*. We discuss below examples of how a process of reification of and participation in clinical reasoning in both educational settings can facilitate the development of clinical reasoning capability in student physiotherapists.

Reification of and participation in clinical reasoning in the academic classroom setting

For participants in Christensen's study (2007), little of their academic programme overtly dealt with understanding clinical reasoning as a means of integrating different areas of learning into their overall approach to decision making in practice. For example, one participant explained:

> We did discuss different approaches to psychological aspects, emotional issues, worrying ... about attending to people's other needs and potential referrals you should make, but I don't think it was ever really discussed in terms of clinical reasoning, it was just like this is something else to put together. And for me personally, I was thinking physical stuff would be clinical reasoning, and then the emotional, touchy feely stuff would be, ... [separate]. I just never really put it together in the same boat until now. (Robin)

Reification refers to the process whereby a community of practice gives form to concepts and experiences central to practice in order to facilitate the shaping of experience by members of a practice community; it results in 'focusing our attention in a particular way and enabling new kinds of understanding' (Wenger 1998, p. 60). Reification may involve the production of 'abstractions, tools, symbols, stories, terms and concepts that reify something of that practice in a congealed form' (Wenger 1998, p. 59). We contend that clinical reasoning, a complex abstract and practice phenomenon, is a key component of practice that can and should be reified in the academic classroom setting. Such overt reification can foster students' paying attention to and learning to communicate clinical reasoning; it has the potential to facilitate experiential learning throughout the whole professional entry education process, but especially during clinical education.

Definitions and models of clinical reasoning can assist this process of reification of clinical reasoning in the academic classroom context.

The explicit exploration of the ways in which clinical reasoning is described in theoretical and research-derived models can allow educators to 'create points of focus around which the negotiation of meaning becomes organized' (Wenger 1998, p. 58). Through this process students learn to cope with the task of making sense of the overwhelming amounts of information that they will face in practice in the context of collaborating with each individual patient. This is consistent with the view of education for capability put forth by Bowden & Marton (1998), who emphasized that 'it is important to make ways of seeing (e.g. making meaning in the context of clinical practice) visible to students' (p. 40).

This finding suggests that overt attention should be directed towards the facilitation of students' understanding of clinical reasoning in general and to understanding the thinking and motivation of all the participants (clinician, patient/client, caregivers, other healthcare team members) in the clinical decision-making process. The students need to understand different clinical reasoning strategies, dialectical thinking, metacognition/reflection and critical thinking processes and the impact of a range of contextual factors (e.g. practice setting, time constraints, economic resources) on clinical reasoning. To achieve these outcomes requires an educational focus on the facilitation of students' understanding of how all of these *parts* influence and are influenced by each other within the *whole* of the clinical reasoning process.

As one example, students could explore the model of clinical reasoning as a dialectical process presented by Edwards and colleagues (Edwards et al 2004, Edwards & Jones 2007). We view dialectical thinking as an important dimension of clinical reasoning capability and as an inherent aspect of capable expert practice. Educators can explore with their students how dialectical thinking could be realized in action, and can facilitate students' attempts to reason through a variety of mock practice scenarios in ways consistent with these models.

Educators can also discuss with their students the connection between clinical reasoning and learning from practice. They can overtly explore opportunities for engaging in metacognition and for application of critical thinking skills in reflecting on their own reasoning and in providing critical feedback on the reasoning of their peers.

In these examples of application of early reified understandings to practice scenarios, it becomes clear that reification of clinical reasoning should not stand alone but requires participation in actual practice-based decision making, to allow students to translate and construct for themselves a deeper understanding of clinical reasoning, and to begin to 'renegotiate its meaning in a new context' (Wenger 1998, p. 68). Although participation in the academic classroom setting is necessarily limited in that it is not a true practice context, it can be likened to the process by which newcomers are gradually brought into practice communities through limited, more peripheral forms of participation (Lave & Wenger 1991).

By overtly facilitating students' understanding and practice of reflective, critical and dialectical thinking skills within clinical reasoning in the academic setting, educators can also guide students towards development of the thinking and learning skills needed for capable reasoning in the clinical education setting. By laying a theoretical foundation through reification of clinical reasoning, and then facilitating a form of participation with clinical reasoning through simulated practice activities in the classroom setting, educators can provide students with opportunities to develop their understanding of the complex nature of clinical reasoning and its link to other components of their education (e.g. theoretical and research knowledge, practical skills, communication skills, professional identity). This can allow students to practise elements of *doing* physiotherapy and *being* physiotherapists in a setting that is far more predictable and less complex than the clinical education setting.

We propose that by facilitating an overt awareness of clinical reasoning and by providing opportunities for controlled practice with complex models of clinical reasoning in the academic classroom setting, educators can explicitly guide students away from any tendencies toward overly reductionistic, linear, or rigid ways of perceiving and thinking in practice. Such rigid ways of framing situations are not congruent with the adaptive, flexible, multifaceted approaches to collaborative

patient-centred reasoning and practice demonstrated by expert physiotherapists (Edwards & Jones 2007, Jensen et al 1999). Acknowledging that 'humans *must* differentiate, interpret, draw analogies, filter, discard, and generalize in order to deal with the vast amounts of information that confront them in every moment' (Davis & Sumara 2006, p. 26) means that educators should foster in students an approach to clinical reasoning that achieves an appropriate balance in the perception and weighting of the relevant factors within a larger complexity perspective (Stephenson 2004).

Complexity thinking prompts the examination of relationships 'between and among different layers of organization, any of which might be properly identified as complex and all of which influence one another (in both enabling and constraining ways)' (Davis & Sumara 2006, p. 26). We see the development of complexity thinking, which we propose as a key dimension of clinical reasoning capability, to be a desirable focus of teaching and learning in professional entry education. 'Complexity thinking helps us actually take on the work of trying to understand things while we are a part of the things we are trying to understand' (Davis & Sumara 2006, p. 16). This is precisely the nature of the work that students must learn to accept if they are to become capable clinical reasoners in the context of collaborative client-centred practice.

Participation in and reification of clinical reasoning in the clinical education setting

Wenger (1998) argued strongly that participation and reification are both intrinsic and complementary to each other in the negotiation of meaning. Participation is the process by which reification is produced and interpreted, and reification enables participants in a community of practice to communicate about and coordinate their perspectives and meanings derived from experiences. According to Wenger (1998), one cannot exist without the other, and their duality is essential to the type of learning newcomers must achieve in order to become full participating members of a community of practice. Through participation, the learning of reified structures and practices is put into action, and through critical reflection they become open to revision and expansion as learners go beyond their initial understandings.

The professional entry education system of physiotherapists (similar to the education systems of all healthcare professions) relies in great part on situated clinical education learning experiences to provide the context and opportunity for students to become novice professional practitioners. As discussed earlier, research participants in Christensen's (2007) study experienced varying opportunities for facilitation of participation in and reflection on clinical reasoning during their clinical education experiences. Overall, the participants reported that the majority of their learning related to clinical reasoning occurred during clinical education, but that the availability and quality of opportunities for facilitation in the clinic were greatly influenced by the characteristics of assigned clinical educators. Clinical educators varied greatly in their awareness of and ability to facilitate clinical reasoning and the thinking and learning skills (reflection, critical thinking, dialectical thinking and complexity thinking) which our research identified as intimately involved in its capable performance.

One participant described the situation as follows:

> And if you haven't one good CI [clinical instructor], then you really haven't learned at all, . . . we're getting a great education, but if you have been just with crummy CIs this entire time, you have no chance of really applying it and using your knowledge, and so . . . you pretty much have wasted this education if you haven't been able to talk it out with someone who really knows how to help you learn and motivate you to learn. I think who you end up becoming as a PT is largely based on who you've had in your past experiences. I think it's really important that everyone gets a really good clinical experience at some point, . . .'cause you'll get bad luck, sometimes people end up with some terrible CIs, so I just think it's really . . . it's really important that we all get a chance to be somewhere good. (Diane)

We propose that within the clinical education setting, capability in clinical reasoning can be facilitated though interaction with skilled clinical educators who are aware of the reified conceptions of clinical reasoning that students bring from the academic classroom setting, and who understand and are skilled in ways of guiding students toward the construction of their own understanding of clinical reasoning through participation and critical reflection in the real world. To achieve this, clinical and academic classroom educators must communicate and coordinate their efforts, overcoming the barriers inherent in being physically and pedagogically separated. A strengthening of the links between educators in the academic and clinical education settings is necessary in order for all students to be facilitated in developing capability in clinical reasoning throughout the whole of their professional education process. Wenger (1998) argued for a balanced pedagogical approach to teaching and learning of complex knowledge: 'An excessive emphasis on formalism without corresponding levels of participation, or conversely a neglect of explanations and formal structure, can easily result in an experience of meaninglessness' (p. 67).

CONCLUSION

For educators aiming to facilitate clinical reasoning capability in their students, this learning process might best be viewed as the development of 'ever more sophisticated ways of interpreting experience. So understood, the most critical aspect of a teacher's role is not provision of information, but participation with learners in the development of strategies to interpret that information' (Davis et al 2000, p. 131). The clinical reasoning of healthcare professionals can be regarded as a complex expression of their negotiation of meaning in practice – their strategy for interpreting and learning from clinical experiences. The intentional provision and facilitation of learning opportunities that guide students toward the development of capability in clinical reasoning is certainly a very important way in which educators can contribute to improving professional entry educational outcomes.

References

American Physical Therapy Association 2003 Guide to physical therapist practice, 2nd edn. American Physical Therapy Association, Alexandria, VA

Bowden J, Marton F 1998 The university of learning: beyond quality and competence. Routledge Falmer, London

Cant R, Higgs J 1999 Professional socialization. In: Higgs J, Edwards H (eds) Educating beginning practitioners: challenges for health professional education. Butterworth-Heinemann, Oxford, p 46–51

Christensen N 2007 Development of clinical reasoning capability in student physical therapists. Unpublished PhD thesis, University of South Australia

Clouder L 2003 Becoming professional: exploring the complexities of professional socialization in health and social care. Learning in Health and Social Care 2(4): 213–222

Davis B, Sumara D 2006 Complexity and education: inquiries into learning, teaching, and research. Lawrence Erlbaum, Mahwah, NJ

Davis B, Sumara D, Luce-Kapler R 2000 Engaging minds: learning and teaching in a complex world. Lawrence Erlbaum, Mahwah, NJ

Edwards I, Jones M 2007 Clinical reasoning and expertise. In: Jensen G M, Gwyer J, Hack L M et al (eds) Expertise in physical therapy practice, 2nd edn. Elsevier, Boston, p 192–213

Edwards I, Jones M, Carr J et al 2004 Clinical reasoning strategies in physical therapy. Physical Therapy 84(4): 312–335

Higgs J, Andresen L, Fish D 2004 Practice knowledge – its nature, sources and contexts. In: Higgs J, Richardson B, Abrandt Dahlgren M (eds) Developing practice knowledge for health professionals. Butterworth-Heinemann, Edinburgh, p 51–69

Jensen G M, Gwyer J, Hack L M et al 1999 Expertise in physical therapy practice. Butterworth-Heinemann, Boston

Lave J, Wenger E 1991 Situated learning: legitimate peripheral participation. Cambridge University Press, Cambridge

Plsek P E, Greenhalgh T 2001 Complexity science: the challenge of complexity in health care. British Medical Journal 323:625–628

Schön D 1987 Educating the reflective practitioner: toward a new design for teaching and learning in the professions. Jossey-Bass, San Francisco

Stephenson R C 2004 Using a complexity model of human behaviour to help interprofessional clinical reasoning. International Journal of Therapy and Rehabilitation 11(4): 168–175

Weidman J C, Twale D J, Stein E L 2001 Socialization of graduate and professional students in higher education: a perilous passage?. Jossey-Bass, San Francisco

Wenger E 1998 Communities of practice: learning, meaning, and identity. Cambridge University Press, Cambridge

World Confederation for Physical Therapy 2004 Declarations of principle and position statements. Online. Available: http://www.wcpt.org 25 June 2004

Zimmerman B J, Lindberg C, Plsek P E 2001 Edgeware: insights from complexity science for health care leaders, 2nd edn. VHA, Irving, TX

Chapter **37**

Speech-language pathology students: learning clinical reasoning

Lindy McAllister and Miranda Rose

INTRODUCTION

In our chapter published in the previous edition of this book (McAllister & Rose 2000) we wrote:

> Writing this chapter posed something of a dilemma because, in general, speech-language pathologists do not talk about clinical reasoning. ... Firstly, speech-language pathologists (educators and clinicians) may well discuss or write about differential diagnosis, problem solving, decision making, critical thinking, professional judgment and diagnostic reasoning; they rarely discuss clinical reasoning. Secondly, the processes involved in clinical reasoning in our profession have been poorly researched and are little understood within the profession. (p. 205)

Since we wrote that chapter, a paradox has emerged. Some discussions of applications of other professions' models of clinical reasoning to speech-language pathology (SLP) models are appearing (McAllister & Lincoln 2004, Young 2001). However, there continues to be no substantial published research into the clinical reasoning practices of our profession. A 2005 search for references to research into clinical reasoning in SLP in academic databases and recent prominent texts on assessment and management of communication and swallowing disorders revealed minimal results. However, references to clinical reasoning are now quite common on university websites that describe their curricula, in professional association publications detailing professional competencies, and in texts

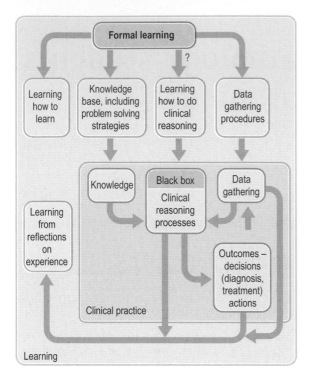

Figure 37.1 Clinical reasoning in speech pathology – the 'black box'

describing clinically-related activities. Thus, while the profession appears to have become alerted to and interested in clinical reasoning as a necessary component of clinical practice, and is now using the term 'clinical reasoning' with greater frequency, it is used on the basis of a paucity of data about the actual clinical reasoning practices taking place in SLP.

SEEKING CLINICAL REASONING IN SLP

In this chapter we make a distinction between clinical decision making (a term more common in SLP) and clinical reasoning. We see clinical decision making as an end-product of clinical reasoning; that is, as the generation of tangible decisions about clinical management. In contrast we see clinical reasoning as the often intangible, rarely explicated thought processes that lead to the clinical decisions we make. We suggest that clinical reasoning utilizes *metaprocesses*, including an awareness or a becoming conscious of what we are thinking and

what thought processes we are using. Reflection in and on action (Schön 1987) has a major role to play in clinical reasoning.

Based on our critical reading of the literature, we could describe the process of clinical reasoning in SLP as the 'black box' of information processing occurring between the input phase of data gathering and the output phase of producing decisions (concerning diagnosis and treatment) and taking action (Fig. 37.1). The reasons for this 'black box' state of affairs lie in the history and operation of our profession wherein clinical reasoning, being (broadly) the thinking associated with clinical practice, was assumed to be a skill that could be absorbed without explication. Kamhi (1998, p. 102), for instance, argued that 'as clinicians become more experienced, they gradually internalise the framework of an assessment protocol and become proficient at analysing and interpreting test information and observational data'. The SLP profession seems to have adopted what Boshuizen & Schmidt (2000) referred to as a content-oriented approach to clinical reasoning. This approach assumes that knowledge and reasoning are interdependent. There is an expectation that with increasing knowledge and clinical experience, students and clinicians will be better able to reason and make clinical decisions. University curricula have concentrated more on knowledge acquisition and skills development while 'issues specific to the decision-making process are relegated to the periphery of discussion' (Records et al 1994, p. 74).

Another focus of our profession has been on outcomes and solving problems in clinical practice. Consider recent sources in the SLP literature: for example, Dodd's 1995 text *Differential Diagnosis and Treatment of Children with Speech Disorder* contains a chapter on a problem-solving approach to clinical management. This problem-solving model begins at the stage of description of the current communication status (after diagnosis). Although it is an excellent model for problem solving in client management, it offers no clues to the clinical reasoning which lies behind the clinical problem solving. The *Pocket Reference of Diagnosis and Management for the Speech-Language Pathologist* (White 2000) contains a wealth of useful information to assist in clinical problem solving or decision making. It does not consider the clinical reasoning thinking processes underpinning diagnosis and management.

Another factor limiting understanding of clinical reasoning in SLP is that it has been seen as a linear or logical process, which obscures the 'messiness' and complexity of clinical reasoning in action. Duffy (1998, p. 96) suggested that the processes of decision making 'became obscured with training that views diagnosis as a linear, test-oriented, and mechanistic process, and that often "teaches" diagnosis by starting with the target disorder (the diagnosis) and then proceeding back to its defining symptoms and signs'. Yoder & Kent (1988) published an influential series of decision-making trees for the diagnosis and management of communication disorders. They stated that the trees were not to be seen as recipes, but rather as a series of guidelines and prompts for the clinician engaged in decision making. 'Cookbooks cannot deal with the unknown or the uncertain, but clinical decision making frequently encounters them' (Yoder & Kent 1988, p. xi). This approach has the advantage of providing guidance without rigidity and recognizing the need for professional judgement as part of decision making. However, the focus is again on the decision steps to be taken rather than on the nature of thinking in which clinicians engage and how they might respond to the prompts provided. The approach reinforces the view that clinical reasoning and decision making are basically linear and logical, whereas we argue that they are not. Further, the responsibility for learning how to think lies with the clinician. It is not made explicit.

EMERGING DIRECTIONS AND CHALLENGES IN SLP CLINICAL REASONING

In their edited text *Differential Diagnosis in Speech-Language Pathology*, Philips & Ruscello (1998) provided a broader picture of the process of diagnosis. Although they referred readers to decision-making trees they moved beyond a formulaic data collection approach to an acknowledgment that 'the speech-language pathologist's curiosity and inquisitiveness drive the process of differential diagnosis. The clinician who accepts diagnostic challenges, is curious about missing information and inconsistencies, constantly questions, and searches for possible answers is most likely to solve puzzles presented by difficult problems' (Philips & Ruscello 1998, p. 3). It is argued here that clinicians need to be aware of missing information and inconsistencies and to be thinking about them, questioning self, the process and the data. In other words, clinicians need to be engaged in metacognition, or thinking about thinking, a key component in the Higgs & Jones (2000) model of clinical reasoning. Kamhi (1998) and Deputy & Weston (1998) have reminded readers of the importance of asking causal questions but cautioned them about assuming linear causality. Asking questions about factors that may or may not cause communication disorders and that contribute to the data obtained in evaluation is an important component of what we would call clinical reasoning.

Records et al (1994) discussed clinical judgment. They emphasized not only the objective aspects of data collection, but also the subjective aspects of the decision-making process; the gut feelings, expertise and insights which are aspects of clinical reasoning. They considered clinical judgment to be a process poorly understood by speech-language pathologists. Scholten (2001) argued that both classroom and clinical experiences can be used to facilitate student clinical reasoning. She suggested that teachers should use authentic problems to develop students' understanding of clinical problems and transfer of theoretical knowledge. However, again, such assertions were based on theory from medical education and student learning in general rather than specific evidence in speech language-pathology.

HOW DO SPEECH-LANGUAGE PATHOLOGISTS REASON?

In the relative absence of direct clinical reasoning research, writers in our discipline have resorted to supposition or analogy, drawing on research in other professions. Campbell (1998) outlined four approaches to diagnostic decision making found in clinical medicine that also apply to SLP: pattern recognition, decision-making trees, diagnosis by exhaustion (collecting all possible data), and hypothetical-deductive reasoning. Duffy (1998, p. 97) stated that 'most good diagnosticians reach conclusions through a hypothetical-deductive strategy, with frequent reliance on pattern recognition'. The paucity of research into decision making and clinical reasoning in SLP does not provide data to test Campbell's or Duffy's assumptions. However, in their reflection on comparisons with reasoning approaches in other disciplines, Campbell and Duffy began to question possible reasoning strategies in SLP.

A promising discussion in our field comes from Hagstrom (2001) who presented a potential framework for using and building theory in clinical action in SLP. Hagstrom wrote about clinical action being guided by theory and proposed Bamberg's (1997) six-element framework of theory analysis as a tool for reflection on practice. Table 37.1 illustrates the six aspects of Bamberg's framework, with typical clinical questions that could be asked in SLP practice. Although Hagstrom did not directly discuss clinical reasoning and made no reference to research examining reasoning in other

Table 37.1 Bamberg's aspects of theorizing in action and their potential applications to speech–language pathology

Aspect	Typical speech–language pathology clinical questions
Domain of inquiry	What knowledge base(s) could/should I be drawing on in working with this client/situation?
Person	Am I working with a client actively engaged in his/her care, or a passive client?
Course of development	Is change for this client/situation likely to happen step by step or can steps be merged or skipped?
Telos	What is the ideological endpoint for me and for my client in this situation?
Mechanism	What is likely to cause change to happen in this client/situation?
Methodology	What type of data should be collected? How will they be collected and documented?

professions, it appears to us that there is a direct connection between her arguments and our discussion of clinical reasoning practices.

OTHER SOURCES OF KNOWLEDGE ABOUT CLINICAL REASONING IN SLP

In the absence of direct research on clinical reasoning in SLP, educators have turned to related fields for suggestions about possible reasoning approaches and strategies. Recently, Norman (2005), writing in medical education, summarized some 30 years of research into clinical reasoning in medicine, the results of which may be of significance for SLP. Norman described the 'expert' medical practitioner as one who utilizes an extensive and multidimensional knowledge base including illness scripts, decision trees, symptom and disease probabilities, semantic qualifiers, basic sciences and experience-based knowledge. The way that these mental representations will be utilized at any one time depends on the nature of the problem/case to be solved, and other factors such as the time available and recent experiences.

Perhaps a useful starting point for investigation of clinical reasoning in SLP is a model of narrative clinical reasoning developed in the field of occupational therapy (Fleming 1991). The model describes 'therapists with three track minds' who use a number of clinical reasoning approaches, depending on the client, presenting problems and contexts. Three main reasoning approaches have been described in occupational therapy: procedural, interactive and conditional. Procedural reasoning emphasizes a client's disease state and disability. Interactive reasoning is concerned with the clients' feelings and clients' perceptions of the intervention they are receiving. Conditional reasoning reflects a concern for clients' disabilities and functioning in the wider context of their daily life, integrating both procedural and interactive reasoning approaches. Given the similarities in values and beliefs about clients and therapy between occupational therapy and SLP, the three-tracked mind approach to clinical reasoning could serve as a useful starting point for SLP research.

In physical therapy, Edwards et al (2004) have presented a rigorous qualitative study of clinical reasoning drawn from the observation and interview of expert physical therapists in daily practice. Edwards et al argued for a dialectical model of clinical reasoning in physical therapy. 'A dialectic is a debate intended to reconcile a contradiction without attempting to establish either view as intrinsically "truer" than the other' (Edwards et al 2004, p. 323). The dialectic in their clinical reasoning model is the tension between the two major types of reasoning observed in their participants, hypothetico-deductive reasoning and narrative reasoning. Expert physical therapists were found to use both of these reasoning types in a highly interrelated way in every clinical task, resulting in a complex and rich reasoning process. The two types of reasoning were observed in a number of reasoning strategies (or behaviours): interaction, procedure, teaching, collaboration, prediction and ethics. The dialectic model of clinical reasoning has great intuitive appeal in terms of its applicability to SLP, as speech-language pathologists work in both acute and non-acute settings which call for different types of clinical reasoning (Mattingly & Hayes-Fleming 1994). However, it remains to be seen just how accurately the model developed by Edwards et al describes the clinical reasoning of speech language pathologists.

TEACHING CLINICAL REASONING IN PROFESSIONAL ENTRY CURRICULA

Considering the historical frame of reference above it is not surprising that there is little evidence or recognition of the need for teaching clinical reasoning in professional entry curricula in SLP. Knowing about how experts reason does not directly explain how to help novices become more expert. In reviewing the literature on educational approaches to facilitating student clinical reasoning Norman (2005, p. 424) wrote:

> Focusing instruction on one processing strategy or another [e.g. pattern recognition] may be less important than engaging students with many problems, which are carefully sequenced to optimize learning and transfer ... central to the acquisition of expertise, both in medicine and many other domains, is the opportunity for

> deliberate practice with multiple examples and feedback, both to facilitate effective transfer of basic concepts and to ensure an adequate experiential knowledge base.

Doyle (1995) in fact argued against having units within an SLP programme entitled 'clinical reasoning', arguing that there is little evidence that a theoretical coverage of the area will generalize to clinical practice. In one of the most influential texts in the area of education of speech-language pathologists, Rassi & McElroy (1992) made no more than passing mention of clinical reasoning and did not advocate its inclusion in SLP curricula. Most programmes (with a few exceptions, see Edwards & Rose this volume) designed to prepare SLP professionals do not include in the curriculum subjects that seek to make the process of clinical reasoning explicit for students. Some curricula do teach decision analysis. Syder (1996), for instance, discussed how by engaging with simulated patients, students' differential diagnosis and complex problem-solving skills could be developed. Since 1999, we have found several more references to clinical reasoning activities in university programmes preparing students for practice (e.g. Cecconi 2005), although the descriptions of many of these examples appear to reflect clinical decision making rather than the metacognitive processing associated with clinical reasoning.

The clinical reasoning in which SLP practitioners undoubtedly engage is rarely discussed or made explicit. Most SLP students develop clinical reasoning abilities without having the process made explicit. However, in any programme there will be at-risk students who have difficulty with the development of clinical competence (Maloney et al 1997). Nemeth & McAllister (1995) suggested that, for at least some of these students, the difficulty lies in how they think about their clinical work. Certainly, as experienced managers of large speech-pathology clinical education programmes, we can attest to the challenges presented by students who 'don't know how to think' about their clinical work. We believe that these students in particular, as well as other students who appear to learn well through knowledge building and experience, benefit from having the processes of clinical reasoning made explicit as a routine part of clinical education. To this end, Rose and colleagues at La Trobe University in Australia have developed a stream within their clinical education programme based on principles of clinical reasoning documented in medicine (see McAllister & Rose 2000). The programme aims to deliberately facilitate clinical reasoning skills from first to final year of their 4-year undergraduate degree. The programme enables students to make meaningful links between their otherwise discrete, encapsulated discipline-based knowledge stores (e.g. voice versus motor speech disorders) and equips them with metacognitive tools to reflect on and develop their practice.

A PROBLEM–BASED LEARNING APPROACH TO TEACHING CLINICAL REASONING IN SLP

In seeking to minimize the theory–practice gap identified by educators in the programme at La Trobe University and to facilitate enhanced clinical reasoning, staff looked for educational approaches and methods that would:

- Make clinical reasoning a more conscious process for students, in the belief that this awareness would facilitate better clinical reasoning in novel or complex situations
- Utilize adult learning and constructivist approaches to learning that recognize prior learning, self-generated motivation to learn, and the learner's personal constructs of the world (Knowles 1990)
- Utilize clinical reasoning processes that stress hypothetico-deductive reasoning (Elstein et al 1978), pattern recognition (Barrows & Feltovich 1987), reflective practice (Schön 1987), client-centred practice (Egan 1990), illness scripts (Schmidt et al 1990) and narrative reasoning (Mattingly 1991)
- Demonstrate similarities in the clinical reasoning process across client disorder type and age group
- Provide explicit opportunities to develop links across student knowledge bases in order to facilitate a more integrated overall knowledge base

- Provide opportunities for metacognitive processing (Higgs & Jones 2000) about the clinical reasoning process
- Provide multiple opportunities to practise reasoning and theory application with realistic clinical cases.

The teaching and learning approach that best incorporates the above principles was thought to be problem-based learning (PBL). For a recent meta-analysis of the effects of PBL see Dochy et al (2003). Students work in the small groups (8–14) and together discuss and solve real-life clinical 'problems' or cases that provide the context and motivation for learning. Students' prior knowledge is activated by working through the cases and elaboration of knowledge is achieved through student-centred discussion. Self-directed learning is emphasized, which further increases the motivation to learn. A PBL case tutorial commonly occurs at the start of the week, followed by independent learning around unresolved issues and attendance at lectures or practical classes, after which the students return to a second PBL case tutorial toward the end of the week. At this tutorial the students review and share their newly acquired knowledge and evaluate solutions to the clinical problem at hand. Through these activities students acquire knowledge in integrated and clinically meaningful networks. The acquisition, clarification and extension of knowledge is achieved largely through clinical reasoning activity, in the actual format that is utilized by practitioners in the field (Best et al 2005).

In 1998, the staff at the School of Human Communication Sciences at La Trobe University agreed to develop and implement a fully integrated problem-based learning (PBL) curriculum in its new graduate-entry Master of SLP degree. Staff and clinical educators in the field reported positive views of these masters degree students' clinical reasoning abilities and a greater flexibility and autonomy in students' clinical reasoning skills, particularly in dealing with novel and complex cases. In 2003, encouraged by the success of the Masters programme, the staff introduced PBL to the 4-year undergraduate programme.

PBL has been partially implemented in a number of SLP programmes throughout the world

(University of Hong Kong, University of Dublin, University of Northern Iowa), although at this time there is little published evidence about its impacts and outcomes in SLP. At La Trobe University, we are currently undertaking a comparative, longitudinal investigation into students' perceptions of learning and the development of professional competence in a cohort of students in the PBL stream and a cohort in the didactic stream which is currently being phased out. We also plan to investigate the clinical reasoning abilities of the participants at the time of graduation and following 12 months of practice. It is hoped that such data will help to illuminate potential effects of PBL on clinical reasoning skills in SLP.

Clinical reasoning opportunities are perhaps maximally available in real-life clinical practicum experiences. However, the ways in which clinical educators and students interact during the practicum are critical to the integrity of the clinical reasoning activity that ensues. Research has highlighted the lack of theory-based discussion undertaken by clinical educators with their students during clinical placements (Kenny 1996, Rose et al 1996). The vast majority of SLP clinical educators have not had undergraduate experiences or graduate units that emphasized clinical reasoning and the metacognitive processes associated with it. It is therefore not surprising that clinical educators have not naturally emphasized such activity with their students.

SUMMARY

In this chapter we have highlighted the confusion in terminology used in discussion of clinical decision making and clinical reasoning in SLP and the limited discussion of clinical reasoning in SLP education and practice. The dominant assumptions in SLP seem to be those of 'knowledge banking', which assumes that clinical decisions are made more easily with more knowledge, and that the making of decisions is a linear and logical process. Little attention is paid to the processes that lead to clinical decisions, that is, clinical reasoning processes. We have presented an argument for making the clinical reasoning process more explicit. Research into the clinical reasoning process in SLP is required. We have discussed curriculum options for SLP students which systematically seek to develop clinical reasoning skills drawing on reasoning strategies from other disciplines and the traditional methods of clinical decision making typically found in the SLP profession. We hope that this chapter will serve as a catalyst for discussion of clinical reasoning in our profession.

References

Bamberg M 1997 Narrative development: six approaches. Lawrence Erlbaum, Mahwah, New Jersey

Barrows H S, Feltovich P J 1987 The clinical reasoning process. Medical Education 21:86–91

Best D, Rose M, Edwards H 2005 Learning about learning. In: Rose M, Best D (eds) Transforming practice through clinical education, professional supervision, and mentoring. Elsevier, London

Boshuizen H P A, Schmidt H G 2000 The development of clinical reasoning expertise. In: Higgs J, Jones M (eds) Clinical reasoning in the health professions, 2nd edn. Butterworth Heinemann, Oxford, p 15–22

Campbell T 1998 Themes in diagnostic decision making. Seminars in Speech and Language 19:3–6

Cecconi C 2005 Evidence-based practice and metacognitive clinical reasoning in clinical education. Paper presented at the American Speech-Language Hearing Association National Convention, November 19, 2005, San Diego, CA

Deputy P, Weston A 1998 A framework for differential diagnosis of developmental phonological disorders. In: Philips B J, Ruscello D (eds) Differential diagnosis in speech-language pathology. Butterworth Heinemann, Boston, p 113–158

Dochy F, Segers M, Van den Bossche P, Gijbels D 2003 Effects of problem-based learning: a meta-analysis. Learning and Instruction 13:533–568

Dodd B 1995 A problem solving approach to clinical management. In: Dodd B (ed) Differential diagnosis and treatment of children with speech disorder. Whurr, London, p 149–165

Doyle J 1995 Issues in teaching clinical reasoning to students of speech and hearing science. In: Higgs J, Jones M (eds) Clinical reasoning in the health professions, 2nd edn. Butterworth Heinemann, Oxford, p 224–234

Duffy J 1998 Stroke with dysarthria: evaluate and treat; garden variety or down the garden path. Seminars in Speech and Language 19:93–98

Edwards I, Jones M, Carr J et al 2004 Clinical reasoning strategies in physical therapy. Physical Therapy 84(4): 312–335

Egan G 1990 The skilled helper: a systematic approach to effective helping, 4th edn. Brooks/Cole, Pacific Grove, CA

Elstein A S, Shulman L S, Sprafka S A 1978 Medical problem solving: an analysis of clinical reasoning. Harvard University Press, Cambridge, MA

Fleming M H 1991 The therapist with the three track mind. American Journal of Occupational Therapy 45:1007–1014

Hagstrom F 2001 Using and building theory in clinical action. Journal of Communication Disorders 34:371–384

Higgs J, Jones M 2000 Clinical reasoning in the health professions. In: Higgs J, Jones M (eds) Clinical reasoning in the health professions, 2nd edn. Butterworth Heinemann, Oxford, p 3–14

Kamhi A 1998 Differential diagnosis of language learning disabilities. In: Philips B J, Ruscello D (eds) Differential diagnosis in speech-language pathology. Butterworth Heinemann, Boston, p 87–112

Kenny B 1996 An investigation of self-evaluation by speech pathology students during supervisory conferences. Unpublished Masters thesis, University of Sydney

Knowles M 1990 The adult learner: a neglected species, 4th edn. Gulf Publishing, Houston TX

McAllister L, Lincoln M 2004 Clinical education in speech-language pathology. Whurr, London

McAllister L, Rose M 2000 Speech-language pathology students learning clinical reasoning. In: Higgs J, Jones M (eds) Clinical reasoning in the health professions, 2nd edn. Butterworth Heinemann, Oxford, p 205–213

Maloney D, Carmody D, Nemeth E 1997 Students experiencing problems learning in clinical settings. In: McAllister L, Lincoln M, McLeod S, Maloney D (eds) Facilitating learning in clinical settings. Stanley Thornes, Cheltenham UK, p 185–213

Mattingly C 1991 The narrative nature of clinical reasoning. American Journal of Occupational Therapy 45:998–1005

Mattingly C, Fleming M H 1994 Clinical reasoning: forms of inquiry in a therapeutic practice. F A Davis, Philadelphia

Nemeth E, McAllister L 1995 Students experiencing difficulties in clinical education: their perspectives. Paper presented at the annual conference of the Australian Association of Speech and Hearing, Brisbane, May

Norman G 2005 Research in clinical reasoning: past history and current trends. Medical Education 39:418–427

Philips B J, Ruscello D 1998 Differential diagnosis in speech-language pathology. Butterworth Heinemann, Boston

Rassi J, McElroy M 1992 The education of audiologists and speech-language pathologists. York Press, Timonium, MD

Records N, Jordan L, Tomblin J B 1994 Clinical judgement: a familiar concept, but a poorly understood process. National Student Speech Language Hearing Association Journal 21:74–81

Rose M, McGartland M, Joffe B 1996 Current supervisory practice. In: Rose M (ed) Proceedings of the 2nd Biennial Conference of the Foundation for Quality Supervision. La Trobe University, Melbourne, p 78–94

Schmidt H G, Norman G R, Boshuizen H P A 1990 A cognitive perspective on medical expertise: theory and implications. Academic Medicine 65:611–621

Scholten I 2001 Teachers' conceptions of their role in improving students' preparation for clinical work in dysphagia. American Journal of Speech Language Pathology 10:343–357

Schön D A 1987 Educating the reflective practitioner. Jossey-Bass, San Francisco

Syder D 1996 The use of simulated clients to develop the clinical skills of speech and language therapy students. European Journal of Disorders of Communication 31:181–192

White P 2000 Pocket reference of diagnosis and management for the speech-language pathologist. Butterworth Heinemann, Boston

Yoder D, Kent R 1988 Decision making in speech-language pathology. Decker, Toronto

Young S E 2001 Clinical reasoning in speech pathology practice: an exploration of relevant models. In: Wilson L, Hewitt S (eds) Proceedings of the Speech Pathology Australia National Conference. Speech Pathology Australia, Melbourne, p 259–265

Chapter **38**

Teaching clinical reasoning in nursing education

Suzanne Narayan and Sheila Corcoran-Perry

Clinical reasoning has been integral to nursing education for decades in both academic and staff development programmes. Beginning in the early 1960s, clinical reasoning was taught as 'the nursing process'. This general process involved linear steps of assessing patient needs, planning and implementing nursing care to meet the identified needs and evaluating outcomes. Research on nurses' clinical reasoning conducted since the late 1970s has revealed the inadequacy of this nursing process construct as a representation of how nurses actually reason and make clinical judgements (Corcoran 1986, Grobe et al 1991, Hurst et al 1991, Tanner 1987). The findings have demonstrated that nurses use a wide range of analytical and intuitive processes as they encounter patient situations that are characterized by complexity, uncertainty, and instability. Therefore, the teaching of clinical reasoning has changed from focusing on a single, linear process to developing a variety of clinical reasoning skills.

Nurses use clinical reasoning to make both autonomous and collaborative interdisciplinary judgements about patient care. The scope of nursing practice includes diagnosing and treating human responses to actual or potential health problems (American Nurses' Association 2003). As participants in the healthcare team, nurses also engage in collaborative judgements regarding the diagnosis and treatment of patients' disease conditions. Given the complexity of clinical reasoning in nursing and the range of healthcare issues involved, nurse educators use many instructional methods to help learners develop the necessary reasoning skills and knowledge base.

In this chapter, we describe five instructional strategies that are used in nursing education to teach aspects of clinical reasoning. They are analogy, iterative hypothesis testing, interactive model, 'thinking aloud', and reflection-about-action. Some of these strategies emphasize cognitive processes while others emphasize knowledge organization. Still others stress both process and knowledge.

ANALOGY

An analogy is defined as 'a resemblance in some particulars between things otherwise unlike, i.e. a similarity' (Jorgensen 1980, p. 2). It is a simple but powerful linguistic tool for developing both creative and critical thinking abilities. Often analogies are used to make the unfamiliar familiar, or to make the familiar unfamiliar (Alexander et al 1987). Nursing educators often use analogies to simplify the mental image of a task, or to view a situation from another perspective (Elsberry & Sorensen 1986). For example, when students are struggling to understand the circulatory system, an instructor might have them imagine that it is a closed system of tubing (blood vessels) with a pump (the heart) to circulate fluid (blood).

The *synectic* model of teaching is a formal instructional approach that incorporates analogies. It has five phases: (1) describe the present situation or problem; (2) present and describe an analogy for the situation; (3) describe the similarities between the analogy and the situation; (4) describe the differences between the analogy and the situation; and (5) re-explore the original situation on its own terms (Joyce et al 2004).

A nursing faculty member used this model to help beginning nursing students develop a simple but powerful mental representation (Corcoran & Tanner 1988). In a medical-surgical setting, the teacher often heard students describe patients in terms of their diseases. To counter these reductionistic perspectives and to develop a sense of patients as whole, indivisible persons, the teacher began with Phase 1 in which she acknowledged the difficulty many people have grasping the concept of holism. In Phase 2, the teacher presented an analogy, setting out jars of baking ingredients which the students identified. The teacher mixed these ingredients in a bowl. The next question was, 'Can I retrieve any of the individual ingredients?' to which the answer was 'No'. Next the teacher revealed a cake, asking the students to describe the analogy. This phase helped students gain insight into the meaning of the term *whole*. They came to view the whole of a cake as something greater than and different from the sum of its ingredients. In Phase 3, the teacher asked the students to describe the similarities between the cake and a whole person. In Phase 4, the teacher asked the students to focus on the differences between a cake and a person. Phases 3 and 4 involved the students' critical thinking abilities as they analysed the similarities and differences between the cake analogy and the concept of a person. In Phase 5, the teacher and students re-examined the concept of holism. They explored the language that would represent a view of persons as holistic beings.

Analogies promote both creative and critical thinking, two processes central to clinical reasoning. Creative thinking abilities are relevant to hypothesis generation during the diagnostic reasoning process, as well as to the generation of possible interventions. For example, analogies can help one visualize multiple interpretations of cues or causes of presenting symptoms. Similarly, analogies can promote both multiple and innovative ways for treating a given condition or situation. The critical thinking abilities promoted by the use of analogies are relevant to hypothesis and treatment evaluation. For example, the generated alternatives and/or treatments must be compared and contrasted for potential effectiveness and efficiency. Therefore, an analogy can be exploited as a conceptual tool for teaching aspects of clinical reasoning.

ITERATIVE HYPOTHESIS TESTING

Recent research in nursing and in medicine provides evidence that clinicians (physicians, nurses and nurse practitioners) use an iterative (repetitive) hypothesis testing approach in their diagnostic reasoning (Burman et al 2002; Elstein et al 1978, 1990; Offredy 1998; Tanner et al 1987). The findings show that clinicians form diagnostic hypotheses based on minimal clinical data, activate hypotheses very early in the process, and use the activated hypotheses as a context for gathering additional relevant data to confirm or eliminate hypotheses. This repetitive approach enables decision makers to cope with the limits of short-term memory because only a few diagnostic hypotheses are kept in working memory at one time. Each hypothesis represents a cluster of cues, a single *chunk*. Such chunks place less demands on working memory than do many pieces of unrelated data. One can then rule in or rule out single hypotheses. Clinicians can use the hypothesized diagnosis to collect additional data to either support or reject it. Or they can compare two or three hypotheses at a time. Also, the diagnostic hypotheses help decision makers to distinguish relevant from irrelevant data, since the classifications of most medical and nursing diagnoses include defining characteristics or critical symptoms. These characteristics or symptoms become the relevant data to collect.

Kassirer (1983) proposed a comparable strategy called *iterative hypothesis testing* for enhancing clinical reasoning. It consists of three phases: asking questions to gather data about a patient, justifying the data sought, and interpreting the data to describe the influence of new information on clinical reasoning.

A nursing staff development instructor used iterative hypothesis testing with a group of telephone triage nurses who wanted to improve their diagnostic reasoning skills. They acknowledged that the goal of triage is proper disposition of patients who call the clinic, that is, referral of the patient to an appropriate healthcare provider at an appropriate time and place (Corcoran-Perry & Bungert 1992). However, they did not feel confident about their approach to triage. One of the nurses, Jim, described a patient, Samuel Morris, who called the clinic indicating that he was feeling unwell and had pain. A member of the group began data collection by asking for the history information on Mr Morris's care plan, indicating that she did not know Mr Morris and wanted some background that might allow her to help him more efficiently and effectively. Jim stated that the care plan indicated a history of degenerative joint disease, hypertension, and obesity. The nurse who requested the data interpreted the new information. She reported that it made her

think of several possible sources of pain, including joint pain associated with his degenerative disease. Another member of the group indicated that she would ask Mr Morris where his pain was. Her justification was that she associated pain with four classic categories of description: location, duration, intensity and distress. Jim quoted Mr Morris's response: 'It feels like it is right under my breastbone'. The nurse who asked for the data interpreted this response by indicating that it made her think immediately of a myocardial infarction (MI). Substernal pain did not seem connected to his degenerative joint condition. The next nurse asked about duration of pain, with the justification that she was pursuing the primary descriptors of pain, as well as classic symptoms of MI. Jim provided the information that Mr Morris's pain had occurred on and off for the past 2 days. It hurt when he took a deep breath. The nurse interpreted that this new information did not fit the classic symptoms of MI and made her think that perhaps he had a recent mechanical injury to his chest. The questioning, justifying, and interpreting continued as the nurses pursued the pain descriptors and tested the competing hypotheses. They learned that Mr Morris could not recall a recent activity that might cause injury, but that his chest felt 'tight' and that he experienced sweating and feelings of indigestion. Concluding that he might be experiencing a life-threatening condition, the group chose to have Mr Morris brought to the emergency room (ER) by ambulance for immediate medical attention. Jim reported that Mr Morris had been brought into the ER and had, in fact, suffered a MI. As the group re-examined their reasoning processes, they became more aware of their previously unconscious use of hypothesis generation and testing. They indicated that Mr Morris's situation helped them refine their knowledge of MI symptoms in elderly persons. They now realized that elderly persons might not experience the sudden, sharp, and intense pain often described by younger persons with myocardial infarctions. As illustrated, iterative hypothesis testing can be used to enhance diagnostic reasoning. It is helpful for discriminating among specific competing hypotheses and for clarifying the defining characteristics which differentiate them.

INTERACTIVE MODEL

The interactive model is a strategy that is designed to teach new knowledge by building on and refining previous learning (Eggen & Kauchak 2006). The model stresses the interactions between and among the learner and new content, what is already known and what is to be learned, text-book knowledge and that gained through practical experience. The conceptual foundation of the interactive model is schema theory (Rumelhart 1977, Rumelhart & Abrahamson 1973, Rumelhart & Norman 1981). Schemata are mental structures that organize knowledge and guide the way we perceive and categorize information from the world around us. Rumelhart and colleagues suggested that people try to make sense of what they encounter on the basis of prior knowledge and experience. Schemata serve as a way to store this information as elaborated networks of interconnected ideas. Schemata are not static. They are active processes that are constantly being re-evaluated for fit and usefulness. When learning occurs, schemata are tuned and refined to accommodate new knowledge.

The interactive model includes three components: advance organizers, progressive differentiation and integrative reconciliation (Ausubel 1963, Ausubel et al 1978). The following example illustrates the use of the interactive model to teach the concept of peripheral oedema. The instructor began by presenting an advance organizer, a blueprint or framework that previewed the material to be learned and connected it to information already familiar to the student. Advance organizers link new information to an existing schema and provide a way to refine the old schema or create a new one. The advance organizer presented a brief statement about the concept of oedema. The instructor then used the process of progressive differentiation to help the students examine the relationships within the new content on peripheral oedema and to link the new content to their previous knowledge about the general concept of oedema. She differentiated peripheral oedema into several types. Then she distinguished each type according to usual cause, nature, pigmentation, ulceration, foot involvement and other relevant characteristics. The example shows how the ideas in the refined schema of peripheral oedema were related to previous ideas in an organized way. This linking of concepts provided a basis to encode the information and to store it in long-term memory. Students' refinement of a schema is not just passive learning of the instructor's schema. Instead, students are actively engaged in forming new relationships among ideas, connecting this new content to previous knowledge and building upon their own existing schema. Finally, the instructor applied integrative reconciliation, the third component of the interactive model, in which the students were actively engaged in recognizing similarities and differences, exploring the relationships between concepts, and making inferences about underlying causes or other critical features.

Recently, nursing educators have used another application of the interactive model, called *concept mapping*, to facilitate students' independent learning of concepts in the clinical setting, in small group work, and in preparing for examinations (All et al 2003, Trausch 2003). A concept map is a visual representation of ideas or concepts and their interrelationships that is similar to an advance organizer.

Learning through the interactive model promotes deep learning, which involves learning for understanding and meaning rather than rote learning of facts and principles (Biggs 1979, Marton & Saljo 1976). Use of this teaching strategy strengthens the content and organization of the knowledge that the nurse employs during clinical reasoning. Furthermore, the interactive model also fosters essential skills that underlie clinical reasoning, including cue and pattern recognition and hypothetico-deductive reasoning.

'THINKING ALOUD'

Thinking aloud is a teaching strategy that is helpful in developing nurses' knowledge and clinical reasoning processes. Originally, thinking aloud was used as a data collection method in research on the cognitive processes people use to solve problems or make decisions (Ericsson & Simon 1984, Newell & Simon 1972). Corcoran and colleagues (1988) suggested that since this method had proved effective in revealing the requisite factual knowledge and its structural organization and the cognitive processes used by research subjects during clinical reasoning, the strategy would also be beneficial in teaching clinical reasoning skills. In this strategy, the nurse is given a particular clinical situation (either real or simulated) and asked to think aloud while making a decision. The thinking aloud verbalizations may be tape-recorded and later transcribed. Analysis of the transcripts reveals the cues to which the nurse attends, the hypotheses or inferences generated and the nursing actions proposed.

This strategy was employed using a transcript of a cardiovascular clinical specialist thinking aloud about a simulated patient case. The clinical specialist shared this transcript with new nurses being oriented to a cardiovascular step-down unit. The situation involved a man who had been transferred from a coronary care unit (CCU) to a step-down unit four days after experiencing a myocardial infarction. His wife was quite concerned about the transfer. Together the clinical specialist and the new nurses analysed the transcript for the cues to which the specialist attended, her interpretations of cues, the hypotheses generated and the nursing actions proposed. With a more advanced level of nurses, the clinical specialist might examine the transcript for the ways in which cues are combined, evidence of ruling hypotheses in or out and the rationale for nursing actions.

The thinking aloud method can be adapted and used to enhance clinical reasoning skills in many situations. Instructors may find it a useful strategy in teaching students in clinical settings. For example, an instructor might ask a student to think aloud as nursing care is planned. The instructor supports and reinforces the student's appropriate use of knowledge and clinical reasoning processes and helps the student become aware of lack of knowledge or errors in reasoning.

Experienced nurses may use the thinking aloud method to enhance their clinical reasoning skills. They could share thinking aloud verbalizations as they make diagnostic or treatment decisions for patients who are particularly challenging or difficult. Thinking aloud may reveal underlying causes of errors in clinical reasoning. Such errors may be revealed through feedback from peers or experts during thinking aloud sessions or by the nurses' enhanced ability to justify clinical inferences and correct their own errors in reasoning.

REFLECTION–ABOUT–ACTION

Reflection-about-action is a strategy for promoting deliberation about one's practice within the context of particular clinical situations (Harris 1993, Schön, 1987). Reflection-about-action occurs when one contemplates prior clinical situations, especially situations that were puzzling, troublesome or particularly interesting (Harris 1993). Since the reflections occur after a particular event, the knowledge gained usually cannot make a difference to the event at hand. However, the new knowledge can influence future clinical reasoning in similar situations.

The theoretical underpinnings for this strategy come from the work of Benner (1984), Schön (1983, 1987) and Harris (1993). All effectively argued for a new epistemology of professional practice. This epistemology conceptualizes professional knowledge as being gained from actual experience in clinical situations. One does not simply apply theoretical knowledge to a clinical situation. Instead, one gains this type of knowledge through the experience of making decisions about clinical situations, particularly situations characterized by complexity, uniqueness, uncertainty, instability, and/or conflicting values (Harris 1993). Clinical reasoning in such situations cannot rely simply on acontextual facts, rules or procedures that were learned in a classroom or from the literature. Instead, much of the required knowledge and the clinical reasoning processes are developed in the experience of practice. However, experience in the usual sense is not adequate. One develops this type of knowledge and skill not from simply doing something, but from *reflecting* on clinical judgements made, feelings generated, and actions taken within the context of particular situations.

Although the clinical setting traditionally has been used as a learning laboratory in nursing education, this site has been considered the place where students develop skill in applying what they already know. It has been assumed that the theoretical knowledge gained in the classroom provides the foundation on which clinical practice is based. However, the work of Benner (1984) and Schön (1983, 1987) has caused many nursing educators to rethink the purposes for using the clinical setting as a site for learning. Instead of conceptualizing clinical activities as opportunities for students simply to apply theoretical knowledge, these educators view such activities as a means for students to develop new and different types of knowledge. This knowledge is integrated with the theoretical knowledge that students bring to their clinical activities and incorporated into their clinical reasoning about particular patient situations.

Reflection-about-action is a strategy that promotes pondering about a particular situation in relation to the environment in which it occurs, as well as the feelings experienced, the judgements made and the actions taken. Consequently, the theoretical and professional knowledge and the reasoning processes implicit in clinical practice can be delineated, elaborated, criticized, and transformed for future practice (Harris 1993). Schön (1987) suggested that clinicians (whether students or professionals) should reflect together on practice, using specific examples in the form of cases or demonstrations.

The following example illustrates how reflection-about-action was used in a senior nursing student's elective clinical experience. The student observed and worked with an expert hospice nurse mentor as she cared for several patients who were experiencing severe pain. At the end of each clinical session, the student and mentor reflected together on how they made clinical decisions about the recurrent, troublesome problem of pain control for particular patients. During these reflections-about-action, the mentor referred to aspects of each patient's condition that she thought contributed to the experience of pain. She attended to multiple, diverse cues and related them to her diagnostic conclusion about the patient's level of pain. The student had noted the same patient concerns, but interpreted them as separate issues. She recognized the cues and generated separate diagnostic hypotheses about each. However, upon hearing the mentor's reflections, the student realized that she had not considered other aspects of the patients' situation as being interdependent and

pain related. As a result of this dialogue, the student gained a greater appreciation for the complex nature of pain as a human experience. As the mentor went on to describe her selection of particular drugs and their dosages to control a woman's pain, the student asked about the 'rules' that the mentor used. When the mentor indicated that she had few rules because each case was unique, the student commented: 'But you made statements that sounded like rules or guidelines. And they were statements that I hadn't read in my textbooks or in the studies that I reviewed about pain control'. When the mentor asked the student what rules she heard, the student said, 'Well, you said things like "Keep it chemically simple", "It is better to increase the dosage than to increase the frequency of an analgesic", and "This woman is likely to have constipation as a side-effect of the analgesic; I should start a laxative to prevent or at least control that."' The mentor was surprised to hear these statements, not realizing that she had made them. Then she shared with the student particular clinical situations earlier in her practice that had made these informal rules (heuristics) meaningful to her.

This illustration exemplifies how reflection-about-action can be an important strategy for enhancing the clinical reasoning of both nursing experts and nursing students. Taking time to ponder particular clinical experiences enables one to gain new insights, to integrate theoretical and professional knowledge with feelings, actions and outcomes, and to use the experience as a basis for clinical decision making in future practice. In this sense, experience is not simply the passage of time, but rather a source of new knowledge, a challenge to clinical reasoning skill and an opportunity to transform one's practice. As Schön (1987) pointed out, reflection is critical for both experienced practitioners' and novices' development, renewal and self-correction.

CONCLUSION

The teaching of clinical reasoning has changed from focusing on a single, linear process to developing a variety of clinical reasoning skills and a broad, well-organized knowledge base. In this chapter we selected five strategies that nursing educators use to teach diverse clinical reasoning skills. There are many other strategies that have been used to enhance nurses' clinical reasoning skills, including computer assisted instruction, use of decision analysis and simulation laboratories for teaching and testing clinical reasoning. Two excellent resources for other educational strategies to promote development of general reasoning skills are *Models of Teaching* by Joyce et al (2004) and *Strategies for Teachers: Teaching Content and Thinking Skills* by Eggen & Kauchak (2006). It is important for educators to develop a repertoire of strategies, beginning with one or two and adding others over time.

References

Alexander P, White C, Haensly P et al 1987 Training in analogical reasoning. American Educational Research Journal 24:387–404

All A, Huycke L, Fisher M 2003 Instructional tools for nursing education: concept maps. Nursing Education Perspectives 24(6):311–317

American Nurses' Association 2003 Nursing's social policy statement, 2nd edn. American Nurses' Association, Kansas City

Ausubel D 1963 The psychology of meaningful verbal learning. Grune and Stratton, New York

Ausubel D, Novak J, Hanesian H 1978 Educational psychology: a cognitive view, 2nd edn. Holt, Rinehart and Winston, New York, p 39

Benner P 1984 From novice to expert: excellence and power in clinical nursing practice. Addison-Wesley, Menlo Park, CA

Biggs J 1979 Individual differences in study processes and the quality of learning outcomes. Higher Education 8:381–394

Burman M, Stepans M, Jansa N et al 2002 How do NPs make clinical decisions? The Nurse Practitioner 27(5):57–64

Corcoran S A 1986 Task complexity and nursing expertise as factors in decision making. Nursing Research 35(2): 107–112

Corcoran S, Tanner C 1988 Implications of clinical judgment research for teaching. In: National League for Nursing (eds) Curriculum revolution: mandate for change. National League for Nursing, New York, p 159–176

Corcoran S, Narayan S, Moreland H 1988 'Thinking aloud' as a strategy to improve clinical decision making. Heart and Lung 17:463–468

Corcoran-Perry S, Bungert B 1992 Enhancing orthopaedic nurses' clinical decision making. Orthopaedic Nursing 11:64–70

Eggen P, Kauchak D 2006 Strategies for teachers: teaching content and thinking skills, 5th edn. Allyn & Bacon, Boston

Elsberry N, Sorensen M 1986 Using analogies in patient teaching. American Journal of Nursing 86:1171–1172

Elstein A S, Shulman L S, Sprafka S A 1978 Medical problem solving: an analysis of clinical reasoning. Harvard University Press, Cambridge, MA

Elstein S A, Shulman L S, Sprafka A S 1990 Medical problem solving: a ten year retrospective. Evaluation and the Health Professions 13:5–36

Ericsson K A, Simon H A 1984 Protocol analysis: verbal reports as data. MIT Press, Cambridge, MA

Grobe S, Drew J, Fonteyn M 1991 A descriptive analysis of experienced nurses' clinical reasoning during a planning task. Research in Nursing and Health 14:305–314

Harris I B 1993 New expectations for professional competence. In: Curry L, Wergin J F et al (eds) Educating professionals: responding to new expectations for competence and accountability. Jossey-Bass, San Francisco, p 17–52

Hurst K, Dean A, Trickey S 1991 The recognition and non-recognition of problem-solving stages in nursing practice. Journal of Advanced Nursing 16:1444–1455

Jorgensen S 1980 Using analogies to develop conceptual abilities. ERIC Reports, #ED 192 820, US Department of Health Education and Welfare, National Institute of Education, Washington, DC

Joyce B, Weil M, Calhoun E 2004 Models of teaching, 7th edn. Allyn Bacon, Boston

Kassirer J 1983 Sounding board: teaching clinical medicine by iterative hypothesis testing. New England Journal of Medicine 309:921–924

Marton F, Saljo R 1976 On qualitative differences in learning: I Outcome and process. British Journal of Educational Psychology 46:4–11

Newell A, Simon H A 1972 Human problem solving. Prentice-Hall, Englewood Cliffs, NJ

Offredy M 1998 The application of decision making concepts by nurse practitioners in general practice. Journal of Advanced Nursing 28(5):988–1000

Rumelhart D 1977 Introduction to human information processing. Wiley, New York

Rumelhart D, Abrahamson A 1973 A model for analogical reasoning. Cognitive Psychology 5:1–28

Rumelhart D, Norman D 1981 Analogical processes in learning. In: Anderson J R (ed) Cognitive skills and their acquisition. Erlbaum, Hillsdale, NJ, p 335–359

Schön D A 1983 The reflective practitioner: how professionals think in action. Basic Books, New York

Schön D 1987 Educating the reflective practitioner. Jossey-Bass, San Francisco

Tanner C 1987 Teaching clinical judgement. In: Fitzpatrick J, Tauton R (eds) Annual review of nursing research. Springer, New York, p 153–174

Trausch P 2003 Student drawing: a clinical learning tool. Nurse Educator 28(2):58–60

Chapter 39

Assessing clinical reasoning

C.P.M. van der Vleuten, G.R. Norman and L.W.T. Schuwirth

CHAPTER CONTENTS

The term *clinical reasoning* is used in varying ways. In this chapter we use it to refer to the mental activities involved in arriving at a diagnosis and a management plan. Thus it is related to activities like history taking or physical examination, which are somewhat distinct.

Typical for the assessment of clinical reasoning is the use of an authentic professional situation as a stimulus format, usually in the form of a simulation representing a professional situation using a paper, a verbal or a practical performance situation. Many representations are possible, ranging from simple to complex, and they can be connected to many different types of response format. Experimentation with all these phenotypes actually reflects the history of clinical reasoning assessment as described in more detail below. It follows very intuitive notions of how clinical reasoning should be assessed, moving towards increasingly more simplified forms of assessment based on growing insights from research and practical experiences. To a large extent, the history of clinical reasoning represents a sobering experience, falsifying many of the original intuitive beliefs. However, this is not uncommon in education research (van der Vleuten et al 2000) and really makes the story worth telling. In doing so, we will limit our discussion primarily to cognitive assessment methods. We acknowledge that clinical reasoning also occurs in performance-based measures such as the Objective Structured Clinical Examination (OSCE) (Petrusa 2002) or methods involving real-life clinical settings (Turnbull & Van Barneveld 2002); but reasoning is first and foremost an activity of the mind.

HISTORICAL PERSPECTIVE

In the 1960s and 1970s there was considerable interest in the development of methods which assessed 'clinical problem-solving skills'. The main thrust was to mimic authentic clinical situations as creatively as possible both in the stimulus and in the response format. This entailed a simulation on paper, and later by computer, of the process by which a doctor took a history, obtained information from the physical examination and made diagnostic, investigational and management decisions.

Undoubtedly the most popular of the many variants was the *Patient Management Problem* (PMP) (Mcguire & Babbott 1967). A typical PMP begins with a variable amount of information about the patient. The student is then requested to collect further data sequentially in either a linear or a branching fashion, typically using a 'rubout' pen that exposes the answer. After collecting history and examination data, ostensibly in the manner and order that would have pertained in the live patient situation, the student may select investigations and/or make diagnostic and management decisions. The pathway of the student is compared to that of an expert or criterion group, and composite scores are determined.

The death knell of PMPs was the finding that performance on one PMP is a poor predictor of performance on another PMP. From a number of studies the correlation across problems was of the order of 0.1–0.3 (Norman et al 1985). This observation appears to undermine one of the original hypotheses underlying the development of problem-solving simulations, i.e. that they measure problem-solving ability. If that were so, correlations between PMPs ought to be high, since those who are better problem solvers should exhibit superior performance across a wide range of problems, independent of specific content knowledge. The explanation of this phenomenon is referred to variously as *content specificity* or *case specificity* (Elstein et al 1978). Interestingly, the finding is not peculiar to PMPs but is also seen for other methods which assess aspects of clinical competence and performance (van der Vleuten & Schuwirth 2005).

One variant that has survived the passage of time is the modified essay question (MEQ), which has been used quite extensively by the medical profession in some parts of the world, both for in-course assessments and for the certification of competence. This reflects, in part, the relative ease of construction of MEQs as compared to PMPs (Feletti & Engel 1980). A typical MEQ once again begins with a case vignette as a stimulus. Students are asked to respond to questions in a short essay format. New information is provided sequentially which relates to differing and evolving circumstances of the same case. Some skill is required to avoid providing cues to earlier or subsequent sections of the MEQ. Few studies are available of the reliability and validity of this method but it has face validity, appears to be acceptable and is practicable (Feletti & Engel 1980, Neufeld & Norman 1985). Nevertheless, there is no reason to presume that the MEQ would be any less vulnerable to the deleterious effect of content specificity than any other format.

Given these limitations, doubt has been cast on the value of any format which involves extensive and lengthy testing with relatively few cases (Swanson et al 1987). In addition, the experience with PMPs has alerted us to our limited understanding of the nature of clinical reasoning. Among other things, it has stimulated research of a more fundamental nature into the cognitive functioning of medical students and doctors (Eva 2005, Norman 2005).

NEW CONCEPTS OF CLINICAL REASONING

In the 1970s and 1980s several studies showed that while expert clinicians systematically outperformed less experienced doctors on a variety of simulations of clinical problem solving (Neufeld et al 1981), there was little difference in the problem-solving process they used. This led to a new direction in fundamental research, guided primarily by methods of cognitive psychology (Eva 2005, Norman 2005, Norman et al 1989, Regehr & Norman 1996, Schmidt et al 1990) (see also Chapters 10 and 20 in this book).

Current understanding would suggest that problem-solving ability is not a separate skill or entity which grows with training and experience, and that it cannot be measured independently of relevant content knowledge. Problem-solving ability appears to be highly dependent on knowledge, not just the amount of knowledge but also its specificity and the way it is structured, stored, accessed and retrieved. This is not to say that knowledge alone is sufficient for efficient and effective clinical reasoning. Higher-order control processes also play an integral role (Bransford et al 1986). But the notion that there is a general, content-independent skill that experts acquire during training is simply incompatible with the evidence. Knowledge – its amount, its kind, and its organization – is central to expertise.

One theory of knowledge organization proposes three different kinds of knowledge relevant to solving clinical problems. The most elementary is knowledge of disease processes and causal relationships, the basic science of medicine. At a later level, students acquire *illness scripts* which are quite literal list-like structures relating signs and symptoms to disease prototypes (Feltovich & Barrows 1984). At the highest level of functioning, the expert uses a sophisticated form of pattern recognition characterized by speed and efficient use of information (Brooks et al 1991, Schmidt et al 1990). It appears that this representation is drawn to a large degree from direct experience with patients, and that pattern recognition is, in fact, recognition at a holistic level of the similarity between the present patient and previous patients (Hatala & Norman 1999).

This is not to indicate that all expert clinical reasoning occurs by pattern recognition. More recent research suggests, not surprisingly, that experts may make use of all kinds of knowledge – basic science, clinical and experiential (De Bruin et al 2005, Norman 2005). If the problem is one with which the person has had considerable previous experience, then it is probably recognized very early by a pattern recognition process. Little active thinking is required and there is a rapid resolution of the problem. However, if no easy solution is evident, more systematic intellectual activities must be brought into play, either formal testing of hypotheses through accumulation and weighting of specific data, or causal reasoning at the level of basic disease mechanisms. An individual will demonstrate a range of approaches, both within and across problems, depending on previous experience and exposure to problems of a similar nature.

To the extent that this view is correct, it is evident that early attempts to assess clinical reasoning were doomed. We cannot consider it a generic process. Instead, we must contemplate the evaluation of several qualitatively different strategies. Some, like pattern recognition, are efficient and indeed may be over in seconds. These strategies will defy any attempt at measurement of the process. Some, like causal reasoning, are focused on detailed reasoning about mechanisms and are little concerned with data acquisition. As a result, they are inadequately captured by a focus on observable behaviours like history taking and physical examination. These issues have serious implications for assessment.

NEW ASSESSMENT DEVELOPMENTS

From the above experiences and empirical findings several things became clear. The first is that assessment must be anchored in case-based material presented in a way that will induce and sample clinical-reasoning activities. The second is that laboriously taking a student through the full data-gathering and investigational phase of a real or simulated clinical case is an inefficient approach when the concern is to evaluate clinical reasoning, simply because of the content-specificity problem and the consequent need to present students with large numbers of cases before satisfactory levels of test reliability can be achieved. For example, it has been shown because of this problem that up to 8 hours of testing time may be required to achieve reliable assessments with PMPs (Norcini et al 1985). Such studies have triggered a search for more cost-effective methods with simpler simulation technologies. We will discuss a number of them. There is one other implication; since there are multiple knowledge representations, each or all of which may be invoked to solve a particular problem, it makes little sense to attempt to identify the specific knowledge or strategy used to solve any problem. It suffices simply to ensure that sufficient numbers of cases have been sampled to differentiate reliably between better and poorer clinical reasoners on the basis of their success rates.

In examining the various contemporary methods, one useful distinction in assessment methods is between stimulus formats and response formats (Norman et al 1996). The *stimulus format* refers to the task that is being presented to a candidate in the assessment. It may be very simple and short, for example a question about the signs and symptoms of a particular disease, or it may be very complex and time consuming. A case scenario or maybe even a video presenting a patient case to the candidate represents an illustration of the latter. The stimulus format is ended with a lead-in question that connects the previous information to required response from the candidate, for example, 'What is the most likely diagnosis?' The *response format* refers to the way the response of the candidate is captured. It could consist of a short menu of options (multiple choice), long extensive (computerized) menus, a short write-in format, a long write-in format (essay-type questions), an oral response (oral examinations) or a behavioural response either in a simulated environment (e.g. OSCE) or in a real-life context.

KEY FEATURE

As a suggestion from a 'think-tank' conference on clinical reasoning, the first Cambridge Conference, the idea emerged to focus on essential elements of a clinical case (Norman et al 1992). The idea was based on the premise that any single case contained much 'dead wood' from a clinical-reasoning perspective. For example, in one case the critical challenge might be to elicit and interpret elements within the history, with little further being added by the physical examination and laboratory investigations. In another case the challenge might be the appropriate selection and interpretation of laboratory results. In other words, it may be possible to focus the problem-solving stimulus. One concrete outcome has been the *key feature* approach developed for the Medical Council of Canada certification examinations as an alternative to PMPs (Page & Bordage 1995, Page et al 1990). In this procedure, clinical situations, as presenting in actual practice, are produced as written case scenarios representing the stimulus format. The key features are identified on the basis of those elements critical to resolution of the problem. Questions relating to the key features are then devised and may be posed in a variety of response formats (e.g. short answer, multiple choice questions (MCQ) or selection from longer menus of options). Such an approach allows a sample of 40–50 cases to be administered in the same time as that required to administer 12–15 PMPs.

Studies so far have indicated improved reliability as compared to the PMP, but still 3–5 hours of testing time is required. Data from the Medical Council of Canada showed that a reliability of 0.80 is reached with approximately 40 cases in 4 hours of testing time (Page & Bordage 1995). Other studies reported slightly worse findings (Hatala & Norman 2002), or slightly better findings (Fischer et al 2005). A recent study has shown that 2–3 items per case is the optimal for achieving maximum reliability (Norman et al 2006); reading time will compromise reliability when fewer items are used and information redundancy will compromise reliability when more items are used. Validity studies investigating correlations with other measures typically show moderate correlations. More compelling are studies that use think-aloud strategies when comparing stimulus formats. They show that case-based stimulus formats elicit other cognitive processes than fact-oriented stimulus formats (Schuwirth et al 2001, Skakun et al 1994). Response formats that use menus instead of write-ins may cue the candidate to both correct and incorrect answers (Schuwirth et al 1996a) with slightly higher scores as a net effect, naturally depending on the number of alternatives in the menu (Schuwirth et al 1995). Score correlations across these response formats, however, are invariantly high (Schuwirth et al 1996a).

A modern variation of the key feature format is the use of computers for test administration, allowing more flexible use of pictorial and audio information (Schuwirth et al 1996b, Fischer et al 2005). Practical information on the construction of key features is readily available (Schuwirth et al 1999, Farmer & Page 2005). The writing of key features requires significant staff input (Hatala & Norman 2002).

MULTIPLE CHOICE QUESTIONS (MCQS)

In their simplest format simulations take the form of *vignette-based MCQs* (Case & Swanson 2002). This is the preferred format of the US National Board of Medical Examiners in their undergraduate licensure examinations. In recent years they completely changed the assessment strategy of their written examinations. All test items used are now vignette-based MCQs. The United States Medical Licensing Examination (USMLE) consists of two parts. Step 2 is the clinical component and is fully patient-based. Short cases are presented that require some form of judgement or decision. This may be related to data gathering, to case management or to any other phase of the clinical problem. For example, instead of asking:

> Ibuprofen belongs to a certain group of NSAIDS. Which group?
>
> a.   Salicylates
> b.   Acetic acid derivatives
> c.   Oxicam derivatives
> d.   Propionic acid derivatives
> e.   Pyrazolinone derivatives

this topic of pain management could be addressed as for example:

> Mr Brown has a carcinoma of the esophagus. The carcinoma has metastasized and curative treatment is not possible. Initially, the disorder caused little pain, which was easily suppressed with nonsteroidal anti-inflammatory analgesics and a weak opioid. Due to more invasive growth of the carcinoma, the pain has increased and the pain management is no longer adequate even at the highest dosage of the current medication. Which is the most indicated next step in the pain therapy in this case?
>
> a.   Adding a tricyclic antidepressant to the present medication.
> b.   Adding a strong opioid to the therapy while discontinuing the weak opioid medication
> c.   Increasing the dosage of the nonsteroidal anti-inflammatory analgesics
> d.   Adding a tranquillizer to the current medication.

After the case presentation the lead-in prompts the candidate to make a choice from a menu.

USMLE Step 1 is on basic sciences, but even there the strategy is to design a reasoning question. Instead of asking:

> Which neurotransmitter/s activate/s the sweat glands?
>
> a.   Only acetylcholine
> b.   Only adrenaline and noradrenaline
> c.   Only adrenaline and acetylcholine
> d.   Only noradrenaline and acetylcholine
> e.   Noradrenaline, adrenaline and acetylcholine.

the topic of temperature control could be addressed as for example:

> Charles and Irene are going to travel through Mexico for 2 months. At Mexico City airport the temperature is no less than 40°C. Their clothes get sticky. They wonder whether they will get used to these temperatures the next few weeks. If one compares the average loss of fluid in litres per day and the loss of salts in g salt/day of the last week for their visit to the first week, what is the most probable result?
>
> a.   both fluid loss and salt loss will have decreased
> b.   both fluid loss and salt loss will have increased
> c.   fluid loss will have increased and salt loss will have decreased
> d.   fluid loss will have decreased and salt loss will have increased

These questions are, with some initial training, relatively easy to write, particularly because they come close to what clinicians do in actual clinical practice. The response format is a menu. The length of the menu does not need to be fixed, but is usually as long as there are meaningful alternatives.

Another MCQ type also proposed by the US National Board of Medical Examiners was Extended Matching Questions (EMQs). Originally this was introduced as a 'pattern recognition test' (Case & Swanson 1993, Case et al 1988). Students are presented with a series of brief case scenarios based on a single chief complaint (e.g. shortness of breath) and must select the most appropriate diagnosis or action from a menu of options. EMQs are relatively easy to construct.

MCQs of the kind described represent clinical reasoning formats in their simplest form. They are characterized by a professionally authentic stimulus format in combination with a closed response format. Reliability is similar to that of normal MCQs (Case et al 1994). Stimulus formats with richer (and longer) vignettes contain more 'measurement information' and contribute better to reliability than other vignettes. Longer menu response formats may appear to be better, but recent evidence suggests no advantage over simple 5-option MCQs (Swanson et al 2005). More complex response formats (e.g. using multiple best answers or allowing logical operators between different elements) and more complex scoring systems (like penalties and partial credit) are not recommended. Simple single best-answer formats and simple scoring systems are advised. In all, simple strategies seem to work best. An excellent manual for writing these MCQs is available (Case & Swanson 2002) and is freely available from the website of the US National Board of Medical Examiners (www.nbme.org).

OTHER CLINICAL REASONING FORMATS

On the basis of cognitive expertise theory, Charlin and his co-workers proposed the Script Concordance Test (SCT) (Charlin et al 2000). Most clinical problems are ill-defined, and experts do not collect exactly the same data and do not follow the same paths of thought. They also show substantial variation in performance on any particular real or simulated case. Their reasoning performance is based on illness scripts that have been shaped through individual training, experience and clinical exposure. Charlin et al challenged existing MCQ-based formats for their characteristic of applying well-known solutions to well-defined problems requiring a unique right solution. The SCT, in contrast, uses ill-defined problems and a method called aggregate scoring (Norman 1985) that takes expert variability into account. A clinical scenario is presented that provides a challenge to the candidate since not all data are provided for solution of the problem. A menu of options is presented from which the candidate may score the likelihood of each option in relation to the solution of the problem on a +2 to −2 scale. An example is:

> A 25 year-old male patient is admitted to the emergency room after a fall from a motorcycle with a direct impact to the pubis. Vital signs are normal. The X-ray reveals a fracture of the pelvis with a disjunction of the pubic symphysis.

followed by a series of questions like:

If you were thinking of	And then you find	This hypothesis becomes
Urethral rupture	Urethral bleeding	−2 −1 0 +1 +2

The scoring reflects the variability experts demonstrate in the clinical reasoning process. Credits on each item are derived from the answers given by a reference panel. The credit for each answer is the number of reference panel members that have provided that answer, divided by the modal value for the item. For example, if on a particular item six panel members (out of 10) have chosen response +1, this choice receives 1 point (6/6), and if three experts have chosen response +2, this choice receives 0.5 (3/6). The total score for the test is the sum of credits obtained on all items.

Numerous studies of the validity of the SCT have been conducted (Charlin & van der Vleuten 2004). Reliability is quite good, showing that a value of 0.80 is reached with approximately 1 hour of testing using about 80 items.

OTHER CLINICAL REASONING ASSESSMENT METHODS

In the recent literature other methods have also been proposed. However, they either have had, as yet, less impact on the assessment field or are supported by only limited research into their measurement properties.

An instrument that has some resemblance to the SCT is a test called the Clinical Reasoning Problem (CRP) (Groves et al 2002). The CRP is intended specifically to assess the *process* of clinical reasoning, not so much the outcome. The stimulus format consists of a clinical scenario including a presentation, history and physical examination. Subjects are asked to nominate the two diagnoses they consider most likely, to list the features that they regard as important in formulating their diagnosis, to indicate whether these features are positively or negatively predictive, and to give a weighting of each. There is not necessarily a single correct answer. Scoring is again done by using information from an expert panel. Reliability of the CRP seems comparable to that of MCQs and moderate correlations are found with criterion variables.

Finally, the Clinical Reasoning Exercise has been designed to assess students' knowledge of the basic mechanisms of disease (Neville et al 1996). The stimulus format presents short clinical presentations, with history and examination data as a stimulus format and a one-paragraph write-in answer as the response format. Approximately 15 cases are required for an acceptable level of reliability (0.78), and consistency of scores across multiple tests is excellent (0.84) (Wood et al 2000). Moderate correlations have been found with a knowledge test.

IMPLICATIONS AND ADVICE FOR THE TEACHER

As has become evident from this review, our success in developing valid measures of clinical reasoning for student assessment has been a sobering experience. Clearly *the* method for clinical reasoning assessment does not exist. It is clear that our intuitive notions of complex clinical simulations are not what we might have expected from them in the first place. Simpler simulation technologies, with capacity for much greater sampling, seem to do a better job. If this is the disheartening reality, what should we as educators do in day-to-day practice? Are there some guidelines that could be developed from the findings so far which would allow us to proceed with some forms of assessment of clinical reasoning, albeit with caution? Unfortunately there are no fixed answers to these questions. For instance, the answer may be quite different for tests which are to be used in undergraduate courses largely for formative purposes than for those used for major postgraduate certifying examinations where high levels of reliability are demanded.

There are several key points we wish to make. First, it is hard to imagine a credible assessment of clinical competence which does not attempt to evaluate clinical reasoning skills. An assessment using less-than-perfect instruments is preferable to no assessment of this component at all. This is an issue of validity which must apply to the whole assessment procedure.

A second compelling argument against discarding our imperfect instruments is the very direct and powerful relationship between assessment and student learning. Academic success is largely defined by examination performance and academic success is what students are seeking. Thus, students will devote much of their energy to identifying and studying what they believe will be in their examination (van der Vleuten & Schuwirth 2005). This impact of examinations on student learning will often be greater than that of the training programme and is sometimes referred to as *consequential validity* (Messick 1995). Such effects must be seen as inevitable, if not desirable. The only answer is to ensure a good match, at least in students' minds, between the assessment procedures and the expected outcomes of the course. Failure to do so may have serious consequences. The bottom line is that a choice for a particular method may be motivated because of its (expected) education effect. For example, in a recent presentation on the assessment programme of a PBL school, the use of the somewhat older modified essay questions was maintained even at the cost of substantial resources because of the beneficial effect on the assessment of the learning of students (Prideaux 2006).

Finally, as this chapter makes clear, many ways to assess clinical reasoning are available and some are quite ingenious and creative. If no single measure is *the* measure, the choice is really yours. Which method appeals to you or your institution? How much effort do you wish to invest in writing simple or more complex stimulus formats? How many resources would you like to spend on the response format? What sort of reliability is required in your setting? What kind of impact do you strive for? What affinity or convention exists in your situation in relation to clinical reasoning assessment? Answers to these questions may vary considerably across different education contexts. A deliberate and motivated choice among the many possibilities that the literature now has to offer is on your agenda. The simpler your selected approach, the more you can rely on existing technologies and procedures and the less you will need to invest in unique solutions.

References

Bransford J, Sherwood R, Vye N et al 1986 Teaching thinking and problem solving: research foundations. American Psychologist 41:1078–1089

Brooks L R, Norman G R, Allen S W 1991 Role of specific similarity in a medical diagnostic task. Journal of Experimental Psychology: General 120(3): 278–287

Case S M, Swanson D B 1993 Extended-matching items: a practical alternative to free response questions. Teaching and Learning in Medicine 5:107–115

Case S M, Swanson D B 2002 Constructing written test questions for the basic and clinical sciences. National Board of Medical Examiners, Philadelphia

Case S M, Swanson D B, Stillman P S 1988 Evaluating diagnostic pattern recognition: the psychometric characteristics of a new item format. Paper presented at 27th Conference on Research in Medical Education, Washington DC

Case S M, Swanson D B, Ripkey D R 1994 Comparison of items in five-option and extended-matching formats for assessment of diagnostic skills. Academic Medicine 69: S1–S3

Charlin B, van der Vleuten C 2004 Standardized assessment of reasoning in contexts of uncertainty: the Script Concordance approach. Evaluation and the Health Professions 27:304–319

Charlin B, Roy L, Brailovsky C et al 2000 The script concordance test: a tool to assess the reflective clinician. Teaching and Learning in Medicine 12:189–195

De Bruin A B, Schmidt H G, Rikers R M 2005 The role of basic science knowledge and clinical knowledge in diagnostic reasoning: a structural equation modeling approach. Academic Medicine 80:765–773

Elstein A S, Shulman L S, Sprafka S A 1978 Medical problem solving: an analysis of clinical reasoning. Harvard University Press, Cambridge, MA

Eva K W 2005 What every teacher needs to know about clinical reasoning. Medical Education 39(1):98–106

Farmer E A, Page G 2005 A practical guide to assessing clinical decision-making using the key features approach. Medical Education 39:1188–1194

Feletti G, Engel C 1980 The modified essay question for testing problem-solving skills. Medical Journal of Australia 1:79–80

Feltovich P J, Barrows H S 1984 Issues of generality in medical problem solving. In: Schmidt H G, De Volder M L (eds) Tutorials in problem-based learning: a new direction in teaching the health professions. Van Gorcum, Assen, p 128–142

Fischer M R, Kopp V, Holzer M et al 2005 A modified electronic key feature examination for undergraduate medical students: validation threats and opportunities. Medical Teacher 27:450–455

Groves M, Scott I, Alexander H 2002 Assessing clinical reasoning: a method to monitor its development in a PBL curriculum. Medical Teacher 24(5):507–515

Hatala R, Norman G R 1999 Influence of a single example upon subsequent electrocardiogram interpretation. Teaching and Learning in Medicine 11:110–117

Hatala R, Norman G R 2002 Adapting the key features examination for a clinical clerkship. Medical Education 36:160–165

Mcguire C H, Babbott D 1967 Simulation technique in the measurement of problem-solving skills. Journal of Educational Measurement 4:1–10

Messick S 1995 The interplay of evidence and consequences in the validation of performance assessments. Educational Researcher 23:13–23

Neufeld V R, Norman G R (eds) 1985 Assessing clinical competence. Springer, New York

Neufeld V R, Norman G R, Feightner J W et al 1981 Clinical problem-solving by medical students: a cross-sectional and longitudinal analysis. Medical Education 15(5): 315–322

Neville A J, Cunnington J, Norman G 1996 Development of clinical reasoning exercises in a problem-based curriculum. Academic Medicine 71:S105–S107

Norcini J J, Swanson D B, Grosso L J et al 1985 Reliability, validity and efficiency of multiple choice question and patient management problem item formats in assessment of clinical competence. Medical Education 19:238–247

Norman G R 1985 Objective measurement of clinical performance. Medical Education 19:43–47

Norman G 2005 Research in clinical reasoning: past history and current trends. Medical Education 39:418–427

Norman G, Tugwell P, Feightner J et al 1985 Knowledge and clinical problem-solving. Medical Education 19:344–356

Norman G R, Brooks L R, Allen S W 1989 Recall by experts and novices as a record of processing attention. Journal of Experimental Psychology: Learning, Memory and Cognition 5:1166–1174

Norman G, Allery L, Berkson I et al 1992 Research in the psychology of clinical reasoning: implications for assessment. Cambridge Conference IV. Cambridge, Office of the Regius Professor, Cambridge University

Norman G, Swanson D, Case S 1996 Conceptual and methodology issues in studies comparing assessment formats: issues in comparing item formats. Teaching and Learning in Medicine 8:208–216

Norman G, Bordage G, Page G et al 2006 How specific is case specificity? Medical Education 40(7):618–623

Page G, Bordage G 1995 The Medical Council of Canada's key features project: a more valid written examination of clinical decision-making skills. Academic Medicine 70:104–110

Page G, Bordage G, Harasym P et al 1990 A new approach to assessing clinical problem-solving skills by written examination: conceptual basis and initial pilot test results. In: Bender W, Hiemstra R J, Scherpbier A et al (eds) Teaching and assessing clinical competence. Groningen, Boekwerk Publications, Groningen, The Netherlands, p 403–407

Petrusa E R 2002 Clinical performance assessments. In: Norman G R, van der Vleuten C P M, Newble D I (eds) International handbook for research in medical education. Kluwer Academic Publisher, Dordrecht, p 673–709

Prideaux D 2006 Constructed response items: MEQs & SAQs. IDEAL Train the Trainer Assessment Workshop. Muscat, Sultanate of Oman

Regehr G, Norman G R 1996 Issues in cognitive psychology: implications for professional education. Academic Medicine 71(9):988–1000

Schmidt H, Norman G, Boshuizen H 1990 A cognitive perspective on medical expertise: theory and implications. Academic Medicine 65:611–622

Schuwirth L W T, van der Vleuten C P M, Donkers H H L M 1995 Computerized long-menu questions, an acceptable un-cue-version. In: Rothman A I, Cohen R (eds) The sixth Ottawa Conference on Medical Education. University of Toronto Bookstore Custom Publishing, Toronto, p 178–181

Schuwirth L W T, van der Vleuten C P M, Donkers H H L M 1996a A closer look at cueing effects in multiple-choice questions. Medical Education 30:50–55

Schuwirth L W T, van der Vleuten C P M, De Kock C A et al 1996b Computerized case-based testing: a modern method to assess clinical decision making. Medical Teacher 18:295–300

Schuwirth L W T, Blackmore D E, Mom E et al 1999 How to write short cases for assessing problem-solving skills. Medical Teacher 21:144–150

Schuwirth L W, Verheggen M M, van der Vleuten C P et al 2001 Do short cases elicit different thinking processes than factual knowledge questions do? Medical Education 35:348–356

Skakun E N, Maguire T O, Cook D A 1994 Strategy choices in multiple-choice items. Academic Medicine 69: S7–S9

Swanson D B, Norcini J J, Grosso L J 1987 Assessment of clinical competence: written and computer-based simulations. Assessment and Evaluation in Higher Education 12:220–246

Swanson D B, Holtzman K A, Albee K et al 2005 Psychometric characteristics and response times for content-parallel extended-matching and one-best-answer items in relation to number of options. Academic Medicine 81(10 Suppl):S52–S55

Turnbull J, Van Barneveld C 2002 Assessment of clinical performance: in-training evaluation. In: Norman G R, van der Vleuten C P M, Newble D I (eds) International handbook of research in medical education. Dordrecht, Kluwer Academic Publishers, p 793–810

van der Vleuten C P M, Dolmans D H J M, Scherpbier A J J A 2000 The need for evidence in education. Medical Teacher 22:246–250

van der Vleuten C P M, Schuwirth L W T 2005 Assessment of professional competence: from methods to programmes. Medical Education 39:309–317

Wood T, Cunnington J, Norman G 2000 Assessing the measurement properties of a clinical reasoning exercise. Teaching and Learning in Medicine 12:196–200

Chapter 40

Using simulated patients to teach clinical reasoning

Helen Edwards and Miranda Rose

CHAPTER CONTENTS

In this chapter we describe how and why we have used simulated patients to teach clinical reasoning. We focus on the reality for teachers and for students of using simulated patients, and on the processes required to make a simulated patient programme work.

Simulated patients were introduced into the medical education literature in a detailed format by Barrows (1971). For Barrows, a simulated patient is a healthy person who has been trained to portray the historical, physical and emotional features of an actual patient. Simulated patients are based on actual case histories, not an amalgam or 'ideal' case developed for teaching or assessment purposes. Lay people, often with prior theatrical experience, are trained to portray all aspects of a real case. After training, the simulated patients are checked for accuracy by an experienced clinician before being used with students. Once trained, simulated patients are used in a structured way in student education, most commonly as a bridge into working in clinics, or in assessment.

Simulated patients have been used in a range of healthcare professions to teach and assess a wide variety of clinical skills – interviewing and counselling, data gathering, performing physical examinations, conducting psychosocial assessments and developing skills in clinical reasoning and decision making. The American Medical Association reported in 2001 that simulated/standardized patients were used in instruction in US medical schools for history taking (106 schools), doctor–patient communication (104), general physical examination skills (93) and specialized physical exams (e.g. gynaecological) (114) (Williams et al 2001). Other examples worldwide include assessing Finnish general practitioners' abilities to conduct first contraception consultations (Peremans et al 2005); educating American medical students to recognize biopsychosocial issues (e.g. family violence) during patient interviews (Elman et al 2004); teaching communication skills to British undergraduate medical students (Rees et al 2004); assessing the professional performance of Scottish community pharmacists (Watson et al 2004); and developing the cultural competence of medical students working with French speaking minority groups in Canada (Drouin & Rivet 2003).

In developing our simulated patient programme we adhered closely to the Barrows model. Other users have modified the original concept, often altering the case, training or presentation to suit their philosophy or circumstances. Recently, excellent innovations with simulated patients have emerged. Kneebone et al (2005) described a successful quasi-clinical education experience for medical students whereby invasive clinical procedures (e.g. insertion of a catheter) were rehearsed with a simulated patient (for the communication and interpersonal skills component) who had an inanimate model attached (for the technical/motor skill component).

REASONS FOR USING SIMULATED PATIENTS

The use of simulated patients has been supported in the literature over many years. Gordon et al (1988) reported that experienced clinicians could not differentiate between real and simulated patients during history taking or physical examination. Students relate well to simulated patients (Sanson-Fisher & Poole 1980). Reporting on a comprehensive assessment programme at Southern Illinois School of Medicine, Vu et al (1992) concluded that the use of simulated patients increased the feasibility, validity, reliability and utility of performance based examinations. Ainsworth et al (1991) used simulated patients in all years of the medical course at the University of Texas for teaching and assessment, in introduction to patient

evaluation, history taking and physical examination skills, integrating clinical skills, clinical clerkship, demonstration of competence, senior assessment and during the postgraduate medicine residency. Wallace et al (2002) focused on use of simulated patients in objective structured clinical examinations and psychiatry. Although papers such as these convince us of the value of simulated patients, it needs to be emphasized that simulated patients are not a replacement for real patients. Rather, simulated patients are an educational tool used to develop and refine students' clinical skills, as they progress to becoming competent practising clinicians.

The most important reason for teachers to use simulated patients is to manage and control aspects of the clinical learning environment, including programming, level of content, environment, ethics and safety, economy and reproducibility. The process of 'time out' and feedback from the simulated patients improves the educational experience for students. Enormous pressure is placed on university programmes to ensure their students meet high preclinical standards (Rose 2005) in the face of reduction in the number of clinical education opportunities for students and the stress of the clinical education role and workplace. Our rationales for developing a simulated patients programme were to better prepare students for clinical settings and to reduce the variability and lack of control in clinical teaching.

MANIPULATING PROGRAMMES AND CONTENT

Using simulated patients enables teachers to programme student/patient interactions to suit the curriculum. Teachers can select a particular case, nominate the time to study that case, and be reasonably assured that the interaction will actually occur at the scheduled time and with the designated case. The teacher can predetermine the level of clinical reasoning involved in the learning activity. In real clinics, plans are frequently disrupted by reality (for example, the patient has disappeared to the X-ray department!). Using simulated patients results in efficient and effective use of teachers' and students' time.

Teachers using simulated patients can be specific about the type of encounter offered to students. This is achieved by manipulating the type and complexity of disorder to be studied, the level of interpersonal and reasoning skill required for a successful interaction, the complexity of the therapeutic/assessment task, the duration of the encounter, and whether the student deals with a part of or the whole of a treatment or assessment session. Novice students can be given a theoretically less complex disorder in their early encounters with clinical reasoning, in order to build confidence. Teachers can match levels of theory acquisition to practice. Rehearsal of specific skills such as interviewing can be achieved without overwhelming students by the complexity of patients' disorders. Teachers may wish to specifically challenge students' interpersonal skills, for example offering them an encounter that will test their ability to keep a patient motivated.

Using simulated patients allows teachers to be prescriptive and to use educational theory to select an encounter that best suits the students' learning needs. Such prescription is in stark contrast to real clinical situations where learning is often haphazard. By manipulating variables, clinical reasoning can be taught in appropriately small chunks, at a pace that matches students' learning and level of experience. Students are still expected to cope with and adapt to the unexpected and to be flexible in the clinical setting, but with simulated patients the teacher can control when and how students have to be flexible.

MANIPULATING THE ENVIRONMENT

Simulated encounters allow control over the type of environment in which clinical encounters take place. Thus at certain times teachers may wish students to have to deal with noisy, distracting or threatening environments, while at other times teachers may create an environment as conducive as possible to a successful encounter. Teachers can set up hospital-like environments, outpatient clinics, home based situations and so on, to best meet the learning goal. By comparison, in the real clinical setting, teachers must deal with whatever happens to be present.

SIMULATED PATIENTS IN ACTION

ETHICS AND SAFETY, ECONOMY AND REPRODUCIBILITY

The use of simulated patients simplifies some aspects of ethics and safety in clinical practice. Since simulated patients do not really have the conditions for which they are being assessed or treated, they can be used for long sessions or exposed to many repetitions of the same procedure, neither of which would be ethical or practical with real patients. It is possible to have a number of students working with one simulated patient, an economic use of time that may reduce expenditure. Teachers can have greater confidence that every student working with a particular simulated patient is receiving the same kind of clinical experience. Simulated patients are trained to accurately reproduce their symptoms, case histories and psychosocial backgrounds across different encounters. They are therefore predictable and consistent over time. Real patients are far from this!

TIME OUT

Using time out in working with simulated patients is of great benefit when teaching clinical reasoning. Students or teachers can call 'time out' at any point during an encounter with a simulated patient, to break from the interaction and seek assistance/feedback/reassurance from peers or the facilitator. During time out the simulated patient freezes, staying in role but not interacting with the student until 'time in' is called. At that point the encounter resumes as though there had been no break in the interaction. Time out is used for discussion, group input, problem solving and reviewing performance. Students are often able to reason creatively about the current situation, resume with new strategies and then complete a more successful encounter, thereby increasing their confidence.

Students can also trial various interventions, call time out, receive some feedback or have time to reflect, and then try again with a different approach. Time out is a rich opportunity for developing clinical reasoning. Details are fresh in students' minds, there is space to reflect and there is the opportunity to resume immediately and try again, rather than having to wait until the next real patient encounter (and perhaps develop some performance or anticipation anxiety in the meantime).

FEEDBACK FROM PATIENTS

At the completion of the encounter, simulated patients can 'de-role' and return as themselves, to give feedback to students on any aspect of the encounter. Students are encouraged to seek specific feedback about their performance, making use of the rich opportunity to develop their clinical reasoning. As issues about the encounter arise, the facilitator or other students may refer to examples from clinical work or theory to assist a student in devising a maximally effective encounter.

EDUCATIONAL FOCUS

The focus in using simulated patients is educational. This contrasts with the mix of education and service delivery that occurs with real patients. In an encounter with a simulated patient students can be encouraged to try different approaches. Students can make mistakes and learn from them without endangering the patient. There are few opportunities for students to experiment in the real clinic, and yet this can be an important learning process for students. It helps students to develop deep approaches to learning and to discover their individual style of working, rather than simply adopting that of their clinical teachers.

A SIMULATED PATIENT IN USE: EXAMPLE 1

When speech pathology students first attempt to diagnose a communication disorder of neurological origin they have to observe and process an enormous amount of information about their clients. In a teaching/learning session it is helpful to be able to present just a part of the overall neurological problem, so that the amount of information to be processed is reduced and students can begin to see some patterns.

The simulated patient

The simulated patient is a 36-year-old unemployed mother of two, on a single parent pension. She sustained a cerebrovascular accident some 3 months ago and a diagnostic CT scan revealed a large area of decreased attenuation in her left frontoparietal region. She presents with a dense right upper limb-hemiparesis and resolving Broca's type aphasia. She is currently an inpatient in a fast-stream rehabilitation centre.

The students and the learning task

Twenty speech pathology students in the third year of their 4-year undergraduate programme are completing their theoretical studies of neurological disorders and are about to enter an off-campus clinical placement in this area. The students' task is accurately to diagnose the communication disorder of the simulated patient using a series of tests, while maintaining rapport and attending to any patient queries.

The teaching session

In a teaching room with a one-way screen, each group of students engages with the simulated patient in turn, endeavouring to perform the required tests. They or the teacher can call time out and leave the room to discuss the situation with the teacher on the other side of the screen. Students in the first group have difficulty obtaining a sample of the patient's speech. During time out a student asks: 'She seems so depressed, I can't get her to talk. What should I do?' The group discusses the need to deal with the patient's emotional problem first and then move on to the speech test. This proves to be an effective strategy.

In comparison, until the patient breaks down crying, the second group does not recognize that she is distressed by failing to complete their test. They need guidance during time out, to break down the task into more manageable parts. During debriefing the patient de-roles and gives this group feedback on how it felt to be assessed, to fail, to not understand the purpose of the testing, and to have deficits so plainly demonstrated. She also gives reinforcement to the students about their interaction styles, their obvious concern for her well-being and their empathy. The students talk about optimal ways of indicating errors in client responses without making clients feel inadequate, and their difficulty in continuing testing when clients are failing. They ask questions about how they could have worded things so that the patient could understand what they were doing.

HOW THIS EXAMPLE FACILITATED CLINICAL REASONING

This example illustrates the richness in learning to be derived from using simulated patients in teaching clinical reasoning. Working with a simulated patient was a powerful way for the students to become aware of and learn to critique their own reasoning. Students could test different approaches or ideas with the simulated patient, receive feedback from their peers and the teacher, and then correct or retrial their approach.

A SIMULATED PATIENT IN USE: EXAMPLE 2

This example focuses on clinical reasoning during history taking with nurses. History taking is central to effective diagnosis and clinical management of clients. Clinicians rely on effective reasoning and decision making during history taking to guide the process, to test the reliability of the data collected and to pay attention to the needs of the client (for example, arranging a break if the process becomes distressing).

Students need to learn how to reason during client interactions and how to make use of the information they obtain for diagnostic and management decisions. Students often experience anxiety when confronted with planning and implementing client interactions in the clinical setting. The aim of the exercise described here is to prepare year 1 nursing students for history taking through practice with simulated patients. It occurs one week before the students' first clinical fieldwork experience.

The exercise allows students to practise history taking and reasoning with simulated patients without a patient suffering any consequences from student mistakes. Further, feedback from the simulated patient, teacher and peers helps develop students' data collection and reasoning abilities. The specific task is for students in small groups to take the patient's history and to explore the reasons behind timing and technique in collecting patient information of an intimate nature.

ORGANIZING THE LEARNING ACTIVITY

To enable 250 students to participate, four simulated patients are used over a 2 day period. The case studies provide a mix of common client scenarios, each combined with a variety of social problems. They include depression, cerebrovascular accident, head injury and arthritis. One teacher is assigned to two simulated patients to introduce the students, monitor the interaction and call time out where appropriate. Students, divided into groups of four, are allocated 20 minutes to conduct the interviews. To help students develop an appreciation of the variety of emotional responses they might experience and the variety of decisions they might need to make during initial interactions with patients, they are not told that the patients are simulated. They believe that a number of patients with a variety of chronic illnesses have agreed to interviews with the students. During the interviews students are asked to assess the patient's reactions to the level of information (general and intimate) obtained, and to document their reasons for the time and techniques they have selected to elicit intimate information. Students document these findings in a journal, together with their feelings.

The majority of students are obviously nervous when entering the interaction. Some repeat in intricate detail the verbal patient description that has been provided by the teacher immediately prior to the interaction. Others seek reassurance that the teacher would be close by if required. The students are introduced to the patients and the interactions begin.

The power of the simulated patients to generate the emotions commonly experienced during nurse–client interactions is continually evident. Helen, rehabilitating from a closed head injury with adynamic affect, proves to be the most difficult for the students. Helen's lack of nonverbal feedback increases the students' unease. There are long periods of silence accompanied by nervous glances between students and teachers. The prolonged periods of silence not only cause unease for the students, but we are tempted to interject to help the conversation from time to time. It requires a constant effort to remind myself that the focus for this is experiential learning and that the confusion and unease the students experience are necessary motivators to encourage them to explore their reasoning, feelings and behaviour. Many of the students assigned to Helen are unable to elicit more than basic information. Other simulated patients exhibiting 'normal' responses help the students feel more at ease. Students elicit more useful data and a greater amount of intimate information from conversations with these patients. In fact, so personal is the information given by Sheila, a woman caring for her sick husband at home, as well as running the family business, that it brings a tear to some students' eyes. Another group of students are convinced that they can actually see the knee swelling described by Patsy (another simulator), even though the knee is normal.

Once it is obvious that a lull has developed in the conversation with a patient, usually about 20 minutes into the exercise, time out is called and the patient is asked to de-role. This event is, for me, the most dramatic. Some students begin to laugh, stating that they feel like they were on 'Candid Camera'. Others become angry, saying that they feel cheated. One student says that she feels she can no longer trust me and that she will not be able to be sure that patients she encounters in her clinical rotation are real. Fortunately the angry students are in the minority, with most students experiencing relief that the patients are simulated.

The sense of relief following the disclosure provides a comfortable platform for the students to discuss their performance and reasoning. Students who have gathered little intimate information relate that they had difficulty deciding when to seek this information because of the absence of appropriate cues. The simulator and teacher help the students explore other possible indicators and techniques for gathering this information. Students who have been more successful can describe the reasons for their timing and use of techniques for data collection. Client cues,

student comfort level, age and sex of the client and severity of the presenting symptoms are commonly identified by this group as factors contributing to their successful reasoning and performance.

The students' written feedback is used to expand upon the feedback discussions. The majority of students are able to identify key elements to be considered when deciding when and how to explore client information of a more personal nature. Students also discuss how they performed in relation to these elements, and how they could make improvements. Some students state that they had not recognized the complexity of this type of clinical decision until completing and analysing the simulated patient session. This observation provides an insight into an important advantage of the use of simulated patients over actual clinical practice: simulated learning experiences more frequently and more readily promote reflection on learning experiences. Such reflection encourages students to turn their experiences into learning.

In this exercise, students' feelings also become the focus for reflection. Students identify a sense of empathy with their patients and compassion for them, even after they have learned that the patients are simulators. The anxiety witnessed by the monitoring teachers is also mentioned in the students' journals. Many question their ability to carry out the interaction prior to the exercise, but later report that they feel more comfortable about performing this task in the future.

EVALUATION

The aim of enabling students to develop their clinical reasoning and interaction skills with patients, buffered by the security of simulation, was met in this exercise. All students stated that they found the exercise to be of benefit, including students who had felt angered by the deception. The interaction provided the vehicle and motivation for students to analyse their clinical reasoning and interactions, and it provided some positive feedback about their existing skills. Journal entries from students' later clinical rotations demonstrated an increased awareness of their own and their colleagues' clinical reasoning and interpersonal behaviour. The client histories collected by the students also demonstrated that desirable learning had occurred, including students' enhanced ability to decide when and how to elicit relevant information.

With the benefits of hindsight we would have informed the students that the patients were simulated. The literature recommends this, asserting that once the interaction begins the student forgets that the patient is simulated. This was advice that we chose to ignore, believing that the experience would be more meaningful and effective if the students thought the patients were real. The anger expressed by some students indicated that this course of action could be detrimental. In fact, the assertion that simulation is forgotten was supported during this exercise. Even though some students had been told by their peers that the patients were simulators, it made little difference to the outcome. One student, for instance, stated in her journal, 'I felt silly at first because she wasn't a real patient, but after a while I forgot as she was very believable'.

Apart from its learning value, this exercise demonstrates how simulated patients can be used in a cost-effective manner with large groups of students. Students were able to explore their reasoning and behaviour in a secure environment and were better prepared for the demands of the real clinical world.

MAKING SIMULATED PATIENTS WORK FOR YOU

The decision to incorporate simulated patients in a teaching programme entails commitment at a number of levels. Our experience suggests that four areas are particularly crucial to successful use of simulated patients: teacher approach, quality control, financial arrangements and organizational commitment.

TEACHER APPROACH

Teachers must be committed to using simulated patients properly. Simulated patients are not like a book that can be borrowed just when needed. They need to be looked after and treated respectfully and

humanely, with consideration for the arduousness of their role. In a recent study, potential burnout and stress of simulated patients was investigated. Results suggested that simulated patients experience stress during role plays of certain symptoms and behaviours. The research underlined the need for careful simulated patient debriefing with experienced teaching staff following simulator sessions (Bokken et al 2004). Such debriefing time requires careful scheduling to fit with teaching commitments.

Teachers must be clear about how they wish to use a simulated patient in their teaching, and what is appropriate training and debriefing for such a teaching session. Students also need to be adequately prepared, to act in an appropriate manner and to take the teaching session seriously. Our experience is that students quickly forget the artificial nature of the encounter and participate in a 'real' way with the simulated patients. Thus, encounters are frequently emotionally evocative for students and simulators and require sensitive facilitation.

QUALITY CONTROL

Simulated patients are used with students at different year levels in a number of courses and settings. A system of quality control is necessary to ensure that simulated patients are trained and used appropriately, and in particular that they perform consistently across time and across different situations. Our quality control strategies include careful selection of the people to become simulators, detailed consideration of possible cases for simulation, systematic training involving a clinician, checking sessions with 'outsiders' as part of training, a user's manual for teachers, feedback sheets from teachers after each session, debriefing between teachers in meetings, and an annual meeting between all teaching staff and simulators.

Researchers at Maastricht University have reported on the development and trial of a simulated patient performance assessment tool (Wind et al 2004). The Maastricht Assessment of Simulated Patients was shown to have good internal validity and reasonable reliability and may be of use in monitoring the quality of simulator performances.

FINANCIAL ARRANGEMENTS

Using simulated patients is a labour intensive and expensive operation. We use a casual employee tutor pay scale for our simulators, and pay for training at the same rate as actual simulation. Other organizations use different pay rates depending how simulated patients are used (e.g. prolonged sessions, giving extensive feedback, particularly taxing roles or undergoing invasive procedures). It is necessary to budget for the use of simulated patients, and although it may be cheaper than operating in the real clinic there can be resistance to adding another expense to the teaching curriculum.

ORGANIZATIONAL COMMITMENT

The final prerequisite for successful implementation is organizational commitment. The infrastructure required to run a successful simulated patients programme is more than an individual or even a small group of staff can expect to provide successfully. A successful simulated patients programme depends on having a bank of appropriately trained simulators. This requires deciding on cases to be simulated, recruiting and training patients, and organizing and monitoring their use. We have found it best to designate one person as the central coordinator of the programme, who can interact with individual simulators throughout their recruitment, training and use. Ker et al (2005) have emphasized the need for appropriate training and care of simulated patients.

CONCLUSION

Using simulated patients to teach clinical reasoning is a particularly rich and flexible teaching approach that allows students to develop skills in a safe, structured environment. Teachers can use simulated patients to help students become aware of how they behave in interacting with clients and how and why they make clinical decisions, and to provide students with a positive view of their capacity for creative clinical reasoning. These skills can be directly transferred into the real clinical setting.

Acknowledgement

The authors acknowledge the contribution of Bill McGuiness to this work. Bill was a co-author in previous versions of this chapter. Work commitments prevented his involvement in this third edition.

References

Ainsworth M, Rogers L, Markus J et al 1991 Standardized patient encounters: a method for teaching and evaluation. Journal of the American Medical Association 266:1390–1396

Barrows H S 1971 The simulated patient. Charles Thomas, Springfield, IL

Bokken L, van Dalen J, Rethans J 2004 Performance-related stress symptoms in simulated patients. Medical Education 38(10):1089–1094

Drouin J, Rivet C 2003 Training medical students to communicate with a linguistic minority group. Academic Medicine 78(6):599–604

Elman D, Hooks R, Tabak D et al 2004 The effectiveness of unannounced standardised patients in the clinical setting as a teaching intervention. Medical Education 38(9):969–973

Gordon J, Sanson-Fisher R, Saunders N 1988 Identification of simulated patients by interns in a casualty setting. Medical Education 22(6):533–538

Ker J, Dowie A, Dowell J et al 2005 Twelve tips for developing and maintaining a simulated patients bank. Medical Teacher 27(1):4–9

Kneebone R, Kidd J, Nestel D et al 2005 Blurring the boundaries: scenario-based simulation in a clinical setting. Medical Education 39(6):580–587

Peremans L, Rethans J, Verhoeven V et al 2005 Adolescents demanding a good contraceptive: a study with standardised patients in general practices. Contraception 71(6):421–425

Rees C, Sheard C, McPherson A 2004 Medical students' views and experiences of methods of teaching and learning communication skills. Patient Education and Counseling 54(1):119–121

Rose M 2005 The cycle of crisis in clinical education: why national-level strategies must be prioritised. Advances in Speech-Language Pathology 7(3):158–161

Sanson-Fisher R W, Poole A D 1980 Simulated patients and the assessment of medical students' interpersonal skills. Medical Education 14(4):249–253

Vu N V, Barrows H, Marcy M L et al 1992 Six years of comprehensive, clinical, performance-based assessment using standardized patients at the Southern Illinois University School of Medicine. Academic Medicine 67(1):42–50

Wallace J, Ranga R, Haslam R 2002 Simulated patients and objective structured clinical examinations: review of their use in medical education. Advances in Psychiatric Treatment 8:342–348

Watson M, Skelton J, Bond C et al 2004 Simulated patients in the community pharmacy setting: using simulated patients to measure practice in the community pharmacy setting. Pharmacy World and Science 26(1):32–37

Williams R, Makoul G, Hawkins R et al 2001 Standardized/simulated patients in medical education. Available http://www.ama-assn.org/ama/pub/category/5373.html 18 Nov 2005

Wind L, van Dalen J, Muijtens A et al 2004 Assessing simulated patients in an educational setting: the MASP (Maastricht Assessment of Simulated Patients). Medical Education 38(1):39–44

Chapter 41

Peer coaching to generate clinical reasoning skills

Richard Ladyshewsky and Mark A. Jones

Novice health professionals who lack clinical experience are challenged to a greater degree than experienced clinicians when faced with the task of clinical reasoning. These novices commonly have a reduced ability to judge the relevance and importance of clinical tasks, especially when contrasted to expert performance (Edwards et al 2004, Jensen et al 2000, Oldmeadow 1996). Novices also tend to make errors in the process of reasoning when attempting to make clinical decisions because of their reliance on hypothetico-deductive reasoning processes (Edwards et al 2004, Jensen et al 2000). This stems from a knowledge base that is being restructured, moving from a predominance of biomedical knowledge to more clinically meaningful patterns (Boshuizen & Schmidt 1995, Carnevali 1995). Boshuizen & Schmidt termed this tendency to make frequent errors an intermediate effect.

The education of novices needs to address the development of their clinical reasoning abilities, including consideration of multiple determinants of health (Jones et al 2000, WHO 2001). They need to value diverse sources of information from the available research evidence as well as the patient's knowledge and views on health and illness. This information is used to develop their professional craft knowledge and skills such as manual handling and communication to facilitate diagnosis and treatment. For continued growth as health professionals they need to value and develop capability in critical reflection (Jensen et al 2000, Schön 1991). In this chapter we discuss the use of peer-centred learning as a method to facilitate the development of clinical reasoning in novice practitioners.

LEARNING FROM PEERS

Learning from peers is sometimes referred to as cooperative learning. Cooperative learning, however, is a broad educational strategy that encapsulates many forms of peer-centred learning. For example, Johnson & Johnson (1978, 1987) and Johnson et al (1981) used the term 'cooperative learning' to describe principles of group learning; that is, learning that is enhanced by group interdependence and individual accountability.

The literature on peer learning and the definitions that emanate from this work are abundant. Gerace & Sibilano (1984), for example, defined peer teaching as collaboration between two people of equal rank working together to solve a problem. Lincoln & McAllister (1993) examined the concept of peer learning in detail and raised an important differentiation between process and procedure. Peer learning is the process, and is related to the outcomes of the collaborative learning experience. In contrast, peer tutoring, peer teaching, peer review and peer evaluation are specific procedures that allow peer learning to occur. The procedure discussed in this chapter to describe the peer learning experience is *peer coaching* (Ladyshewsky 2000). It is an educational procedure in which peers coach one another through clinical experiences using demonstration, observation, collaborative practice, feedback/discussion and problem solving.

MODES OF LEARNING AND PEER COACHING (PC)

EXPERIENCE–BASED LEARNING

Clinical experience is a significant part of novice practitioners' learning. Clinical experiences are used to restructure biomedical knowledge into more meaningful clinical patterns, which ultimately guide practice (Boshuizen & Schmidt 1995, Carnevali 1995). For example, clinical patterns attended to by physiotherapists comprise more than biomedical diagnostic information. Therapists, as a result of their clinical experience, also develop and revise clinical patterns relating to physical, environmental and biopsychosocial factors. These factors all contribute to the development and understanding of patients' problems, and thus are integrated into clinical patterns of management strategies, clinical patterns for recognizing safety precautions and contraindications, and clinical patterns related to judging prognoses.

The importance of experiential learning for the cognitive structures of learners has been described by numerous authors (e.g. Barker-Schwartz 1991, Boud 1988, Brown et al 1989, Graham 1996, Higgs 2004, Kolb 1984). Boud (1993) argued that learners construct newer forms of knowledge and understanding using their previous experiences as a template. These experiences are influenced not only by the novice practitioner's underlying knowledge base, but also by the social and cultural context of the learning situation. Brown et al (1989) described learning that encompasses both physical and social contexts as 'situated' learning. Learning in these real-life situations allows concepts to evolve because the situation, and the negotiations and discussions that occur with others, recast the information into a more densely textured form (Graham 1996). That is, knowledge acquired in the context for which it will be used (i.e. clinical practice) is made more meaningful and accessible (Rumelhart & Ortony 1977, Schön 1987, Shepard & Jensen 1990).

Boud (1988, 1993) challenged educators to put more emphasis on how students learn from complex experiences. On the basis of constructivist learning theory, which states that learners construct their own unique forms of knowledge, it can be argued that more attention needs to be paid to learning from experience (Boud 1993, Brown et al 1989, Mezirow 2000). Strategically engaging the learner in the actual learning experience, therefore, is one method of enhancing learning.

Quite often during the course of a clinical education experience a novice practitioner is exposed to a wide variety of patients and problems. Hopefully, some of this experience is translated into learning and the novice practitioner's competence is improved. More often than not, however, novice practitioners do not gain as much as they could from the patient management experience, particularly if they have poor self-evaluation skills. Boud (1988) described a strategic approach to learning from experience as a series of three stages, generalizable to any learning experience.

The first stage involves returning to the experience so that the learner can recapture as many parts of it as possible. The second stage involves attending to conceptions about performance, and reflecting on the conceptions that arose during the experience. Recognizing these conceptions helps learners to understand how they influence their specific interpretations and general understanding. The third stage involves re-evaluating the experience, where the new experience is related to prior experiences and new knowledge is reorganized using a variety of cognitive and metacognitive strategies such as association, integration, validation and appropriation (Boud 1988). *Association* involves connecting ideas and feelings which are part of the original experience to existing knowledge. *Integration* involves processing these associations to see if there are patterns or linkages to other ideas. *Validation* involves testing the internal consistency of these emerging concepts in relation to existing beliefs and knowledge. And *appropriation* involves making this new knowledge an integral part of how one acts or feels.

The influence of experiential learning and the use of discussion to enhance cognitive processing are present in the theoretical perspectives of other educational theorists. Belenky and colleagues (1986) described two concepts: connected knowing and separate knowing. Although both forms of knowing are important, connected knowing is a preferred educational orientation because it includes the sharing of common experiences and discussion of the feelings that inform ideas. Separate knowing is an orientation to learning that is characterized by impersonal and objective reasoning, commonly referred to as critical thinking. Barker-Schwartz (1991) argued that learning activities involving discussion of experiences and illustration of theory in practice will promote connected knowing. This same notion is emphasized in the literature on transformative learning, where critical discourse is promoted as essential for testing the validity of one's construction of meaning (Mezirow 2000). Peer coaching, which promotes observation of theory in practice, collaborative practice, feedback/discussion and problem solving, can be used to promote this connection.

The use of PC appears to provide a rich opportunity for novice practitioners to more actively engage themselves in the learning experience. This is consistent with current conceptions of the complexity of clinical reasoning, in particular, *dialectical reasoning*. In the dialectical model, clinical reasoning has been described as a process 'that moves between those cognitive and decision-making processes required to optimally diagnose and manage patient presentations of physical disability and pain (hypothetico-deductive or instrumental reasoning and action) and those required to understand and engage with patients (narrative or communicative reasoning and action)' (Edwards et al 2004, p. 328). The development of more robust clinical knowledge and reasoning frameworks becomes possible because of the opportunities to refine and restructure knowledge in consultation with others.

LEARNER-MANAGED LEARNING: DEVELOPING LEARNING STRATEGIES, USING METACOGNITION

Bandura (1971, 1997) discussed perspectives on social learning theory, and described three kinds of reinforcement that influence learning outcomes. The first is *direct external reinforcement*. Under this form of reinforcement, people regulate their behaviour on the basis of the consequences they experience directly. The second is *vicarious reinforcement*, which occurs by observing the experiences of others and then modifying one's own behaviour based upon the consequences just observed. Thirdly, *self-administered reinforcement* involves regulating one's behaviour according to standards. The nature of PC provides rich opportunities for these three types of reinforcement to occur. For example, feedback from a peer may help novices to recognize certain consequences of their behaviour or their failure to recognize a standard of behaviour required.

In a review of adult learning theory, Mezirow (1981) discussed technical, practical and emancipatory knowledge, three forms of empirical knowledge identified by Habermas (1972). Mezirow described them as three approaches to learning, and discussed their influence on the generation of knowledge. He argued that most educational methods emphasize the first two perspectives, which focus on the provision and evaluation of knowledge and skills. Mezirow felt they ignored the emancipatory perspective. Emancipatory learning 'involves an interest in self-knowledge, that is, the knowledge of self-reflection. . . . Insights gained through critical self-awareness are emancipatory in the sense that at least one can recognize the correct reasons for his or her problems' (Mezirow 1981, p. 5). Mezirow argued that metacognition or personal awareness about knowledge enhances cognition.

Emancipatory learning can be promoted by encouraging discussion and dialogue with peers and by participating in and leading learning groups (Mezirow 1981). This helps learners to identify real problems involving power relationships, institutional ideologies that are embedded in myths and their own feelings, for example. Mezirow argued that by critiquing these psycho-cultural perspectives, alternative meaning perspectives can be created. This type of emancipatory learning is critical in clinical reasoning, particularly if one considers the importance of personal knowledge in pragmatic/ethical reasoning (Edwards et al 2005, Jones & Rivett 2004, Neistadt 1996, Schell & Cervero 1993). These forms of reasoning involve considering the moral, political and economic dilemmas in clinical practice.

The above discussion illustrates the importance of learning how to learn and the use of *metacognition*. Metacognitive skills are cognitive skills necessary for the management of knowledge and other cognitive skills (Biggs 1988). Metacognition involves being aware of one's cognitive processes and controlling them (Higgs & Titchen 1995). Skills in metacognition have been shown to enhance problem-solving and learning (Biggs 1988). Thus, academic programmes designed to enhance students' capacity to generate and acquire new knowledge and to enhance their clinical reasoning abilities need to develop students' metacognitive skills (Higgs & Jones 2000, Jones et al 2000, Lincoln & McAllister 1993, Rivett & Jones 2004, Terry & Higgs 1993, Tichenor et al 1995).

Although independent metacognition and 'reflection-in action' (Schön 1991) can be used by an individual practitioner, peers can heighten the cognitive and metacognitive experience by consciously engaging in specific discussion at each stage of the experience (Higgs & Titchen 1995, Jones 1995). Peer coaching is a particularly useful method to facilitate metacognition because of the joint problem-solving activities that take place between peers (Terry & Higgs 1993). This metacognitive activity can lead to enhanced clinical reasoning skill and greater levels of competency (Higgs & Jones 2000).

PEER COACHING IN CLINICAL EDUCATION PROGRAMMES

One of the reasons for encouraging PC in the clinical education setting is that clinical educators may not always be available to assist novice practitioners. Time pressures and workloads may make it difficult for supervisors to explore clinical reasoning in action with students. Peer coaching can relieve supervisors of some of this responsibility, particularly with more straightforward clinical problems (Goldenberg & Iwasiw 1992). Costello (1989) found that a significant amount of learning occurred between peers as part of the 'hidden' curriculum. Claims by students that they were taught most by other students, compared to instructors and ward personnel, have also been reported in the literature (Lewin & Leach 1982).

Even with good supervisor availability, novices may still not ask their superiors for support because of fear of negative appraisal. May & Newman (1980) pointed out that effective problem-solving is most likely to occur in an environment where students are free to test out their thinking skills, explore alternatives and discover approaches that may or may not match other clinicians' solutions. However, in situations where novice performance is subject to continuous evaluation, novices may be reticent to test out their thinking with their supervisors (Erickson 1987). Boud (1988) described learning partnerships as one strategy to overcome such reticence.

Fostering peer discussion in the clinical setting promotes exposure of learners' thoughts and arguments and allows discussion and restructuring of knowledge to take place (Regehr & Norman 1996). This can be facilitated by having students work with the same patient over the course of a placement and by having them see other patients with similar or dissimilar diagnoses (Cohn 1989, Grant et al 1988). The discussion that emanates from such experiences should enable students to create stronger relational structures in their knowledge base, leading to better encapsulation of their knowledge and more finely tuned clinical patterns and prototypes (Bordage & Lemieux 1986, Rivett & Jones 2004). Resnick (1988) contended that the collective problem-solving that occurs in PC leads to insights and solutions that would otherwise not occur, as it brings to light misconceptions that have been directing novice practice.

Several examples of peer-centred learning are described in the health sciences education literature. These learning strategies have been used in classrooms and in clinical settings with good results. Graham (1996), for example, conducted a qualitative study of ten physical therapy students in an entry level Master of Physical Therapy programme. One of the key themes to emerge from this study was the value of discussion. Discussion with peers was seen to be a key conceptualization strategy. Students stated that they would study course content initially, and then engage in a discussion with peers to boost their comprehension.

Iwasiw & Goldenberg (1993) studied peer learning among nursing students using a surgical dressing change procedure. They measured the cognitive and psychomotor gains of nursing students taught by peers and those taught by nursing instructors. Cognitive gains were significantly higher for the peer-taught group, and psychomotor gains, although not significant, showed greater improvement among the peer-taught group. DeClute & Ladyshewsky (1993) compared the clinical competency scores of physiotherapy students in a peer-centred learning placement to the scores of those in an individual learning placement. Clinical competency scores of the peer group were significantly higher across all performance dimensions. Ladyshewsky (2002, 2004) also found that peer coaching resulted in a more thorough clinical intervention and enhanced students' clinical reasoning performance.

Other studies in the health sciences, more descriptive in nature, report the social and affective benefits of peer-based learning (Claessen 2004, Costello 1989, DeDea 1996, Gerace & Sibilano 1984, Haffner-Zavadak et al 1995, Ladyshewsky

1993, Lincoln & McAllister 1993, Tiberius & Gaiptman 1985). Some of these additional benefits include enhanced individual effort among learners, more positive communication, greater intercollegial support, efficient use of teaching resources, a shift from extrinsic to intrinsic motivation to learn, higher educational achievement, increased opportunities for learning and greater practice using critical thinking skills.

PREPARATION FOR PEER LEARNING

Coaching skills may need to be developed by novice practitioners before engaging in a peer learning experience. Before they can capitalize on the potential benefits of PC, learners may need to develop skills in leadership, communication, trust building, decision making and conflict management, which are all important elements of both adult learning and skilled clinical reasoning (Goldenberg & Iwasiw 1992, Johnson & Johnson 1987). Students also may require assistance in determining how to work as a dyad during a shared patient experience. Ladyshewsky (2004) reported that during a shared patient encounter, students may experience role confusion that can interfere with the provision of timely feedback and support during the patient encounter. This occurs because students do not have the skills to work collaboratively and give feedback in the presence of a patient. Lincoln & McAllister (1993) added that teaching of learning theory and practice in peer learning is an essential part of preparation for peer learning. An understanding of how to optimize learning not only enhances students' ability to maximize their learning experiences and outcomes, but also equips them with valuable strategies to promote patient learning, which is an essential skill for all health professionals. Development of these cooperative learning skills in students is particularly important in health sciences students, who may be reticent to support one another because they have had to compete vigorously to enter professional schools (Lynch 1984). Sharan (1980) similarly pointed out that students accustomed to years of individual competition for grades are not likely to engage in mutual assistance automatically.

For a successful peer learning experience to take place, positive interdependence, individual accountability and group processing ability need to be present (Johnson 1981; Johnson & Johnson 1978, 1987; Ladyshewsky 2006; Slavin 1990). *Positive interdependence* means that there is a cooperative goal structure in place and learners perceive that they can attain their goals only if the other learners with whom they are linked also obtain their goals. In clinical practice, this may mean outlining specific cooperative learning objectives or delineating joint tasks. Students must also be held *accountable* for their participation; otherwise the learning outcomes of the group are compromised. Ladyshewsky & Varey (2005) described in detail an eight-stage model for peer coaching relationships that can be used to assist students in structuring the relationship. These eight stages encompass: assessment and trust building; planning (time and place); formalizing process and scope; defining purpose and goals; clarifying facts and assumptions; exploring possibilities; gaining commitment to actions; and offering support and accountability. Failure to meet the objectives within each of these eight stages compromises the overall effectiveness of the PC strategy. Lastly, learners should also explicitly be given the opportunity to engage in face-to-face *group interactions*. Otherwise, they may not actively approach their peer for support because of concerns that the instructor may interpret it as a sign of weakness.

PEER COACHING: AN EXAMPLE

Two novices are given the joint responsibility to evaluate a patient with a neuromuscular disorder.

The novices are encouraged to discuss their ideas and plans for the evaluation openly with each other, as well as to ask open-ended questions of one another such as, 'What are the reasons for doing these tests?', 'What sort of findings will result?' and 'What do they mean?'. Knowledge gaps may also be identified as part of this reciprocal coaching process. In some cases, the novices may be able to assist one another in working through a knowledge gap. In other cases, the pair may need to consult their supervisor or do additional research to bridge the knowledge gap.

CONCLUSION

Actively engaging novice practitioners in their learning is a key component of professional education, and one that needs to be reinforced in professional preparation programmes. Implementing learning models that encourage novice practitioners to learn alongside their peers can enhance the potential for increased clinical competence and reasoning. Peer learning strategies such as the PC approach described in this chapter can enrich the depth of the clinical learning experience and heighten the metacognitive aspects of novice practitioners' learning. These are important educational imperatives for developing high-level cognitive outcomes such as concept identification, analysis of problems, judgement and evaluation. The PC approach to clinical learning should be encouraged as a model of professional development for novice practitioners.

References

Bandura A 1971 Social learning theory. General Learning Press, New York

Bandura A 1997 Self efficacy: the exercise of control. W H Freeman, New York

Barker-Schwartz K 1991 Clinical reasoning and new ideas on intelligence: implications for teaching and learning. American Journal of Occupational Therapy 45 (11):1033–1037

Belenky M, Clinchy B, Goldberger N et al 1986 Women's ways of knowing: the development of self, voice, and mind. Basic Books, New York

Biggs J 1988 The role of metacognition in enhancing learning. Australian Journal of Education 32:127–138

Bordage G, Lemieux M 1986 Some cognitive characteristics of medical students with and without diagnostic reasoning difficulties. Paper presented at the 25th Annual Conference of Research in Medical Education, New Orleans

Boshuizen H, Schmidt H 1995 The development of clinical reasoning expertise. In: Higgs J, Jones M (eds) Clinical reasoning in the health professions. Butterworth-Heinemann, Oxford, p 24–32

Boud D 1988 How to help students learn from experience. In: Cox K, Ewan C (eds) The medical teacher, 2nd edn. Churchill Livingstone, London, p 68–73

Boud D 1993 Experience as the base for learning. Higher Education Research and Development 12(1):33–44

Brown J, Collins A, Duguid P 1989 Situated cognition and the culture of learning. Educational Researcher 18(1):32–42

Carnevali D L 1995 Self-monitoring of clinical reasoning behaviours: promoting professional growth. In: Higgs J, Jones M (eds) Clinical reasoning in the health professions. Butterworth-Heinemann, Oxford, p 179–190

Claessen J 2004 A 2:1 clinical practicum, incorporating reciprocal peer coaching, clinical reasoning, and self-and-peer evaluation. Journal of Speech-Language Pathology and Audiology 28(4):156–165

Cohn E 1989 Fieldwork education: shaping a foundation for clinical reasoning. American Journal of Occupational Therapy 43(4):240–244

Costello J 1989 Learning from each other: peer teaching and learning in student nurse training. Nurse Education Today 9:203–206

DeClute J, Ladyshewsky R 1993 Enhancing clinical competence using a collaborative clinical education model. Physical Therapy 73(10):683–689

DeDea L 1996 The process, design, and implementation of an alternative, collaborative approach to clinical education using the 3:1 supervisory model. Paper presented at the 12th International Congress of the World Confederation for Physical Therapy, Washington, DC

Edwards I, Jones M, Carr J et al 2004 Clinical reasoning strategies in physical therapy. Physical Therapy 84(1):312–335

Edwards I, Braunack-Mayer A, Jones M 2005 Ethical reasoning as a clinical-reasoning strategy in physiotherapy. Physiotherapy 91:229–236

Erickson G 1987 Peer evaluation as a teaching-learning strategy in baccalaureate education for community health nursing. Journal of Nursing Education 26(5):204–206

Gerace L, Sibilano H 1984 Preparing students for peer collaboration: a clinical teaching model. Journal of Nursing Education 23(5):206–209

Goldenberg D, Iwasiw C 1992 Reciprocal learning among students in the clinical area. Nurse Educator 17(5):27–29

Graham C 1996 Conceptual learning processes in physical therapy students. Physical Therapy 78(8):856–865

Grant R, Jones M, Maitland G 1988 Clinical decision making in upper quadrant dysfunction. In: Grant R (ed) Physical therapy of the cervical and thoracic spine. Churchill Livingstone, New York, p 51–80

Habermas J (trans J J Shapiro) 1972 Knowledge and human interest. Heinemann, London

Haffner-Zavadak K, Konecky-Dolnack C, Polich S et al 1995 Collaborative models. PT Magazine February, p 46(trans. J J Shapiro)54

Higgs J 2004 Educational theory and principles related to learning clinical reasoning. In: Jones M A, Rivett D A (eds) Clinical reasoning for manual therapists. Butterworth-Heinemann, Edinburgh, p 379–402

Higgs J, Jones M 2000 Clinical reasoning in the health professions. In: Higgs J, Jones M (eds) Clinical reasoning in the health professions, 2nd edn. Butterworth-Heinemann, Oxford, p 3–14

Higgs J, Titchen A 1995 Propositional, professional and personal knowledge in clinical reasoning. In: Higgs J, Jones M (eds) Clinical reasoning in the health professions. Butterworth-Heinemann, Oxford, p 129–146

Iwasiw C, Goldenberg D 1993 Peer teaching among nursing students in the clinical area: effects on student learning. Journal of Advanced Nursing 18:659–668

Jensen G M, Gwyer J, Shepard K F et al 2000 Expert practice in physical therapy. Physical Therapy 80(1):28–43

Johnson D 1981 Student-student interaction: the neglected variable in education. Educational Researcher 1:5–10

Johnson D, Johnson R 1978 Cooperative, competitive, and individualistic learning. Journal of Research and Development in Education 12(1):3–15

Johnson D, Johnson R 1987 Research shows the benefits of adult cooperation. Educational Leadership 45:27–30

Johnson D, Maruyama G, Johnson R et al 1981 Effects of cooperative, competitive, and individualistic goal structures on achievement: a meta-analysis. Psychological Bulletin 89(1):47–62

Jones M 1995 Clinical reasoning and pain. Manual Therapy 1:17–24

Jones M A, Rivett D A 2004 Introduction to clinical reasoning. In: Jones M A, Rivett D A (eds) Clinical reasoning for manual therapists. Butterworth-Heinemann, Edinburgh, p 3–24

Jones M, Jensen G, Edwards I 2000 Clinical reasoning in physiotherapy. In: Higgs J, Jones M (eds) Clinical reasoning in the health professions, 2nd edn. Butterworth-Heinemann, Oxford, p 117–127

Kolb D 1984 Experiential learning: experience as the source of learning and development. Prentice-Hall, Englewood Cliffs, NJ

Ladyshewsky R 1993 Clinical teaching and the 2:1 student-to-clinical instructor ratio. Journal of Physical Therapy Education 7(1):31–35

Ladyshewsky R 2000 Peer assisted learning in clinical education: a review of terms and learning principles. Journal of Physical Therapy Education 14(2):15–22

Ladyshewsky R 2002 A quasi-experimental study of the differences in performance and clinical reasoning using individual learning versus reciprocal peer coaching. Physiotherapy Theory and Practice 18(1):17–31

Ladyshewsky R 2004 The impact of peer coaching on the clinical reasoning of the novice practitioner. Physiotherapy Canada 56(1):15–25

Ladyshewsky R 2006 Building cooperation in peer coaching relationships: understanding the relationships between reward structure, learner preparedness, coaching skill and learner engagement. Physiotherapy 92(1):4–10

Ladyshewsky R, Varey W 2005 Peer coaching: a practical model to support constructivist learning methods in the development of managerial competency. In: Cavanagh M, Grant A, Kemp T (eds) Evidence-based coaching. Volume 1: Theory, research and practice in the behavioural sciences. Australian Academic Press, Bowen Hills, p 171–182

Lewin D, Leach J 1982 Factors influencing the quality of wards as learning environments for student nurses. International Journal of Nursing Studies 19(1):125–137

Lincoln M, McAllister L 1993 Peer learning in clinical education. Medical Teacher 15(1):17–25

Lynch B 1984 Cooperative learning in interdisciplinary education for the allied health professions. Journal of Allied Health 13(2):83–93

May B, Newman J 1980 Developing competence in problem solving. Physical Therapy 60(9):1140–1145

Mezirow J 1981 A critical theory of adult learning and education. Adult Education 31(1):3–24

Mezirow J 2000 Learning to think like an adult: core concepts of transformation theory. In: Mezirow J (ed) Learning as transformation: critical perspectives on a theory in progress. Jossey-Bass, San Francisco, p 3–33

Neistadt M 1996 Teaching strategies for the development of clinical reasoning. American Journal of Occupational Therapy 50(8):676–684

Oldmeadow L 1996 Developing clinical competence: a mastery pathway. Australian Physiotherapy Journal 42(1):37–44

Regehr G, Norman G R 1996 Issues in cognitive psychology: implications for professional education. Academic Medicine 71(9):988–1000

Resnick L 1988 Learning in school and out. Educational Researcher 16(9):13–20

Rivett D A, Jones M A 2004 Improving clinical reasoning in manual therapy. In: Jones M A, Rivett D A (eds) Clinical reasoning in manual therapy. Butterworth-Heinemann, Edinburgh, p 403–431

Rumelhart D, Ortony E 1977 The representation of knowledge in memory. In: Anderson R C, Spiro R J, Montague W E (eds) Schooling and the acquisition of knowledge. Lawrence Erlbaum, Hillsdale, p 99–135

Schell B, Cervero R 1993 Clinical reasoning in occupational therapy: an integrative review. American Journal of Occupational Therapy 47(7):605–610

Schön D 1987 Educating the reflective practitioner. Jossey-Bass, San Francisco

Schön D 1991 The reflective practitioner: how professionals think in action. Ashgate Publishing, London

Sharan S 1980 Cooperative learning in small groups. Recent methods and effects on achievement, attitudes, and ethnic relations. Review of Educational Research 50 (2):241–271

Shepard K F, Jensen G M 1990 Physical therapist curricula for the 1990s: educating the reflective practitioner. Physical Therapy 70(9):566–577

Slavin R 1990 Research on cooperative learning: consensus and controversy. Educational Leadership 47(4):52–54

Terry W, Higgs J 1993 Educational programmes to develop clinical reasoning skills. Australian Physiotherapy Journal 39(1):47–51

Tiberius R, Gaiptman B 1985 The supervisor-student ratio: 1:1 versus 1:2. Canadian Journal of Occupational Therapy 52:179–183

Tichenor C J, Davidson J, Jensen G M 1995 Cases as shared inquiry: model for clinical reasoning. Journal of Physical Therapy Education 9(2):57–62

World Health Organization 2001 ICF Checklist Version 2.1a, Clinician form for international classification of functioning, disability and health. Online Available http://www.who.int/classification/icf/checklist/icf-checklist.pdf, April 15, 2002

Chapter 42

Using open and distance learning to develop clinical reasoning skills

Janet Grant

INTRODUCTION

Health sciences education is a distributed process with students located in different sites at different times. Consistency, quality assurance and cost-effectiveness of education are of paramount importance and this presents challenges to the profession. Distance learning demonstrates its strengths in such circumstances and many would believe that this will be the next paradigm shift in health sciences education, democratizing educational provision, improving access to the resources of more advantaged schools and building transparency and accountability into the process of educational development.

WHAT IS DISTANCE LEARNING?

Health sciences education is, in practice, a distributed system. Clinical practice is central to training and so students and trainees learn wherever there are patients. And patients are distributed across the community and within hospitals. Far from wondering how distance learning can teach medicine, the more relevant question is: How can health sciences education be conducted effectively without distance learning techniques? As it is used in the UK Open University, which was the world's first distance learning university, distance learning may be defined as: individual study of specially prepared learning materials, usually print and sometimes e-learning, supplemented by integrated learning resources, other learning experiences, including face-to-face teaching and practical experience, feedback on learning and student support.

Distance learning provides a rich and planned experience for learners that is quality assured, flexible and cost-effective. Often distance learning is equated with e-learning. But it is much more, as Figure 42.1 shows.

Firstly, there is a learning management system which, these days, is usually the electronic framework in which all the other elements hang. Information technology is then called a virtual learning environment (VLE). But it could equally be a management system based on central office functions if computing power is unavailable. Within this system, students can be offered a variety of carefully planned, developed and quality assured elements (Grant 2001) which ensure curriculum coverage. Electronic (or print) elements can be:

- interactive learning resources
- library resources
- synchronous and asynchronous discussions and teaching events
- portfolios
- curriculum maps, learning records and logbooks
- formative and summative assessments
- clinical problems and clinical reasoning guides and exercises
- progress tracking through a personal curriculum map and mentor.

Face-to-face elements can include tutorials, clinical supervision, skills labs, residential and elective events and assessments. These elements require careful planning and integration but many, such as the unpublished clinical problem solving exercises which we use as the basis of current workshops, are already available in print form. Distance learning components, then, can be divided into

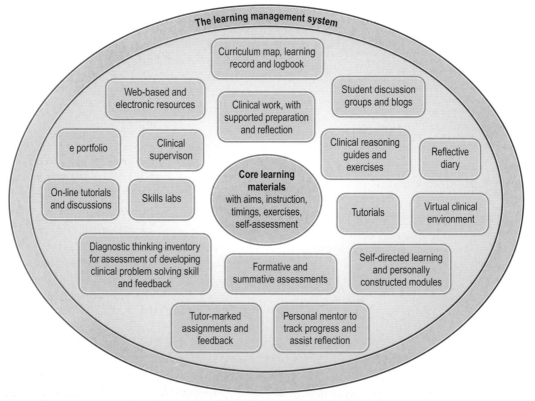

Figure 42.1   The components of a distance learning programme, organized within a learning management system

three main types, each of which has its role to play: (a) traditional paper-based approach; (b) electronic learning (e-learning); and (c) mobile learning (m-learning using, for example, hand-held computers for continuing professional development, as described by Walton et al 2005).

Specially constructed, traditional paper-based learning with learning activities is still used widely, often in conjunction with e-learning as a 'blended approach'. E-learning is able to offer:

- resource-based learning
- peer learning
- instructor- or student-led learning
- collaborative and problem-based learning.

The medium can offer a rich virtual learning environment made up of blogs (open web-log diaries) and wikis (participant-led glossaries), structured conferencing, instant messaging and e-portfolios. So e-learning is more than structured course materials. E-learning itself can also replicate the less formal interactions between students and teachers, as McConnell (2006) explains: 'students and teachers do "meet"; they meet in virtual learning environments (VLEs) through the use of computers' (p. 1).

However, although students are enthusiastic about e-learning, they also wish to retain some printed text which offers active learning, problem solving and feedback (Clarke et al 2005, Donnelly & Agius 2005, Markova et al 2005, Urquhart et al 2002). And we should not forget that there is still the concern that having learning materials exclusively on-line or reliant on computer-based software might penalize those who cannot afford or access computers, those who are in remote areas with only unreliable dial-up connections, and those who are not computer literate. But distance learning allows the use of print as well as more technology-based media, and it may well be that different modalities are equally as effective in achieving learning objectives associated with clinical reasoning (Lysaght & Bent 2005).

It is apparent that distance learning can fill gaps in community settings, allow those who have limited access to specialist teachers to study, and, with the new technological developments, may eventually become the preferred method for teaching in undergraduate, postgraduate and continuing education settings.

CAN DISTANCE LEARNING TEACH CLINICAL MEDICINE AND HEALTH SCIENCES?

Learning in the health sciences has much in common with learning in other disciplines: these professions have a base of knowledge, skills and attitudes which are combined and applied in clinical problem solving. So if distance learning can enable students to learn engineering, or biological sciences, or offer teacher training courses, as the Open University does in the UK, then surely distance learning can teach clinical medicine.

But the health professions are different from these other disciplines in some fundamental ways:

- Health sciences education involves patients and unpredictable events and opportunities for learning.
- Health sciences students are distributed across a wide range of practice locations.
- Solving clinical problems is both the main outcome of health sciences education and its main learning experience.
- Students and postgraduates learn in the real context of patient care. This requires supervision. Yet this context also means that learners must act alone in their interactions with patients and be properly prepared to do this safely and to reflect on it afterwards to ensure that it has its full learning effect.

Feasibility studies conducted in the Open University and more recently in other universities have shown quite clearly that distance learning is a powerful support to these complex processes. Figure 42.2 shows some of the potential applications of distance learning techniques in a clinical setting.

MODELS AND DESCRIPTIONS OF THE CLINICAL PROBLEM SOLVING PROCESS

To design and implement distance education to teach clinical problem solving we need to understand this phenomenon. The literature provides many models and descriptions of clinical reasoning and problem solving, as discussed in previous chapters. Researchers have chosen either to describe

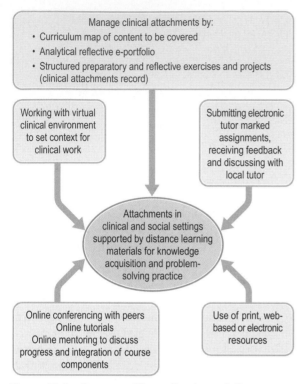

Figure 42.2 Some specific applications of distance learning techniques in a clinical context

or to model the clinical problem-solving process. Descriptions are based in cognitive psychology and try to portray what is going on inside the head of the clinician, whereas models tend to find another way of representing the process, usually in terms of statistical or algorithmic frameworks. But teaching based on statistical or algorithmic models such as Bayes' theorem (Gill et al 2005) can only ask students to use a formula which will overlay their own cognitive processing of the data. We therefore propose to advocate strategies that will help students to enhance their thinking processes by preparing for and reflecting on experience.

DESCRIPTIONS BASED ON COGNITIVE PSYCHOLOGY

Overall, although cognitive psychology researchers have chosen to use different terms to describe what is happening inside the head of the student or clinician who is trying to work out what, if anything, is wrong with a patient, the overall picture is much the same. It is one which has the following main characteristics:

- individuality of thinking based on memories built up from past experience of patients and cases
- case-specific expertise based on a 'bank' of cases built up through experience
- increasing accessibility of the right part of memory, with increasing experience of clinical problem solving, as a result of more appropriate organization of knowledge
- organization of information in memory as a key to efficient clinical problem solving
- clinicians reverting to the use of basic science to solve the problem from first principles, when knowledge based on clinical experience fails.

FUNDAMENTAL FACTORS IN IMPROVING CLINICAL PROBLEM SOLVING

Our own original research (Gale & Marsden 1983; Grant & Marsden 1990, 1991) is in line with the other cognitive models and descriptions and has been used as the basis of teaching for improved clinical problem solving (Gale-Grant & Marsden 1986). The work has been successfully used to analyse clinical decision making in other fields such as dentistry (Maupomé & Sheiham 2000). We have shown that five processes are important in helping students and clinicians to understand and improve their diagnostic thinking process:

1. The organization of clinical memory

Reflection and experiences in accessing memories helps to develop the ease and flexibility of thinking based on appropriate organization of memory stores that characterizes the more experienced clinician (Grant & Marsden 1987, 1988). Distance learning must offer enhancement of the knowledge base, guidance in the use of knowledge to solve clinical problems, and ways to reflect on and analyse that process.

2. Individuality of thinking

As clinicians develop, their personal memory stores become more individual, developed, appropriate and tailored through use and clinical practice (Grant & Marsden, 1987, 1988).

3. Gaining access to memory

When students or clinicians are presented with clinical information, they make sense of it by recognizing for themselves certain personally important pieces of information. These individually-relevant *forceful features* act as the key point of access to memory structures and allow clinicians to make sense of that clinical information. It is clear that effective diagnostic thinking is an individual thing; easy diagnoses are not those where the forceful feature is indisputable but rather where there is scope for individualized ways of looking at the problem.

4. Responding to clinical information

Students and clinicians are thinking actively from the very beginning of the clinical interview (Gale & Marsden 1984). They may: make pre-diagnostic interpretations of available information (e.g. there is a myocardial problem); make a diagnostic interpretation (e.g. acromegaly); or (in the absence of forceful features) focus on the quality of the information and consider what further inquiries are needed to move the decision making forward.

Of particular interest here is recognizing that clinical reasoning is much more an interpretive process than a purely logical or formulated one. For instance, Montgomery (2006) regards clinical medicine as an 'interpretive, science-using practice' and this view is supported by our and others' research. It is useful for teachers to help students to recognize their own thinking patterns, forceful features and memory structures so they can critique and develop them to become appropriate for the reasoning tasks they face.

5. Mechanisms of error

Reasoning errors can be classified into three main types: becoming set or trapped into an inappropriate way of seeing the data, making incorrect interpretations, and misinterpreting the relevance of information. There is, perhaps, too much unreasonable moral panic about such 'errors' and biases which might simply be a normal or unusual part of the thinking process, but which clinicians should

know about (Eva & Norman 2005, Klein 2005), and evidence suggests that knowing about them does improve performance (Round 1999). Instead, because clinical problem solving is case-specific and person-specific, with different content and types of reaction to clinical information, there is no one reasoning system that can be taught. Distance learning, therefore, must link in with the wide clinical experience of students and trainees to help them see the variety of their thinking, to monitor the errors they make and to be aware of the successful heuristics they can use.

HOW CAN DISTANCE LEARNING FACILITATE THE DEVELOPMENT OF CLINICAL PROBLEM–SOLVING SKILLS?

Clinical problem solving is the core of clinical practice. To facilitate this skill is to facilitate the practice of health professionals. It is on the five process aspects of thinking described above, common to all students and clinicians, that distance learning support can be focused, along with the technical and content-based support that distance learning can offer so well. Clinical problem solving does not have to be taught as such; it simply has to be revealed.

There have been many approaches over the years to teaching clinical problem-solving skills, the most widespread of which are integrated and problem-based curricula. Others have, for example, offered special seminars (Struyf et al 2005) or special cognitive skills training (Lavelle 1978), and there were early attempts to use computer-assisted training for clinical problem-solving (De Dombal 1979). These mainly fell by the wayside, however, perhaps not surprisingly since research suggests that this is a skill that cannot be taught (Schuwirth 2002) as it is a natural function of dynamic thinking; it can only be facilitated by allowing students and clinicians to understand their own thinking processes and to monitor the types of approach they take, the errors they make and the strategies they might use to improve their performance.

Our distance learning approach is therefore one that assumes that the learners are in a clinical environment or other professional workplace and that we can: help them to prepare; sensitize them to key aspects of the situation and of their performance; guide them to reflect systematically on that; help them to understand the dynamic of strategies used to collect and process patient or client-related data (such as the clinical interview) and their cognitive reactions to and influences on it; and help them to find strategies to improve their performance.

We follow Schuwirth's (2002, p. 695) advice that 'educational interventions for clinical reasoning should be based on providing the learner with feedback rather than on teaching a generic strategy'.

Eva (2005) also agrees that orienting students to 'multiple reasoning strategies' and 'flexibility regarding the ways by which solutions to clinical problems can be derived' is the most productive and evidence-based approach. Computer-mediated environments have already been used to facilitate such reflection in a clinical setting (Cooner & Dickmann 2006).

We are not the first to argue that distance learning can support the development of clinical reasoning (see Medélez Ortega et al 2003) but, as Spencer (2006, p. 591) points out, clinical teaching lies at the heart of medical education at both undergraduate and postgraduate levels: 'It is the only setting in which the skills of history taking, physical examinations, clinical reasoning, decision-making, empathy, and professionalism can be taught and learned as an integrated whole.' And yet, as Spencer points out, because this is the site of practice as well as learning there are problems of time, competing pressures on the teacher who is also the responsible clinician and difficulty in planning in an unpredictable clinical environment. Despite this, the real workplace environment is most suited to the successful application of the experiential learning cycle (based on the work of Kolb et al 1979) that is the basis of acquiring the expertise to solve clinical problems. Simply helping students to learn more effectively from their workplace experience by asking them to reflect on it and to make links between different elements will develop the deep learning style which, in turn, has been shown to correlate with more effective clinical reasoning (Groves 2005).

The substantial body of research into clinicians' thinking processes indicates clearly that expertise is a function of reflection on experience (Grant & Marsden 1990, Jensen et al 2000, Schmidt et al 1990). Others (Bradley 2005, Klein 2005) have suggested that students and clinicians should be made aware of their own thinking processes. Sobral (2000) has likewise shown that improved quality of reflection is associated with a more positive learning experience and may be conducive to enhanced diagnostic ability as measured by the Diagnostic Thinking Inventory (Bordage et al 1990). It is in guiding this cycle that distance learning can play a fundamental role in the development of clinical problem-solving skills. It has already been shown (Ryan et al 2004) that an online clinical reasoning guide can be highly effective in the context of problem-based learning and we envisage that a similar document, especially if interactive and based on the main and shared features of clinical thinking, could play an important supportive role for students and clinicians in their areas of clinical attachment.

Given evidence that clinicians are often unaware of the thinking processes they use (Dunn et al 1996), guiding such reflection is of paramount importance. Figure 42.3 shows interventions that can be made using distance learning techniques. These can assist planning through exercises and resources. Professional experience itself can be recorded and analysed using logbooks, diaries and other records. Materials that ask the learner to reflect on the clinical encounter, on feelings, processes, problems and strategies, backed up by analytical instruments such as the Diagnostic Thinking Inventory and other rating scales, can then be used. Finally, learners can use this process to develop personal concepts and understanding of their own clinical problem-solving processes.

A DISTANCE LEARNING STRATEGY TO ASSIST THE DEVELOPMENT OF EFFECTIVE CLINICAL PROBLEM SOLVING

We have seen that:

- There is no one accurate and correct model or description of clinical reasoning

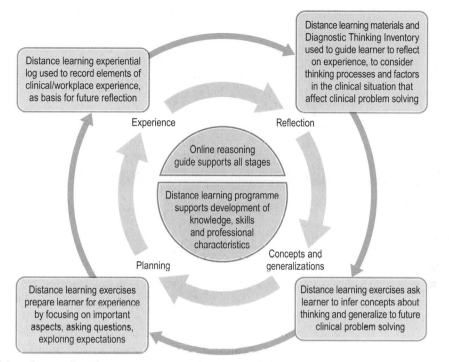

Figure 42.3   Using distance learning to support experiential learning

- Clinical problem solving is context-bound and domain-specific (Schuwirth 2004)
- Clinical problem solving is idiosyncratic in that different experts will follow different routes to reach the same solution to a clinical problem and this individuality increases with increasing expertise
- Skill and accuracy increase with increasing experience and reflection on experience
- A sound basis of knowledge, skill and clinical experience is required to underpin the effective development of clinical problem-solving acumen.

These factors seem to suggest that we should not be teaching students to use a particular method of clinical problem solving; instead we should be ensuring that students have the opportunity to use their knowledge and skills in the context of many different clinical problems, that they should accumulate extensive clinical experience and that they should be helped and guided to reflect on that experience so that they can consciously identify their own approaches to clinical problem solving,

understand the sorts of errors they make and the problems they encounter in thinking about clinical information, be aware of the internal connections they access in their memories, and do all this in the context of the clinical encounter. This has already been shown to be an effective pedagogical approach (Groves et al 2002).

The educational strategy, then, is to reveal and stimulate conscious and systematic analysis of the student's personal experience of clinical problem solving. It has been noted (Cuello-Garcia 2005) that 'revealing or visualizing the thinking involved in making clinical decisions is a challenge', but it is the challenge that must be taken up. Distance learning is an effective medium for this approach.

THE DIAGNOSTIC THINKING INVENTORY

Online tests of clinical reasoning have already been applied with some success in specialties (Sibert et al 2005). The Diagnostic Thinking Inventory developed by Bordage et al (1990) is a validated psychometric instrument which reveals the structure and flexibility of thinking in clinical problem solving. It has been widely used in medical and health professional education for research and to help students understand their thinking processes (Groves et al 2002, 2003). Such an instrument would be highly effective for self-report or as the basis of online mentoring for distributed students when combined with self-reports of clinical encounters.

WHAT DOES THE FUTURE HOLD?

It is clear that distance learning is not only an appropriate medium for health sciences education and for the facilitation of clinical problem-solving skills; it is a necessary medium. We have shown that there are myriad potential interventions that distance learning techniques can offer and there is gradually accumulating a positive body of experience and research that gives encouragement to distance learning in clinical education.

The current approaches to facilitating clinical problem-solving skills can be translated into distance learning formats. It will take a partnership between distance learning designers and health sciences educationalists to convert this potential into a new era of practice. Distance learning requires careful design to ensure active learning and reflection. It requires careful planning to ensure relevance and integration with clinical experience.

Distance learning is now mainstream and brings predictable, quality-assured education and support to students who are distributed across geographical distances and located in different sites. Its techniques are many and varied and its development methods incorporate quality assurance (Grant 2001). Distance learning must be carefully planned and developed whether it is by electronic (Curry & Smith 2005) or more traditional media (Grant 2001). If designed and implemented well (Mehotra et al 2001), distance learning can deliver almost all the outcomes required by traditional courses. It is cost-effective, quality assured, monitorable and student oriented. Where students are learning the central skill of clinical problem solving, they deserve to be supported by distance learning techniques and materials.

References

Bordage G, Grant J, Marsden P 1990 Quantitative assessment of diagnostic ability. Medical Education 24:413–425

Bradley C P 2005 Commentary: can we avoid bias? British Medical Journal 330:784

Clarke A, Lewis D, Cole I et al 2005 A strategic approach to developing e-learning capability for healthcare. Health Informatics and Libraries Journal 22(2):33–41

Cooner D, Dickmann E 2006 Assessing principal internships and habits of mind: the use of journey mapping to enhance reflection. Innovate 2(4). Online. Available: http://www.innovateonline.info/index.php?view=article&id=217 18 June 2006

Cuello-Garcia C 2005 Sharing the diagnostic process in the clinical teaching environment: a case study. Journal of Continuing Education in the Health Professions 25(4):231–239

Curry M, Smith L 2005 Twelve tips for authoring on-line distance learning medical post-registration programmes. Medical Teacher 27(4):316–321

De Dombal F T 1979 Computers and the surgeon. Surgery Annals 11:33–57

Donnelly A B, Agius R M 2005 The distance learning courses in occupational medicine – 20 years and onwards. Occupational Medicine 55:319–323

Dunn T G, Taylor C A, Lipsky M S 1996 An investigation of physician knowledge-in-action. Teaching and Learning in Medicine 8(2):90–97

Eva K W 2005 What every teacher needs to know about clinical reasoning. Medical Education 39(1):98–106

Eva K W, Norman G R 2005 Heuristics and biases – a biased perspective on clinical reasoning. Medical Education 39(9):870–872

Gale J, Marsden P 1983 Medical diagnosis: from student to clinician. Oxford University Press, Oxford

Gale J, Marsden P 1984 The role of the routine clinical history. Medical Education 18:96–100

Gale-Grant J, Marsden P 1986 Medical students as adult learners: implications for an innovative short course in the clinical curriculum. Medical Teacher 8(3):243–251

Gill C J, Sabin L, Schmid C H 2005 Why clinicians are natural Bayesians. British Medical Journal 330:1080–1083

Grant J 2001 Distance learning: a response to overcome current challenges in medical education? Towards Unity for Health 4(October):21–23. WHO/EIP/OSD/NL/A/2001.2.

Grant J, Marsden P 1987 The structure of memorised knowledge in students and clinicians: an explanation for diagnostic expertise. Medical Education 21:92–98

Grant J, Marsden P 1988 Primary knowledge, medical education and consultant expertise. Medical Education 22:173–179

Grant J, Marsden P 1990 Quantitative assessment of diagnostic ability. Medical Education 24(5):413–425

Grant J, Marsden P 1991 Diabetes care in general practice. Lilly Diabetes Care Division, Oxford

Groves M 2005 Problem-based learning and learning approach: is there a relationship? Advances in Health Sciences Education 10:315–326

Groves M, Scott I, Alexander H 2002 Assessing clinical reasoning: a method to monitor its development in a PBL curriculum. Medical Teacher 24(5):507–515

Groves M, O'Rourke P, Alexander H 2003 The association between student characteristics and the development of clinical reasoning in a graduate-entry, PBL medical programme. Medical Teacher 25(6):626–631

Jensen G M, Gwyer J, Shepard K F et al 2000 Expert practice in physical therapy. Physical Therapy 80(1):28–43

Klein J G 2005 Five pitfalls in decisions about diagnosis and prescribing. British Medical Journal 330:781–784

Kolb D A, Rubin I M, McIntyre J M 1979 Organizational psychology: an experiential approach, 3rd edn. Prentice-Hall, Englewood Cliffs, NJ

Lavelle S M 1978 Information processing by medical students. Medical Education 12(Suppl):108–109

Lysaght R, Bent M 2005 A comparative analysis of case presentation modalities used in clinical reasoning coursework in occupational therapy. American Journal of Occupational Therapy 59(3):314–324

McConnell D 2006 E learning groups and communities. Society for Research into Higher Education and Open University Press, Maidenhead

Markova T, Roth L M, Monsur J 2005 Synchronous distance learning as an effective and feasible method for delivering residency didactics. Family Medicine 37(8):570–575

Maupomé G, Sheiham A 2000 Clinical decision-making in restorative dentistry: content-analysis of diagnostic thinking processes and concurrent concepts used in an educational environment. European Journal of Dental Education 4(4):143–152

Medélez Ortega E, Burgun A, Le Duff F et al 2003 Collaborative environment for clinical reasoning and distance learning sessions. International Journal of Medical Informatics 70(2–3):345–351

Mehotra C M, Hollister C D, McGahey L 2001 Distance learning: principles for effective design, delivery, and evaluation. Sage Publications, Thousand Oaks, CA

Montgomery K 2006 How doctors think: clinical judgement and the practice of medicine. Oxford University Press, Oxford

Round A P 1999 Teaching clinical reasoning – a preliminary controlled study. Medical Education 33(7):480–483

Ryan G, Dolling T, Barnet S 2004 Supporting the problem-based learning process in the clinical years: evaluation of an online clinical reasoning guide. Medical Education 38(6):638–645

Schmidt H G, Norman G R, Boshuizen H PA 1990 A cognitive perspective on medical expertise: theory and implications. Academic Medicine 65.611–621

Schuwirth L W T 2002 Can clinical reasoning be taught or can it only be learned? Medical Education 36(8):695–696

Schuwirth L W T 2004 Assessing medical competence: finding the right answers. Clinical Teacher 1(1):14–18

Sibert L, Darmoni S J, Dahamna B et al 2005 Online clinical reasoning assessment with the Script concordance test: a feasibility study. BMC Medical Informatics and Decision Making 5:18. Online. Available: http://www.biomedcentral.com/1472-6947/5/18 18 Jun 2006

Sobral D T 2000 An appraisal of medical students' reflection-in-learning. Medical Education 34(3):182–187

Spencer J 2006 Learning and teaching in the clinical environment. British Medical Journal 326:591–594

Struyf E, Beullens J, Van Damme B et al 2005 A new methodology for teaching clinical reasoning skills: problem solving seminars. Medical Teacher 27(4):364–368

Urquhart C, Chambers M, Connor S et al 2002 Evaluation of distance learning delivery of health information management and health informatics programmes: a UK perspective. Health Informatics and Libraries Journal 19.146–157

Walton G, Childs S, Blenkinsopp E 2005 Using mobile technologies to give health students access to learning resources in the UK community setting. Health Informatics and Libraries Journal 22(2):51–65

Chapter 43

Cultivating a thinking surgeon: using a clinical thinking pathway as a learning and assessment process

Della Fish and Linda de Cossart

CHAPTER CONTENTS

INTRODUCTION

We have, over the last 4 years, been developing in the UK a new approach to teaching and assessing clinical thinking and professional judgement for surgeons in particular and doctors in general (De Cossart & Fish 2005, 2006; Fish & De Cossart 2006, 2007). We began this work by conducting a detailed and robust analysis of the complexities of clinical practice, of the way senior clinicians conduct themselves in practice and of how they make difficult clinical decisions. Through this we came to see a huge range of invisible influences that shaped their success as clinicians in maximizing patient care in hospital settings.

We believe we form a unique combination of a widely experienced consultant surgeon working with a senior educator whose expertise is in the practice of teaching and with a long-term interest in the development of professional judgement (Fish & Coles 1998). This has, we believe, enabled us to explore and clarify our differing perspectives and harmonize them into an educational enterprise that enables doctors to uncover, explore, articulate and therefore develop those elements of their practice that are invisible. We have coined the term *invisibles* in respect of all this, because the focus of this work is on both the implicit elements of practice and those aspects of the tacit that can be identified. We do not use *tacit*, because some of the tacit is inevitably ineffable (see De Cossart & Fish 2005, Schön 1987) and also because the term apparently excludes the implicit.

Our newly developed suite of six 'heuristics' provides devices to prompt exploration and increase understanding of what drives visible behaviour and feeds observable behaviour (see Fish & De Cossart 2007). These focus on: the importance of the context of the decision making; the kind of person the doctor is; the drivers of the doctor's professional practice; the forms of knowledge that are brought up in thinking about the patient; and the clinical thinking processes that lead to a specific professional judgement (see also De Cossart & Fish 2005, Fish & De Cossart 2007). We believe that in this we offer medicine a new language and framework in which to discuss, develop and assess the thinking processes which lead doctors to complex decisions.

THE CONTEXT IN WHICH WE HAVE SHAPED THESE IDEAS

In contextualizing this work, we recognize five perspectives as background to this chapter.

1. THE CHANGING WORKING AND EDUCATIONAL CONTEXT FOR DOCTORS IN THE UK

In the past, surgeons spent many hours in their work environment reflecting on, analysing and developing their practice, mainly orally, in harness with a senior clinician and also with their peers. Such learning conversations, however, rarely led to robust written records of the development of the learner's clinical thinking and professional judgement.

Today, two major changes (one in education and one in service requirements) have rendered this approach obsolete. In education, the introduction of more specific curricula for postgraduate medicine have highlighted the importance of recording the learner's progress and the possible uses of this learning record over the doctor's career. In service terms, the new ways of working in the UK, specifically because of the European Working Time Directive, have meant that doctors must learn faster and, given the current litigious climate, must focus more on being articulate about their professionalism, values, intentions, decision making and patient management (Royal College of Physicians 2005).

Indeed, by 2009 the hours of work for all UK doctors will be reduced to 48 per week. This virtually halves the time spent in practice and therefore the time available for postgraduate medical education, since doctors' main learning opportunities occur entirely within their working hours. Interestingly, these issues are also beginning to emerge in the USA where in New York State the hours per week have recently been reduced to 80.

2. THE CHARACTER OF CURRENT TEACHING AND ASSESSMENT IN POSTGRADUATE MEDICINE, AS REQUIRED BY NEW GOVERNMENT INITIATIVES

The current elements that are required for assessment (and therefore for learning) in the new educational programmes for postgraduate doctors in the UK use methods ('Tools of the Trade') which attend mainly to the visible components of practice. These were aimed initially at the early years of postgraduate medicine but are already being pushed into more advanced training programmes. This is cause for concern, since they were unchallenging even for the most junior doctors in their simplistic characterization of real practice, and we believe that they are simply inappropriate for specialist doctors who are being developed to engage in the highly complex care of patients both in hospitals and in the community.

This foundation curriculum has come about because in the early 21st century the Department of Health (DoH), through the initiatives 'Modernising Medical Careers' and 'A Firm Foundation', set out to update and reform medical education and training and shorten the time between entry to medical school and acquisition of a Certificate of Completion of Training (CCT) (DoH 2002, 2003, 2004). As a result, newly graduated doctors are now required to undertake a compulsory 2 years of generic clinical work (Foundation Years 1 and 2 (F1 and F2)), designed to expose them to a wide range of clinical practice and ensure that they are able to recognize and initiate management of the acutely sick patient. This foundation programme is based upon the idea that all aspects of medical practice can be broken down into a series of competencies.

There is now a requirement that these competencies are tested at frequent intervals by four devices known collectively as *Tools of the Trade*. These tools are: the personal assessment tool (MINI PAT); the clinical examination tool (Mini CEX), which focuses on the processes related to the clinical examination of patients; the DOPS (which is concerned with the doctor's ability to complete clinical procedures correctly); and Case-based Discussion tool (CbD), which tests seven competencies of the doctor's consideration of the patient case, each of which is given a very broad definition (e.g. 'professionalism') and is assigned one tick box. All these tools are designed to be optically read by computer, and record most of their details in tick boxes. The specialty programmes currently being developed to follow the foundation programme are likely to include a core and a specialty element. They too, worryingly, enshrine these four limited tools.

Each of these Tools of the Trade is based upon some research (which seems to give them credibility beyond previous assessment processes). But most of this research was conducted in cultures other than the UK and largely in undergraduate contexts. In fact there is no sound evidence that these tools are appropriate either for the selection or for the in-programme assessment of postgraduate doctors in Britain. Neither do they support the development and the detailed assessment of professionalism, clinical thinking or professional judgement. Indeed, they depend heavily upon only what is observable in the clinical setting and make no demands on trainees to reach beyond the basics on which they are repeatedly tested. For this reason we see them as necessary but not sufficient in the foundation years, and as needing to be replaced in the specialty years with something that does more justice to the nature of real clinical practice.

3. THE CONTEXT OF DECISION MAKING IN MEDICINE

We believe that Tools of the Trade encourage a reductionist approach to clinical practice in doctors of the future which not only minimizes the importance of professional judgement but also ignores previous work on decision making in medicine.

A review of this literature shows three broad approaches. Statistical models (for example those based on the Bayes theorem) have supported decision making in medicine and the way it is taught by some since the 1960s (see White & Stancombe 2003); illness scripts have been favoured by some (Schmidt et al 1992); and pattern recognition by others (Patel & Groen 1986). None of these seems to have been developed beyond the original concepts, and we do not see evidence that they attend adequately to clinical practice in its more complex forms. However, it is our contention that the dimensions of decision making they attend to and a critical exploration of their ideas (based on what happens in real practice) ought to have informed the content of Tools of the Trade.

Our critique of these approaches is that they have traditionally focused postgraduate learners on diagnosis and on their underlying factual (propositional) knowledge, driving postgraduate learning in medicine more and more in the direction of learning clinical factual knowledge. All of this has emphasized a formulaic approach to teaching and assessment, which does not attend to the complexities of clinical practice, the need for doctors to develop wide-ranging exploration of the patient case and to provide for individual patients a carefully constructed management plan which takes account of all the human factors as well as the scientific ones and which is the mark of a wise professional. Indeed, in the more recent literature we have found reference by both clinical and lay writers (Demar et al 2006, Eraut & Du Bouley 2000, Montgomery 2005, White & Stancombe 2003) to the inappropriateness of the tyranny of algorithms and protocols and their dangerous exclusion of doctors' discretion to move outside them.

It is true that more recently there have been broader approaches to medical decision making in the work of Atkinson (1995), Cox (1999), Dowie & Elstein (1988), Downie & Macnaughton (2000) and White & Stancombe (2003). While we applaud this trend towards drawing on science together with the humanities and arts to understand and illuminate the thinking processes involved, we believe that even here the basic conception of medical decision making to which these new approaches are directed has been too narrow.

It is our contention then that much work on medical decision making is flawed because often the ideas have been developed from theory to practice, overlooking the complexities of real clinical practice and highlighting only the easily definable aspects of it. We see evidence that this approach is creating doctors who are fearful of stepping beyond clearly defined boundaries learned in the classroom (at medical school and hospital induction programmes). We find it deeply disturbing that doctors are being restricted by such systems and becoming fearful and unable to use their discretion safely for the benefit of the patient.

4. THE CONTEXT IN WHICH WE HAVE DEVELOPED OUR IDEAS

It was these matters of concern that led us to investigate the work of wise and successful doctors and surgeons in the clinical setting, and by this means to develop our ideas about both the processes of clinical thinking and the nature of professional judgement. Further, we have developed ways of using this knowledge by creating new educational activities that enable doctors at all stages to articulate the invisible elements of their practice and also to provide concrete written evidence of their developing understanding of that practice (of how they learn it, and of their responsibilities to the patient and society).

5. THE COMPONENTS OF THE CLINICAL THINKING PATHWAY: PROVIDING A LANGUAGE AND FRAMEWORK FOR EDUCATING DOCTORS

By mapping the thinking processes of working surgeons and doctors as focused on clinical problems, we produced the clinical thinking pathway shown in Figure 43.1. This pathway begins with formulating a complex clinical problem. *Complex problem* as construed by the surgeon, alone or in consultation with patients and colleagues, here contrasts with medical or surgical decisions, the relatively simple answers to closed questions about fairly uncomplicated clinical activities. Complex problems draw upon the surgeon's (patients' and colleagues') values, beliefs and experience, and then trigger the need for clinical reasoning. This seeks, through

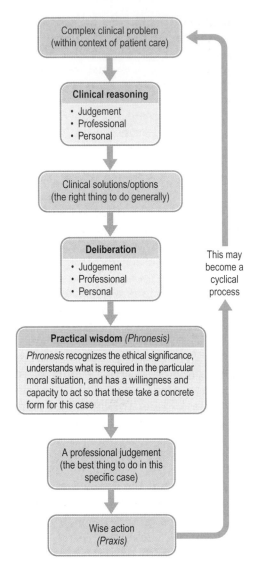

Figure 43.1   Clinical thinking: the key elements and their basic relationship (see De Cossart & Fish 2005, p. 137)

neutral logic and scientific knowledge, which are not contextualized to the patient, to identify and explore those elements and actions that will be significant in the resolution of the problem. This in turn leads to an objectified and generalized clinical conclusion or conclusions about what is the right thing to do generally in such cases.

Doctors then need to situate this generalized logic and adapt this neutral clinical solution to the needs of the specific individual patient within the particular clinical context. They do so by engaging in deliberation which weighs, prioritizes and responds to the context-specific demands and pressures. These emanate from the patient's needs; the clinician's views, vision, abilities, knowledge; and the requirements and possibilities of the particular managing authority. Practical wisdom (or what Aristotle called *phronesis*) then helps the practitioner to focus on and understand the particular ethical dimensions and moral situation of this individual patient. This thinking process leads to a professional judgement, which is a decision about the best action to be taken in this particular patient's interests. It is the end result of the whole process of clinical thinking. Where practical wisdom has been harnessed to consider the moral and ethical issues, the resulting activity can be referred to as wise action or what Aristotle called *praxis* (see Carr 1995, p. 71). Each stage, together with its associated decision making, must of course be kept under frequent review.

Although they are presented in simple terms in Figure 43.1, none of the thinking processes endemic to clinical reasoning and deliberation is actually simple. At all points, the salient features involved need to be identified, the significance of various elements needs to be weighed, and the meaning of even the most scientific of evidence needs to be interpreted. Further, all human situations are constantly evolving, and there is always a need for professionals to continue to respond to developments and to refine or reconsider their conclusions. In response, the professional practitioner's vital capacity to exercise personal professional judgement comes into play at all points along the pathway. It enables the surgeon to deal with the complexity, the competing demands and the ambiguities which often arise in evolving human interaction. Unlike the (public) professional judgement referred to above, which is the end product of the whole process of clinical thinking, this personal professional judgement is an ability to weigh up competing elements, ideas, and actions and to adjudicate between conflicting but equal priorities. Thus the personal professional judgement of the clinician lies at the core of medical practice.

We see these key elements and their basic relationship as the foundation of any kind of clinical thinking (although of course some elements will be present in greater or lesser degrees depending on the nature of the problem). Thus, this general pathway can be used to explore such thinking, whether it is focused on the process that leads from the first outpatient consultation to an agreed treatment plan, is concerned with the thinking that leads to wise action within the treatment itself, or is seeking the resolution of wider clinical issues.

DISTINGUISHING BETWEEN CLINICAL REASONING AND DELIBERATION

The two main forms of reasoning within clinical thinking (clinical reasoning on the one hand and deliberation, or practical reasoning, on the other) are greatly contrasting in nature. In its simplest and purest form, clinical reasoning construes the complex clinical problem as a technical one. It then operates through a formula to solve a clinical problem (comes to a clinical conclusion) by using a straightforward set of rules, with the assumption that what counts as evidence would be agreed by everyone.

A key example of clinical reasoning (generally referred to as *diagnostic reasoning*) involves coming to a working diagnosis. From this viewpoint, clinical reasoning can be seen as a biomedical process which distinguishes the disease from the patient and regards the problem as to do with malfunctioning parts of the patient. It is a technical problem, requiring technical competence from the practitioner. It is based on rigorous logic and order, collects predictable categories of evidence, and uses a formulaic approach to reach a clinical decision. It claims a scientific basis, and stems from a world view that sees facts as objective, precise and absolute, and 'truth' as 'out there', waiting to be discovered. It assumes that scientific theory can be directly translated into practice. And it is deliberately devoid of moral and ethical concern.

Newly qualified doctors are usually unaware that there is any more to clinical thinking than the simple version of clinical reasoning. But even in the most technical of patient cases, investigations must be selected, evidence must be interpreted and explanations found for it, and judgements must be made about when enough evidence is at hand. This may well require other versions of clinical reasoning beyond the traditional diagnostic/scientific reasoning with its hypothetico-deductive base, such as narrative reasoning and interactive reasoning. At postgraduate level in medicine then, clinical reasoning takes on a more complex form and is illuminated at various points by personal/professional judgement. Nonetheless, it still follows a logical order, still sees the problem and its solution in broadly scientific terms, and thus can fairly readily be made overt by surgeon educators and shared with and developed in their learners. It can then be assessed orally and in writing.

In contrast, deliberation always recognizes the complexity at the core of clinical thinking and sees clinical problems as humane problems which are inevitably characterized by messiness and uncertainty and which require an echoing human response from the practitioner. Deliberation holds as an open question what would count as evidence in respect of its arguments. It thus needs to draw on professionals' personal judgement processes and practical wisdom to produce a professional decision, which in turn leads to a wise action. Beginning doctors are often shocked to discover the central importance of deliberation.

A key example of deliberation is the process which turns a working diagnosis into a treatment plan for a particular patient, and which has been agreed by that patient and others involved. Deliberation, then, is grounded in the professional's humanity and is concerned with the patient's social being in the world. It calls upon imagination and compassion in practitioners to help them understand how patients are seeing and feeling and thus to interpret more sensitively what they want and need. It involves the artistry of practice. It draws on knowledge of science and life, sensitivity to language, understanding of social interaction and recognition of what is involved at a human level in constructing a history. Further, it admits the existence of emotional elements in the patient's story and the practitioner's response. It sees disease as a breakdown of the patient's social world, and crucially recognizes that the meaning of any situation is likely to be construed differently by each of the different people involved in it. (That is, it acknowledges both the social construction of knowledge and multiple versions of reality.)

Deliberation is based on pragmatic and practical reasoning in which human and equally competing priorities vie for attention, in an order that must arise from the particulars of the problem and will therefore be different for different patients. It thus eschews formulae for thinking, using instead an investigative approach to unearthing all the pertinent elements, and a reflective and critical approach to prioritizing and weighing them up. It is based on a view of the world as complex, ambiguous and uncertain. It works from practice to theory. Typically, it involves clinicians in appreciating patients' experiences of illness, such as their feelings and fears about being ill, their ideas about what is wrong with them and the basis of those ideas, the impact of the problem on their lives, their expectations about what should be done, and their sense of control or powerlessness in relation to their situation (see Higgs et al 2004). Practical wisdom is what enables practitioners to focus on and be sensitive to the moral and ethical dimensions involved.

We wish to make it clear, however, that this model (like all diagrams) simplifies and reduces real-life complexities. For example, we do not see these processes as solitary activities leading to decisions by lone professionals. Nor do we see them as necessarily happening within a short and simple linear time scale. We also recognize with White & Stancombe (2003, p. 14) that 'case formulations often remain unarticulated in encounters with patients . . . and may not exist as single events produced spontaneously on discrete occasions . . . [but] emerge gradually over time and through conversation with colleagues'. We also recognize that the clinical setting involves multi-professional teams, so that decision making itself is a collective organizational activity. Further, we acknowledge that in human interaction, one person's way of making meaning out of a situation can never precisely match another's.

In De Cossart & Fish (2005, Chapter 7) we have further elaborated on the issues and pressures that doctors need to consider during both clinical reasoning and deliberation, and have delineated a range of the kinds of judgement that doctors make. These include the following forms of judgement: hasty, habitual, tactical, strategic, and professional (see Table 43.1).

Table 43.1   The kinds of judgements we make in practice

Kind of judgement	Visible response	Assessment description
Hasty	Knee-jerk reaction	Unsatisfactory/unprofessional
Habitual	Going through motions	Automatic/practitioner as automaton
Tactical	Selects tactics known to please	Basic practical response/practitioner as apprentice
Strategic	Accepts problem, but chooses what is easiest for self	Considered response/ practitioner as senior technician
Professional	Enquires into problem and what is needed for the best for patient, can do this (checks), and then does it	Enlightened response/practitioner as professional working on the basis of practical wisdom

A DISTILLATION OF OUR EXPERIENCES IN USING THIS PATHWAY WITH POSTGRADUATE DOCTORS

What we offer in this pathway, then, is a framework which can be used either in a linear or a three-dimensional fashion that allows weaving around various points as the case becomes complex and more demanding. (We like the image of the helicoid rather than a spiral to describe this because it is like a helix, but is screw-shaped – a curve on a developable surface – and is therefore unlike a spiral which can become a straight line when the surface is unrolled into a plane. See Figure 43.2.)

OUR EXPERIENCE IN USING THE HEURISTICS, INCLUDING THE CLINICAL THINKING PATHWAY

A wide range of educational activities, seminars, educational pilots and programmes have fed into our distillation of the lessons we have learned from using the clinical thinking pathway (amongst the rest of the heuristics):

The learning processes

In all these seminars we taught most sessions (with a few pragmatic exceptions) as a team of educator and clinician. In this we used the expertise and strengths of each professional. Behind the scenes the educator led the shaping of the preparation, the careful adjustment of aims for each session, ensured that the writing was responded to on time

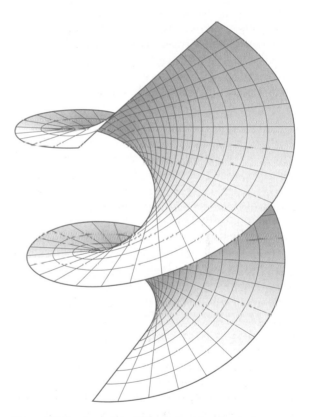

Figure 43.2   A model of the helicoid pathway

and kept records, while the clinician kept an eye on the clinician participants and the feedback from the clinical setting. In the classroom, the educator taught the invisibles and how to write reflectively, while the clinician took charge of the discussion of complex cases and used the invisibles to help learners to think through an entire surgical operation.

In all the educational programmes we helped learners to develop a critique of case-based discussion, introduced the invisibles and particularly the clinical thinking pathway, illustrated its use in enriching the discussion of a case, helped learners to develop reflective written accounts of their clinical thinking, provided examples of good reflective writing using the pathway, and helped them to change their view of 'learning to learn' in the clinical setting.

In terms of assessment, we illustrated how the invisibles could be used to enrich the assessments required by Tools of the Trade. We required learners to bring to an assessment panel one case-based discussion form (which was evidence of their having already been assessed on this case in the clinical setting) together with a subsequently written reflection on that case using the invisibles. Their task on the day was to discuss their written reflection in terms of: (a) the key insights the case generated that reinforced their learning; and (b) an evaluation of the use of the case. This case was the third of four pieces of writing the students completed, either between sessions of the course or with help in class. These writing tasks offered a further means of assessment because they provided a means for students to demonstrate their developing insight during the course. Evaluations indicated that these strategies helped students to see how they could give better evidence of their professional development in both formal and informal assessment settings.

WHAT WE HAVE LEARNED AS A RESULT

At a detailed level we learned that teaching and assessing clinical reasoning is far more demanding than at first appears, and that working as an educator/clinician team makes everything more possible because each brings a different capability to the task and sees the needs of the programme from a different (but relevant) perspective. We came to see that seminar sessions in a programme need to be mandatory (which is true for teachers as well as learners), and that assessment of the educational attainments (as distinct from the clinical attainments) of trainees must be part of formative and summative assessment. We saw that the spaces and activities between sessions are important for maturation and that continuity can be achieved across a series of seminars by being determined! We noted that teaching trainees nudges consultants into thinking (that such consultant teachers themselves need a sheltered practicum in which to learn) and that the teaching we have done has infected the ground because trainees now see clinical decision making differently.

We came to see the need to insist on proper backup, which (some) deaneries are not prepared for (in terms of registers, resources, communication with learners between sessions). We discovered that many learners have had bad experiences of reflective practice and that it is better to talk about reflective learning and 'clinical reflective writing'. Individual response to their writing does motivate highly. It is also vital to set a supportive and safe environment in which learners can take risks, enjoy being outrageous, creative and exploratory (for example, many said they enjoyed the chance to find their OWN preferred approach to the writing).

Most importantly, we have learned that what we attempted can be achieved. We attempted to develop young clinicians' insight into the complexities of their practice, and to help them to articulate and explore what drives their practice. This can and does change how they structure their thinking about patients, and offers a language that they quickly come to use naturally. Despite concerns from system managers that the cost is too great, we would argue that doctors cannot afford NOT to engage with these ideas, given the way the 'invisibles' can enhance clinical thinking and improve patient safety and care.

References

Atkinson P 1995 Medical talk and medical work: the liturgy of the clinic. Sage Publications, London

Carr W 1995 For education: towards critical educational inquiry. Open University Press, Buckingham

Cox K 1999 Doctor and patient: exploring clinical thinking. University of New South Wales Press, Sydney

De Cossart L, Fish D 2005 Cultivating a thinking surgeon: new perspectives on clinical teaching, learning and assessment. tfm Publishing, Shrewsbury

De Cossart L, Fish D 2006 So just how do surgeons think? Hospital Doctor 27 April:20–21

Demar C, Doust J, Glaziou P 2006 Clinical thinking: evidence communication and decision making. Blackwell Publishing, London

Department of Health 2002 Unfinished business. Department of Health, London

Department of Health 2003 Modernising medical careers. Department of Health, London

Department of Health 2004 MMC The next steps the future shape of foundation, specialist and general practice training programmes. Department of Health, London

Dowie J, Elstein A (eds) 1988 Professional judgment: a reader in clinical decision making. Cambridge University Press, Cambridge

Downie R S, Macnaughton J 2000 Clinical judgement: evidence in practice. Oxford University Press, Oxford

Eraut M, Du Bouley P 2000 Developing the attributes of medical judgement and competence. University of Sussex, Brighton

Fish D, Coles C (eds) 1998 Developing professional judgement in health care: learning through the critical appreciation of practice. Butterworth-Heinemann, Oxford

Fish D, De Cossart L 2006 Thinking outside the (tick) box: rescuing professionalism and professional judgement. Medical Education 40(5):403–404

Fish D, De Cossart L 2007 Educating the wise practitioner: teaching, learning and assessment at the core of medicine. Royal Society of Medicine, London

Higgs J, Jones M, Edwards I et al 2004 Clinical reasoning and practice knowledge. In: Higgs J, Richardson B, Abrandt Dahlgren M (eds) Developing practice knowledge for health professionals. Butterworth-Heinemann, Edinburgh, p 181–199

Montgomery K 2005 How doctors think: clinical judgement and the practice of medicine. Oxford University Press, Oxford

Patel V L, Groen G J 1986 Knowledge-based solution strategies in medical reasoning. Cognitive Science 10:91–116

Royal College of Physicians 2005 Doctors in society: medical professionalism in a changing world. Royal College of Physicians, London

Schmidt H G, Boshuizen H P A, Norman G R 1992 Reflections on the nature of expertise in medicine. In: Keravnou E (ed) Deep models for medical knowledge engineering. Elsevier, Amsterdam, p 231–248

Schön D 1987 Educating the reflective practitioner. Jossey Bass, New York

White S, Stancombe J 2003 Clinical judgement in the health and welfare professions: extending the evidence base. Open University Press, Maidenhead

Chapter **44**

Teaching clinical reasoning and culture

Elizabeth Henley and Robyn Twible

Many countries today demonstrate cultural, ethnic and linguistic diversity, especially developed countries such as Australia, Canada, the UK and the USA where migrants or children of migrants constitute a substantial part of the population. Some developing countries such as Indonesia, India, and even Fiji and the Solomon Islands have historically been composed of diverse cultures.

In a multicultural society the provision of health care involves many interactions among people whose needs and views on what constitutes health care may differ vastly and may also differ from those of the service provider. These differences can pose problems for both provider and recipient, if care is not taken to facilitate the delivery of therapy services. An important aspect of effective multicultural interaction is consideration of the extent of similarity between people's cultures. When people from different backgrounds come together in a clinical interaction, that interaction is influenced by many cultures, and the overlap of knowledge and influence between the participants will vary from one situation to another (Fitzgerald 1992). In some cases, the amount of commonality will be great; in others, especially if the participants come from cultures with very different healthcare beliefs and healthcare delivery systems, the overlap will be much less. The less overlap there is among participants' cultures, the more challenging it will be for the therapist to effect a successful outcome within the cultural interaction.

Since therapy interactions provide the setting for many different forms of complex multicultural interactions, it is advisable for students in the health sciences to learn how to use sound clinical reasoning within cultural contexts. This chapter deals with the teaching of clinical reasoning within the context of therapy education which promotes cultural awareness, cultural sensitivity and cultural competence.

DEFINITION OF CULTURE

Everyone has a *culture* which influences all aspects of daily life. Culture should not be seen as something external to a person; rather it is an integral part of each person. As in all clinical reasoning situations, it is critical to put practice and models of practice into context. It is important therefore, in this instance, to determine a working definition of culture and what it constitutes. Culture is the learned, shared patterns of perceiving and adapting to the world which are reflected in the learned, shared beliefs, values, attitudes and behaviours characteristic of a society or population (Fitzgerald 1991). Culture is more than tradition; it is dynamic, evolving continuously.

Another important factor to be recognized is that diversity within cultures is often as great as diversity across cultures. Often there is no right or wrong answer in client–therapist interactions. Therapists need to understand that the people with whom they interact have different values, attitudes, beliefs and behaviours; if you understand your own values, attitudes and beliefs you will be more readily able to understand and respect individuals whose values, attitudes and beliefs are different from yours. Each person must be viewed from an individual perspective, and an open, sensitive reasoning process can be used to facilitate client–therapist interactions.

Before we explore the clinical reasoning process and the concept of culture, it is important to clarify the distinction between culture and concepts of ethnicity and race. *Race* refers to the biological characteristics of people, involving genetic, anatomical and structural differences (Riggar et al 1993). *Ethnicity* is distinct from race, in that ethnicity describes the characteristics of a group of people that provide the group with common markers or a sense of belonging. These markers may include

linguistic, behavioural, or environmental factors (Fitzgerald 1991).

Finally, interpreting culture in its broadest sense, we can speak of the different cultures of women and men, of youth and age, as well as the cultures of different societal groups. Then it is clear that cultural considerations should lie at the core of all clinical reasoning applications.

CULTURE AND HEALTH

The need for health professions to address issues of culture has been widely discussed in the literature (Dyck 1989, French 1992, Garan 2005, Krefting 1991, Parasyn 2005). A workshop manual (Garan 2005) which explores cultural diversity for health workers is an excellent resource for any therapist who is interested in 'mapping the development of cultural health care'. This manual provides not only useful tools (e.g. a checklist for cultural competence) but also an extensive list of contacts and valuable relevant resources (e.g. website references). Kinebanian & Stomph (1992), in describing the dilemmas of occupational therapists in the Netherlands dealing with immigrant clients, have provided guidelines to help therapists discover their own biases and adapt their services for an increasing number of clients from different cultures.

Others, such as Parasyn (2005) and Krefting (1991), have highlighted issues of culture related to physiotherapy and occupational therapy, discussing the benefits of incorporating cultural competency into clinical practice and community development activities. Cultural awareness and competency may then appropriately guide therapists towards modifying therapy interventions in ways which are sensitive to clients' needs. Fitzgerald (1992) further suggested that a lack of knowledge is often not the issue or problem, as knowledge can be gained through education. Rather, the problem lies in a lack of acknowledgment of alternative beliefs and lack of awareness of cultural differences. Fitzgerald (1992, p. 38) pointed out that 'in every clinical interaction there are at least three cultures involved: (a) the personal or familiar culture to the provider,

(b) the culture of the client or patient, and (c) the culture of the primary medical system'.

Robison (1996) devised a cultural competency index and used it to highlight some deficits among physiotherapists in their management of clients from another culture. Issues in intercultural interactions were related to the values of the therapists as well as the values of the clients, a fact that many therapists did not recognize. Interestingly, it was found that therapists from migrant backgrounds did not necessarily score more highly on Robison's cultural competency index than those from non-migrant backgrounds. Generally, therapists with a poor understanding of their own value system created problems from both client's and therapist's perspective. This poor understanding produced negative stereotyping and bias towards people from different cultural backgrounds. In addition, the therapists who expressed assimilationist, ethnocentric or dispassionate attitudes often lacked understanding and tended to display hesitancy towards treating people from different cultural backgrounds.

In summary, cultural differences in intercultural interactions have the potential to create confusion and even conflict. Unsuccessful interactions may be characterized by a lack of satisfaction with the interaction in both therapist and client. Successful intercultural interactions are characterized by mutual satisfaction, effective communication and positive therapy outcomes (Meadows 1991).

EDUCATIONAL CONSIDERATIONS

Cultural values play a significant role in influencing the reactions, beliefs and even outcomes of therapy (Robison 1996). Education about cultural issues, therefore, needs to be embedded throughout the curriculum and should permeate all aspects of the educational process. 'No one exposure alone will be adequate to ensure learner growth in terms of increased cultural awareness' (Carpio & Majumdar 1992, p. 6). It is the type and method of education that are crucial in improving competency (Carpio & Majumdar 1992, Robison 1996).

Today, all education programmes should prepare therapists to work in multicultural environments, and a primary objective of educators should be to develop cultural competency in their students and graduates. It is evident from the definition below that cultural competency is an essential ingredient of effective clinical reasoning in intercultural contexts.

Cultural competency has been defined as 'the ability of individuals to see beyond the boundaries of their own cultural interpretations, to be able to maintain objectivity when faced with individuals from cultures different from their own and be able to interpret and understand behaviours and intentions of people from other cultures non-judgementally and without bias' (Walker 1991, p. 6). The first step in developing cultural competency is recognizing and understanding the client as a person first and foremost (Robison 1996, Twible & Henley 1998). From this starting point, students should develop a compassion for their fellow human beings and a cultural attitude. Therefore educators must strive to encourage students in this behaviour, and ultimately to produce therapists with knowledge-seeking behaviours who are willing to explore their clients' *stories* or *histories*. Parasyn (2005, p. 8) described this skill as maintaining a state of 'openness, listening and sponging [absorbing], questioning and ... engaging in all that is happening around you'. Everybody should be culturally competent.

At one time or another in everyday interactions in service provision, all therapists interact with people from backgrounds that are culturally and linguistically different from their own. In an educational institution, therefore, consideration must also be given to the cultural competencies of the education providers, for they are the ones who will undoubtedly exert influence over the learning of their students. Faculty who are culturally aware are most likely to incorporate cultural content in their teaching activities and to model culturally appropriate behaviours. It is important that all educators, not just those who specialize in cultural issues, incorporate cultural awareness into their teaching. Garan (2005) provided a checklist for cultural competence that is an excellent screening tool for educators and students alike, to ensure that culturally sensitive practices and values permeate throughout the educational organization.

CULTURAL REASONING

Enhancing self-monitoring skills facilitates effective clinical reasoning (Carnevali 1995, Refshauge & Higgs 1995). One way of enhancing self-monitoring skills is for novice reasoners to systematically apply a series of questions or an organizational framework to thinking activities (see Bridge & Twible 1997 for an example). Cultural awareness, knowledge acquisition, and use of knowledge about cultures are critical elements of effective clinical reasoning and should be part of the organizational framework. Table 44.1 illustrates the interrelationships between clinical reasoning and cultural competency. Parallels exist in these processes in the tasks of problem sensing and cultural awareness, knowledge acquisition, and the use of this knowledge in reasoning and decision making as a guide for clinical intervention and behaviour.

As novice reasoners, students should be taught to consider culture routinely throughout their interactions with clients (that is, during assessment, intervention and evaluation). One educational strategy is to link culture to the existing clinical reasoning teaching, so that it pervades all aspects of the curriculum and is incorporated into all case study analyses undertaken. Factors that need to be considered include the social and cultural background of the client, the beliefs and values in the client's culture (and how they differ from the therapist's beliefs and values), as well as the limitations of the therapist and the environment in which the service is being provided (Fitzgerald et al 1995).

Table 44.1   Interrelationship between clinical reasoning and cultural competency terminology

Clinical reasoning	Cultural competency
Issue/problem sensing or noticing	Cultural awareness
Knowledge acquisition	Cultural knowledge acquisition
Making clinical decisions (e.g. issue/problem validation, treatment choices) as the basis for clinical intervention	Making cultural decisions as the basis for behaviour

In reasoning situations, novice learners often make errors because cues are missed or underpinning knowledge is absent. A means of checking current knowledge and understanding is essential, because clinical intervention should be based upon an informed judgement concerning the client's condition or potential dysfunction (Bridge & Twible 1997). In intercultural interactions, cues may be missed because the therapist does not pick up a cultural prompt (an indication that consideration of culture is particularly important) or the therapist does not have culture-specific knowledge related to the particular client.

The two most difficult areas for novices in the clinical reasoning process are 'issue/problem sensing' and 'issue/problem validation or intervening' (Neistadt 1992, Rogers & Holm 1991). Discussing the cultural clinical reasoning process, scholars (e.g. Fitzgerald et al 1996, Garan 2005, Robison 1996) describe 'cultural awareness competency' and 'knowledge competency' (cf Table 44.1). The intervening step of knowledge acquisition or cultural knowledge acquisition poses few problems for students. Students' difficulties lie firstly in recognizing the need to acquire the knowledge and secondly in applying that knowledge effectively in clinical decision making as part of the therapy process. Therefore it is imperative in curricula to address both cultural awareness and the application of cultural knowledge, in order to promote effective cultural reasoning.

Cultural awareness or issue/problem sensing

The critical factors in *cultural awareness* are acknowledgement of alternative beliefs and awareness of cultural differences. Development of this knowledge and awareness needs to be fostered in students.

Most people have beliefs about the cause of an illness, what kind of illness it is, the natural course that the illness will take, and how it should be treated. The sources we draw upon to inform us about our state of health and to explain it to others have been classed as popular, professional and traditional (Kleinman 1980). On the basis of these sources of ideas and information, different explanatory models are formed to describe or explain illness and disability. The models used by health practitioners (i.e. professional models) are frequently different from those used by their clients (i.e. lay models). It is often difficult to match the therapist's perception of a particular illness or disability with the client's understanding or experience of it. The disparity is likely to be even greater when the client and the health professional come from different cultural backgrounds. Thus, any clinical interaction can involve perspectives from multiple cultures and several systems within each culture. One of the skills that therapists regularly use to gain information regarding clients' beliefs and cultural influences is the history-taking process.

Narrative reasoning and history taking are an integral part of the therapist–client interaction. It is during history taking that the therapist actively listens to the client's story and establishes a relationship with the client. When therapists incorporate information from the affective and knowledge domains of the client's story into future clinical decisions, they set the scene for a culturally appropriate client-centred approach to service provision.

Cultural influences should routinely be considered within clinical narratives, since cultural awareness enables therapists to identify what knowledge needs to be acquired. To facilitate student learning of the cultural clinical reasoning process, case stories with a cultural component should be incorporated into undergraduate tutorial sessions; role-plays and use of critical incident methodology (Fitzgerald et al 1995) are strategies that have been used successfully. Simulation experiences, such as BaFa BaFa (Shirts 1977) and NaZa NaZa (Newfields 2001) also have been used successfully to improve cultural awareness in students; Newfields (2001) considered that the focus of 'learning-by-doing' engages learners more fully and moves them to a deeper level of cross-cultural understanding. Perhaps the greatest benefit in such simulations is that participants gain a deeper perspective of their own values and tolerance for diverse positions. Such simulation exercises do not help students to cope with all types of intercultural conflict, but do focus their ideas.

Cultural knowledge acquisition

If students perceive that their current clinical knowledge base is lacking, they usually know how to acquire the necessary knowledge from available literature. For cultural information, there are two other important sources: (a) cultural informants or brokers, and (b) clients and family members and other community members of the cultural group.

Fitzgerald et al (1995), Garan (2005) and Parasyn (2005) have provided valuable guidance to assist in the development of cultural knowledge. They have outlined key principles to consider in acquiring cultural knowledge, frameworks for exploring cultural issues relevant to individual practitioners and the client population, and have suggested guidelines for developing department policy for the treatment of clients from culturally diverse backgrounds (Box. 44.1). The therapist assimilates all available sources of knowledge, and validates the information for the current situation. Invariably, the more valid or relevant the level of knowledge invoked, the greater the confidence the therapist will have in that knowledge and the smaller the degree of uncertainty (Figure 44.1).

Using cultural knowledge appropriately, or validation of issues and problems

Cultural knowledge can be used to determine appropriate modes of communication and forms of assessment of clients when conducting observation of their performance of functional activities and physical examination. In addition, cultural knowledge informs students as they develop working hypotheses, validate assessment findings and select and implement a management programme having considered the implications, assessed the risks and determined the expected outcomes. The focus in validation of issues and problems is on the examination of discrepancies between the original clinical image and the real and gradually unfolding clinical scenario (Bridge & Twible 1997), and this validation process incorporates the application of cultural knowledge. Parasyn (2005) also strongly advocated the use of cultural brokers as critical in the successful application of community development activities. When working in countries other than their own,

Box 44.1 Key principles to consider in acquiring cultural knowledge

- Gather culturally relevant information
  - the published literature
  - cultural informants or brokers
  - clients, family members and other community members of the cultural group
- Validate that information in light of the presenting situation to avoid cultural stereotyping
- Consider the impact of therapy domains of concern and concepts, for example:
  - personal space
  - communication issues and language, especially expression of and language of emotions, cultural protocols
  - time and space
  - gender roles
  - beliefs and practices associated with health, illness, disability and healing
- Examine your own beliefs, values and attitudes
- Appreciate that interactions are part of a dynamic reciprocal process
- Find a common base from which to work
- Determine the goals from the perspective of all participants
- Select interventions that consider cultural restrictions or taboos, common practices and available resources
- Engage in continual assessment of the level and appropriateness of cultural knowledge
- Substitute joys and challenges for problems and frustrations

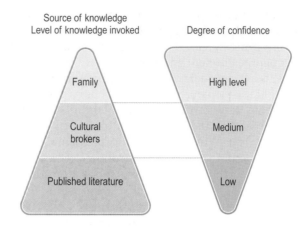

Figure 44.1 Hierarchy of knowledge sources for cultural decision making

REASONING STRATEGIES TO FACILITATE CULTURAL COMPETENCY

Workshops have been recognized as useful means of providing awareness training, since they challenge the values and biases of health workers, educators and students (Fitzgerald et al 1996, Garan 2005). Such workshops often use critical incident methodology (Brislin et al 1986, Brislin & Yoshida 1994) and explanatory models (Kleinman 1980) as reflective frameworks to identify cultural issues and to understand clients' perceptions of health, illness and service delivery. Others use checklists for cultural competence as a starting point to creating a favourable cultural environment, to ensure that all members of the organization, be they cleaners, administrative staff or health providers, are culturally aware and culturally competent (Garan 2005).

A CASE STUDY: FIELDWORK EXPERIENCE – 'OPERATION INDIA AND BEYOND'

Since 1995, students from the University of Sydney have engaged in a fieldwork programme which provides a good example of the implementation of cultural reasoning. This programme involves student fieldwork placements in community-based rehabilitation (CBR) projects in rural and

therapists often enter communities blindly; cultural brokers are an essential reference group of people who can teach the 'interloper' about the values, beliefs, norms, ways of doing, ways of thinking, ways of seeing and ways of understanding, all of which are crucial to working within the realms of community development (Twible & Henley 1998).

remote villages in southern India, Fiji, Maldives, Bangladesh and Tonga. Principal goals of the programme are to foster students' awareness of the place of cultural understanding in clinical practice and to develop their cultural competency.

In the preparatory phase, students participated in a series of workshops and other activities designed to enhance their cultural competency. During the programme a variety of activities further fostered students' cultural awareness and their capacity to engage in 'cultural reasoning'. These activities ranged from the life experiences involved in travelling to remote areas of a country quite different from their own to living in unfamiliar environments and interacting with people whose lives were culturally dissimilar to their own. In addition, the students learned a great deal about performing the tasks of clinical reasoning and clinical practice in the context of the local people's culture.

When the students were interviewed after their placements, it was apparent that the fieldwork experience highlighted for them the impact of interaction with the host country's culture on their cultural competencies. Though Lightfoot (1985) suggested that experience with diverse cultures is important, findings from our fieldwork experiences highlighted that it may be the *type* of experience that results in enhancement of aspects of cultural competency. That is, people can be exposed to cultural differences, but exposure alone does not necessarily improve one's cultural competency (Robison 1996). A cultural interaction that allows the therapists to experience different cultures positively arises from the development of skills in cultural awareness and acknowledgement of alternative beliefs.

Students reflected that in order to provide effective therapy, they had to seek knowledge specific to the host culture (from local cultural brokers) and consider the cultural factors that would have an impact on therapy. Examples of such factors included feeding activities which occurred exclusively with use of the right hand, the procedure for toileting which involved squatting, and the impact of the students' clothing on the level of respect gained from the staff and villagers. The students reported that personal values and assumptions were often in conflict with local community values concerning health care.

Interestingly, we can report that many of the physiotherapists and occupational therapists who participated in 'Operation India and beyond' experiences have continued to develop their knowledge and skills in cultural competence. Some have completed higher degrees in international health, seeking international development work through government and non-government agencies in health promotion as well as therapy-related activities (see e.g. Parasyn 2005); some have worked as youth ambassadors in developing countries (Tonga, Samoa, Solomon Islands, Sri Lanka); still others have used their cultural competency skills in working with linguistically and culturally diverse groups in Australia (Garan 2005). Many have chosen community practice as their preferred option for employment because of its culturally diverse clientele. In most situations, these therapists are used by their peers to take on the most culturally challenging and complex clients and are recognized as a 'cultural resource'.

CONCLUSION

The varied situations in which graduates work demonstrate the importance of understanding the unique nature of culture, both as a concept and as part of the reality of all of the participants involved in the processes of clinical reasoning and clinical practice. It is important to recognize that each individual presents differently and that assumptions cannot be applied to all people associated with a particular group. Clinical competencies, communication skills, cultural strategies, a culturally aware attitude and compassion are significant factors that have been identified as common across all intercultural clinical interactions, whether at home or abroad. As Robison (1996, p. 141) argued, 'when empowered with competent practices, a cultural attitude and a sense of compassion, therapists can successfully interact with people from any cultural background in any country, whether it be outback Australia or an urban hospital. For globally competent therapists, the context is not an obstacle.'

References

Bridge C E, Twible R L 1997 Clinical reasoning: informed decision making in practice. In: Christiansen C, Baum C (eds) Occupational therapy: enabling function and well being, 2nd edn. Slack, Thorofare, NJ, p 158–179

Brislin R W, Yoshida T 1994 Improving intercultural interactions: modules for cross-cultural training programs. Sage, Thousand Oaks, CA

Brislin R W, Cushner K, Cherri C et al 1986 Intercultural interactions: a practical guide. Sage, Newbury Park, CA

Carnevali D L 1995 Self-monitoring of clinical reasoning behaviours: promoting professional growth. In: Higgs J, Jones M (eds) Clinical reasoning for the health professions. Butterworth-Heinemann, Oxford, p 179–190

Carpio B A, Majumdar B 1992 Experiential learning: an approach to transcultural education for nursing. Journal of Transcultural Nursing 4(1):4–11

Dyck I 1989 The immigrant client: issues in developing culturally sensitive practice. Canadian Journal of Occupational Therapy 56(5):248–255

Fitzgerald M H 1991 The dilemma – race? ethnicity? culture? The Rehabilitation Journal 7(2):5–6

Fitzgerald M H 1992 Multicultural clinical interactions. Journal of Rehabilitation Apr/May/June:1–5

Fitzgerald M H, Mullavey-O'Byrne C, Twible R L et al 1995 Exploring cultural diversity: a workshop manual for occupational therapists. School of Occupational Therapy, University of Sydney

Fitzgerald M H, Mullavey-O'Byrne C, Clemson L et al 1996 Enhancing cultural competency: training manual. Transcultural Mental Health Centre of NSW, Sydney

French S 1992 Health care in a multi-ethnic society. Physiotherapy 78(3):174–179

Garan N 2005 Multicultural awareness resource kit: mapping the development of cultural health care. Queensland Multicultural Communities Council Gold Coast Inc, Ashmore, QLD

Kinebanian A, Stomph M 1992 Cross cultural occupational therapy: a critical reflection. American Journal of Occupational Therapy 46(8):751–757

Kleinman A 1980 Patients and healers in the context of culture. University of California Press, Berkeley, CA

Krefting L 1991 The culture concept in the everyday practice of occupational and physical therapy. Physical and Occupational Therapy in Pediatrics 11(4):1–16

Lightfoot S C 1985 The undergraduate: culture shock in the health context. Australian Occupational Therapy Journal 32:118–121

Meadows J L 1991 Multicultural communication. Physical and Occupational Therapy in Pediatrics: Quarterly Journal of Developmental Therapy 11(4):31–42

Neistadt M E 1992 The classroom as a clinic: applications for a method of teaching clinical reasoning. American Journal of Occupational Therapy 46(9):814–819

Newfields T 2001 NaZa NaZa: A classroom adaptation of a cross-cultural training simulation. Journal of Nanzan Junior College 29(Dec):107–129

Parasyn C 2005Aharenmen! Who better understands a community than those who live in it! International Conference in Engaging Communities Brisbane, QLD: August 14–17. Online. Available: http://www.engagingcommunities2005.org 28 December

Refshauge K, Higgs J 1995 Teaching clinical reasoning in health science curricula. In: Higgs H, Jones M (eds) Clinical reasoning for the health professions. Butterworth-Heinemann, Oxford, p 105–116

Riggar T F, Eckert J M, Crimando W 1993 Cultural diversity in rehabilitation: management strategies for implementing organizational pluralism. Journal of Rehabilitation Administration 17(2):53–61

Robison S 1996 Exposure and education: the impact on the cultural competency of physiotherapists. Honours thesis, School of Physiotherapy, University of Sydney

Rogers J C, Holm M B 1991 Occupational therapy diagnostic reasoning: a component of clinical reasoning. American Journal of Occupational Therapy 45(11):1045–1053

Shirts R G 1977 BaFa BaFa: a cross culture simulation. Simulation Training Systems, Del Mar, CA

Twible R L, Henley E C 1998 Field training for occupational therapy and physiotherapy students in developing countries – the India experience. ActionAid Disability News 9(1):17–21

Walker M L 1991 Rehabilitation service delivery to individuals with disabilities: a question of cultural competence. OSERS News in Print 6–11

Chapter **45**

Teaching clinical reasoning to medical students

Ann Sefton, Jill Gordon and Michael Field

Clinical reasoning is the process by which health practitioners evaluate and make decisions on the diagnosis and management of a patient. It is of particular importance when a patient presents with what has been described as an ill-structured problem (Barrows & Feltovich 1987). The development of clinical competence is dependent on increasingly refined and elaborated medical knowledge (Schmidt et al 1990) and judgement (Round 2001). The critical endpoint of the reasoning process will result in decisions, often based on exploration of a range of possibilities that may include further history, physical examination or investigation.

Both the nature of the learning (whether in traditional or in problem based programmes) and the timing of clinical experience need to be considered in helping medical students learn clinical reasoning. In addition to experiencing a particular curriculum, students are also developing within a broader framework of professionalism (Mann et al 2005). Medical students initially try to understand patients who may present with a bewildering, unsorted array of complex information (clinical, personal, social, emotional) of uncertain relevance. In the early stages, students have only limited knowledge on which to build their reasoning. They are often anxious about the appropriateness and effectiveness of their communication skills in seeking and clarifying relevant information. The challenge for teachers is to encourage the ordering and prioritizing of information based on the most cogent elements; the generation, testing and refining of hypotheses; and the formulation of clear, specific, answerable diagnostic or therapeutic questions.

What are the most appropriate strategies to achieve these aims and how are they best made explicit to students?

CLINICAL REASONING AND ITS COMPONENTS

The idea of a 'generic' form of clinical reasoning is appealing (Schuwirth 2002). However, it has been noted that clinical reasoning is both domain-specific and idiosyncratic. The challenge for medical educators is not only to make explicit the processes of reasoning (Kassirer 1989, 1995), but also to help students identify the relevant and necessary content information and efficient ways of retrieving these data.

Reasoning alone is inadequate for clinical decision making; knowledge and understanding of basic mechanisms of human function (both normal and abnormal) are essential. Basic biomedical sciences must be linked to clinical and epidemiological information. Data from several sources must be organized into coherent representations of disease processes (Boshuizen & Schmidt 1992, Schmidt et al 1990). Recently, debate has centred around the effectiveness of different methods to tie the acquisition of knowledge more securely to the development of clinical reasoning. As Round (2001) has noted, relevant perspectives include psychology, clinical psychology, clinical practice and clinical education. She questions whether teachable cognitive skills can exist independently of their context. Nendaz & Bordage (2002) also ask whether teaching reasoning separately from content can be successful.

EXPERTISE

One research approach has been to identify the components of expert diagnostic and management skills. A diagnosis often represents an explanation of an illness (Elstein 1995), implicitly emphasizing the need for mechanisms of health and disease to be understood. Although hypothetico-deductive reasoning was for years seen as the commonest form of diagnostic reasoning, it now may be considered a relatively weak conceptual approach (Coderre et al 2003). Neufeld et al (1981) suggested

that skills of practitioners and students are attributable to experience rather than to superior reasoning. Associations of symptoms and signs generate patterns that experts recognize quickly; for students, the patterns have little meaning. Increasing medical knowledge must be 'chunked' for manageability (Schuwirth 2002) and integrated into logically organized and elaborated 'pattern recognition' structures or 'illness scripts' (Schmidt et al 1990) in order to aid rapid, accurate and relevant retrieval.

Effective clinical reasoning is based on iterative information gathering, a process in which hypotheses are framed, tested, modified or discarded (Kassirer 1995). This process requires skills in communication and physical examination, as well as the selective ordering and interpretation of investigations, using the best evidence available (Sackett et al 1997).

A BROADER VIEW OF CLINICAL REASONING

Much of the research on clinical reasoning has focused on diagnosis, while management, comprising by far the greater part of patient care, has been relatively neglected. Management requires more than understanding the processes of disease, mechanisms for repair and means of alleviating symptoms. Technical expertise must be combined with a deep and empathic understanding of the patient's perspectives and needs that derives from face to face encounters requiring effective communication. Students therefore need longitudinal experiences if they are to see how the clinical reasoning process contributes to patient care over time.

Teaching needs to include a number of common elements: observations are made, and information – often disorganized and not expressed in medical terms – is collected; the data are ordered into more or less formal hypotheses based on existing medical knowledge and experience; further inquiry seeks clarification; diagnostic possibilities are identified that can be eliminated; a plan is developed for further investigation and/or immediate management. An experienced clinician often undertakes some of those processes in parallel, rather than sequentially. Given the reports of significant errors in over- or under-estimating probabilities (see Round 2001), explicit discussion of those biases with students as they gain experience could contribute to some improvement in the transfer of clinical reasoning skills.

WHAT CAN TEACHERS DO?

In teaching clinical reasoning, medical teachers must determine overall curricular goals, identify essential content and design the processes for learning which will best support the development of an effective medical professional. Not all teachers acknowledge the need to make educational strategies explicit to students, and some have little insight into inconsistencies in their own performance. However, we argue that it is *essential* to focus explicitly both on the processes of clinical reasoning itself and on the educational methods that support its development. Students need to be engaged actively as informed partners.

Structuring experience using templates and algorithms

For the novice with limited knowledge, the parallel processing and chunking of related information is restricted; some structure to information gathering is essential. Templates with rigorous steps are initially useful to ensure that essential information is not missed, but rigid adherence is inefficient in the long term. When templates or algorithms are used uncritically, students may fail to recognize priority issues and to develop appropriately structured knowledge for rapid responsiveness (Schmidt et al 1990). A recent approach to diagnostic problem representation (Nendaz & Bordage 2002) has been shown to enhance students' capacity to describe and recall problems more effectively, although interpretation was not improved. Strategies of this kind seem to be effective for students early in their clinical studies. Round (2001) notes that using algorithms – although they can be effective – is seen as too time consuming.

Reflection and feedback

Grant (1989) has encouraged students to share experiences and articulate the processes they use to work through diagnostic problems. In a supportive and safe atmosphere, her students express themselves honestly and receive specific, sensitive feedback; they also observe and model the strategies of others. Schuwirth (2002) has also stressed the essential importance of feedback. Perhaps the most significant benefit is the development of metacognitive skills so that self-aware learners identify their thinking processes and monitor their progress. The strategy may well appeal to those who are convinced of the individuality of mental processes or who question the notion of imposing a single best reasoning process.

Teaching clinical reasoning in traditional curricula

Most medical schools define a certain number of preclinical years focusing on basic sciences, and a number of clinical years where students interact with patients, illness is emphasized and clinical reasoning introduced. The transition can be difficult for a number of reasons. Students learn science by hypothetico-deductive reasoning from first principles (Niaz 1993), processes that are appropriate to the biomedical or physical sciences (Patel and Kaufman 1995). In contrast, such strategies are used by skilled medical practitioners only when problems are particularly difficult or obscure (Norman et al 1994). Students find it hard to reason backwards when confronted with patients with ambiguous symptoms and signs (Barrows & Feltovich 1987, Patel et al 1991).

When individual subjects are taught in isolation, little information is transferred between them. Thus the conceptual linkages necessary for effective clinical problem solving (Schmidt et al 1990) are not readily established. The recent information knowledge explosion within existing disciplines and the inclusion of new topics (e.g. molecular biology, intracellular signalling) has increased the overload of medical curricula, militating against the thoughtful reflection required for deep understanding. Pushed to master an increasing volume of facts, students resort to surface learning at the expense of critical analysis and thinking. When assessments value recall, students are discouraged from reasoning at all (Ramsden 2003). The resulting deficiencies hamper the later development of effective clinical reasoning when basic and clinical subjects must be interrelated.

Attempts to overcome these difficulties generally rely on the importation of basic biomedical sciences into the clinical teaching arena and the importation of clinical cases into the biomedical sciences. Some medical sciences lend themselves to presentation from the perspective of the abnormal (e.g. endocrine excess and deficiency help in understanding normal balances and controls; the function of neuroanatomical structures is illustrated by lesions). Such examples can introduce students to aspects of clinical reasoning. Since fewer medically qualified staff now teach in the early years, conceptual links between basic and clinical sciences are less accessible to the teachers and thus to the students. In traditional programmes, specific approaches to integrating clinical experiences and basic sciences include those of Coles (1990), in which basic science examinations were delayed until after the first clinical attachments, and Patel & Dauphinee (1984), in which students learned some basic science during clinical years. In both examples, students had elaborated their knowledge and were better able to retrieve and use basic information in clinical settings.

Hospital and community settings can be used to provide clinical examples of important concepts for students in early years of traditional programmes. At their best, such experiences provide not only a sense of relevance to the basic studies but also opportunities for students to see and model aspects of clinical reasoning. To be effective rather than tokenistic, however, the exposure must be well planned and students must be actively engaged rather than passive onlookers. The aims must be explicit and directly related to other concurrent learning.

Problem–based learning

Problem-based learning (PBL) appears to offer substantial advantages in the health professions. Those who introduced PBL at McMaster University included clinical thinking as a high priority (Neufeld & Barrows 1974). PBL removes the separation between basic sciences and clinical applications; students use the vocabulary of both and integrate their understanding across discipline boundaries. PBL encourages reasoning in the context of discussion of the problems (Engel 1992) with the support of a facilitator (Barrows 1983). Models of clinical reasoning are frequently used as a framework for PBL discussion (Barrows 1985, McPherson & Murphy 1997, Neame 1989), making the process more explicit. The small group tutorial provides a safe environment in which issues brought into discussion are scrutinized. Evidence suggests that the clinical reasoning skills of such students are enhanced (De Vries et al 1989, Groves et al 2002, Patel et al 1991). In some PBL schools, early clinical contacts with patients reinforce the students' learning. Further, explicit tutorials in clinical years can be designed to enhance the reasoning processes (Mandin et al 2000, Ryan et al 2004).

Content and coverage are important. If students are to develop a strong base of clinically elaborated knowledge (Patel et al 1991) or 'illness scripts' (Schmidt et al 1990), they need to be exposed to a variety of common and important clinical presentations and problems. Specialized teaching hospitals for clinical education can emphasize students' exposure to the rare, complex and life threatening. Computers can be used to track and map content, allowing teachers to demonstrate how their topic contributes to an integrated understanding of medicine (Field & Sefton 1998).

Teaching methods have been criticized in both traditional programmes (e.g. Neame 1989) and problem-based curricula (e.g. Patel et al 1991). A specific learning unit (Van Gessel et al 2003) has been shown, however, to be successful in the transition between early PBL classes and the clinical setting. Faced with an array of models of clinical reasoning, and demands from content experts, how do planners embark on a problem-based approach? We suggest that it is useful to select one model of clinical reasoning (e.g. Kassirer 1989) and base the tutorial discussion on it. The precise model is less important than its generic use as a framework to structure the flow of interaction and encourage the development of metacognitive skills. It later serves as a fallback strategy in complicated clinical situations, when Bayes' theorem or other strategies can be introduced.

Many PBL programmes are 'hybrid' in the sense of providing structured sessions which support the learning actively generated by the problems (Armstrong 1998, Sefton 1997). Not only self-direction but the processes of identifying cues and searching for associations and explanations are muted or even subverted if problems are encountered only *after* formal study of the elements. Introducing disciplines followed by cases to illustrate applications has long been a feature of some traditional programmes, whether subject-specific or more integrated. That strategy fails to exploit the power of active inquiry learning, and its effectiveness in supporting problem solving rather than stimulating interest has not been extensively reviewed and evaluated. The danger of such strategies is that they may be seen as 'optional extras', not allocated the essential time that students need for independent learning and consolidation.

Computers, evidence-based medicine and clinical reasoning

Current imperatives exert pressure on doctors to practise medicine efficiently and cost-effectively (Towle 1998). Guidelines are advocated, encouraging optimal use of resources. Patients (as well as students) now have unprecedented access to information from the internet (Carlile & Sefton 1998, Ward et al 2001). It is imperative that students learn to respond to changing expectations and pressures in using technology to support their reasoning. Thus they must frame appropriate questions, access relevant information, appraise it critically and apply the data to clinical decisions (Straus et al 2005). A variety of resources is available (www.cebm.net, www.cebm.utoronto.ca, www.ebmny.org) and essential information can be accessed to guide clinical judgment and monitor practice. The availability of large databases, library resources and other information for students as well as for practising doctors has significant implications for medical education (Coiera 1997). By encouraging a critical and evidence-based approach, access to online information is revolutionizing medical practice and decision making (Craig et al 2001), and there is evidence that the skills can be introduced very early into problem-based programmes (Carlile et al 1998) as well as during the clinical years (Zebrack 2005).

Computer programs are now being specifically designed to encourage students' diagnostic reasoning skills (Bryce et al 1998). Standardized and 'realistic' clinical situations can offer students and teachers insights into the processes of clinical thinking. A student's reasoning path through each problem can be tracked and recorded, without risking harm or embarrassment to a patient. The sequential steps are accessible to student and teacher, who can review and discuss the process in detail. Areas of strength are recognized and concerns identified, enhancing the student's metacognitive skills. Remedial assistance can be designed as needed.

LEARNING CLINICAL REASONING IN PRACTICE SETTINGS

Regardless of experiences in the early years of a medical curriculum, students quickly recognize certain fundamental differences in cognitive approach once they enter practice settings more or less fulltime. Experienced clinicians, as teachers and de facto role models, may appear to 'short circuit' the reasoning process in routine encounters with patients. Skilled clinicians use such abridged strategies in the efficient pursuit of a final diagnosis (Coderre et al 2003, Glass 1996, Kassirer 1989, Kassirer & Kopelman 1991, Newble & Cannon 1994, Ridderikhoff 1991, Round 2001). They typically establish an early context for continuing investigation and management by invoking one or more initial working diagnoses, often arrived at by the recognition of a familiar set of data from a background of extensive knowledge of clinical features and prevalence of disease. In contrast to the formal process of problem-based learning, many rules of thumb, shortcuts or 'heuristics' (Kassirer & Kopelman 1991) which are not formally taught as such are used to recognize clinical patterns. Moreover, clinicians will be observed frequently to discard, replace and revive hypotheses as data accrue, seemingly making 'intuitive' judgments on the utility of specific tests or interventions. It is not surprising that many students rethink their approach to clinical problems in acquiring this practice style. They may feel caught between the admonition to be thorough and systematic in gathering, recording and presenting clinical data on the one hand and the pressure to reach efficient but appropriate diagnostic endpoints on the other. While they are exhorted to avoid 'premature closure' in the diagnostic process, they may feel that senior practitioners do it regularly.

This dilemma in the transition to clinical settings is resolved by implementing an educational model in which the underlying basis of real world clinical reasoning is made explicit. Teaching formats used for decades in ward environments have not been successful in achieving this aim. The traditional case presentation, in which all the data concerning a patient's admission are assembled and delivered without interruption, is unlikely to lead to significant insights by any students present into how diagnostic and management decisions were made. Even less useful are fact-based 'topic tutorials' in which textbook summaries of specific diseases are presented.

Specific approaches appear to promote better acquisition of clinical reasoning. First, the structure of clinical case presentations can change so that 'iterative hypothesis testing' is modelled (Kassirer 1983). Here the student in possession of the details of the case releases only small packets of information to a group of peers, who form appropriate hypotheses and justify the need for further specific data on this basis. The clinician acts as a supportive facilitator of the interactions among the students, injecting where necessary the knowledge base or 'experience' needed to reject some directions of inquiry and reinforce others.

Second, as an extension of the basic problem-based learning approach, Ryan et al (2004) report the use of an online reasoning guide to support students who take turns to present a patient. In collaborative tutorials, this guide supports the process of reasoning and prompts students to evaluate critically their peers' and clinicians' reasoning.

A third strategy calls for more explicit use of Bayesian analysis in justifying the use of clinical and investigative data (Kassirer & Kopelman 1991, Glass 1996). Bayesian analysis is an epidemiological approach based on a theorem in probability theory named after Thomas Bayes (1702–1761). In clinical decision analysis, it is used for estimating the probability of a particular diagnosis given the appearance of some symptom, sign or test result in a specific patient (Last 1995). Although the formalities of this approach are not familiar to some practising clinicians, they make implicit use of the principles (to a greater or lesser extent) in interpreting individual items of clinical information, and in ordering diagnostic tests, based upon long familiarity with their utility and performance. Since students cannot have instant access to this experience-based behaviour pattern, they should be encouraged to seek the underlying data justifying the use of specific pieces of information for confirming or rejecting a diagnosis. To this end, basic textbooks of clinical epidemiology (Straus et al 2005) and targeted journals such as *ACP Journal Club* from the Canadian Medical Association and Evidence-based Medicine (www.evidence-basedmedicine.com) are invaluable adjuncts to appropriate training in the principles of evidence based medicine as they apply to clinical practice.

CONCLUSION

Regardless of the model of curriculum, if clinical reasoning is incorporated as an explicit goal, it is necessary to include appropriately staged teaching strategies and effective feedback to students. Students must be encouraged and rewarded by assessments which measure their development of reasoning skills as well as knowledge as they progress from novice to expert. These conclusions imply substantial commitments to communication with students and adequate staff development, so that all are aware of the values assigned to the process of clinical reasoning.

References

Armstrong E G 1998 The Harvard Medical School curriculum: a hybrid model of problem-based learning. In: Boud D, Felletti G (eds) The challenge of problem-based learning. Kogan Page, London, p 45–52

Barrows H S 1983 Problem-based, self-directed learning. Journal of the American Medical Association 250:3077–3080
Barrows H S 1985 How to design a problem-based curriculum for the preclinical years. Springer Publishing, New York

Barrows H S, Feltovich P J 1987 The clinical reasoning process. Medical Education 21:86–91

Boshuizen H P A, Schmidt H G 1992 On the role of biomedical knowledge in clinical reasoning by experts, intermediates and novices. Cognitive Science 16:153–184

Bryce D A, King N J, Graebner C F et al 1998 Evaluation of a diagnostic reasoning program (DxR): exploring student perceptions and addressing faculty concerns. Journal of Interactive Media in Education 1, http://www-jime.open.ac.uk/98/1/

Carlile S, Sefton A J 1998 Healthcare and the information age: implications for medical education. Medical Journal of Australia 168:340–343

Carlile S C, Barnet S, Sefton A J et al 1998 Medical problem-based learning supported by intranet technology: a natural student-centred approach. International Journal of Medical Informatics 50:225–233

Coderre S H, Mandin P, Harasym H et al 2003 Diagnostic reasoning strategies and diagnostic success. Medical Education 37:695–703

Coiera E 1997 Guide to medical informatics, the internet and telemedicine. Chapman and Hall, London

Coles C R 1990 Elaborated learning in undergraduate medical education. Medical Education 24:14–22

Craig J C, Irwig L M, Stockler M R 2001 Evidence-based medicine: useful tools for decision making. Medical Journal of Australia 174:248–253

De Vries M W, Schmidt H G, De Graaff E 1989 Dutch comparisons: cognitive and motivational effects of problem-based learning on medical students. In: Schmidt H G, Lipkin M Jr, De Vries M W, Greep J M (eds) New directions for medical education. Springer-Verlag, New York, p 230–238

Elstein A S 1995 Clinical reasoning in medicine. In: Higgs J, Jones M (eds) Clinical reasoning in the health professions. Butterworth-Heinemann, Oxford, p 49–59

Engel C E 1992 Not just a method but a way of learning. In: Boud D, Felletti G (eds) The challenge of problem-based learning. Kogan Page, London, p 23–33

Field M J, Sefton A J 1998 Computer-based management of content in planning a problem-based medical curriculum. Medical Education 32:163–171

Glass R D 1996 Diagnosis: a brief introduction. Oxford University Press, Melbourne

Grant J 1989 Clinical decision making: rational principles, clinical intuition or clinical thinking? In: Balla J I, Gibson M, Chang M (eds) Learning in medical school: a model for the clinical professions. Hong Kong University Press, Hong Kong, p 81–100

Groves M, Scott I, Alexander H 2002 Assessing clinical reasoning: a method to monitor its development in a PBL curriculum. Medical Teacher 24(5):507–515

Kassirer J P 1983 Teaching clinical medicine by iterative hypothesis testing: let's preach what we practice. New England Journal of Medicine 309:921–923

Kassirer J P 1989 Diagnostic reasoning. Annals of Internal Medicine 110:893–900

Kassirer J P 1995 Teaching problem-solving – how are we doing? New England Journal of Medicine 332:1507–1509

Kassirer J P, Kopelman R I 1991 Learning clinical reasoning. Williams and Wilkins, Baltimore

Last J M 1995 A dictionary of epidemiology, 3rd edn. Oxford University Press, Oxford

McPherson J, Murphy B 1997 Preparing problems for an integrated, problem-based curriculum. In: Henry R, Engel C, Byrne K (eds) Imperatives in medical education. Faculty of Medicine and Health Sciences, University of Newcastle, p 180–191

Mandin H, Jones A, Woloschuk W et al 2000 Helping students to learn to think like experts when solving clinical problems. Academic Medicine 75:1043–1045

Mann K V, Ruedy J, Millar N et al 2005 Achievement of non-cognitive goals of undergraduate medical education: perceptions of medical students, residents, faculty and other health professionals. Medical Education 39:40–48

Neame R L B 1989 Problem-based medical education: the Newcastle approach. In: Schmidt H G, Lipkin M Jr, de Vries M W, Greep J M (eds) New directions for medical education. Springer-Verlag, New York, p 112–146

Nendaz M R, Bordage G 2002 Promoting diagnostic problem representation. Medical Education 36:760–788

Neufeld V, Barrows H 1974 The McMaster philosophy: an approach to medical education. Journal of Medical Education 49:1040–1050

Neufeld V R, Norman G R, Feightner J W et al 1981 Clinical problem-solving by medical students: a cross-sectional and longitudinal analysis. Medical Education 15(5):315–322

Newble D, Cannon R 1994 A handbook for medical teachers, 3rd edn. Kluwer Academic Publishers, Bordrecht

Niaz M 1993 Problem solving in science. Journal of College Science Teaching 23:18–23

Norman G R, Trott A L, Brooks L R et al 1994 Cognitive differences in clinical reasoning related to postgraduate training. Teaching and Learning in Medicine 6:114–120

Patel V L, Dauphinee W D 1984 Return to basic sciences after clinical experience in undergraduate medical training. Medical Education 18:244–248

Patel V L, Kaufman D R 1995 Clinical reasoning and biomedical knowledge: implications for teaching. In: Higgs J, Jones M (eds) Clinical reasoning in the health professions. Butterworth-Heinemann, Oxford, p 117–128

Patel V L, Groen G J, Norman G R 1991 Effects of conventional and problem-based medical curricula on problem-solving. Academic Medicine 66:380–389

Ramsden P 2003 Learning to teach in higher education. Routledge, London

Ridderikhoff J 1991 Medical problem-solving: an exploration of strategies. Medical Education 25:196–207

Round A P 2001 Introduction to clinical reasoning. Journal of Evaluation in Clinical Practice 7:109–117

Ryan G, Dolling T, Barnet S 2004 Supporting the problem-based learning process in the clinical years: evaluation of an online clinical reasoning guide. Medical Education 38(6):638–645

Sackett D L, Richardson W S, Rosenberg W et al 1997 Evidence-based medicine: how to practice and teach EBM. Churchill Livingstone, New York

Schmidt H G, Norman G R, Boshuizen H P A 1990 A cognitive perspective on medical expertise: theory and implications. Academic Medicine 65:611–621

Schuwirth L W T 2002 Can clinical reasoning be taught or can it only be learned? Medical Education 36(8):695–696

Sefton A J 1997 From a traditional to a problem-based curriculum: estimating staff time and resources. Education for Health 10:165–178

Straus S E, Richardson W S, Glasziou P et al 2005 Evidence-based medicine: how to practice and teach EBM, 3rd edn. Churchill Livingstone, Edinburgh

Towle A 1998 Changes in health care and continuing medical education for the 21st century. British Medical Journal 316:301–304

Van Gessel E, Nendaz M R, Vermeurlen B et al 2003 Development of clinical reasoning from the basic sciences to the clerkships: a longitudinal assessment of medical students' needs and self-perception after a transitional learning unit. Medical Education 37:966–974

Ward J P T, Gordon J, Field M J et al 2001 Communication and information technology in medical education. Lancet 357:792–796

Zebrack J R, Anderson R C, Torre D 2005 Enhancing EBM skills using goal setting and peer teaching. Medical Education 39:513–514

Chapter 46

Using case reports to teach clinical reasoning

Darren A. Rivett and Mark A. Jones

CHAPTER CONTENTS

Case-based learning has traditionally been a key element in the education of health professionals. The case conference and written case reports were used in medicine to teach students and share clinical experiences with colleagues long before the advent of most if not all of the allied health professions. In the last few decades clinical cases have formed the focus of problem-based learning (PBL) curricula in medicine, physiotherapy, occupational therapy and other health professional entry level programmes (Barrows & Tamblyn 1980). The shift to PBL and various other case-based modes of education has maintained the high profile of the humble case report and kept it on the educational 'centre stage', largely in recognition of the pivotal role of clinical reasoning in the development of clinical competence and the critical role of the case report in fostering reasoning skills (Cockburn & Polatajko 2004, Rivett & Jones 2004). Skills in clinical reasoning can only be developed in the context of clinical cases, and case reports are an invaluable means of promoting the acquisition of such skills (McKenzie 2000). Students perceive the immediate relevance of case-based learning to clinical practice, thus stimulating their interest and motivation for deep learning and advanced reasoning (Sandstrom 2006).

In contrast, the present paradigm of evidence-based practice (EBP) has seen the relegation of the clinical case as a research tool and the ascension of what is arguably an unhealthy obsession with randomized controlled trials (RCTs) and systematic reviews (see Smith & Pell 2003 for a witty and provocative criticism of the latter). Although the latter types of studies are commonly regarded as higher and case reports and case series as lower in the hierarchy of evidence (Sackett et al 2000), it should be considered that all types of evidence and study design have their individual strengths and weaknesses. Case reports may have limited generalizability, but RCTs are further removed from the individual and clinical reality. Jenicek (1999) noted that although case reports may represent one of the lower levels of evidence, they often constitute the first line of evidence. Importantly, case reports suggest areas for future research and can therefore be viewed as a form of communication from clinician to researcher (Domholdt 2005), in addition to providing some justification for resources for higher-level research. Accordingly there has been an impassioned call in the journals of several disciplines to retain case reports and to recognize that their strengths help compensate for the weaknesses of RCTs (and vice versa); that is, case reports and RCTs are complementary forms of evidence (Ellis & Adams 1997, Farmer 1999, Himmelhoch 2003, Rothstein 1993, Vandenbroucke 2001). Farmer asserted that 'while the anecdote cannot be used to derive general principles neither do the rules derived from averaged group observations have meaning at an individual level' (p. 93).

There is a real temptation for clinicians to abrogate their responsibilities to individual patients by uncritically adopting clinical guidelines or protocols derived from the results of RCTs and systematic reviews, without having first determined whether the recommended course of management is appropriate for an individual patient, the unique presentation and the clinical context (Jones et al 2006). Case reports or series have the advantage over RCTs of providing a detailed description of the patient(s) and their clinical presentation, enabling clinicians to determine the similarity of their actual patient's features with those described in the case(s), and thus providing a form of 'individualized evidence' for that patient's management decisions. It should be noted that Sackett et al (2000) described EBP as the integration of best research evidence (basic science and patient-centred clinical research) with clinical expertise and patient values. Without clinical expertise, which in turn depends on clinical reasoning ability,

EBP becomes nothing more than an exercise in cookbook, recipe-driven health care (Jones et al 2006).

DEFINING THE CASE REPORT

The case report can commonly be found in professional journals or texts under a variety of titles including case history, diagnostic dilemma, clinical notes, clinical problems and treatment report. A case report is defined as 'systematic documentation of a well-defined unit: usually a description of an episode of care for an individual, but sometimes an administrative, educational, or other unit' (Domholdt 2005, p. 149). More simply, it is a reflective, insightful and detailed description of clinical practice. Cases that share common features constitute a case series.

The terms *case report* and *case study* are often used interchangeably. However, many authors differentiate between them. The case study is actually a qualitative research design used to describe and analyse the uniqueness and complexity of a case within its various contexts (Domholdt 2005). For example, Jensen et al (1999) chose the case study design to investigate expert physical therapy practice, in particular the clinical reasoning of clinical experts. To a greater degree than with case reports, case studies provide a rich and substantial description of the matter under study, generally until saturation has been achieved (Jensen et al 1999).

Case reports should also be clearly differentiated from the single-case experimental design study. With the single-case design, a prospective detailed description is provided of a single case or series of similar cases in which a relationship between measurable outcomes and a treatment intervention is investigated. Usually this is undertaken using an AB or an ABAB design in which A represents a baseline or non-treatment phase and B represents the treatment phase (Hicks 2004). The design uses a systematic process of introduction and withdrawal of an intervention to evaluate its effects in a controlled manner (Domholdt 2005). This process potentially provides a means to determine whether any observed clinical changes are the result of the treatment or of natural resolution. As a research tool, the single-case design has the advantage of focusing on individual(s) and their unique clinical presentation, although its predictive power is limited beyond the individual(s) described. It is therefore more controlled (as subjects act as their own control) and more systematic than a case report and is not retrospective in nature, although occasionally a case report may actually incorporate a single-case design study.

Case reports can have several aims (Hennekens & Buring 1987):

- communicating new clinical concepts or procedures, or challenge existing theories
- flagging unusual clinical presentations (e.g. acquired immunodeficiency syndrome (AIDS) and Alzheimer's disease were first described in case reports (Farmer 1999, Hennekens & Buring 1987)).
- describing and providing preliminary research evidence for new clinical tests or treatment interventions, including adverse and beneficial effects
- acting as a vehicle for professional development
- fostering in both students and clinicians the development of clinical reasoning skills such as pattern recognition.

The last point is critical for the development of clinical reasoning skills. Case reports provide a valuable resource for teaching and learning skills in clinical reasoning and critical analysis (Tichenor et al 1995), and in particular for helping students build cognitive schemata or clinical patterns (Prion 2000). The use of the case report in learning 'accelerates acquisition of the pattern-rich, situation-specific and readily recallable heuristic knowledge of experienced clinicians' (Scott 2000, p. 291). The remainder of this chapter focuses on this latter role of case reports in their various forms.

ADVANTAGES OF THE CASE REPORT

Case reports have many attributes that naturally fit the teaching of skills in clinical reasoning. A clearly described and well designed case report provides an integrative learning opportunity in the context of the clinical problem: biological sciences, behavioural and social sciences, professional knowledge, ethical issues and context-specific problems can all be incorporated in the learning experience. A case report can be an accurate description of a real-life clinical encounter, or it can be somewhat contrived or designed to bring about a particular learning outcome.

The best case reports require active participation and engagement of the learner, with some inclusion of prompts to facilitate self-directed learning (Lawrence 1998). This typically involves activities such as responding to questions strategically located throughout the text. Questions can be designed to elicit students' clinical reasoning at a particular stage of the unfolding case, prior to the author's reasoning becoming evident (see Jones & Rivett 2004 and Spencer 1998 for examples). They may also require students to pause, consult a reference source, peer or mentor, in order to answer knowledge-based questions and to permit the clinical reasoning process to proceed using the newly acquired knowledge, while promoting self-directed learning. In addition, visual or auditory cues (e.g. referral letters, X-rays, auscultatory sounds or photographs) requiring active interpretation can be introduced at appropriate points in the recounting of the case. Such activities can of course be undertaken individually or in the small group learning situation in which peer support and reciprocal learning help promote clinical reasoning skill acquisition, akin to PBL in small groups (Ladyshewsky et al 2000a). In the group learning situation the stimulated discussion may require students to put forward and defend their clinical reasoning about a particular case. They can also learn from their teacher upon articulation of the teacher's thinking processes, and upon modelling of exemplary clinical reasoning behaviours (Prion 2000).

The best case reports are based on authentic cases, ensuring that students are exposed to experiences they will likely encounter in clinical practice and providing a richness of interpersonal and contextual detail (Cox 2001, Lysaght & Bent 2005). Case reports offer a number of advantages compared to using real patients (Barrows & Tamblyn 1980). These advantages, although not applicable to all case report formats, can be summarized as follows:

- The level of complexity and the nature or focus of the case can be tailored and progressed for the stage and learning needs of the student.

- All students are exposed to the same predetermined learning experiences with pre-selected clinical presentations, whereas real cases are somewhat unpredictable.
- Ready availability facilitates self-paced and self-directed learning, as well as flexibility of learning, i.e. case reports are available on demand and are portable.
- Reviewing of the case can be undertaken on multiple occasions until mastery is achieved.
- Accompanying resources can be provided or referenced to enhance the learning potential of the case.
- There is no risk to the patient or the student; that is, it is a safe learning environment where errors can be made with minimal consequences.
- Feedback is immediately available.
- Case reports help to prepare and instil confidence in the student for the real-life clinical setting.

DISADVANTAGES OF THE CASE REPORT

Although there are many benefits to using case reports in promoting the learning of clinical reasoning skills, there are some limitations to the various formats of case reports (Barrows & Tamblyn 1980). These limitations are lessened when the case and its format more closely approximate or simulate real-life clinical practice. The traditional written case report in particular suffers from several limitations, including:

- realism is compromised
- clinical assessment skills may not be challenged
- information may only be provided via text and so certain cues may be absent (e.g. verbal intonation, facial expressions, responses to palpatory tests)
- the clinical reasoning of the author may inhibit the thinking and decision-making of the student and limit the information available in the case
- the consequences of a student's clinical reasoning and related actions cannot be evaluated unless they coincide with those of the author.

The use of other formats for case reports helps to overcome some of these limitations.

FORMATS OF CASE REPORTS

The traditional narrative report at the back of a professional journal has been the typical format of a case report. However, formats for case reports have evolved over recent times, particularly in response to case-based curricula and as new technologies have become available. Nevertheless, all types of case reports have the potential to foster the development of cognitive and metacognitive clinical skills (awareness and monitoring of one's thinking and learning processes (Jensen & Shepard 2002)), including the identification and correction of errors of reasoning and gaps in knowledge. Case report formats range from simple written paper cases to challenging simulated patients. At present there is little or no evidence to suggest that the choice of format used to present cases has any significant influence on the attainment of clinical reasoning learning objectives by students (Lysaght & Bent 2005). It would therefore be desirable to use a variety of case formats to cater for different student learning preferences (e.g. visual versus auditory learners) and to avoid staleness of learning experiences due to format repetition.

WRITTEN CASE REPORTS

Written case reports can provide a detailed real-life description of an actual clinical experience. Depending on the aim, written case reports may or may not include a description of the thought processes of the clinician either during or at the end of the case. Students striving to improve their clinical reasoning may benefit from being exposed to the written description of an expert clinician's ongoing reasoning processes in relation to a particular case. However, students may also benefit from the delayed provision of such information until they have had the opportunity to read and consider the essential clinical data themselves, thus affording an opportunity to compare their thoughts and interpretations to those of the expert clinician, effectively a form of delayed feedback. In some cases it may be possible to provide clinical information serially or sequentially rather than all at once, enabling students to interpret each piece of data in the light of previous findings (and before receiving the next) and to decide on the appropriate next action, whether it be an inquiry strategy or a treatment intervention. Moreover, questions designed to promote reflective inquiry and meta-cognitive skill development can be interspersed among the clinical data (see Jones & Rivett 2004 for examples).

Written case reports are inexpensive, readily available and easily accessible, and can be used as an individual learning tool or in a group-learning situation (e.g. in a journal club). Students can use written case reports whenever and wherever they desire, and can seek assistance from the literature or from colleagues at any stage in relation to the case.

For practising clinicians, writing up and perhaps publishing a case report fosters reflective inquiry and thus the advancement of their clinical reasoning skills. Swisher & Page (2005) noted that writing a case report provides an opportunity for clinicians to examine and reflect on their clinical observations and reasoning, share their work with others, and contribute to improved patient care and professional knowledge. As Jensen & Shepard (2002, p. 110) highlighted, 'reflection is the element that turns experience into learning'. Regrettably, some journals no longer publish case reports, considering them to represent low-level evidence in the EBP paradigm. Such a decision ignores the other benefits of published case reports, most notably their contribution to the development of clinical reasoning skills and the related critical role of clinical expertise in implementing the scientific evidence (Jones et al 2006, Sackett et al 2000). The potential case report author is referred to McEwen (2001) for a step-by-step procedure on writing a case report.

ORAL CASE REPORTS

Case reports can also be disseminated in oral format at professional conferences or in-service seminars. In a similar manner to written case reports in journals or texts, oral case report presentations can describe the reasoning process of the clinician either as the case unfolds or at its conclusion. Slides or overhead transparencies can be used progressively to unveil the clinical findings and subsequent actions, and to prompt the audience to engage with the case using stimulatory questions.

A novel means of using case reports in a group situation is the *fish-bowl* learning format. This is described in detail elsewhere (Carr et al 2000, Higgs 1990), but essentially it involves a panel comprised of two parts mediated by an intervening moderator. One part of the panel consists of several students who together act as the clinician by attempting to reason their way through a presented clinical case. The other part consists of several experts, both clinical and from underpinning disciplines or other relevant professions (e.g. physiology, law). The case itself is presented by other students who role-play the patient (and sometimes carer) for the interview and progressively provide the results of physical tests and responses to treatment on overhead transparency or slide. The case is based on a real patient seen by the presenting students in the clinical setting, although a fictitious case can be used if necessary. The moderator helps to ensure that the session reaches its learning goals in a timely fashion.

The fish-bowl format permits multiple viewpoints to be shared, as students and expert clinicians each describe their reasoning processes and justify their decisions, as well as through challenging the reasoning of other participants. The students may benefit from being exposed to clinical experts modelling appropriate clinical reasoning behaviour, either as they 'think aloud' during the problem-solving process or upon reflection. The expert clinicians can also provide immediate constructive feedback to students on their evolving clinical reasoning processes and associated decisions as the case unfolds. In this way, the clinical reasoning of both experts and students is made explicit. In addition, the students presenting the case benefit from detailed reflection upon their real-life clinical experience.

AUDIOVISUALLY RECORDED CASE REPORTS

The use of a videotaped recording of an actual clinical experience, whether partial (e.g. patient interview) or more complete, has several additional advantages to paper-based case reports. In addition to the interaction between clinician and patient, the recording can include interviews with the clinician, who recalls significant moments and reflects upon clinical reasoning at key junctures in the unfolding case (for an example see the DVD by Sexton et al 2005). Videotaped patient encounters can be paused at critical points during playback to enable the teacher to highlight examples of clinical reasoning behaviour as they pertain to the clinical case. These may include pivotal points in decision making or errors in reasoning or data elicitation (Scott 2000). Text captions can be included to help overcome any speech interpretation problems.

COMPUTER–BASED CASE REPORTS

By combining several media (e.g. text, audio, video, graphics and photographs) with the facility of programming varying responses depending on inputted decisions, computers have dramatically opened up the possibilities available to contribute to the development of clinical reasoning skills. Case reports can be accessed in CD-ROM format or via the internet. This medium promotes student interactivity with the case report, arguably producing a learning experience more similar to that of a health professional with an actual patient than the earlier formats of case reports.

The greatest advantage of computer-based case reports is that case information can be selected by users in a non-linear fashion (i.e. they can navigate at will, as in the clinical setting), with responses to interrogative questions or to physical tests immediately available. Web-based case reports can also be linked to other resources (e.g. online journal articles, virtual discussion groups) and CD-based case reports can be accompanied by additional resources (e.g. relevant anatomical or histological images, copies of self-report questionnaires). In addition, questions (and answers) pertaining to the case may be embedded at key points to test and improve content knowledge and understanding of the case presentation, thereby expanding the reality and versatility of the modified essay question case report assessment sometimes used in health science education (Newble et al 2000). A score indicative of the student's performance in managing the case, as well as from answering any related interpretive or content-specific

questions, can be produced unobtrusively during the learning exercise to provide further feedback (McGrath et al 2001).

There is some evidence that computer-based case learning is well received by students and at the very least produces learning outcomes comparable to alternative methods (Kraemer et al 2005, Sakowski et al 2001, Schneiders & Rivett 2000). However, it can have the disadvantage of cueing the student if only a limited range of navigational options is provided. This case report format also requires access to a modern computer (and possibly a high-speed internet connection) and a degree of technical sophistication. At present there are not many case-based programmes available for non-medical health professionals, probably due to the high cost and substantial time required for production.

SIMULATED CASE REPORTS

The simulated (or standardized) patient is a form of case report that overcomes many of the limitations of the basic written case report. Actors can be trained to simulate almost any real-life clinical scenario or actual patient case required for learning, with varying degrees of complexity, and produce a high level of clinical realism and acceptable performance reliability (Ladyshewsky et al 2000b, 2000c). This case format is flexible in that the simulated patient can be assessed by a student, a small group of students or by the teacher modelling clinical reasoning skills. However, care must be taken to provide the actor with no more information than a lay person would normally understand or know, to help ensure realism of performance.

There are many advantages to using simulated patients. First, they are available as required, and all findings about the clinical presentation are known in advance to the teacher, thus ensuring that each student receives a standardized learning experience. Second, in addition to clinical reasoning skills, various non-reasoning skills can be developed, including interviewing, counselling and physical examination protocols. Third, simulated patients can tolerate repeated examination by students (Barrows & Tamblyn 1980) and 'time-out' can be called by the student or the teacher to permit discussion and reflection without any limitation. Fourth, many ethical and safety concerns entailed in using real patients for learning are overcome by the use of simulated patients. Finally, students receives immediate, real-time feedback as to the consequences of their clinical decisions and actions, during both assessment and treatment. In addition, the actor can provide further objective feedback to students, especially regarding interpersonal and manual handling skills.

Although a simulated patient can provide a high degree of case replication, significant time and money are required to script the case and train the actor. Some physical findings cannot be simulated by actors, nor can some tests and treatments be safely performed, somewhat limiting the scope of problems and procedures available to be simulated. High fidelity computerized mannequins and other such simulation training devices can to some extent compensate for these limitations, and thus these two types of simulation can be used in a complementary manner. That is, mannequins and other electromechanical simulators can in some cases mimic certain physiological features that cannot be realistically portrayed by simulated patients.

Alternatively, a student can role-play a patient recently encountered in the clinic to another student (or group of students) acting as the clinician. This format has the advantage of not requiring any scripting, training or additional resources, but is patently a less realistic scenario to the examining student than using an unknown actor.

CONCLUSION

Clinical reasoning is an essential skill on the road to clinical expertise, but it requires deliberate cultivation and regular attention. While real-life clinical practice is critical for the development of reasoning skills and the organization of a sound knowledge base, the case report can also be used successfully to achieve this end. Although case reports have many roles, the promotion of learning in the clinical context remains paramount and undiminished in the EBP paradigm. There is a growing variety of formats available for student interaction with a case report, each bringing advantages and disadvantages to the learning experience while helping ensure that individual student learning needs are met. Thus the case report can be viewed as a uniquely valuable and complementary learning tool to traditional clinical education in the advancement of clinical reasoning skills in students.

References

Barrows H S, Tamblyn R M 1980 Problem-based learning: an approach to medical education. Springer, New York

Carr J, Jones M, Higgs J 2000 Learning reasoning in physiotherapy programs. In: Higgs J, Jones M (eds) Clinical reasoning in the health professions, 2nd edn. Butterworth-Heinemann, Oxford, p 198–204

Cockburn L, Polatajko H 2004 Using the divergent case method. Medical Education 38:550–551

Cox K 2001 Stories as case knowledge: case knowledge as stories. Medical Education 35:862–866

Domholdt E 2005 Rehabilitation research: principles and applications, 3rd edn. Elsevier Saunders, St Louis

Ellis S J, Adams R F 1997 The cult of the double-blind placebo-controlled trial. British Journal of Clinical Practice 51:36–39

Farmer A 1999 The demise of the published case report – is resuscitation necessary? British Journal of Psychiatry 174:93–94

Hennekens C H, Buring J E 1987 Epidemiology in medicine. Little Brown, Boston

Hicks C 2004 Research methods for clinical therapists: applied project design and analysis, 4th edn. Churchill Livingstone, Edinburgh

Higgs J 1990 Fostering the acquisition of clinical reasoning skills. New Zealand Journal of Physiotherapy 18:13–17

Himmelhoch J M 2003 On the usefulness of case studies. Bipolar Disorders 5:69–71

Jenicek M 1999 Clinical case reporting in evidence-based medicine. Butterworth-Heinemann, Oxford

Jensen G M, Shepard K F 2002 Techniques for teaching and evaluating students in academic settings. In: Shepard K F, Jensen G M (eds) Handbook of teaching for physical therapists, 2nd edn. Butterworth-Heinemann, Boston, p 71–126

Jensen G M, Gwyer J, Hack L M et al 1999 Expertise in physical therapy practice. Butterworth-Heinemann, Boston

Jones M A, Rivett D A 2004 Clinical reasoning for manual therapists. Butterworth Heinemann, Edinburgh

Jones M, Grimmer K, Edwards I et al 2006 Challenges in applying best evidence to physiotherapy. Internet Journal of Allied Health Sciences and Practice 4(3):Online.http://ijahsp.nova.edu/articles/vol4num3/jones.htm 12 January 2007

Kraemer D, Reimer S, Hörnlein A et al 2005 Evaluation of a novel case-based training program (d3web.Train) in hematology. Annals of Hematology 84:823–829

Ladyshewsky R, Baker R, Jones M 2000a Peer coaching to generate clinical-reasoning skills. In: Higgs J, Jones M (eds) Clinical reasoning in the health professions, 2nd edn. Butterworth-Heinemann, Oxford, p 283–289

Ladyshewsky R, Baker R, Jones M et al 2000b Reliability and validity of an extended simulated patient case: a tool for evaluation and research in physiotherapy. Physiotherapy Theory and Practice 16:15–25

Ladyshewsky R, Jones M, Baker R et al 2000c Evaluating clinical performance in physical therapy with simulated patients. Journal of Physical Therapy Education 14: 31–37

Lawrence D J 1998 Foreword. In: Spencer P (ed) Case studies for manual therapy: a problem-based approach. Churchill Livingstone, New York, p vii–viii

Lysaght R, Bent M 2005 A comparative analysis of case presentation modalities used in clinical reasoning coursework in occupational therapy. American Journal of Occupational Therapy 59(3):314–324

McEwen I 2001 Writing case reports: a how-to manual for clinicians, 2nd edn. American Physical Therapy Association, Alexandria, VA

McGrath D, Maulitz R, Baldwin C D 2001 An active learning framework that delivers clinical education case studies on the web. Academic Medicine 76:548

McKenzie L 2000 Teaching clinical reasoning in clinical education: orthoptics. In: Higgs J, Jones M (eds) Clinical reasoning in the health professions, 2nd edn. Butterworth-Heinemann, Oxford, p 270–275

Newble D, Norman G, Vleuten C 2000 Assessing clinical reasoning. In: Higgs J, Jones M (eds) Clinical reasoning in the health professions, 2nd edn. Butterworth-Heinemann, Oxford, p 156–168

Prion S 2000 The case study as an instructional method to teach clinical reasoning. In: Higgs J, Jones M (eds) Clinical reasoning in the health professions, 2nd edn. Butterworth-Heinemann, Oxford, p 174–183

Rivett D A, Jones M A 2004 Improving clinical reasoning in manual therapy. In: Jones M A, Rivett D A (eds) Clinical reasoning for manual therapists. Butterworth-Heinemann, Edinburgh, p 403–431

Rothstein J M 1993 The case for case reports (editor's note). Physical Therapy 73:492–493

Sackett D L, Straus S E, Richardson W S et al 2000 Evidence-based medicine: how to practice and teach EBM, 2nd edn. Churchill Livingstone, Edinburgh

Sakowski H A, Rich E C, Turner P D 2001 Web-based case simulations for a primary care clerkship. Academic Medicine 76:547

Sandstrom S 2006 Use of case studies to teach diabetes and other chronic illnesses to nursing students. Journal of Nursing Education 45:229–232

Schneiders A G, Rivett D 2000 Evaluation of a computer assisted learning (CAL) program for clinical reasoning in manipulative physiotherapy. In: Singer K P (ed) Proceedings of the International Federation of Orthopaedic and Manipulative Therapists conference. International Federation of Orthopaedic and Manipulative Therapists, Perth, p 395–399

Scott I 2000 Teaching clinical reasoning: a case-based approach. In: Higgs J, Jones M (eds) Clinical reasoning in the health professions, 2nd edn. Butterworth-Heinemann, Oxford, p 290–297

Sexton M, French H, McCreesh K et al 2005 Fundamental techniques of physiotherapy examination and treatment of the lumbar spine. DVD. Clinics in Motion, Dublin

Smith G C S, Pell J P 2003 Parachute use to prevent death and major trauma related to gravitational challenge: systematic review of randomised controlled trials. British Medical Journal 327:1459–1461

Spencer P 1998 Case studies for manual therapy: a problem-based approach. Churchill Livingstone, New York

Swisher L L, Page C G 2005 Professionalism in physical therapy. History, practice and development. Elsevier Saunders, St Louis

Tichenor C J, Davidson J, Jensen G M 1995 Cases as shared inquiry: model for clinical reasoning. Journal of Physical Therapy Education 9(2):57–62

Vandenbroucke J P 2001 In defense of case reports and case series. Annals of Internal Medicine 134:330–334

Chapter 47

Using mind mapping to improve students' metacognition

Mary Cahill and Marsha Fonteyn

This chapter introduces a teaching strategy known as mind mapping and examines its relationship to critical thinking and metacognition. We demonstrate how this strategy can improve the way your students think and learn, and present a pilot study examining the use of mind mapping as a tool to improve the metacognitive skills of nursing students.

A mind map or concept map is a graphic representation of information or the thought processes of an individual (Buzan & Buzan 1996, Novak & Gowin 1984). There are several approaches to teaching students how to build mind maps. In some instances, especially in natural science education, a group of related words or concepts is presented to the student accompanied by a lecture and the students are then asked to create a mind map. The concepts or words are connected with arrows and sometimes there are words along the arrows such as 'leads to', 'causes', 'is related to', 'becomes', 'is needed for' (Jegede et al 1990, Novak 1990, Okebukola & Jegede 1989). In other instances, an idea or a concept is placed centrally on a piece of paper and students participate in an activity similar to brainstorming, making multiple outward connections from that central point to elucidate how ideas or concepts are related (Dorough & Rye 1997, Novak & Gowin 1984, Regis et al 1996).

We were particularly interested in whether mind mapping could improve the critical thinking and metacognitive abilities of nursing students. The importance of teaching nursing students critical thinking skills, and the applicability of critical thinking to the generation of clinical decisions resulting in favourable patient outcomes, have been documented in the nursing literature (Alexander & Giguere 1996, Baker 1996, Conger & Mezza 1996, Degazon & Lunney 1995, Fonteyn 1995, Oermann 1997, Whiteside 1997). Degazon & Lunney (p. 271) refer to critical thinking as a 'multidimensional cognitive and perceptual process, including intuition, that involves reflective thought for decision making'. They assert that critical thinking is correlated with nursing competence, and that in order to advance to higher levels of clinical competence, ever increasing and sharpened critical thinking skills are needed. Alexander & Giguere (p. 16) maintain that the development of critical thinking skills in nursing education fosters 'therapeutic nursing interventions that promote the health of the whole individual'; they define critical thinking as an 'analytic process addressing not only problem solving but also the ability to raise pertinent questions and critique solutions'.

Teaching of a purely linear, reductionist type of reasoning style provides nursing students with only some of the skills they will need to arrive at prudent clinical decisions. Critical thinking allows decisions to be made through a more reflective and multidimensional thinking process. Students are thus provided with the skills necessary to weigh the importance and relevance of large amounts of data, consider alternatives and options, and ultimately arrive at sound and logical decisions (Baker 1996, Degazon & Lunney 1995, Oermann 1997). Fonteyn (1995, p. 60) views critical thinking and clinical reasoning as the essence of nursing practice, stating that 'it is intrinsic to all aspects of care provision, and its importance pervades nursing education, research and practice'. She stresses the need for the teaching of critical thinking in nursing curricula, in order to produce graduate nurses with the skills necessary to function effectively and competently in the ever-changing, demanding and increasingly complex healthcare setting.

A closely aligned concept, often equated with critical thinking, is metacognition. This term 'refers to an awareness of our own cognitive processes (thinking and learning abilities) or knowing about what we know' (Gordon & Braun 1985, p. 2). 'Metacognition, broadly speaking, is identified as that body of knowledge and understanding that reflects on cognition itself. Put another way, metacognition is that mental activity for which other states or processes become the object of reflection. Thus, metacognition is sometimes referred to as thoughts about cognition, or thinking about thinking' (Yussen 1985, p. 253).

The educational psychologists Gavelek & Raphael (1985), in their investigation of metacognitive processes, described two critical areas of learning where metacognition plays a key role. The first area relates to the active role of learners in guiding their own learning processes. It is metacognitive self-knowledge which enables students to function as independent learners. The second area in which metacognition plays a key role is in the concept of transfer. Metacognition is the central way in which learners are able to apply, consider, modify and reflect upon cognitive activity across varying tasks. Indeed, it is this process which allows learners to gain a deeper understanding and awareness of the interactive nature of the learning process. Degazon & Lunney (1995, p. 271) define metacognition as 'the ability to recognise, analyse and discuss thinking processes', and suggest that as learners increasingly focus on their thinking processes, their metacognitive abilities likewise improve. They state that due to the nature of metacognition as a tool for self-modification, development of this skill 'provides a basis for growth as a thinking professional' (p. 272).

Many of the tenets of mind mapping find their roots in Ausubelian (Ausubel 1963) learning theory. According to this theory, human thinking and understanding are based not only on understanding concepts, but also on understanding the relationships between concepts. In other words, concepts do not exist in isolation, but rather depend on others for meaning. Ausubel distinguished between rote learning and meaningful learning. Meaningful learning occurs when learners take new concepts and incorporate or relate them to concepts or knowledge structures already possessed. Thus learners can widen and enhance their existing knowledge domains. Rote learning, on the other hand, involves an arbitrary assignment of new concepts or knowledge into the present cognitive structure, without consideration of how this new knowledge may relate to, enhance or advance the learner's existing cognitive structure.

Okebukola & Jegede (1988, p. 490) contended that concept mapping is an effective way to attain meaningful learning because 'each concept depends upon its relationships to many others for meaning'. Heinze-Fry & Novak (1990) compared students who learn meaningfully to those who employ rote learning. They argued, 'in contrast to students who learn by rote, students who employ meaningful learning are expected to retain knowledge over an extensive time span and find new, related learning progressively easier' (p. 463).

Proponents of the mind map as an educational aid point to the similarities between the radiant, associative nature of the brain and the graphic representation of knowledge through a mind map. Buzan & Buzan (1996) describe the highly complex biochemical pathways and architecture of the brain, asserting that the internal brain pathways function associatively and radiantly, and that any outward expression of this internal structure, such as mind mapping, serves to enhance creativity, learning and higher orders of thinking. They suggest that association is one of the major ways to improve memory and creativity, and that 'it is the integrating device our brains use to make sense of our physical experience, the key to human memory and understanding' (p. 100). They discuss the inadequacies of traditional note taking as a means to learn, organize and create, saying that 'by its very nature, the linear presentation of standard notes prevents the brain from making associations, thus counteracting creativity and memory' (p. 50).

Learning theorists Novak & Gowin (1984), in their classic text *Learning How to Learn*, encouraged the use of mind mapping as a way of representing relationships between concepts. These authors maintained that the best way to help students to learn meaningfully is to allow them to see explicitly the nature of the relationships between concepts as they exist within and outside their minds. They pointed to the mind map as a means of externalizing relationships and connections between concepts and ideas. They described the mind map as a 'visual road map showing some of the pathways we may take to connect meanings of concepts' (p. 15). Additionally, Novak & Gowin asserted that in the process of drawing mind maps, new relationships and new

meanings between concepts may arise or become evident in ways that were not readily apparent prior to construction of the mind map.

A large body of research has emerged from the science education field, examining the efficacy of mind mapping as an educational tool. Findings indicate that mind mapping increases achievement, decreases perceived anxiety and promotes meaningful learning. Regis et al (1996, p. 1088) reported positive outcomes from using the mind map as a 'metacognitive tool to help chemistry teachers and learners to improve teaching and learning'. Barenholz & Tamir (1992) compared learning and achievement outcomes for 'mappers' vs. 'non mappers' in a high school microbiology programme. They found that post-test scores compared with pre-test scores were higher for those in the 'mapping' group. Jegede et al (1990) investigated the usefulness of mind mapping as a means of decreasing student anxiety and increasing achievement in biology. Based on pre- and post-test scores on both achievement and anxiety scales, mind mapping, as compared to traditional instruction, was found to enhance learning and decrease anxiety within the context of biology study.

Heinze-Fry & Novak (1990) found that meaningful learning was enhanced using mind mapping. The students in their study described mind mapping as 'an integrated educational experience', and said it helped them 'make sense out of the material' (p. 471). Additionally, students in this study reported that mind mapping gave them insight into how they learned and helped to clarify connections.

Okebukola & Jegede (1989) investigated the usefulness of mind mapping as a way to decrease perceived anxiety in the study of ecology and Mendelian genetics. They found a significant decrease in anxiety and perception of subject difficulty among students employing mind mapping compared with a control group. The authors contended that one of the mechanisms accounting for these results was the acquisition of meaningful learning. If students are unable to understand a subject, especially one traditionally perceived as difficult, they are likely to exhibit higher levels of anxiety and perceive greater subject difficulty. On the other hand, if students can identify the intricate relationships and connectedness between concepts and ideas, a greater depth of understanding is attained. Okebukola & Jegede remarked, 'by making the student feel comfortable when working within intricate and interconnected systems of thought, concept mapping could be said to depress anxiety levels toward such intricate and originally perceived as difficult concepts' (p. 90).

Study of the nursing literature reveals some information about using mind mapping as an educational tool. Irvine (1995) discusses whether concept mapping could be used to promote meaningful learning in nurse education. This nurse educator describes how the focus of nursing education has shifted from rote learning to methods that help students learn how to learn. Rather than merely transmitting facts, nursing education has become more concerned with facilitating learning. Irvine maintains that the information nurses will need to contend with continues to increase in both size and complexity, and promoting meaningful and effective learning is thus an issue of importance. She suggests that mind maps be used as a metacognitive strategy to promote meaningful learning in nursing education.

All & Havens (1997) encourage the use of mind maps to help nursing students approach and make sense of large amounts of highly technical and complex text book material. They advocate mind mapping as a means of enhancing understanding of classroom activities and helping to organize data obtained before and after the clinical day. They discuss the obsolescence of rote learning in nursing education, and advocate the use of alternative methods of learning which promote the development of the sound critical thinking skills that nurses will need to deal effectively with the complex clinical situations they encounter in their practice.

A MIND MAPPING PILOT STUDY

The use of mind maps was introduced to a group of nine nursing students during a 15-week clinical practicum at a large American teaching hospital. The students were in their third year of a 4-year baccalaureate nursing programme. For this clinical practicum, the students did not come into the hospital the day before clinical to receive a patient

assignment and review that patients' charts; and they did not develop nursing processes (written care plans) for each patient to guide their care on the following day. Fonteyn & Flaig (1994) have challenged nursing educators to question their continued use of this traditional strategy that may not be as effective for developing students' metacognitive skills as other teaching strategies, such as clinical logs and mind maps.

For this practicum, each student arrived in time for the morning report and was assigned to work with one of the registered nurses (RNs) on duty, who then gave the student a patient assignment. After report, the student quickly looked up the essential information needed to care safely for the patient(s), and then proceeded to do a complete assessment on each patient. From this assessment, the student identified priority problems to be addressed that day, determined a plan of care, and then articulated these findings to the RN and the clinical staff. Thus, instead of using a deductive approach to patient care, the students utilized a more inductive methodology, combining new pieces of data with those previously acquired, thereby furthering their understanding of the patient case as the shift progressed.

For the first 10 weeks of the clinical practicum, students recorded their thoughts about each patient case in a clinical log which they completed at the end of each clinical week and handed to their clinical instructor for review and feedback. We recommend reflective writing in clinical logs as a means of improving students' metacognition (Fonteyn & Cahill 1998). During the last 5 weeks of the semester, instead of writing in clinical logs, students drew a graphic representation of their thinking about a patient case, a mind map, after having been provided with some explanatory information about mind maps from their clinical instructor. The mind maps were intended to illustrate the mental organization of the students' thoughts about their plan of care for a particular patient.

Figure 47.1 is an example of a student's mind map. The central focus of this mind map is the patient's medical diagnosis, and the map shows other major concepts as equally important. These include: assessment, report, nursing interventions and goals. Data related to each of these primary concepts radiate to form a cluster of associated details.

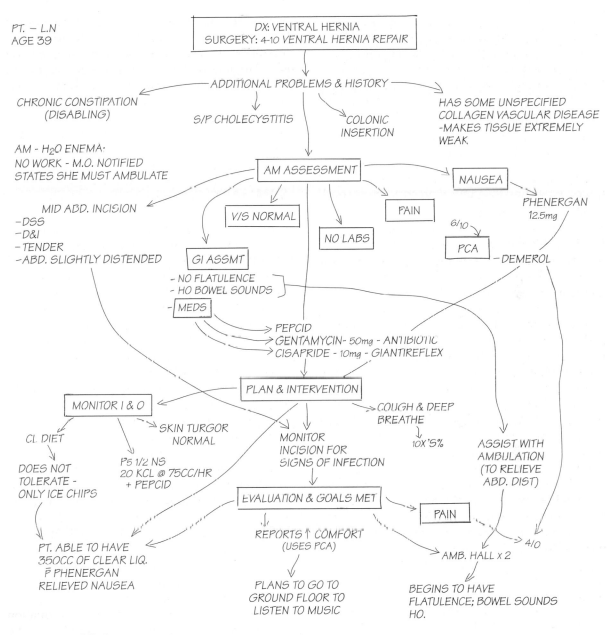

PT. – L.N
AGE 39

DX: VENTRAL HERNIA
SURGERY: 4-10 VENTRAL HERNIA REPAIR

ADDITIONAL PROBLEMS & HISTORY

CHRONIC CONSTIPATION
(DISABLING)

S/P CHOLECYSTITIS

COLONIC
INSERTION

HAS SOME UNSPECIFIED
COLLAGEN VASCULAR DISEASE
-MAKES TISSUE EXTREMELY
WEAK

AM - H_2O ENEMA·
NO WORK - M.O. NOTIFIED
STATES SHE MUST AMBULATE

AM ASSESSMENT

NAUSEA

PHENERGAN
12.5mg

MID ABD. INCISION
-DSS
-D&I
- TENDER
-ABD. SLIGHTLY DISTENDED

V/S NORMAL

PAIN

NO LABS

6/10

PCA

– DEMEROL

GI ASSMT

- NO FLATULENCE
- HO BOWEL SOUNDS
- MEDS

PEPCID
GENTAMYCIN- 50mg - ANTIBIOTIC
CISAPRIDE - 10mg - GIANTIREFLEX

PLAN & INTERVENTION

MONITOR I & O

COUGH & DEEP
BREATHE

SKIN TURGOR
NORMAL

MONITOR
INCISION FOR
SIGNS OF INFECTION

10X'S%

ASSIST WITH
AMBULATION
(TO RELIEVE
ABD. DIST)

CL. DIET

DOES NOT
TOLERATE -
ONLY ICE CHIPS

P5 1/2 NS
20 KCL @ 75CC/HR
+ PEPCID

EVALUATION & GOALS MET

PAIN

PT. ABLE TO HAVE
350CC OF CLEAR LIQ.
P̄ PHENERGAN
RELIEVED NAUSEA

REPORTS ↑ COMFORT
(USES PCA)

AMB. HALL x 2

4/0

PLANS TO GO TO
GROUND FLOOR TO
LISTEN TO MUSIC

BEGINS TO HAVE
FLATULENCE; BOWEL SOUNDS
HO.

Figure 47.1   Mind map

Students' completed mind maps were examined with their clinical instructors so that students could improve their thinking about future patient cases. During this activity, the instructor posed a series of questions to elucidate how patient data were structured and interrelated in the student's thoughts that were graphically represented in the mind map. The questions included:

- What is the quality and quantity of data included in your mind map? What does this tell you about your thinking?
- What is the quality and quantity of data omitted from your map? What does this tell you about your thinking? What data are missing that might be important to the case? Why do you think these data are missing?

- What data are linked and what is the significance of these connections?
- What data are not linked and what is the significance of this?
- What other questions arise from examining your map?
- Overall, what have you learned from examining your mind map that could help improve your thinking about future patient cases?

Students' perceptions of how their thinking had improved during this clinical practicum were evaluated using a 'Thinking Assessment' instrument. This tool comprised 10 Likert Scale questions assessing the extent to which students perceived that various activities improved their thinking. Data collected from nine student evaluations were analysed and represented by an average ranked score (out of a possible 5.0) and a percentage of agreement (out of 100%) with each response. Results indicated that students' thinking about patient data and care had improved a great deal. (The average response score was 4.9 (out of 5) or 98% and 4.2 or 84% respectively, for the first two questions.) Students' comments supported these findings, e.g. 'I'm finally able to make sense of all the pieces of the puzzle, to form relationships [among pieces of data]'.

Students considered that their confidence in their thinking had improved considerably since the beginning of the semester (the average score for this question was 4.2 or 84%). In comparing three different cognitive tools (written nursing care plans, clinical logs and mind maps) with regard to how well each improved their thinking, students' response scores indicated they considered that mind maps improved their thinking more than care plans (average score of 4.4 or 88%) and more than clinical logs (average score of 4.2 or 84%).

SUMMARY

Learning is an interactive, dynamic process. Providing students with learning techniques which will reflect the way in which their minds perceive and connect information helps them to become more creative and efficient in their learning. Mind mapping assists students to understand how they link related data for meaning and understanding, and encourages creative and divergent thinking.

Mind mapping shows promise for enhancing the reasoning and metacognitive skills of students, and for decreasing anxiety and fear towards subjects often perceived as difficult. The description of the use of mind maps in a clinical practicum confirms the value of this unique and creative tool. We encourage the use of this metacognitive teaching strategy and suggest its use in nursing education as a means to enhance the learning and critical thinking abilities of nursing students.

References

Alexander M K, Giguere B 1996 Critical thinking in clinical learning: a holistic perspective. Holistic Nursing Practice 10(3):15–22

All A C, Havens R L 1997 Cognitive/concept mapping: a teaching strategy for nursing. Journal of Advanced Nursing 25:1210–1219

Ausubel D P 1963 The psychology of meaningful verbal learning. Grune and Stratton, New York

Baker C R 1996 Reflective learning: a teaching strategy for critical thinking. Journal of Nursing Education 35(1): 19–22

Barenholz H, Tamir P 1992 A comprehensive use of concept mapping in design instruction and assessment. Research in Science and Technology Education 10(1): 37–52

Buzan T, Buzan B 1996 The mind map book. Plume/Penguin, New York

Conger M M, Mezza I 1996 Fostering critical thinking in nursing in the clinical setting. Nurse Educator 21(3): 11–15

Degazon C E, Lunney M 1995 Clinical journal: a tool to foster critical thinking for advanced levels of competence. Clinical Nurse Specialist 9(5):270–274

Dorough D K, Rye J A 1997 Mapping for understanding. Science Teacher 64(1):37–41

Fonteyn M E 1995 Clinical reasoning in nursing. In: Higgs J, Jones M (eds) Clinical reasoning in the health professions. Butterworth-Heinemann, Oxford, p 60–71

Fonteyn M E, Cahill M 1998 The use of clinical logs to improve nursing students' metacognition: a pilot study. Journal of Advanced Nursing 28(1):149–154

Fonteyn M, Flaig L 1994 The written nursing process: is it still useful to nursing education? Journal of Advanced Nursing 19:315–319

Gavelek J R, Raphael T E 1985 Metacognition, instruction, and the role of questioning activities. In: Forrest-Pressley D L, MacKinnon G E, Waller T G (eds) Metacognition, cognition, and human performance, vol 2. Instructional practices. Academic Press, Orlando, p 103–136

Gordon C J, Braun C 1985 Metacognitive processes: reading and writing narrative discourse. In: Forrest-Pressley D L, MacKinnon G E, Waller T G (eds) Metacognition, cognition, and human performance, vol 2. Instructional practices. Academic Press, Orlando, p 1–75

Heinze-Fry J A, Novak J D 1990 Concept mapping brings long term movement toward meaningful learning. Science Education 74(4):461–472

Irvine L M C 1995 Can concept mapping be used to promote meaningful learning in nurse education? Journal of Advanced Nursing 21:1175–1179

Jegede O J, Alaiyemola F F, Okebukola O J 1990 The effect of concept mapping on students' anxiety and achievement in biology. Journal of Research in Science Teaching 27(10):951–960

Novak J D 1990 Concept mapping: a useful tool for science education. Journal of Research in Science Teaching 27(10): 937–949

Novak J D, Gowin D B 1984 Learning how to learn. Cambridge University Press, New York

Oermann M H 1997 Evaluating critical thinking in clinical practice. Nurse Educator 22(5):25–28

Okebukola P A, Jegede O J 1988 Cognitive preference and learning mode as determinants of meaningful learning through concept mapping. Science Education 72(4): 489–500

Okebukola P A, Jegede O J 1989 Students' anxiety towards and perception of difficulty of some biological concepts under the concept mapping heuristic. Research in Science and Technological Education 7(1):85–92

Regis A, Albertazzi P G, Roletto E 1996 Concept maps in chemistry education. Journal of Chemical Education 73(11):1084–1088

Whiteside C 1997 A model for teaching critical thinking in the clinical setting. Dimensions of Critical Care Nursing 16(3):152–165

Yussen S R 1985 The role of metacognition in contemporary theories of cognitive development. In: Forrest-Pressley D L, MacKinnon G E, Waller T G (eds) Metacognition, cognition, and human performance, vol 1. Theoretical perspectives. Academic Press, Orlando, p 253–283

Index

Q